The Aids Epidemic

The Aids Epidemic

Private Rights and the Public Interest

Edited by Padraig O'Malley

Beacon Press Boston

Beacon Press
25 Beacon Street
Boston, Massachusetts 02108

Beacon Press books
are published under the auspices of
the Unitarian Universalist Association of Congregations.

The material in this volume first appeared as a special
issue of the *New England Journal of Public Policy,*
volume 4, no. 1 (Winter/Spring 1988)
First published by Beacon Press in 1989

Printed in the United States of America

96 95 94 93 92 91 90 89 8 7 6 5 4 3 2 1

Library of Congress Cataloging-in-Publication Data
The Aids epidemic.
First published as a special issue of the New
England Journal of Public Policy, v. 4, no. 1
(winter/spring 1988)
1. AIDS (Disease)—Government policy—United
States. 2. AIDS (Disease)—United States—Moral
and ethical aspects. 3. AIDS (Disease)—Social
aspects—United States. I. O'Malley, Padraig.
RA644.A25A3615 1989 362.1′969792′00973 88-47890
ISBN 0-8070-0600-9
ISBN 0-8070-0601-7 (pbk.)

Contents

Acknowledgments

The AIDS Epidemic: Private Rights and the Public Interest first appeared as a special issue of the *New England Journal of Public Policy* in May 1988. Although some of the articles have a New England orientation, the questions they raise and the problems they pose are not region-specific and cannot be resolved in a regional context. Of the many people who made this book possible, three deserve special acknowledgment: Betsy Anne Youngholm, who was managing editor of the *New England Journal of Public Policy* AIDS issue, Candace Chick, who was responsible for design, and Toni Jean Rosenberg, copy editor extraordinaire. Thanks for encouragement and support also go to Edmund Beard, director of the John W. McCormack Institute of Public Affairs, University of Massachusetts at Boston, which publishes the *New England Journal of Public Policy,* and to Robert Corrigan, former chancellor of the University of Massachusetts at Boston. Finally, particular tribute is due to the book's contributors, who gave unstintingly of their time to prepare their manuscripts despite hectic schedules and the demands of their professional lives, which are devoted, for the most part, to increasing our understanding of AIDS and to the care of persons with AIDS.

Editor's Note

Padraig O'Malley

"I am afraid that the picture . . . that will develop during the four days to come will be frightening, even more frightening than we have expected," Dr. Lars Olaf Kallings of Sweden's National Bacteriological Institute told the gathering of 7,500 scientists and media reporters in his keynote address to the Fourth International Conference on AIDS held in Sweden in June 1988. His sense of a coming catastrophe was hardly misplaced, and it is now unquestionably, even if belatedly, accepted that the AIDS epidemic is a public policy matter of perhaps unparalleled importance, with a likely impact of overwhelming consequence well into the twenty-first century. The epidemic raises fundamental questions regarding the nature of individual freedom, our responsibilities to others, the always delicate balance between private rights and public interest, and society's obligation to its "out" groups—those members it has stigmatized, discriminated against, ridiculed, and treated as less than full and equal citizens. Indeed, it requires us to ask whether society can discharge its responsibilities in this regard without discarding some of its essential myths about itself.

These are questions which in the best of times we tend to avoid, because they raise issues about the nature of our most deeply rooted fears and anxieties and the role of repression and denial in the conduct of private morality and public affairs—issues that we find discomforting at best and highly disconcerting at worst.

There is hardly an area of public policy that does not fall within the purview of the epidemic, and as the extent of infection and the illnesses associated with it multiply geometrically over the coming years, our cultural, social, religious, educational, financial, and political networks and institutions will be called upon to examine their practices and policies and to address what is found wanting. The purpose of *The AIDS Epidemic: Private Rights and the Public Interest* is partly to facilitate that task.

AIDS has become encumbered by the trappings of metaphor. In *Illness as Metaphor,* Susan Sontag writes that "any disease that is treated as a mystery and acutely enough feared will be felt to be morally, if not literally, contagious. . . . Contact with someone afflicted with a disease regarded as a mysterious malevolency inevitably feels like a trespass; worse, like the violation of a taboo." But what Sontag wrote about cancer—that it "is felt to be obscene—in the original meaning of that word: ill-omened, abominable, repugnant to the senses"—is even more pertinent to our forebodings about AIDS. AIDS satisfies our predilection for punitive notions of disease. There is AIDS as "the killer disease," and there is the "war" against AIDS—allusions that evoke disturbing feelings of unease and dread. Ostensibly, the illness is the culprit, but it is also the AIDS patient who is held to account and to whom blame is imputed, whether implicitly or explicitly. Hence the voices of Fred Garnett, Ron McAvoy, Kevin Brown, Richard Broussand, Tema Luft, and Matilda, the persons with AIDS (PWAs) who gave witness on behalf of their illness at the Third International AIDS Conference in Washington, D.C., in June 1987. These are strong and vibrant voices, resonant with the possibilities of their own lives—not the voices of victims. But there are other voices, the voices of the ill who are without adequate care, who are treated as outcasts, who struggle to maintain some dignity amid the most extreme circumstances of adversity, who are physically deprived, psychologically isolated, denied the compassion we would extend to suffering animals, and who look only for some affirmation of their own humanity before it ceases. We must pay heed.

In the last year, the epidemiology of AIDS in the United States has changed significantly. The evidence now suggests that the once-feared explosion into the general population of HIV—the human immunodeficiency virus that appears to lead inexorably to AIDS in people who become infected with it and are left untreated—will probably not occur, although the evidence is by no means certain; that the rate of new infections among gay men has declined to the point where the virus may have stopped spreading in this community; and that more and more, new cases of infection are being found among drug addicts, their sexual partners, and their babies.

AIDS, therefore, is becoming increasingly a disease of the poor, of blacks and Hispanics, of women, and of children—the population groups we have traditionally neglected and forgotten—rather than of the middle-class white gay men who were primarily afflicted during the epidemic's early years. And since infected intravenous drug addicts appear to be less geographically mobile than many of the infected gay men, AIDS is increasingly becoming a disease that manifests itself in communities with high concentrations of minorities.

Indisputably, despite the reduced spread of HIV among homosexual men, the upsurge in AIDS and AIDS-related disease and the toll of death associated with acquired immunodeficiency syndrome will continue to wreak their devastation: as many as one in every thirty American males between the ages of twenty and fifty are probably infected with the virus. Federal officials now believe that about 20 to 25 percent of the nation's estimated 2.5 million homosexual men and 25 percent of its almost 1 million intravenous drug users have the virus, and that overall between 945,000 and 1.4 million people may be infected. Recent setbacks in the search for a vaccine make the likelihood of a cure in the near future more remote. And recent research shows that the virus sometimes has a special cunning, an ability to make itself invisible to the immune system—and thus to any currently available detection test—in an undetermined number of people it infects. The evidence suggests that unless a cure is found, all of the persons already infected will eventually develop AIDS and die—a human catastrophe of immense consequence.

As of September 1988, some 74,500 cases of AIDS had been reported in the United States, and approximately 42,000 of these persons had died. However, the Centers for Disease Control estimates that the number of new cases alone in 1991 will exceed 52,000, and it projects a cumulative total of 270,000 cases by the year 1991, with perhaps 180,000 deaths, 365,000 cases by 1992, and 453,000 cases by 1993. The actual case loads may be 20 percent higher because there are many undiagnosed cases.

Heterosexual spread of the disease has confined itself almost exclusively to the sexual partners of people who contracted the disease through established modes of transmission: sharing contaminated needles or other drug-injection equipment, receiving infected blood products before the spring of 1985, or engaging in male homosexual intercourse. There is little evidence that heterosexually active people with no known risk factors for AIDS for either partner will spread the disease to each other. In November 1987, the Centers for Disease Control projected that approximately 0.021 percent of this country's estimated 142 million heterosexuals without specific identified risks (30,000 people) are infected. However, the growing number of infected addicts and their sexual partners in the primary and secondary transmission groups, and hence the reservoir of HIV-infected heterosexuals, will inevitably increase the likelihood of transmission to other groups as the epidemiological process works itself out. Women, who consistently account for 6 to 7 percent of AIDS cases, constitute an overall 27 percent of cases in those groups into which a woman can be assigned, a percentage that is on the increase. The total number of pediatric AIDS cases reported to the Centers for Disease Control was 1,185 in September 1988; this number is expected to increase to over 3,000 by 1991. The burden of AIDS cases has been greatest in the Middle Atlantic and Pacific states, where in the metropolitan areas of New York City, San Francisco, and Los Angeles the original cases of AIDS were recognized. The six-year cumulative incidence rates in these two regions are approximately twice the national average and three to four times the rate in New England.

Much has been written about the nation's slow response—nonresponse, some would argue—to the AIDS epidemic and the absence of strong federal leadership. Although the picture has improved in the past year, efforts to contain the disease remain for the most part belated, disjointed, occasionally misguided, and too often inadequate. The President's Commission on AIDS, which published its report in June 1988, addresses some of these problems. It calls for a dramatic increase in federal expenditure on AIDS education, research, and care, new legislation to prevent discrimination against persons infected with the AIDS virus, and a wide range of programs to curb the infection's spread among intravenous drug users and their families.

Much of the problem, of course, has to do with the nature of the disease and the manner in which it first manifested itself. "AIDS requires," Marshall Forstein writes in this volume, "that we take the most difficult, most emotionally charged concerns of our civilization and within the extremes of existing values, morals, social structures, and economics cut through to the essential tasks involved in halting a sexually transmitted disease." Thus, the prolonged silence, especially at the federal level, is due to the fear of addressing the fundamental issues of sexuality, especially homosexuality, and drug addiction. The fear- and anxiety-propelled irrational responses, such as calls for quarantining AIDS patients, and even all HIV-infected individuals, are related to what drug use and sex symbolize and mean in our culture. Forstein raises the issue that still bedevils us: "How does a society begin to address the medical and psychological needs of homosexually oriented people who are intentionally invisible within the fabric of American life, and whose basic civil rights are not clearly guaranteed by the Constitution," especially when many states regard the very sexual activity that is associated with the transmission of the disease as criminal? Moreover, as Forstein argues, there is "something quite different about sex than almost any other human activity which psychologically makes our culture respond regressively and often punitively," and "the association of sex and death, now profoundly etched in our consciousness, and the basic fears of intimacy and sexual expression which have always been a part of our society have created special barriers to the development of coherent, reasonable approaches to this disease.'' Similarly, the conflict around drug addiction ''represents an underlying psychological ambivalence about whether an individual is to blame for his or her addiction or whether, in fact, it is a disease.'' We are still, it seems, susceptible to the proposition that disease can be cured by willpower.

The situation is changing, albeit slowly—far too slowly for those who already have the virus. Above all, there is no well-thought-out, rational policy, and the federal government continues to neglect issues of prevention, civil rights, and health care. Increasingly, state and local governments have been left to fend for themselves. The result is a fragmentation of effort, a mishmash of guidelines, widely varying policy, disparity in distribution of services, and a set of often unsettling contradictions. For example, condoms are distributed free to homosexual men in New York City jails but are contraband in New York State prisons; Connecticut requires applicants to be tested for the AIDS virus for life insurance purposes but New York does not.

Of course, the AIDS epidemic cannot be considered only within the context of the United States. The disease has already appeared in 160 countries, with a worldwide estimate of 150,000 cases through 1987. The World Health Organization (WHO) expects 150,000 new cases to be reported in 1988, bringing the world case load up to 300,000 by the end of that year. But that, unfortunately, is not the worst prediction. WHO estimates that 5 million to 10 million people are infected with HIV, perhaps 3 million in Africa, in which case anywhere from 500,000 to 3 million new cases of AIDS will develop within the next five years in people already carrying the virus.

In the face of the international disaster posed by the epidemic, we will be forced to examine the nature of our global interdependence and the appropriateness of our concepts of national autonomy. We must examine the foolhardiness of implementing short-term measures that give the appearance of benefit but that are in fact inimical to the public interest, and we are compelled to address the overriding need for cooperation, consultation, and joint action among nations. Already, countries are moving to protect their own perceived interests, however narrowly they may be defined. Thus, in the United States, illegal aliens who are applying for permanent residence under the revised resident alien laws are required to be tested for HIV. If they test positive, they are denied residence and are deported to their country of origin, although it is all but certain that they became infected in the United States. In short, the United States is becoming an exporter of the AIDS virus. In China, Japan, India, the Soviet Union, several Soviet bloc nations, Belgium, and Germany, all foreign students are required to take AIDS blood tests. If they test positive, they are sent home. Such measures invite retaliatory responses on the part of other governments, actions undertaken not as a matter of sound policy but simply to reciprocate in kind.

The last words belong to Camus, from *The Plague*. Dr. Rieux, when the epidemic has ended, resolves to compile his chronicle so that

> he should not be one of those who hold their peace but should bear witness in favor of those plague-stricken people; so that some memorial of the injustice and outrage done them might endure; and to state quite simply what we learn in a time of pestilence: that there are more things to admire in men than to despise.
>
> None the less, he knew that the tale he had to tell could not be one of a final victory. It could be only the record of what had had to be done, and what assuredly would have to be done again in the never ending fight against terror and its relentless onslaughts, despite their personal afflictions, by all who, while unable to be saints but refusing to bow down to pestilences, strive their utmost to be healers.

List of Terms

Acquired immunodeficiency syndrome (AIDS). A disease caused by a virus known as HIV, in which the body's immune system is seriously damaged, leaving it vulnerable to infections and some rare cancers that ultimately result in death.

AIDS-related complex (ARC). ARC patients have some symptoms of AIDS, but not the "full-blown" (or "frank") disease. Symptoms may include unexplained swollen glands or fever, weight loss, or persistent diarrhea.

Antibody. A unique protein produced by blood plasma cells to counteract or kill some specific infectious agents — viruses and bacteria.

Antibody-positive. A blood test result showing that a person has been infected with HIV at some time and has developed antibodies to HIV. It does *not* mean that a person has AIDS.

Antigen. A substance that is foreign to the body and that stimulates the formation of antibodies to combat its presence.

Asymptomatic "carrier." A person who has had an infectious organism within the body but who feels or shows no outward symptoms.

Asymptomatic infection. The ability of certain organisms, such as viruses, to get inside a person's cells without resulting in clinical signs or symptoms that tell the person that he or she is infected.

AZT. Azidothymidine, an antiviral drug that has been shown to prolong life in AIDS patients.

Cofactors. Agents or other factors that are necessary to increase the probability for development of a disease when the basic causative agent of that disease is present.

ELISA. Enzyme-linked immunosorbent assay test for antibody.

Epidemiology. The study of relationships among various factors thought to determine the frequency and distribution of diseases in humans.

Exposure. The act or condition of coming in contact with but not necessarily being infected by a pathogenic agent.

Hemophilia. A hereditary blood condition found in males, in which even minor bodily injuries can be followed by prolonged bleeding.

HIV. The virus that causes AIDS. Formerly referred to as LAV or HTLV-III.

HIV-antibody screening test. A test whose purpose is to reveal the presence of antibodies to HIV. It is used on all donated blood and organs and in all medical and clinical testing programs. It is also used at alternative or anonymous test sites. If antibodies are detected, it is assumed that the individual or organ is infected.

Idiopathic thrombocytopenic purpura (ITP). A persistent decrease in blood platelets, of unknown cause, resulting in bruising of skin and tissues.

Immune system. A system within the body which helps the body resist disease-causing organisms such as germs, viruses, or other infectious agents.

Immunosuppressed. A state of the body in which the immune system defenses do not work normally — usually as a result of illness or the administration of certain drugs used to fight cancer or prepare the body to accept transplanted donor organs.

Incubation period. The interval between infection and the appearance of the first symptom. (See "Latency.")

Infected. The state of the body in which a part of it has been invaded by a pathogenic agent that ordinarily multiplies and causes harmful effects.

Intravenous drugs. Drugs injected by needle directly into a vein.

Kaposi's sarcoma. A tumor of the blood vessels most frequently seen in the skin or mucous membranes and associated with AIDS.

Latency. A period when the virus is in the body but rests in an inactive, dormant state. (See "Asymptomatic infection.")

Lentivirus. This is a subgroup of the retroviruses. HIV belongs to this subgroup. Generally, viruses of this group replicate slowly and tend to form latent and chronic infections in their hosts.

Lymphocytes. Specialized white blood cells involved in the immune response.

Morbidity. The degree of symptomatic illness associated with an infectious organism.

Opportunistic infections. Those diseases which are caused by agents that are frequently present in our bodies or environment but which cause disease only when there is an alteration from normal healthy conditions — for instance, when the immune system becomes weak or damaged.

Pathogen. Any disease-producing microorganism or substance.

Perinatal. Occurring in the period during or just before or after birth.

PGL. Persistent generalized lymphadenopathy. A persistent swelling of the lymph nodes. In AIDS, a condition of long-term generalized lymph-node swelling characteristic of the so-called AIDS-related complex.

***Pneumocystis carinii* pneumonia (PCP).** An opportunistic infection of the lung which results in a diagnosis of AIDS.

Prevalence. The total number of persons in a given population with disease at a given point in time — usually expressed as a percentage.

Prognosis. Prediction of course and end of a disease, and outlook based on these factors.

Retrovirus. A genus of viruses which contains the enzyme reverse transcriptase and which requires the synthesis of proviral DNA for its replication.

Seroconversion. The point at which antibodies to specific antigens are produced by B lymphocytes and become detectable in the blood. "Conversion" refers to change from a negative to positive status, or vice versa.

Seronegative. Resulting in a negative reaction to a blood test — the HIV antibody test(s). If high-risk, a person cannot be assumed to be uninfected on the basis of a negative test.

Seropositive. Producing a positive reaction to a blood test — the HIV antibody test(s). A person who has a positive and confirmatory test is presumed to be both infected and infectious.

Syndrome. A set of signs and symptoms that occur together.

Vaccine. A preparation of killed, living attenuated, or living virulent organisms or part of microorganisms which can be administered to produce or increase immunity to a particular disease.

Viruses. Submicroscopic pathogens that grow and reproduce only inside living cells, thus causing disease.

Western blot. Confirmatory test for antibody.

Human Retroviruses

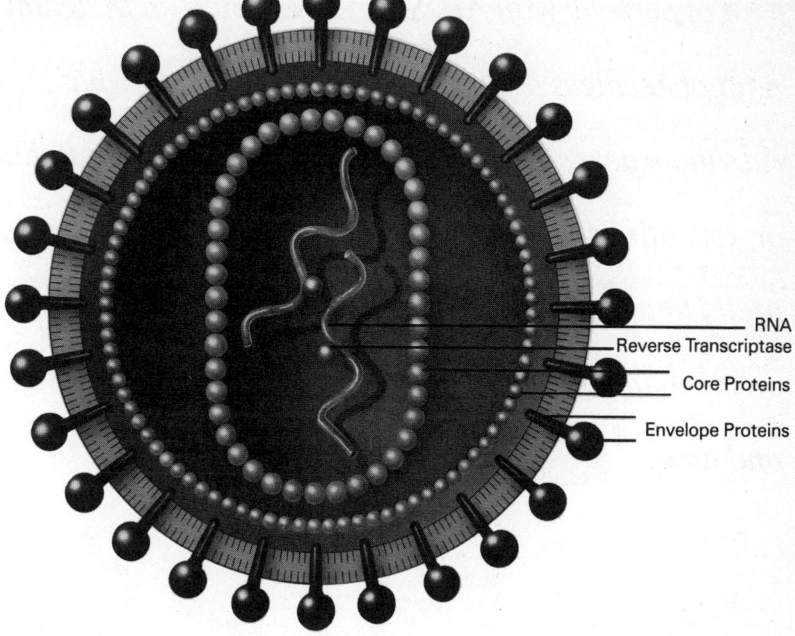

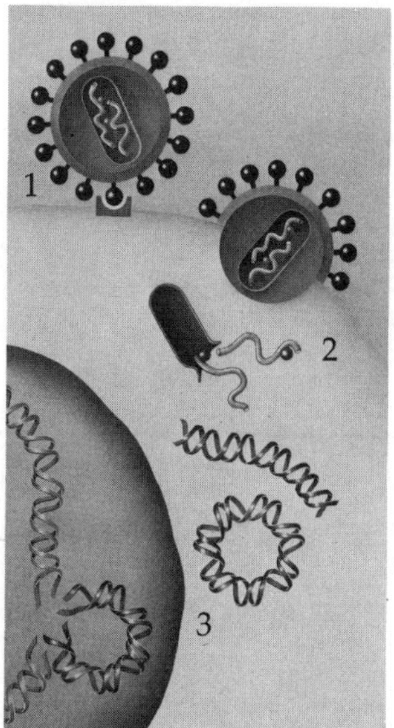

Life Cycle of Retroviruses

1. Binding of virus to target cell.
2. Uncoating of virus and transcription of viral RNA to DNA by reverse transcriptase.
3. Viral DNA circularization and integration into host genome.
4. Transcription and protein synthesis.
5. Assembly of viral proteins and RNA at cell surface.
6. Budding of mature viral particle from host.

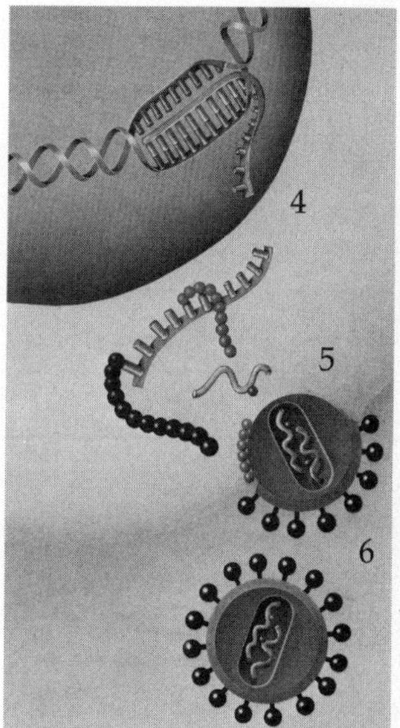

"Emotionally, the disease has taken a very serious toll on me. I got very deeply involved with AIDS organizations. I've seen a lot of persons with AIDS and I've seen a lot of death. A lot of needless death. And I've seen a lot of what I'd call ridiculousness, on the part of government and individuals and organizations over things that were pretty self-destructive and pretty unimportant, and I think that that's what's weighed harder on me than my own personal experience, which has gone up and down."

AIDS: An Overview

Loretta McLaughlin

"We stand nakedly in front of a very serious pandemic, as mortal as any pandemic there ever has been," said Halfdan Mahler, director-general of the World Health Organization (WHO). "I don't know of any greater killer than AIDS, not to speak of its psychological, social and economic maiming. Everything is getting worse and worse with AIDS and all of us have been underestimating it, and I in particular. We're running scared. I cannot imagine a worse health problem in this century." When asked to compare AIDS to other epidemics, such as smallpox, that have infected and killed over the course of history, Mahler said he "could not think of anything else that matched the estimates that one hundred million people will be infected with AIDS within ten years of its discovery."[1]

In the years immediately before the world learned of the baffling and deadly new disease that would come to be called AIDS, there were forewarnings that something truly ominous was stirring.

In late 1979, young New York City men, some of them in prime physical condition, had begun to manifest vague but debilitating symptoms. The men's ailments, at first, did not seem very worrisome. Lymph glands in their neck, groin, or under their arms became swollen — and, curiously, stayed that way, although this common sign of infection is usually temporary. The men also intermittently had sore throats, transient fever, and brutal night sweats. Some had a dry cough, muscle aches, shortness of breath. They complained of being unduly tired, and many, inexplicably, lost a considerable amount of weight. They seemed to have a strange and persistent flu that they didn't ever completely get over. They also seemed chronically run-down and open to one infection after another. They had only one thing in common: they were all homosexuals. And so the syndrome was gratuitously labeled gay-related immune deficiency (GRID), or the gay disease.

Soon, some of these men, whose smouldering illness kept worsening, began to develop different symptoms — peculiar purplish spots on their arms, legs, torso, face. Their doctors had rarely, if ever, seen such blemishes — and never on young healthy men. They appeared to have a skin cancer called Kaposi's sarcoma (KS). While the young men's KS was virulent, the cancer typically had been a chronic affliction of elderly middle-European Jewish men and aged Italian men. It had been slow growing and seldom killed. Portentously, an unexplained but even more aggressively malignant form of KS had recently

Loretta McLaughlin is deputy editor of the editorial pages of the Boston Globe *and is a long-time medical news writer on AIDS.*

turned up in central Africa. In the United States, KS had occasionally been seen in patients who were undergoing chemotherapy for some other form of cancer. These instances of KS were associated with the patients' immune system being impaired by the cancer treatment. As a result, the KS in the New York men was thought of as an "opportunistic" disorder — one that took advantage of a person's immune defenses being down. The men's run-down state also was thought to account for the fungal infection (candida, familiarly called thrush) that often appeared in their mouths, and the gross cold sores (herpes simplex) that sometimes spread across their faces. These, too, were signs that what should have remained bland infections were opportunistically flourishing in the absence of a sound immune system. Strangely, all of these patients also were homosexual. So, the KS syndrome in the young New York men, whose immune systems were obviously out of kilter, though no one knew why, was first labeled Kaposi's sarcoma and opportunistic infections (KS/OI). Or the gay cancer.

During the same period, in California, a handful of cases of *Pneumocystis carinii* showed up — a rare and exotic form of pneumonia. The organism that causes this pneumonia is a truly primitive agent, a protozoan, which in evolutionary terms dates back to the first single-celled animals from which life derived. It is found everywhere in the world and is one of countless microbes that are carried by most people. Normally, these microbes remain innocuous, in that they are kept suppressed in the human system. Yet, in late 1979 and 1980, *Pneumocystis carinii* pneumonia was diagnosed in five young men in Los Angeles. All had the same sort of pre-pneumonia syndrome of fever, malaise, cough, and thrush which had been troubling the New York City KS cases and the GRID patients. Studies of the California men showed that they, too, had impaired immune systems. They all also were homosexual. Now there was "the gay pneumonia, PCP."

What first attracted the attention of the federal Centers for Disease Control (CDC) in Atlanta, Georgia, was a flurry of requests from the Los Angeles doctors for samples of a drug, pentamidine, that was effective against the pneumonia. The drug was needed so rarely that the nation's entire supply was stored at the CDC.

The first public inkling of the five pneumonia cases came in the June 5, 1981, issue of the *Morbidity and Mortality Weekly Report (MMWR),* the CDC's widely disseminated monitor of infectious disease and deaths in the United States. Less than a month later, on July 3, the CDC was reporting the phenomenal appearance of Kaposi's sarcoma in New York City — twenty-six KS cases over a thirty-month period. The same July report importantly noted that six of these twenty-six persons had also developed *Pneumocystis carinii;* there also were ten additional cases of the exotic pneumonia in Los Angeles and six in the San Francisco Bay area. Two of the ten in Los Angeles also had KS, strongly suggesting a link between the cancer and the pneumonia. All the cases still were among homosexuals. By the end of August, there were seventy more patients with both conditions from the same three cities.

Nearly a year passed before the early-phase condition, defined for no apparent reason as generalized lymphadenopathy, or chronic swollen glands, was acknowledged on May 21, 1982, by the CDC as an emerging health problem among American homosexual males; fifty-seven cases were cited. This report noted too that the men's immune systems were abnormal. And by June 11, a second cancer, lymphoma, a rare cancer of the lymph glands, which are key players in the immune system, was added to the roster of disorders related somehow to the swollen gland syndrome in gay men. Sexual transmission was raised as a possibility, as was the use of sexually stimulating "poppers" or other illicit drugs.

It was this year-long association of an emerging new illness with homosexual men — and only homosexual men — that underlies the ease with which the illness that was to become AIDS was medically and politically ignored as a major health problem. As U.S. Rep. Henry Waxman (D-Calif.) had said earlier in April, "There is no doubt in my mind that, if the same disease had appeared among Americans of Norwegian descent, or among tennis players, rather than gay males, the responses of both the government and the medical community would have been different." Noting that copious attention, money, and research had been poured into solving the mystery of a form of pneumonia that in 1976 had struck an American Legion convention in Philadelphia, Representative Waxman concluded, "What society judged was not the severity of the disease but the social acceptability of the individuals affected with it."[2] Yet there were early indicators, had they been heeded, that a medical storm was brewing which eventually would blow across the country — and the world — leaving no corner untouched.

As early as July 9, 1982, the first appearance of the new disease was noted outside the male homosexual community. That day, the CDC reported that the same syndrome — the Kaposi's cancer, the *Pneumocystis carinii* pneumonia, and the severe opportunistic fungal and viral infections — along with an old infection, tuberculosis — had appeared among thirty-four Haitians newly residing in the United States. They, too, were mysteriously immunocompromised. It was a startling development, which the CDC in its low-key style referred to as a "new phenomenon."[3] Nearly all the Haitian patients were heterosexual. The CDC report also noted that an unusual form of KS had recently been observed in Port-au-Prince (Haiti). Though time would reveal that the cases in the Haitians were misconstrued — causing them cruel and unwarranted discrimination — the central point was that the disease had appeared in heterosexual patients, so the cause of its spread was not limited to male homosexual practices. It was an early warning of things to come.

Although the information was not substantial enough to be published, word of other complications and of the transmission of the new disease to other groups was arriving virtually month by month at the CDC. Addicts who used, and often shared, needles to inject narcotics directly into the bloodstream were afflicted. So were the first handful of the nation's twenty thousand hemophiliacs who rely on a product called Factor VIII, extracted from pools of donated blood, to stem their inherited tendency to bleed internally. The new disorder also had been linked to a blood transfusion. A blood recipient had become sick after receiving blood from a donor who later had become sick himself.[4] The nation's leading blood banks, to their later regret, imprudently resisted facing up to the danger this posed for the nation's blood supply. Babies born to mothers who were drug-addicted or who were the sexual partners of needle-using addicts were also falling ill, signifying that the disease could be passed during pregnancy or childbirth. The pattern of the cases all supported the single idea that a new virus, an extraordinarily deadly virus, was loose. The pattern also indicated that the mysterious virus could be transmitted sexually or via blood, much the same as the hepatitis B virus. Questions immediately arose as to whether the new disease could be passed to health workers, as hepatitis can be, from needle sticks with contaminated blood. Infectious-disease experts were relieved that there were no signs the new disease was "contagious," like measles or flu, which spread on airborne particles wherever people congregate. Nor did it seem to be easily "infectious," like mononucleosis, the high-school and college-age disease that is marked by unrelieved fatigue and that can be spread through casual contact, through kissing, or by drinking from the same glass or Coke bottle. Nonetheless, infectious-disease experts, early in the AIDS outbreak, were privately frightened about the prospects for sexual and blood-borne spread. Some of the infections these patients were developing were horrendous — some almost never seen before, except in animals. Further, in some patients, the disease seemed to directly attack the brain. Doctors and nurses were struck by the intensity of the patients' illness; these were among the sickest patients ever seen in a lifetime of providing medical care.

Terribly worrisome would be the prolonged incubation period — now known to extend from two to ten years — when an infected person could look and feel well while harboring the virus and could unwittingly pass it to others. This lengthy symptom-free but infectious stage, a long period of silent transmission, is incredibly dangerous. Without knowing it, the CDC by mid-1982 had already learned the disease's primary target groups and the most salient of its broad clinical ramifications. The final characteristic of the disease was its deadliness: it seemed to eventually kill without exception.

The era of AIDS had dawned. The syndrome was first defined and given its name in the CDC's September 3, 1982, weekly morbidity and mortality report: "This group of clinical entities, along with its specific immune deficiency, is now called acquired immune deficiency syndrome (AIDS)."[5] By that time, there were 593 confirmed cases in the United States, and 243 were already dead. As of February 1988, nearly seven years into the epidemic, yet probably still nearer the beginning than the end, the worst fears of those early days had been realized. Nearly 55,000 cases of AIDS had been logged, and 30,000 had died of AIDS in the United States. A broader definition of AIDS now includes twenty-four infections and ten cancers. The definition also now covers the sickest of those patients with a chronic progressive form of AIDS called ARC (AIDS-related complex) and three other conditions when they develop in people infected with the AIDS virus: dementia, tuberculosis, and a profound, irreversible, eventually fatal weight loss called "wasting" syndrome.[6]

A great deal of scientific progress has been made — more learned, more rapidly than ever before about a single virus. But few doubt that more could have been done had more research funds become available sooner. Too little has yet been done in any coherent or comprehensive way through public education to limit the spread of the disease; to prepare the public for the onslaught of cases that are already in the pipeline; or to rally funds, prepare facilities, or organize the means to deliver medical care to the tens of thousands in the United States and the millions across the world who will need AIDS care in the immediate years ahead.

On the plus side, the cause of AIDS is now known, officially designated human immunodeficiency virus (HIV). A more cunning virus is hard to imagine. It has more genetic material with which to constantly redesign its surface than any other known. It can and does change somewhat, individuate, in virtually each person infected. When activated, it can replicate by making copies of itself many times faster than any other known virus. And, like a fifth column agent, it attacks the very cells in the human system which call forth and orchestrate the defenses that each person relies on to protect against disease.

Discovery of the virus in 1983 by a French team at the Pasteur Institute in Paris — an achievement later duplicated by an American team at the National Cancer Institute — led fairly quickly to development of a test. An indirect test, in that it detects antibody response to the virus rather than the virus itself, was officially released on March 2, 1985. Henceforth, blood could be protected. Though it was loudly argued that the test did not specifically indicate a person was carrying the virus, the finding that a person once infected apparently remains so forever signifies that a positive AIDS antibody test actually does diagnose infection. Thus, those who are infected can be identified. Search for treatment already has elucidated one medicine (AZT) that can at least prolong life for AIDS victims, though it is highly toxic. Dozens of other drugs or treatment approaches are under study. A cure still seems remote, considering the virus's capacity to make itself part of the genetic material of its human host and to take sanctuary in the brain, where most drugs do not reach, or not at full strength. A vaccine is being sought, but the capacity of the virus to change and in other ways to outwit the immune response upon which vaccine protection is predicated diminishes the likelihood that an effective vaccine will soon be available.

From all indications, AIDS will be with us for a long time to come. "AIDS is out of the box," says Dr. James Chin of California, a World Health Organization consultant whose primary work is maintaining global surveillance of the disease. "Even if we had an effective vaccine to protect new cases today, it is something the world would have to live with over the next century." Before it is conquered, AIDS has the potential to disrupt the social and political equanimity of the United States and to wreak havoc on less fortunate parts of the world.

AIDS is seen as a slow plague, one that will probably take a generation to unfold. The United States' capacity to bear this new health burden, though it will be strained, is light-years ahead of that of Third World countries, where the annual outlay for health care amounts to a few scant dollars per person, or less. Yet it is in Third World nations, most notably so far in Africa, the Philippines, the Caribbean, and Central and South America, that the AIDS epidemic is spreading rapidly. These are areas already beset by other dire health, economic, and social problems — from malaria, tuberculosis, and parasitic disorders to malnutrition and poverty, illiteracy and industrial backwardness, rampant population growth and financial dependency.

With the very first case, AIDS was an epidemic. In modern epidemiology terms, that designation applies to any unusual outbreak of a disease, even one more case than should be expected. Because the disease never existed before, AIDS, then, was automatically an epidemic. Though the subject is in dispute, some think that the disease originated in Africa. A virus that is highly similar to the human AIDS virus is found in green monkeys in Africa, though it does not make the monkeys sick. And the first evidence of AIDS — identified much later — were traces of the virus which were coaxed out of human blood samples (stored and frozen for research purposes) collected in Kinshasa, Zaire, in 1959. Though co-exposure to malaria confused the AIDS status of some early blood samples, sporadic cases of what are now known to be AIDS-related diseases clearly date back to the mid-1970s in central and east Africa. Among the earliest victims was a Danish woman surgeon working in Zaire, whose first signs of illness, as was later reported in the British medical journal *Lancet,* began as early as 1973.[7] (A 1969 case is under study in the United States.)

Though it is unproven and probably unprovable where and when the AIDS virus first mutated and infected humans, there is more than theoretical reason for wishing it could be known. If AIDS began in Africa, then it is reasonable to look at the African experience with AIDS as providing some timetable of the epidemic, despite many differences in our experience with the disease.

Currently, the World Health Organization estimates that about fifty thousand cases of AIDS have occurred in Africa, though the official number is only about one-eighth that high. More telling, as a measure of the scope and spread of the disease on that continent, are the crude gauges of the number of Africans who are infected with the AIDS virus.

WHO roughly estimates that more than 3 million Africans may be infected with the AIDS virus — as 10 million people may be worldwide — though the actual numbers could be twice as high. The hardest hit countries are still concentrated in central and east Africa, even though AIDS has now spread throughout the continent. Further, a second AIDS virus, HIV-2, has been found extensively in west Africa; a third, labeled SBL 6669 V-2, was identified in west Africans being treated in Sweden; and a fourth virus that causes AIDS-like disease has been isolated from Nigerian cases. African and World Health Organization specialists, along with European and American medical teams, have carried out blood samplings in capital cities among prostitutes, blood donors, adult and pediatric patients, pregnant women, and health workers at large public hospitals and clinics in many central and east African nations. Updated surveys indicate that up to 20 percent of men and women in the twenty- to forty-year-old age group and 10 percent of hospitalized children in some urban areas are already infected with the AIDS virus.[8] At some large maternity clinics, 20 to 25 percent of pregnant mothers are infected and infant mortality from AIDS alone is high. The findings are difficult to assess, because it is unknown whether those who are using hospitals are sicker or just better informed; thus the groups studied may be selectively high for AIDS. In various cities, however, 1 to 18 percent of the blood donors are positive for AIDS.[9] Other studies indicate that hospital workers are infected at about the same rate as the patients, not from taking care of them but from the same cause as the patients. Infection rates among African female prostitutes range from 27 to 88 percent.[10] Every new sampling shows higher figures, a rate of AIDS infectivity that is still rising at about 1 percent a year. Hard-won gains against a multitude of health problems in Africa threaten to be undone by AIDS. "Millions of deaths occur every year in the Third World because of diseases that could be prevented by vaccines," says WHO director-general Mahler. "Now AIDS comes along and there is the risk it will overshadow all the other diseases."[11]

AIDS is different in terms of symptoms and patterns of spread in Africa than in the United States, which may partially account for why it went unrecognized there so long. One form the disease takes in Africa was labeled "slim disease" — an irreversible wasting away. These AIDS patients look as if they are starving to death for lack of food, and some were confused with those who truly had. Other African AIDS cases, as elsewhere, manifest the viral, fungal, and bacterial infections that their previously healthy immune systems had held in check. AIDS also allows latent tuberculosis to reestablish itself. Recent samplings found that 40 percent of patients in TB sanitaria were infected with AIDS.[12] In countries where underlying TB infection is widespread, the arrival of a disease that can activate TB has a ripple effect. AIDS is such a disease, and while it is not spread casually, TB is, raising the specter of renewed infection with TB among coworkers, family members, community contacts, and health care teams. Further, with AIDS, many patients have severe reactions to anti-TB drugs. Exotic fungal infections that are naturally more prevalent in equatorial countries add to the AIDS burden in such climates. A Massachusetts Institute of Technology study suggests that the speed at which a person infected with the AIDS virus converts from silent to overt disease is governed by the frequency of other infections. If this is so, then Third World people whose lives are peppered with the diseases that thrive in heat, humidity, and squalor are in terrible jeopardy.

In Africa and elsewhere in the Third World, AIDS is indisputably a heterosexual disease, spread primarily through ordinary sexual intercourse, as well as in pregnancy from mother to child, and by breast feeding. As Halfdan Mahler points out, these modes of transmission "touch on the most intimate contacts of family life."[13] Thus, interrupting the spread of AIDS in the Third World will be exceedingly difficult. The incidence of standard sexually transmitted diseases (STDs) also is very high, and these infections often are inadequately treated (there and here), leaving multitudes of STD victims prone to secondary infection with AIDS. Lack of disposable hypodermic needles and syringes contributes to the spread of AIDS in the Third World. Needles are scarce and must be reused; often, they are inadequately sterilized, even though household bleach readily kills the AIDS virus. In some STD clinics, it is common practice for a large syringe to be filled with multiple doses of antibiotics. When the same syringe needle is used to inject a row of patients, if one patient is infected with AIDS, the infection may be passed to the rest — as with needle-using drug addicts in U.S. cities. Pressure-gun injections are also now suspected of being able to spread AIDS. Blood transfusions remain a serious source of AIDS transmission. Testing blood for AIDS currently costs $5 to $10, an impossible expense. New, simple, and inexpensive blood tests will soon be available, but they are less sensitive. Moreover, with the discovery of additional AIDS-causing viruses, tests will have to detect all of them. With limited electric power, there is little opportunity to freeze and store blood. In most of the world, blood drawn in the morning is often transfused before nightfall — "so urgently needed," says one CDC physician, "it is often still warm."[14] Demand for blood is high in Africa and wherever children are prone to sickle-cell anemia, malaria, and parasitic diseases that thin the blood.

The heterosexual spread of AIDS has many catch-22 characteristics in Africa and other Third World countries. High-risk groups, outside of prostitutes and long-distance truck drivers, are not easy targets of prevention campaigns. In many of these countries, polygamy is legal as well as religiously and culturally sanctioned. A polygamous husband with AIDS risks transmitting it to more than one wife: the availability as well as the acceptance of contraception is limited; condoms are the least favored means. In Africa, the average woman bears more than six children. If she is infected, her progeny are likely to be infected during pregnancy or childbirth. Outside the First World, breast feeding is predominant; infected mothers can transmit the AIDS virus in breast milk. Immunization with live virus vaccines, such as for polio, measles, and mumps, carries new risks. Given to AIDS-infected children who inefficiently make antibody, the virus-laced vaccines may give them the actual disease; immunizing other children who may shed live virus from the vaccine may also expose an AIDS-infected child in the family to the infection. Choices with a high social cost lie ahead: cutting back treatment for STDs versus paying for higher priced sterilization procedures; limiting breast feeding versus providing needed nutrition; curtailing immunization versus controlling childhood diseases; restricting blood transfusion versus maintaining life support.

While there was nothing that African nations could have done in the absence of knowledge about AIDS to protect their already hard-pressed people, heroic efforts are now under way. Almost every African nation has appointed an AIDS advisory commission, and education campaigns are gearing up. Yet, on top of intrinsic social problems, many African nations are caught up, directly or indirectly, in political, military, and economic upheaval that involves great movements of troops, workers, displaced families, and refugees. Vast numbers of tradesmen, truckers, food suppliers, and camp followers crisscross the continent, moving back and forth from city to village to encampments. There also is constant relocation of workers from the countryside along the roads and railroad tracks into cities and a consequent mushrooming of slums and informal households. The AIDS virus now travels with all of it.

There is great anxiety that some African countries may lose a key segment of their young adults, along with part of the next generation of children. In one capital city, the rate of infection is about 30 percent among the educated young men — the group that carries out much of the city's daily business and commerce. Professor Charles Myers of the Harvard Institute for International Development (HIID) estimates that by 1995, AIDS will have killed so many productive young adults in Zaire that the nation's gross national product may drop by 8 percent — the equivalent of a $292 billion loss in GNP for the United States. "The mind boggles at the numbers," Myers said of his projections of the impact of AIDS on many central African countries. "On economic grounds alone, the case for very high levels of preventive expenditures — even if success is limited — is extremely strong."[15] Currently, the World Health Organization estimates that it will need $1.2 billion in extra funds to combat AIDS in countries that do not have enough to do it themselves. Yet, the United States is not fulfilling its share of the bargain, despite long-established policy in support of WHO. Dr. William Foege, former head of the CDC, notes that the United States spends on its own health care "in seventy minutes of one day" the $61 million that was assessed as its share of the 1986 WHO budget. Only $10 million has been paid, "while the Soviet Union, China, Japan, and the Western European countries have all paid in full. I am personally embarrassed that our government has weakened the chances of solving the world AIDS problem," Foege says.[16] It will prove to be extremely costly economizing in the long run.

I have devoted considerable attention to AIDS in Africa because more is known about what is happening there. But the AIDS factors and forces at work in Africa apply widely across the Third World. Brazil now ranks second to the United States in incidence of AIDS among single countries in the Western Hemisphere. Though the official number of cases there is two thousand, the actual number is probably ten times greater. The Brazilian government says it is testing donated blood in public hospitals, but some 90 percent of blood for transfusion is collected and sold by private companies, which have not been testing at all, according to U.S. AIDS experts who recently visited there.[17] Other factors in Brazil which are singularly relevant to AIDS spread are the nation's week-long, sexually wanton, pre-Lenten *Carnivale;* religious bans on condom use in an overwhelmingly Catholic nation; surveys that point to a bisexual spread of AIDS ten times greater than in Western Europe; and a well documented, culturally accepted practice of anal intercourse by heterosexuals.[18]

Though Haiti's tally of cases is unofficially set at about fifteen hundred, Haiti's case rate is estimated to be higher, about thirty per one hundred thousand — twice that of the United States as a whole. As here, cases are congregated in cities. Dr. Jean Pape, a Haitian physician who is a member of the Cornell University Medical School faculty, has been researching AIDS in Port-au-Prince since 1982. His research suggests that 10 percent of the adults in urban areas, 66 percent of the city prostitutes (many from the neighboring Dominican Republic), and 3 percent of Haitians in rural areas are infected with the AIDS virus. In a culture where folk medicine predominates, AIDS may also be spread through ritualistic cutting and "injection" of innocuous substances on dirty needles. In the most impoverished nation in the hemisphere, haunted by starvation and now caught up in political turmoil, the prospects for controlling AIDS are dim.

No Central or South American country is without AIDS, nor any island of the Caribbean. And not the Latin American country of Mexico, which appears on its way toward a significant AIDS problem. The effects of sporadic AIDS-prevention campaign blitzes are not long lasting. In many of the countries, strong anti-American protests are being voiced. Many see the United States as the source of their AIDS problem — as is also felt in Europe — believing the disease is spread not only by the U.S. members of the international jet set — American gay males and heterosexual swingers — but also by AIDS-contaminated blood and blood products from the United States.

Informal reports from Cuba indicate that AIDS-infected military personnel returning from Angola are being "held" at one end of the island, where they may be joined by family members if they so wish. Two Cuban hospitals have established AIDS wards, and the Cuban government has established a new AIDS prevention and control program, according to Radio Marti, which operates under the direction of the U.S. Information Agency.

In the Philippines, outbreaks of AIDS have centered in bars and brothels frequented by U.S. servicemen. Beyond trying to cope with their own incipient AIDS problem or to ward off its taking root — especially in Asian countries, where AIDS has appeared later and only minimally — some countries are taking drastic steps to identify and ship home any foreigners found to be harboring the AIDS virus. In China, Japan, and India (as well as the Soviet Union, several Soviet Union bloc nations, Belgium, and Germany), all foreign students already are required to take AIDS blood tests. If the tests are positive, the students' scholarships are revoked and the students are sent home. Since many foreign students in these countries are Africans, concern is growing that AIDS is being used as a new foil for racism. Thailand and Iraq mandate that all visitors — and natives returning from abroad — be AIDS-tested. Belgium is considering the same for visitors from African countries. China is weighing a law that would require any foreign visitor who planned to stay for six months to undergo medical examinations for AIDS.

Similarly, the United States has now made an AIDS test a prerequisite for the 530,000 to 600,000 immigrants seeking permanent residence each year in this country. There is bitter irony in the newly ordered AIDS testing of the estimated 2 million to 4 million illegal aliens who may hope to remain in the United States under the revised resident alien law. If they have been residents here since before 1982 — which the law now requires them to prove — the great probability is that they became infected here. If sent back to their native countries, they will take AIDS — and the potential for spreading it — with them. In San Salvador, health officials are alarmed that hundreds of thousands of Salvadorans now living in the United States will be deported and will bring an AIDS epidemic home with them. All seven cases of AIDS which had been registered in El Salvador by May 12, 1987, were in Salvadorans who contracted AIDS in the United States and "came back to their country to die," says Dr. Lidia de Nieto, a member of the nation's Health Ministry.[19] While great attention was paid to the U.S. decision to test all recruits for military service as well as all members of the armed forces, almost none was given to U.S. State Department testing that began on January 1, 1987, of all Foreign Service personnel and their dependents, including thousands of members of the Peace Corps and the U.S. Agency for International Development. The Foreign Service chapter of the American Federation of Government Employees has filed suit to protest such "routine" testing; court documents revealed that seventeen Americans in the Foreign Service had already contracted AIDS and that five of them had died. AIDS thus has become a new job hazard for Americans working overseas, particularly where there is risk of being injured, requiring transfusions, and getting the AIDS virus from contaminated blood. The future significance of AIDS as a deterrent, not only to government foreign service, including the Peace Corps, but to the army of missionary workers across the world, is scarcely recognized. Nor has the portent of the disease been evaluated in terms of international trade and world economics, political, and even military operations. Kenya has requested that U.S. naval ships no longer allow their crews to disembark at Mombasa; the Philippines have linked their AIDS problem to bar girls working near the U.S. naval base at Subic Bay or Clark Air Base north of Manila, the largest installations used by U.S. forces outside the United States. Very slowly but surely, AIDS is moving into these larger contexts. This past March, an international conference (at the Barbican Center, London, organized by the London School of Hygiene and Tropical Medicine) on the global impact of AIDS met to assess the social, economic, and political AIDS issues, including travel restrictions, employment problems, population dynamics, and volunteer work.

Nowhere has AIDS become so much a part of daily life as in Europe, where the pattern of the outbreak most closely resembles the U.S. pattern. Though they have far fewer cases (eight thousand cases in twenty-seven countries) than the United States, European countries moved quickly into public education campaigns. Direct mailings have gone out to a vast number of households; anti-AIDS messages emblazon subway walls, billboards, taxicabs, and buses; radio, TV, and newspapers carry public service announcements. Near U.S. military bases, AIDS is still commonly referred to as the "Yankee" disease. Yet, despite early efforts, there are indications from Europe that the education campaigns are gaining only limited response in changing personal sexual behavior.

The story of AIDS is far different in the United States, one of its most tragic characteristics being the needless loss of time in the beginning. Many forces, blindly or deliberately, converged to permit the AIDS virus to take a deep hold in this country before any meaningful steps were taken to combat it. Since time is the great enemy in the fight against AIDS, this important, early advantage was lost.

The central failure concerning AIDS is that it was not — and still is not in some quarters — perceived as what it fundamentally is: a disease with potential for destruction of great magnitude, not a form of supernatural retribution. The overriding focus of early social and political attention was its male homosexual spread — too often on judgmental, moralistic terms.

AIDS origin here, primarily among homosexual men, made the disease not only distasteful but dismissable to many, most notably the Reagan White House, which has been unduly influenced by ultraconservative fundamentalists. Representative Waxman is on solid ground when he says, "I am convinced that had the first victims of AIDS been members of the Chamber of Commerce, the Reagan Administration would have responded immediately and forthrightly. Because the male homosexual population was first affected by AIDS, the Reagan Administration thought of this group as dispensable and didn't respond as quickly as it could have and should have. The Administration has handled this whole thing in an irresponsible way. As a matter of fact, I think that when people look back historically at the Reagan Administration, aside from the huge deficit that we have run up over the last six years, the other comment on this Administration will be its failure to deal with the AIDS crisis, which unfortunately will have gotten out of hand and affected maybe millions of people."[20] To the credit of the gay male community, it organized much needed, early support services and was the first to generate self-help, safer sex materials. But the homosexual stigma that was attached to AIDS was the factor, above all others, that fostered political and social neglect, while encouraging the expression of pseudo-religio-political prejudice and vindictiveness. The "gay" label also permitted a paucity of funding and a transference of attention to nonmedical economic and social issues — mandatory blood testing, insurance screening, job discrimination, health benefit eligibility, entitlement to Social Security Disability coverage. Though these issues are significant, the effect was diversionary — a begging of the question: What should the United States be doing to combat the greatest threat to public health in modern times?

None of the major public policy issues surrounding AIDS has yet been resolved.

Essentially these issues can be broadly summarized under three headings: mobilizing to fight the disease, through funding and organizing research and medical care; civil rights, in the sense of safeguards against discrimination within the conflict between public and private rights; and prevention, through education and public health programs.

Mobilizing to Fight the Disease

When the proposed $790 million AIDS budget for FY'88, which covers research, epidemiology, public health services, and information programs, is included, the federal government will have spent or allocated $1.676 billion for AIDS since mid-1981. (On February 18, details of the FY'89 federal budget indicated an administration request for $1.7 billion for all AIDS-related federal programs, including the U.S. Public Health Service [PHS], Medicare and Medicaid, the Department of Defense, and the federal Bureau of Prisons.) The glaring flaw in that funding picture is that the sum did not even amount to $100 million prior to FY'85 — four years into the epidemic. It also should be noted that in each fiscal year since 1983, it has fallen to the Congress to increase the AIDS budget by 76 to 115 percent over the previous year, markedly exceeding the administration's request.[21]

Nearly $485 million in additional monies is budgeted for 1988 to underwrite the federal share of Medicaid, Medicare, Social Security, and Veterans Administration costs for the care and support of AIDS patients, and for massive, mandatory AIDS-testing programs for recruits and members of the armed forces, Job Corps enrollees, Foreign Service employees, and federal prisoners.

Through the end of 1987, individual states had allocated an additional $200 million, primarily for support services and education, though some funds for research were specified. Five states alone (California, New York, Florida, New Jersey, and Massachusetts) accounted for 85 percent of this money.[22]

Insofar as AIDS research is concerned, a number of problems stem from the lack of clear policy. Until 1988, funding was woefully inadequate. Even next year, federal funds for research will approximate only half a billion dollars — the remaining $250 million is earmarked for education and prevention. Whatever excuses may be offered for early failure to recognize the need to fully fund AIDS research, none remain. In October 1986, the National Academy of Sciences (NAS) and the Institute of Medicine (IOM) concluded in their joint study on AIDS that funding for AIDS research should be set at a billion dollars a year by 1990 — two years hence — and, further, that another billion dollars should be spent for public education and prevention, through a combination of federal, state, and private funds. Moreover, NAS-IOM underscored the need for such funds to be new funds — not siphoned from existing Public Health funds, as has chronically been the case in previous years.[23]

A second research problem, in the view of some scientists, has been the lack of a comprehensive, coherent approach to AIDS research. While it is agreed that new knowledge is needed to understand the AIDS virus and its biologic activity in humans — knowledge that can come only from basic research — it is nonetheless arguable that the components of that research can be far better focused and integrated. The National Institutes of Health (NIH) could and should better coordinate in-house and externally assigned work and industrial projects. Much more could be done to bring together the groups involved in these projects. NIH is still authorizing research without first consulting the teams most likely to do the work. While NIH has identified the major lines of research — vaccines, anti-AIDS drugs, and virus investigations — it has not fully asked the research community what it sees as the best approach, the best targets, or the best way to organize. Among those scientists who subscribe to the view that greater coordination is both possible and necessary is Dr. David Baltimore, a Nobelist in medicine and physiology who received the prize for his work in virology, and director of the Whitehead Institute at the Massachusetts Institute of Technology.

One research area that has become better coordinated is the testing of new anti-AIDS drugs under the aegis of the National Institute of Allergy and Infectious Diseases. Such evaluations are now under way at nineteen centers across the country. While much has been done and fresh efforts are being made to enlist the nation's front-line scientists in the research drive to unravel the mystery of AIDS, the public policy issues of how large the federal commitment to AIDS research should be, how fast it can be deployed, and how that research will be organized — perhaps even targeted — are yet to be fully aired or addressed.

Of at least equal importance is the public policy issue of assuring all AIDS patients medical care, and how that care is to be funded. Estimates of the direct medical care costs of AIDS vary widely. The best guess most widely cited is $8.5 billion to $16 billion a year by 1991, calculated for the Centers for Disease Control by economist Anne Scitovsky of the Palo Alto Medical Foundation/Research Institute and her colleague Dorothy Rice of the University of California at San Francisco.[24] Their projections, however, are based on 1985 and 1986 data and on a U.S. Public Health Service forecast that estimates the United States will experience 270,000 cases of AIDS by 1991. Dr. Stephen Joseph, New York City health commissioner, has stressed that in 1991 alone, there will be more new AIDS cases than cumulatively in all the years from 1980 to the present. These projections do not reflect the unexpectedly large explosion of AIDS infectivity in needle-using drug addicts (or any significant spread of AIDS into the heterosexual population), which makes the upper estimate of $16 billion by 1991 more likely. Further, a forecast by the Rand Corporation, a California think tank, considers the PHS projection (of 270,000 cases between 1981 and 1991) low and offers a mid-to-high-range estimate of 400,000 to 750,000 cumulative cases in that period.[25] Rand says its mid-range estimate would boost medical costs for AIDS to $38 billion by 1991.

For comparative purposes, even the low estimate of $8.5 billion a year for AIDS in 1991 rivals or exceeds the medical costs associated with other major health care expenditures: by 1991, $8 billion for caring for auto accident victims; $4.9 billion for digestive cancers; and $3.9 billion for lung cancer.[26]

While $8.5 billion to $16 billion in AIDS medical costs adds only a small percentage increase to the national health care expenditure, it should be kept in mind that AIDS is a completely new cost burden. Further, most AIDS patients are young adults, who historically are in an age group with the lowest medical expenses. Moreover, the costs will not be evenly distributed, any more than the patient load will be. Though U.S. AIDS cases have been concentrated in five major cities (Los Angeles, San Francisco, New York, Houston, and Miami), the CDC predicts that 80 percent of the growth by 1991 will occur outside these areas. Nonetheless, the heaviest case loads will continue in cities, and a disproportionate number of cases will increasingly be among minorities, who dominate the populations of inner-city, urban poor.

Some 50 million Americans have inadequate health care coverage, and 30 million under the age of sixty-five have none.[27] The federal Health Care Financing Administration estimates that 40 percent of AIDS patients' care is currently being paid under federal/state Medicaid programs, though in some inner-city areas the figure rises to nearly 80 percent. To be eligible for Medicaid, of course, AIDS patients must first be impoverished.

The availability of Medicare for AIDS patients, under Social Security Disability coverage, is relatively meaningless. Disabled AIDS patients must "qualify" first by having made payroll contributions; then, they must prove that they are unable to work for a continuous period of at least twelve months. Though the eligibility period for receiving cash benefits has been shortened, patients must wait an additional twenty-four months for Medicare benefits.[28] Only 1 to 3 percent of AIDS patients live long enough to qualify for Medicare, though this could change if new therapies prolong survival.

In view of these medical-cost calculations, the AIDS epidemic requires new public policy on how the costs are to be met. Private insurance pools have been recommended, as have other publicly financed reimbursement strategies. But it is clear that only the federal system can deal with the huge expenditures that AIDS care will entail, and that only federal policy can set the course. The health care system in the United States is disjointed and uneven, owing to the disparate mechanisms under which it is funded, and many health care delivery planners believe that it cannot withstand the financial burden that will be imposed upon it by AIDS. Many of these planners feel that only a national health insurance program, drawing on the widest base possible, will be able to aggregate and dispense sufficient funds in timely enough fashion to meet the challenge of AIDS.

Almost all studies so far have limited their consideration to overt AIDS, according to the old CDC definition. The broader definition put into effect in September 1987, which includes seriously ill ARC patients and other AIDS-related conditions, is expected to raise all estimates by at least 15 percent.[29] Further, new analyses of New York City's experience find that 46 percent of patients hospitalized with AIDS infections are chronic ARC patients, many of whom become sick and die without ever having met official AIDS definitions. The CDC itself has said that its AIDS figures may be underreported by 40 percent. Whatever the actual case loads ultimately prove to be, they are much more likely to be higher, not lower, than current analyses indicate.

Money is not the only AIDS medical care problem. Shortages of nurses and of appropriate facilities, such as hospices for dying AIDS patients and inpatient services for those with dementia, further complicate the picture. Studies indicate that AIDS patients require at least 40 percent more nursing care than other medical/surgical or pediatric patients. This translates into eight or more hours of direct nursing care per day. At these high levels of care, it is estimated that at least thirteen thousand additional nurses will be needed for AIDS patients alone by 1991, at a time when nurses will still be critically scarce. The nursing requirements also preclude the possibility that many AIDS patients will be able to be cared for in nursing homes, since the patients need far more nursing care than is available in a skilled nursing facility. Studies have further shown that AIDS patients, because of physical and mental disabilities, also place high demands on social services. While models for flexible, alternative approaches to AIDS care (most notably developed in San Francisco), such as residences, hospices, and home care, should be pursued, they are not readily available. Shortages in home care staff and in funding for home care already are tying up services for the elderly. A new (October 1987) Massachusetts Hospital Association study identified the "most pressing" gaps in the health delivery system as the unavailability of secure inpatient psychiatric services for AIDS patients suffering neurological and other mental disturbances; an inadequate number of drug abuse programs, particularly methadone treatment centers; and a shortage of home health and hospice services, which already "appear seriously strained."[30]

What is certain is that there will be no quick fix for the medical care requirements of AIDS patients. The hardest hit states already are reaching the limits of their financial ability to cope with the disease. States may be a "laboratory" for devising better medical delivery responses, but AIDS is a national health crisis and the major responsibility for funding and for gearing up the health delivery system to respond lies with the federal government. Such action is fraught with difficulty. Yet, public policy decisions on AIDS medical care issues cannot be avoided much longer.

Civil Rights

At the heart of public policy considerations concerning AIDS is the conflict between individual rights and the need to protect the public health. The AIDS outbreak here began and persists in three groups — homosexual men, drug addicts, and prostitutes — who, regrettably, are classic targets of discrimination and neglect.

Though pockets of public hysteria over AIDS have calmed down as confidence grows that the disease is not casually transmitted, it should be remembered that there were sporadic early and continuing calls from some political-fundamentalist groups for quarantine, including the recommendation that Boston Harbor's Peddocks Island, the former home of a now-abandoned leprosy sanatorium, be used as the site. The 1986 political campaign waged by Lyndon LaRouche in California embodied similar ugly proposals.

Artificial importance has been given the topic of mandatory blood tests for AIDS, as if by identifying all AIDS virus carriers, some easy solution for dealing with the epidemic would emerge. Copious energy has been devoted to the issue of AIDS testing, hardening the lines between advocates and opponents. As Adlai Stevenson said of nuclear weaponry, "There is no evil in the atom," only in what society does with it.[31] So it is with AIDS testing: the problem lies in the use made of it. No problem would exist at all were it not for the stigma that some have assigned to AIDS. In despicable judgments, AIDS is dismissed as a disease of the sexually perverted, depraved junkies, and pariah prostitutes who deserve what they get. Though more subtly expressed, stigma still misshapes much of society's — and the government's — response to AIDS.

The second social force feeding reaction to AIDS is fear. AIDS patients have been evicted from apartments and fired from their jobs; a few have even been ousted from hospitals. Even when the AIDS victims have been children, surely unwitting victims of the disease, fear has turned otherwise reasonable adults into brute-faced protestors, refusing to allow AIDS children to attend school, shunning them and their parents, and even acting out violently against them. Despite the protection afforded by standard precautionary measures, some doctors, dentists, and nurses have refused to care for AIDS patients, and some undertakers have refused to bury them.

Fear and the prejudice born of fear are one thing. Toleration of discrimination against AIDS patients and carriers is another. Education can minimize fear and defuse prejudice, but law and the enforcement of law are needed to prevent future AIDS discrimination.

Such legal protection falls within the realm of public policy. While some states have specifically outlawed AIDS discrimination, here, too, there is need for a national stance. U.S. Sen. Edward Kennedy (D-Mass.) and Rep. Henry Waxman are cosponsoring federal legislation to ban discrimination against people with AIDS, to guarantee confidentiality of AIDS-related records, and to assure privacy. Their bill was filed on June 23, 1987, in the aftermath of the Third International Conference on AIDS, during which police in Washington, D.C., donned heavy, yellow rubber gloves in a fear-mongering reaction to a march by AIDS victims. Though two hearings have been held on the bill, no action is expected until later this year. Some of the delay stems from a persistent, negative undercurrent about AIDS, abetted by the Reagan administration's political position that such legal protection is a state matter. Until destigmatizing legal protection is in place, progress on the whole roster of civil rights issues concerning AIDS will be stalled. These reach into the rights of homosexuals to fair and impartial treatment; of drug addicts and prostitutes to life-saving preventive and curative services; of prisoners whose AIDS infectivity can diminish their prospects for release; of military personnel whose careers may be thwarted because of their AIDS status; of public and private employees to job equity; of children to attend school; and of all people with AIDS to obtain housing, social services, and adequate and compassionate medical care.

Alongside these rights stand the conflicting issues of whether those in sexual contact with AIDS carriers are entitled to know they have been placed at risk; whether insurance companies should be allowed to test applicants; the limits under which public health officials can detain AIDS carriers who deliberately continue behavior that can transmit the infection to others; and how workers in direct care or contact with AIDS patients and AIDS carriers are to protect themselves from infection.

These are formidable public policy issues, ones that are "unlikely soon to be met," says Dr. Harvey Fineberg, dean of the Harvard School of Public Health. As a guideline, he urges that the least restrictive means be sought to protect the community and that a graded series of responses be devised before public policy steps are taken "that run the risk of infringing upon the rights of individuals."[32] A national agenda of AIDS-related civil rights issues needs to be set.

Prevention

Of all the sorry aspects of the AIDS epidemic in the United States, none is sorrier than the slow and inept efforts of the federal government to prevent the spread of the infection. While it is impossible to calculate how many people acquired the infection because they did not know how not to — or, more to the point, had not been told in persuasive ways how to avoid doing so — the number has to be very large, and it is still growing.

The nub of the problem, of course, is that to educate the public about safer sex as a modality for preventing AIDS entails informing people about sexual matters. Sex education is a topic that the U.S. government historically, and this administration particularly, has shrunk from, as if the subject itself were a carnal sin. Beneath the torrents of hypocritical preaching about the need to be sensitive to religious teachings, family values, and traditional morals, the basis for much of the resistance has been the viewpoint that those who violate the bounds of chastity and fidelity should pay for their transgressions. On such terms, AIDS can be dismissed as a form of moralistic retribution, visited upon the willful or, at least, the weak. However desirable strong moral codes may be for the conduct of society, they are weak weapons for combating a disease like AIDS, especially in an era marked by sexually frank commercialism and increasingly open sexual behavior.

Arguments against telling people how to prevent AIDS through the use of condoms rest on the same questionable point that has precluded telling teenagers about responsible (pregnancy-avoiding) sexual behavior: the fear that it would encourage the very behavior that was not wanted — promiscuity — even though extensive pilot programs prove otherwise. The barriers to educating the American public about AIDS are nowhere clearer than in the brouhaha that erupted in 1986 when television networks were confronted by public service announcements that used the word *condom.* Condoms are more openly spoken of now, though still more frequently on news broadcasts than in public service ads.

It was Rock Hudson's death that drove the message home as nothing else had. But until 1986, the source of AIDS preventive education remained almost exclusively the gay male community. AIDS action committees and other similar forums assembled and distributed the first and only booklets, posters, and fliers that advised people how to continue to engage in sexual activities — more safely. Since these messages were directed to homosexual men, they were not generally regarded as appropriate for heterosexuals, though safer sex practices apply universally. Heterosexuals went on blindly unconcerned for a prolonged period, and government agencies did little to instruct them otherwise.

The number of AIDS cases reached a dramatic height (sixteen thousand) in January 1986,[33] and the infection was making inroads among intravenous drug users and prostitutes in major cities. These latter groups not only were largely heterosexual, but also were seen as bridges for the spread of AIDS to the broad general public. Transfusion cases were growing, and more than two-thirds of the estimated twenty thousand seriously afflicted hemophiliacs in the United States had acquired the infection through contaminated blood products.[34] In early 1986, the National Academy of Sciences and the Institute of Medicine decided to undertake a special assessment of the problems and to propose an appropriate national response. Public pressure for action was mounting.

In February 1986, President Reagan called for a report on AIDS from the U.S. surgeon general, Dr. C. Everett Koop. A spokesperson for the U.S. Public Health Service at that time estimated that the report would be ready by May or June, but it was not issued until two weeks before the NAS-IOM report; many felt the timing was deliberate to counteract the complaint that the president had yet to comment or act directly on AIDS.[35] Koop's thirty-six-page, plainspoken report about the medical facts and sexual aspects of AIDS drew heavy fire from the fundamentalist religious contingent and from ultraconservative congressional and White House factions. His pamphlet remained, until October 1987, the only major administration document on AIDS. It has yet to be distributed directly to American households. An influential opponent of sexually specific AIDS education in the schools and of Koop's report is the stolidly conservative U.S. secretary of education, William Bennett. Further, Bennett's former associate Gary Bauer now heads the Domestic Policy Council in the White House. In the aftermath of the Third International Conference on AIDS in June 1987, Congress appropriated $20 million for a mailing of Koop's report to every American household. Instead, a folder was prepared for Dr. Otis R. Bowen, U.S. secretary of health and human services, by the CDC as part of its so-called America Responds to AIDS project. In his introduction, Bowen calls the response "inspiring."[36] With only scant reference to condoms and none to homosexuality, the folder advocates the sharing of family moral and religious values, monogamous relationships, and, for teenagers, saying no to illicit drugs and no to sex. This booklet was to substitute for Koop's forthright report. Some 45 million copies are "targeted" for distribution by states, local health departments, YMCAs, and selected corporations. Congress has officially requested the General Accounting Office to investigate "the Administration's failure" to carry out Congress's mandate to mail AIDS data to every household;[37] other countries, including Great Britain, have done such mailings. The administration, meanwhile, had indicated that it intends to use the $20 million for other purposes. A different pamphlet is now being readied for household mailing this summer, Bowen says, and the U.S. Public Health Service plans to comply with the congressional mandate. Rep. Gerry Studds (D-Mass.) contends that "the White House blocked the widespread distribution of Koop's report, even now, because it deemed the information within the report too explicit for the general public. The Administration's abject failure to fulfill its public health responsibilities now verges on criminal negligence."[38]

While the squabbling over Koop's and Bowen's reports continues — a reflection of the AIDS policy struggle within the White House — cities and community organizations are left to try to combat the spread of AIDS on a local level. Cities like New York, San Francisco, Los Angeles, and Miami have gone public with the AIDS message — on billboards, buses, rapid transit ads, and through extensive use of news media. Some states, including Massachusetts, are sending out their own household mailings and have prepared classroom curricula on AIDS (the CDC is now preparing its version). But there's a lot of slippage between the teaching guides and their use. Communities control what is taught in their schools, and many have denied the introduction of AIDS materials. Though a few cautionary spot announcements have been prepared, federally and at the state level, the broadcast media have largely been slow to use them. The CDC regularly issues medical advisories on AIDS infection control, but these do not reach broad public audiences.

Yet, continuing surveys show that Americans are highly aware of AIDS. Radio and TV news features and documentaries, and stepped up reporting and special AIDS sections in newspapers and magazines, along with plays and movies, have been the purveyors of AIDS information for the public. Among the difficulties in such an arrangement are the information, language, and cultural impediments, and the hit-or-miss nature of the public's reading and viewing habits. Further, the degree of public attention paid the topic of AIDS, as is true of most subjects, waxes and wanes with little consistency.

In terms of public policy, the United States has failed so far to address the need for massive, persuasive, public education aimed at prevention on any long-term basis. Not only has the federal government failed to spell out in precise language the nature of the disease, but it has not yet even recognized that it lacks a mechanism for speaking directly to the public. In Europe, Mexico, Canada, and Australia, as in China and India and Soviet bloc nations, the governments have direct avenues for public communication — through socialized health services and socialized radio and television. Although they are helpful, mailings to households, public health agencies or community organizations do not begin to address the need to persuade people to change their behavior. This involves more than an occasional booklet. What is needed in the United States is some new, direct line of communication — from the federal or state government, or both, to the citizenry. To continually update information about AIDS, as it changes, requires a ready means of getting the information out — quickly, thoroughly, accurately. This is the AIDS education public policy issue that demands immediate attention.

Some still would have it that AIDS has struck like a freak storm, blowing across areas of the world that lie powerless in its path. AIDS, indeed, may be a new whirlwind, but its impact is worsened by the pervasive social neglect that now leaves the United States in a weakened position to cope with it. AIDS is extracting a heavy penalty for our failure to overcome homophobia, drug addiction, and prostitution; to establish a credible system for funding health costs and providing health care; to attract, train, and fund sufficient medical and research personnel and to keep pace with the need for advanced research laboratories; to create an adequate network of home care, nursing home care, hospices, and health communication; to surmount the barriers that place inner-city minorities at risk for every successive medical-social hardship; and to accept the validity of public sex education. That is the landscape onto which AIDS has moved, a setting ill-prepared for its assault.

Though lack of presidential leadership does not fall neatly into a category of public policy, national mismanagement of the AIDS epidemic does. As early as 1984, Congress's Office of Technology Assessment chided the handling of the AIDS outbreak.[39] As recently as August 1987, the U.S. General Accounting Office, in a Briefing Report to Sen. Lawton Chiles, chairman of the Senate Subcommittee on Labor, Health and Human Services, Education and Related Agencies and of the Senate Budget Committee, presented the views of a broad range of American experts on AIDS. It expressed deep concern about a general lack of federal leadership, citing a "patchwork" of federal and state funding for AIDS prevention programs and cumbersome processes for awarding research grants. It also concluded that "within the context of current health policy-making . . . the federal response to AIDS appears uncoordinated and insufficient."[40] Six years into an epidemic of the proportion and severity of AIDS, this conclusion borders on an indictment of the Reagan administration, which has held the reins of federal power since 1981: AIDS played out "on their watch." The latest Reagan ploy has been the naming of an AIDS Commission, originally predominated by AIDS amateurs, to report on the ramifications of the epidemic. Although the commission leadership has been strengthened and is making a diligent effort to assess the AIDS outbreak and the response to it, it is late in the day to do so.

To all appearances, Congress is now taking AIDS out of the administration's hands. Despite the gloomy predictions, it is still possible to marshal the great scientific might and vast social resources of the nation. "To have an impact on what happens in the mid-1990s," warns Dr. Stephen Joseph of New York City, "we will have to take action now."[41] The ultimate public policy question regarding AIDS is whether enough public will and government support can be mustered to act in time. The leviathan of AIDS will not wait.

Perspective

Two rules of thumb are helpful for understanding the AIDS phenomenon.

The first has to do with the pace of infection. It holds that although it takes years for the first 1 percent of a population to become infected, after that a doubling phenomenon sets in — whether the doubling time is six months, a year, or more. Studies of a large cohort of homosexual men show that it took several years for 1 percent of the group to become AIDS-infected, as they were by 1978. It then took only one more year to double to 2 percent, and another year to reach 4 percent. The percentage reached into the teen figures by 1980, the mid-20 percents by 1981. By 1982, 47 percent (almost half) were infected. This happened before there was much awareness of AIDS and little change in behavior to contain its spread. Today the number infected in that group is around 78 percent.

The other rule of thumb relates to how many persons infected with AIDS will convert to illness, and how soon it will happen. At first it seemed that only some few would convert; others would be spared. In the beginning, the conversion rate seemed to be 1 to 2 percent a year, then 3 to 5 percent a year, then 5 to 10 percent. The conversion rate seemed to slow down between the third and fifth years. Now, it appears that after the fifth year of infection, the number of those who convert to illness seems to speed up again. Of eighty-eight California men who have been infected with the AIDS virus for seven years, 90 percent have fallen ill. Rather than escaping the disease state of AIDS, it seems more likely to be a matter of time. Incubation may extend far longer than ten years. These two indices of AIDS — spread of infection and conversion to illness — are of vital importance. The first suggests that if the spread of AIDS is not kept below a critical point, it will continue largely because there will be so many AIDS-infected people available for sexual or blood-related contact with the noninfecteds. In other words, as the pool of virus grows, so does the likelihood of encountering it. The second index, of conversion, indicates that the ultimate number of AIDS cases may be nearly all of those persons now infected. Cases today are a snapshot of the spread of AIDS two to seven years ago. Future cases will be a reflection of failure to act, now.

Details of the AIDS epidemic and the extent to which it was mismanaged on almost every front are documented in a new book, And the Band Played On: Politics, People, and the AIDS Epidemic, *by Randy Shilts, a reporter for the* San Francisco Chronicle *who has been writing about AIDS since 1982. The book stands as an indictment of the interlocking process whereby the early spread of AIDS can be traced to the fractious divisiveness within the male homosexual community; an imperious lack of interest by major science centers; the torpid response of public health officials, voluntary blood banks, state and federal agencies, and most elected officials; and the brittle resistance of the Reagan administration.*

Notes

1. Halfdan Mahler, director-general, World Health Organization, Address to the United Nations, November 20, 1986.
2. U.S. Rep. Henry Waxman (D-Calif.), chairman, U.S. House of Representatives Subcommittee on Health and the Environment, at hearing held at the Gay and Lesbian Community Services Center, Hollywood, California, April 13, 1982.
3. Centers for Disease Control, Atlanta, Georgia. "Opportunistic Infections and Kaposi's Sarcoma among Haitians in the United States." *Morbidity and Mortality Weekly Report* 31 (July 9, 1982): 53–61.
4. Donald Drake, "A Mystery in the Blood," *Philadelphia Inquirer,* January 2, 1983.
5. Centers for Disease Control, Atlanta, Georgia. "Hepatitis B Virus Vaccine Safety: Report of an Inter-Agency Group." *Morbidity and Mortality Weekly Report* 31 (September 3, 1982): 465–467.
6. Centers for Disease Control, Atlanta, Georgia. "1987 Revision of the CDC Surveillance Case Definition for Acquired Immune Deficiency Syndrome." *Morbidity and Mortality Weekly Report.* Special supplement, August 14, 1987.
7. Dr. Ib Bygbjerg, State University Hospital, Copenhagen, Denmark. Letters to the Editor, *Lancet,* April 23, 1983.
8. Personal reporting, AIDS in Africa conference, Naples, Italy, October 1987.

9. Ibid.

10. Ibid.

11. Halfdan Mahler, director-general, WHO, Geneva, Switzerland, news wire services, Feb. 14, 1987.

12. Personal reporting, AIDS in Africa conference.

13. Ibid.

14. Loretta McLaughlin, *Boston Globe,* op-ed page, July 10, 1986.

15. Richard Knox, *Boston Globe,* June 8, 1987, p. 41. Reporting on Third International Conference on AIDS, Washington, D.C., June 1–5, 1987.

16. News wire services, Washington, D.C., June 30, 1987.

17. Personal interviews, October 1987.

18. Richard Parker (Department of Anthropology, University of California at Berkeley), "Acquired Immunodeficiency Syndrome in Urban Brazil." *Medical Anthropology Quarterly* 1, no. 2 (June 1987): 155–175.

19. Annie Cabrera, Associated Press, El Salvador, May 12, 1987.

20. U.S. Rep. Henry Waxman, "Governance Colloquium on AIDS." *Governance: Harvard Journal of Public Policy* (Summer–Fall 1987): 43–47.

21. U.S. General Accounting Office, *AIDS Prevention: Views on the Administration's Budget Proposals.* Washington, D.C., August 12, 1987.

22. Ibid.

23. Institute of Medicine-National Academy of Sciences. *Confronting AIDS: Directions for Public Health, Health Care, and Research.* National Academy Press, Washington, D.C., October 1986, p. 33.

24. A. A. Scitovsky and D. P. Rice, "Estimates of the Direct and Indirect Costs of Acquired Immunodeficiency Syndrome in the United States, 1985, 1986 and 1991," *Public Health Reports* (January–February 1987): 5–17.

25. Anthony Pascal, chief author, et al., Rand Report on AIDS, prepared for the federal Health Care Financing Administration, released June 3, 1987, Rand Corporation, Palo Alto, California.

26. Jesse Green, Madeleine Singer, Neil Wintfeld, Kevin Schulman, and Leigh Passman of New York University Medical Center, *Health Affairs* (journal of Project HOPE Health Sciences Education Center, Millwood, Va.) 6, no. 3 (Fall 1987): 19–31.

27. Institute of Medicine-National Academy of Sciences. *Confronting AIDS,* p. 165.

28. Ibid.

29. Greater New York Hospital Association survey, June 1987.

30. Report of the AIDS Task Force of the Massachusetts Hospital Association, September 1987. Parts II and III.

31. Adlai Stevenson, speech as Democratic presidential candidate, Hartford, Connecticut, September 18, 1952. "Nature is neutral. There is no evil in the atom — only in men's souls."

32. Dean Harvey Fineberg, "Public Health and Private Rights: Health, Social and Ethical Perspectives." *Proceedings of AIDS International Symposium,* New York City, 1986, Hummler Plenum Press.

33. Centers for Disease Control, Atlanta, Georgia. AIDS updates.

34. Centers for Disease Control, Atlanta, Georgia. "HIV Infection and Pregnancies in Sexual Partners of HIV-Seropositive Hemophilic Men — United States." *Morbidity and Mortality Weekly Report* 36, no. 35 (September 11, 1987): 593–595.

35. Personal reporting, June–October 1986.

36. Otis R. Bowen, M.D., secretary, U.S. Department of Health and Human Services. "An Important Message for All Americans." Introduction to *What You Should Know About AIDS,* prepared under contract for the Centers for Disease Control as part of its America Responds to AIDS project.

37. U.S. Rep. Gerry Studds (D-Mass.), *Weekly Report to the People* (of the Tenth Congressional District of Massachusetts), October 2, 1987.

38. Ibid.

39. "Review of the Public Health Service's Response to AIDS." A Technical Memorandum, Office of Technology Assessment, Washington, D.C. U.S. Congress OTA-TM-H-24, February 1985.

40. U.S. General Accounting Office, *AIDS Prevention.*

41. Bruce Lambert, *New York Times,* November 12, 1987, sec. B, p. 2.

Aseptic meningitis. Non-pus-producing inflammation of the lining of the spinal cord and the fluid that surrounds it by viruses or other organisms.

Chemotherapeutic agent. A treatment for an infection or malignancy.

Cytomegalovirus. A virus that is very common and may result in a mononucleosis-like illness in young adults and that can be transmitted sexually. In persons with depressed immune function, this virus can reactivate and cause invasive disease of the eyes, lungs, bowels, and other vital organs.

Dementia. Organic loss of intellectual function.

Disseminated viral infection. The ability of certain viruses to spread throughout an infected individual's body, causing dysfunction of several different organ systems.

Encephalopathy. Any degenerative brain disease.

Epstein-Barr virus. The virus that causes mononucleosis. In individuals whose immune systems are not functioning, this virus may reactivate from a latent stage and cause fevers and invasion of specific organs, and may contribute to the development of lymphomas (lymph gland cancers).

Herpes simplex. A virus that can be chronic and latent and that most typically causes blisters around the mouth or genitals. It is sexually transmitted.

Histologic pattern. The microscopic arrangement of cells characteristic of specific organs and disease states.

Host immune response. The ability of an individual to respond to infectious agents, or to cells that become malignant, in order to protect the individual from developing severe infection or malignancy.

Iatrogenic. Caused inadvertently by a physician, as in an untoward illness or medical problem.

Glossary continued on page 56

The Clinical Spectrum of HIV Infections: Implications for Public Policy

Kenneth H. Mayer, M.D.

The term acquired immunodeficiency syndrome (AIDS) is a definition developed by the Centers for Disease Control to explain the epidemic of immunosuppression first seen in the United States among gay and bisexual men and intravenous drug users in the early 1980s. It is now known that the human immunodeficiency virus (HIV) is the necessary agent for the compromise of the immune system which results in AIDS; however, there is a wide range of manifestations associated with HIV infection. Individuals with AIDS tend to have severe opportunistic infections or malignancies, and the vast majority of individuals die within two years after the diagnosis. At least a fourth of the individuals with HIV infection in one study were found to remain asymptomatic after seven years of infection. Between the long period of asymptomatic infection and the development of life-threatening opportunistic infections, individuals may develop subacute manifestations of HIV infection. Some individuals may develop constitutional symptoms, without any other medical explanation. The clinical use of tests of immunologic function as well as newer tests that may describe the type of HIV infection, such as the serum antigen test, may enhance the ability of clinicians to give infected patients more specific information as to their prognosis. As newer therapies are developed, the utilization of newer diagnostic tests may allow for staging more rational treatment plans. The data suggesting increasing efficacy of Azidothymidine (AZT), as well as the development of newer chemotherapeutic agents, may lead to more widespread HIV testing in order to detect infection at early stages and intervene with specific therapies. Use of the test as a means of altering behavior remains controversial. The development of newer therapies is hindered by the need to avoid exposing HIV-infected individuals to agents that subsequently turn out to be harmful, such as HPA-23 and Suramin. But this must be balanced with the urgent need of individuals to try promising therapeutic agents. Preliminary data suggest that individuals who are treated with AZT at earlier stages of HIV infection may do better; thus, there may be a move in the future to treat people with AZT. The clinical dilemma will persist for some time to come, and the cost of care for individuals with AIDS and HIV infection will be extremely high. Although the illness is frequently fatal, it is most appropriate to be considerate of

Dr. Kenneth H. Mayer is assistant professor of medicine at Brown University and at Memorial Hospital in Pawtucket, Rhode Island, and is research director at the Fenway Community Health Center in Boston.

the individual's desire to have more aggressive therapies, given the variability of HIV infection for each person and the fact that new therapeutic breakthroughs are being made every day.

The AIDS epidemic is profoundly affecting the general public regarding issues of social policy, ranging from the sexual counter-revolution to how one deals with primeval fears of contagion in the age of instant global transport. Medical clinicians comprise one of the groups that have had to respond most to the multiple conundra associated with this epidemic. They were also among those individuals who initially recognized that something new was occurring with the disease in the early 1980s. Nosology is that branch of medical science which deals with the classification of diseases, and at the outset of what is now perceived as a global problem, the new epidemic was a clinically complicated nosological question. Young males, predominantly gay men with multiple sexual partners, as well as a few intravenous drug users, in a discrete number of cities — that is, New York City, San Francisco, and Los Angeles — were perceived to be developing illnesses associated with deranged immunoregulation. The first published report in the medical literature regarding what is now known as the AIDS epidemic was in the *Morbidity and Mortality Weekly Report*, a newsletter of the Centers for Disease Control (CDC), which described several cases of *Pneumocystis carinii* pneumonia in Los Angeles.[1] The authors noted that all of the infected individuals were exposed to cytomegalovirus and wondered whether this virus could be playing a role that could explain why homosexually active males were developing a disease previously associated with individuals who were iatrogenically immunocompromised or malnourished. The subsequent reports of Kaposi's sarcoma,[2] which may occur in immunocompromised individuals, and the appearance of *Pneumocystis carinii* in individuals who presumably could have been infected via contaminated needles, helped to buttress the possibility that a specific infectious agent that could be transmitted sexually and via blood was resulting in the epidemic of immunosuppression. However, for several years an ongoing debate raged, with at least three sides. Some felt that this epidemic was due to a new infectious agent; some thought it was due to agents already present which might have undergone evolution (such as cytomegalovirus, or a combination of infectious agents); and others felt that the epidemic represented a burnout of the immune system, because high-risk individuals tended to be exposed to multiple agents, drugs, and other nonspecific antigens that tended to overwhelm their host defenses. Subsequent elucidation of the retroviral etiology of HIV infection,[3, 4] which was abetted by careful epidemiological studies linking new risk groups and helping to develop a very tight case that HIV was the etiologic agent,[5] has not necessarily diminished the diagnostic and therapeutic questions facing clinicians today. More than six years into the epidemic, clinicians still cannot accurately tell individuals who are infected with HIV when and whether they will develop AIDS and whether they should take Azidothymidine (AZT) or one of the other, less studied treatment regimens.

Definition of the Clinical Spectrum of the Epidemic

When the epidemic of immunodeficiency was first recognized in the early 1980s, the Centers for Disease Control was given the responsibility of trying to define a process whose origin was unclear, whose etiology was unknown, and whose natural history was uncharted. Fortunately, the revolution in immunologic understanding and diagnostic techniques which had occurred in the late 1970s allowed for the conceptualization that a major cell that regulated many aspects of host immune response, the T-helper lymphocyte, was numerically depleted and functionally impaired. All the individuals with this type of impairment manifested one or another of an increasing number of atypical infections and neoplasms.[6] The aggregation of a specific type of immunologic impairment, specific distinctive and atypical types of illnesses, in individuals with specific risk behaviors, allowed the Centers for Disease Control to evolve a case definition of what came to be known as the acquired immunodeficiency syndrome. The dilemma that these investigators faced was how to define this process that was still so unclear without lumping into it individuals whose infections or neoplasms, or both, were due to other causes while at the same time not leaving out the increasing numbers of individuals with some evidence of T-helper lymphocyte immunologic impairment. At an early point in time, the CDC decided to take a narrow-based approach in which cases reported which related to the epidemic would be those of the sickest individuals who did not have other reasons for immunosupression but who had one of a specific laundry list of clinical syndromes that were distinctively atypical in individuals whose immune systems were intact.[7] This approach was extremely effective in picking up individuals who had the classic signs of immunologic impairment and conditions which were the most commonly seen in the course of the epidemic, such as *Pneumocystis carinii* pneumonia and Kaposi's sarcoma. Neither of these conditions occurred with any significant frequency in individuals who were not immunosuppressed or elderly, or both.

However, other individuals developed illnesses that were not specific to immunocompromised individuals, but the severity of their manifestations suggested that they were immunologically impaired. For example, herpes simplex infection around the mouth or

Table 1

Summary of Centers for Disease Control (CDC) Classification System for HIV Infections

Group I.	Acute infection
Group II.	Asymptomatic infection*
Group III.	Persistent generalized lymphadenopathy
Group IV.	Other disease
Subgroup A.	Constitutional disease
Subgroup B.	Neurological disease
Subgroup C.	Secondary infectious diseases
Category C-1.	Specified secondary infectious diseases listed in the CDC surveillance definition for AIDS‡
Category C-2.	Other specified secondary infectious diseases
Subgroup D.	Secondary cancers‡
Subgroup E.	Other conditions

*Patients in groups II and III may be subclassified on the basis of a laboratory evaluation.

‡Includes those patients whose clinical presentation fulfills the definition of AIDS used by the CDC for national reporting.

the perirectal area is not an uncommon infection of homosexually active males who have multiple partners, but the persistence of perianal ulcerations around the rectum in the setting of immunologic abnormalities seen in blood tests was highly suggestive of the wider spectrum of the epidemic. Even more difficult for the clinician were individuals who had persistent wasting syndromes accompanied by significant weight losses, persistent fevers, and malaise, who despite extensive medical evaluations did not have specific infectious agents always identified as the source of their problems. Other individuals who are at high risk to develop AIDS continue to be well for long periods of time with asymptomatic immunologic abnormalities, or may show evidence only of persistent generalized lymph gland swelling associated with blood test abnormalities.[8, 9] Astute clinicians in the cities where the epidemic was first appreciated noted that individuals often progressed from asymptomatic conditions to those of lesser severity to the more severe opportunistic infections. Others noted that certain processes were more common in individuals with specific risk characteristics; for example, homosexually active males were more likely to have Kaposi's sarcoma than individuals who were intravenous drug users.[10]

Even before HIV was delineated as the etiologic agent, clinicians and epidemiologists expanded their vision of the epidemic to incorporate the concept of the iceberg, with those conditions defined as AIDS representing the tip of the iceberg. Progression from asymptomatic high-risk status to full-blown opportunistic infections helped to develop this concept. Even more convincing was the delineation of the similar spectrum of degrees of immunocompromise among individuals who had received blood transfusions from individuals who had subsequently developed AIDS, and among individuals from other nations who did not have any history of homosexual activity or intravenous drug use. The development of an intellectual model of a process that resulted in immunocompromise, with opportunistic infections and neoplasms subsequently supervening, was validated once HIV was isolated, and appropriate seroepidemiologic studies were undertaken which confirmed the increased prevalence of this virus in individuals with AIDS and related symptom complexes.

One might ask, Why should the arbitrary definition of AIDS continue to be reported when one can actually monitor the prevalence of the causative agent itself? Although infection with HIV is necessary for an individual to develop AIDS, it is still not clear whether all individuals who are HIV-infected will ultimately develop the full-blown syndrome. The best data that bear on this issue are derived from a hepatitis B vaccine study that took place in San Francisco from 1978 to 1980 at a clinic for sexually transmitted diseases which is run by the city health department. Of the gay and bisexual men who were found to be infected with HIV between 1978 and 1980, more than one-third developed CDC-defined AIDS by 1987, and approximately 25 percent remain completely asymptomatic.[11] The range for individuals in the middle zone includes asymptomatic immunologic abnormalities; persistent generalized lymphadenopathy; minor opportunistic infections such as thrush and zoster; and the presence of persistent constitutional symptoms. We must be careful about generalizing from this cohort, since prior to recognition of the AIDS epidemic in the early 1980s, there was no widespread education as to what constituted safer sexual practices. If repeated exposures to HIV or other sexually transmitted viruses such as cytomegalovirus and Epstein-Barr virus result in synergistic immunosuppression with the initial HIV infection, then the rates of progression from asymptomatic HIV infection from the men in this cohort could represent a worst-case scenario. However, no single study of homosexual or heterosexual exposure has indicated that unsafe sex after initial HIV infection results in more rapid immunocompromise, and thus the data generated from this cohort can be utilized as a point of reference despite such sexual practices.

The finding that a substantial number of individuals who are HIV-infected develop full-blown AIDS does not mean that a separation in reporting of AIDS is not useful at the present time. Individuals who do not have AIDS may need to utilize many health care services, including multiple laboratory tests, medical evaluations of recurrent minor opportunistic infections, and counseling and support services. Individuals with AIDS tend to have much more severe medical illnesses; thus, monitoring the increasing number of individuals who frequently require intensive, tertiary services is a useful way to monitor health care utilization and to assist planners in projecting what types of resources it will be necessary to deploy as the epidemic continues to progress. AZT is the first drug that has been shown to assist in extending life in individuals with AIDS or with the ill-defined AIDS-related complex (ARC), a term that usually relates to constitutional symptoms associated with HIV infection. It is not known at the present time whether AZT will ultimately forestall the progression to AIDS of many individuals whose HIV infection is rapidly progressing. ("Ill-defined" is used here as a descriptor because specialists do not agree on the definition of AIDS, and therefore various articles and other writings refer to different levels of morbidity.) If current projections by the Centers for Disease Control are correct, between 1 million and 1.5 million Americans are currently infected with HIV, and by 1991 more than a quarter million of them will have developed CDC-defined infections or neoplasms that are now described as one of the conditions defined as AIDS.[12]

The Wide Spectrum of HIV Infection

Intimate sexual contact with an HIV-infected partner or the sharing of contaminated needles does not invariably result in HIV infection. In a prospective study of homosexually active male partners conducted in Boston, more than one-third of the partners were discordant (that is, one partner was seronegative and the other, seropositive) despite possible high-risk anal exposures to infected ejaculate on the part of the susceptible seronegative partner.[13] Whether certain individuals are intrinsically more able to resist infection with HIV or whether some infected individuals are less capable of transmission is not clear at the present time. Some lines of data suggest that individuals may become more efficient in the transmission of HIV infection the longer they carry the virus. This observation has been made concerning hemophiliacs and their spouses;[14] concerning homosexually active male partners; in the recipients of infected blood;[15] and in perinatal studies.[16]

Once an individual has become infected with HIV, it most often takes between three and twelve weeks to develop detectable antibodies. The vast majority of individuals have detectable markers for HIV infection by six months, although there are rare individuals who have not developed HIV antibodies after several years of follow-up. Newer diagnostic tests, such as the detection of serum antigen, may permit demonstration that an HIV exposure has occurred prior to the development of antibody. At the time of seroconversion, individuals may manifest a number of symptoms, including a mononucleosis-type syndrome; rashes that may be hivelike or maculopapular; an aseptic meningitis; and unexplained fevers.[17, 18] However, many individuals, perhaps most, may remain completely asymptomatic for several years after becoming HIV-infected. In response to the increasing understanding of the wide spectrum of HIV infection, the CDC has developed a classification system (see table 1) which describes individuals with acute infection, asymptomatic infection, and persistent generalized lymphadenopathy, as well as those who have clinically significant HIV infection, that is, opportunistic neoplasms and infections, neurological syndromes, or constitutional symptoms, or a combination of these.[19] The individuals in the first three groups of the CDC classification system have highly variable courses. For example, some persons may have persistent HIV-related lymphadenopathy for many years without any other subsequent untoward sequelae.[20] However, once individuals develop systemic complaints and constitutional symptoms, there may be a rapid progression to more severe complications of HIV infection which are subsumed under the acronym AIDS (see tables 2 and 3).

Individuals who have early HIV infection present difficult decisions for clinicians regarding questions of appropriate interventions to prevent them from further immunocompromise. Several studies are now under way in the AIDS Treatment Evaluation Units (ATEUs) that are funded by the National Institutes of Health (NIH). These studies will attempt to determine whether asymptomatic seropositive individuals will benefit from receiving AZT. However, it may take several years to answer this question. In the meantime, many worried individuals who are aware that a subsequent clinical decline is a frequent outcome of long-standing asymptomatic infection try to obtain drugs through black markets — drugs that may be homemade, such as AL-721, or that may be smuggled in from Mexico, such as Ribavirin. Another dilemma for clinicians concerns the decision about how aggressively to diagnostically evaluate individuals with generalized lymphadenopathy. At the early phase of the epidemic, many clinicians were more likely to do lymph node biopsies on patients who had persistent swollen glands, even in the absence of constitutional signs. It has subsequently emerged that without the evidence of hematologic or clinical abnormalities, biopsy most often results in finding a lymph node whose histologic pattern is termed "reactive follicular hyperplasia," a pattern that tells the health care workers only that the lymph gland is "turned on," without conveying any specific prognostic information.[21]

Whether or not an individual has swollen lymph glands, the onset of so-called constitutional symptoms — that is, persistent fevers, chills, sweats, weight loss, and malaise — is generally a negative prognostic sign.[22] Obviously, individuals with HIV infection may have any of these symptoms for other reasons, some of which may or may not portend the onset of an opportunistic infection. Very often, HIV-positive individuals and their clinicians are in a state of worried anticipation once these types of symptoms supervene. An episode of influenza can be emotionally upsetting and result in unnecessary diagnostic studies in anxious seropositive persons. The chronicity of symptoms, generally lasting more than a month, may be a sign that the HIV infection has resulted in a new state of more severe immunocompromise and susceptiblity to opportunistic infection. Individuals with constitutional symptoms generally need to have an extensive medical workup, since some of the conditions they have may be treatable and may be more amenable to therapy if diagnosed early. However, HIV infection itself can result in any of these symptoms, as well as a wide range of neurological findings, though some individuals may undergo expensive workups without obtaining a definitive answer. However, one cannot take the attitude that if the workup initially is negative, there is no use in repeating it if further symptoms develop. Unfortunately, once an individual undergoes a diminution in the ability of the immune system to respond to specific infectious processes, then there is a propensity for developing multiple infections, and thus each new sign or symptom has to be evaluated independently of prior symptom complexes. This possibility for serial infections, sometimes with multiple agents, tends to make the medical management of individuals with HIV infection particularly labor-intensive and costly. The clinician must always balance the aggressiveness of the clinical workup against appropriate therapeutic options for individuals with the AIDS-related complex, but more often than not, it is desirable to proceed with the latest diagnostic tests, since isolation of specific organisms or the definition of specific clinical conditions can lead to appropriate therapy and may result in an improved quality of life for the patient.

The opportunistic infections that individuals develop with AIDS may be due to organisms that are ubiquitous in a specific environment, so that *Pneumocystis carinii* pneumonia is much more common in North America and Europe than in Africa, whereas cryptococcal meningitis and *Isospora belli* enteritis are much more common there. Other opportunistic infections represent reactivation of chronic latent viruses that may have been acquired at earlier ages as the result of intimate contact, such as herpes simplex, cytomegalovirus, and Epstein-Barr virus. However, in individuals with AIDS and severe immunodeficiency due to HIV, these viruses may reactivate in particularly virulent forms, so that chronic, persistent perianal ulcerations may be due to herpes simplex,[23] or cytomegalovirus may result in colitis, blindness, or a refractory pneumonia, syndromes associated with this virus which are seen only in severely debilitated hosts.[24] One conundrum in individuals with AIDS is that with appropriate medical technology, most of these

Table 2

Opportunistic Infections Indicative of a Defect in Cellular Immune Function Associated with AIDS

A. **Helminthic Infection**
   1. Strongyloidiasis (disseminated beyond the gastrointestinal tract)*
B. **Protozoan Infection**
   1. *Pneumocystis carinii* pneumonia
   2. Disseminated toxoplasmosis, or toxoplasma encephalitis, excluding congenital infection
   3. Chronic cryptosporidium enteritis (> 1 month)
   4. Chronic *Isospora belli* enteritis (> 1 month)
C. **Fungal Infection**
   1. Candida esophagitis, bronchopulmonary candidiasis*
   2. Cryptococcal meningitis, or disseminated infection
   3. Disseminated histoplasmosis*
D. **Bacterial Infection**
   1. Disseminated (not just pulmonary or lymphatic) *M. avium-intracellulare* or *M. kansasii*
   2. Extrapulmonary tuberculosis*
E. **Noncongenital Viral Infection**
   1. Chronic (> 1 month) mucocutaneous herpes simplex
   2. Histologically evident cytomegalovirus infection, including liver or lymph node
   3. Progressive multifocal leukencephalopathy

*Not listed in original CDC definition of AIDS but subsequently added.

Table 3

Opportunistic Malignancies Indicative of a Defect in Cellular Immune Function Associated with AIDS

Neoplasm

1. Kaposi's sarcoma (in a person less than sixty years old)
2. High-grade, B-cell non-Hodgkin's lymphoma*
   A. Burkitt's lymphoma
   B. Undifferentiated non-Hodgkin's lymphoma, immunoblastic sarcoma
3. Primary brain lymphoma

*Not listed in original CDC definition of AIDS but subsequently added.

opportunistic infections or neoplasms can be diagnosed, and most of them can be treated. However, the recurrent succession of these debilitating diseases is analogous to the Hydra monster of Greek mythology, which grew back two heads for every one that was cut off. It is this succession of diseases that causes the ultimate mortality from AIDS.

The problem for the patient, the clinician, and society at large is how to determine when the diminishing returns of each new intervention mandate a less thorough investigation of the cause of new complaints. Although individuals who have had their third episode of *Pneumocystis carinii* pneumonia are much less likely to survive than those who have had their first, this kind of information only gives probablistic odds, and does not address the question for each individual of whether life extension at specific junctures promotes human dignity or human suffering.

Infection with HIV may result in neurological disease after initial seroconversion but more often manifests itself later in the course of HIV infection, though specific neurological sequelae may be seen at any point in time.[25] The most dramatic findings include dementia, encephalopathy, and neuropathies, which may involve either muscles or sensation, or both, as well as involvement of the spinal cord.[26, 27] Individuals with HIV infection may be more anxious or depressed, or both, because of the knowledge of their status and because of the social stresses attendant upon being a member of a high-risk group and carrying a life-threatening virus, but independent of these other behavioral modifiers, HIV infection may alter psychological and neurological functions early in the course of the illness. Thus, health care planners must integrate the psychosocial and neuro-behavioral needs of individuals with HIV infection in the calculations of the societal costs of infection, which have thus far been estimated to add as much as $8 billion to $16 billion to the cost of health care in the United States by 1991.[28]

Immature immune systems appear to be even more susceptible to the ravages of HIV infection, presumably because there are no immunologic reserves that have developed over several decades of successfully fending off environmental challenges.[29] Although a consensus among experts does not exist regarding the frequency with which offspring of HIV-infected mothers will be infected themselves, there is general agreement that it is a substantial figure, possibly the majority of live births.[30] These children may be born to mothers who are addicted to drugs or are from disadvantaged socioeconomic environments, or both, and who have to cope with their own HIV infections with all those associated medical problems. Children born with HIV infection may encounter difficulties in placement if their mothers and families are unable to care for them. Thus, the problem of pediatric AIDS, which has grown rapidly in several major metropolitan areas — particularly New York, northern New Jersey, and Miami — raises additional medical, sociological, and ethical concerns for the development of public policy.

Clinical Management Issues: Diagnostic Concerns

The first major clinical use of the HIV antibody test was for the purpose of screening donated blood in order to protect the blood supply.[31] In the first few years of the test's utilization, a wide-ranging public debate occurred in which some individuals were proponents of using the test to screen the entire population, or subgroups of the population, such as individuals seeking marriage licenses; health care professionals; and individuals entering hospitals or being prepared for major surgery. Opponents of these more liberal indications for use of the HIV antibody test pointed out that despite the test being progressively improved and despite the ability to utilize independent corroboration with other more sophisticated tests such as the Western blot, testing for antibodies still seemed to produce an unacceptably high number of false positives, particularly in low prevalence areas, even though the use of a corroborative test substantially reduces the number of false positives.[32, 33] Another concern voiced by opponents of large-scale testing of the general population was that even if all individuals identified as seropositive were truly infected with HIV, once they were identified as seropositive there would be no effective therapies available to offer them. They would have knowledge that they were at increased risk for AIDS and would be at risk for many types of discrimination if the information could not be absolutely protected, with no prospect for reversing their infection. However, over the past year, clinical studies indicate that AZT is efficacious in prolonging life in individuals with AIDS and AIDS-related symptoms,[34] raising new questions of when to test. At the present time, AZT has not been shown to be effective in preventing AIDS in asymptomatic HIV-seropositive individuals, but the studies that are currently under way to evaluate this possibility could radically alter the clinical indications for HIV antibody screening. If AZT or any other antiretroviral drug is shown to prevent immunocompromise in asymptomatic seropositives, the argument could run that proactive HIV testing would be useful so that more individuals could be diagnosed and treated before the onset of irreversible clinical disease.

The argument that the detection of early infection may help prevent subsequent spread into the general population and may reduce morbidity has been the basis for much of current public health policy with regard to other sexually transmitted diseases. Since at the present time AZT looks promising but has not yet been shown to be effective for treating asymptomatic persons, there is much turmoil regarding this issue. Up to one-third of persons with AIDS or ARC who take AZT for more than several months have needed repeated transfusions, and there are those who feel that AZT is a highly toxic drug. Since the data suggest that individuals with lesser degrees of immunocompromise may tolerate the drug better, some rationale exists for earlier treatment. However, one does not know whether HIV could become resistant to AZT over long periods of time, since the drug only suppresses the virus's ability to replicate, and does not kill the virus or remove it from the body; other chronic viruses (for example, herpes simplex) can develop resistance to suppressive therapeutic agents.

Other clinical indications for the knowledge of an individual's HIV and immunologic status are emerging. For example, in children, the use of live virus vaccines, even though the organisms utilized in the vaccines are avirulent, could result in an HIV-infected immunocompromised child becoming very ill with a disseminated viral infection that the vaccine was designed to avoid. Family members may be in high-risk groups themselves and could be susceptible to serious infections from viruses that were excreted by asymptomatic children who had been recently vaccinated. Thus, the public is left with a fairly volatile situation, in which no proven interventions have been shown to alter the natural history of HIV infection in asymptomatic individuals, though several interventions are on the horizon. Individuals who are infected with HIV may benefit from knowing about this if they are going to be exposed to new infectious agents; however, one must be cautionary in noting that these are theoretical concerns, not ones that are currently standard medical practice. It is clear that as the medical advances continue — and one can only hope that they proceed at a rapid pace — then HIV diagnostics will be increasingly more useful. The test itself will have more meaning for individuals when clinicians have something to offer them. In the meantime, the public debate about these issues should help to educate both policymakers and clinicians as to the need to be very clear in their own minds why they want individuals to be screened for HIV.

HIV screening's use as a tool for the modification of high-risk behaviors, and thereby as a tool to decrease the spread of the retrovirus, is one of the major reasons that policymakers have felt the screening should be more widely available. In a context of a program of intensive education about risk behaviors, HIV testing may be helpful for specific individuals. Yet it is difficult to generalize about the efficacy of HIV testing itself, since very few individuals undergo antibody testing without receiving some form of counseling, which may be more relevant to potential behavior changes.

The substantial changes in high-risk behaviors by the gay and bisexual men in one Boston study were similar whether individuals were antibody-positive or -negative and whether or not they knew their test results.[35] On the basis of studies in which individuals enter as volunteers, are given guarantees of confidentiality, and are not under scrutiny by public health officials, it is particularly hard to generalize about the effect of mandating that people know their HIV antibody test results. One can only wonder whether mandatory testing could serve merely to intensify the development of an underground that could be more refractory to the educational messages available in studies, community-based testing sites, and other institutions that offer the test without coercing individuals to participate. The maintenance of a dialogue between the patients and their providers can allow for mutually reinforcing decisions as to when it is appropriate to perform HIV testing and what kinds of support the patient will subsequently need in order to maintain safer sexual practices and to receive appropriate medical follow-up.

Therapeutic Concerns

Another major dilemma for clinicians taking care of individuals with AIDS and HIV infection relates to the pace of clinical trials. At the present time, most persons with HIV infection are not receiving medication to counteract the progressive immunocompromise associated with HIV. Most newly available drugs for treating HIV infection will be tested in the ATEUs and Clinical Studies Groups (CSGs), which are federally funded and centrally coordinated to perform multicenter clinical trials. A consortium of Harvard Medical School–affiliated hospitals (Massachusetts General, Beth Israel, New England Deaconess) is the only such treatment site in New England. The ATEUs have begun several protocols utilizing AZT and are planning more studies to look at newer antiretroviral drugs. Since the criteria for inclusion in a specific clinical study must be fairly rigid, and since many individuals may fall between the cracks in terms of the progression of their specific problems, a large underground has already developed to procure medications from Mexico and overseas in order to give individuals with AIDS and symptomatic HIV infection the opportunity to make their own decisions about whether they would want to receive a specific drug. Of great concern to clinicians is the fact that treatment with the first two highly publicized agents (Suramin and HPA-23) which act against the HIV-specific enzyme, reverse transcriptase, turned out to be more toxic than the untreated HIV infections would have been. Thus, in the absence of meticulous basic research, individuals may become more impressed by the merchandising of purported panaceas and thereby expose themselves to potential harm. By the same rationale, early HIV testing may be useful because an individual may be at a better point to take action that can prevent a more rapid decline in immunologic function. Many clinicians are concerned that drugs may not be tested soon enough on less symptomatic, seropositive persons. Many asymptomatic individuals, perceiving themselves to be at increased risk for developing symptomatic HIV infection in the near future, are clamoring to receive AZT or other, less studied agents, and they indicate that they do not want to sit and wait while their immunologic function inexorably declines. If many of these minimally symptomatic individuals had taken HPA-23 or Suramin, they would have caused themselves more harm than benefit. Thus, the federal health authorities feel that in studying new and promising agents, they must balance the progressively increasing gravity of the epidemic against the need to conduct studies in a careful and organized fashion.

Many hopes have been raised regarding drugs besides AZT, such as Ribavirin, Ampligen, Phosphonoformate, and a host of other compounds.[36, 37, 38] Many of these drugs are now undergoing initial clinical trials, but the process can be a long and arduous one. First, investigators must develop a hypothesis as to why a specific agent may work in a test tube and must demonstrate the efficacy of the compound against HIV-infected cells. Initial studies in humans have to evaluate the pharmacokinetic properties of the drug as well as its toxicities. Then, studies have to show that in human beings a specific drug may have efficacy against HIV infection. The traditional investigational gold standard has been to test a candidate drug in humans against a placebo in a randomized, controlled fashion, utilizing subjects that are selected to be similar in terms of infection and disease characteristics. Many of the promising reports about agents other than AZT do not involve randomized, controlled trials and thus are often a series of anecdotes. The erratic nature of HIV infection makes noncontrolled trials difficult to interpret, since some individuals may remain asymptomatic for as long as nine years after HIV infection, while others may develop AIDS within a year after seroconversion. Individuals with Kaposi's sarcoma, in particular, constitute a subgroup that in the absence of opportunistic infections may remain quite well, with fairly intact immunologic function, for long periods of time.

The clinical end points that are used to evaluate the efficacy of particular therapies are still not standardized. If death is utilized as an end point, one has to follow a large cohort of individuals with fairly advanced HIV infection in order to establish an adequate difference between a new therapy and a placebo. This was done in the case of the trial of AZT, but the data in that study indicated that individuals who had ARC tended to benefit more from AZT than those with AIDS. This would suggest that AZT would be better utilized in individuals who might have earlier stages of HIV infection. However, the AZT trial in asymptomatic HIV-seropositive individuals may have to go on for at least three years before it can be established whether treatment with AZT has a sufficiently large protective effect to warrant the toxicities that may be encountered in the course of therapy. If one does not use death as an end point, but rather opportunistic infections, the cohort size must still be large and homogeneous at the outset in order to produce meaningful data that can establish the efficacy of a specific agent. The clinical and laboratory criteria, which are needed to include individuals in specific cohorts and to assess the effectiveness of specific agents, have not yet been routinely standardized. For example, some individuals feel that the presence of thrush is a particularly bad prognostic sign,[39] whereas others are more concerned by the persistence of constitutional symptoms. It is not clear whether one can compare an asymptomatic person with thrush to a person who has lost significant weight and who has persistent fevers, chills, and sweats and multiple hematologic abnormalities. In the lab, the most useful immunologic criterion for inclusion in a specific group that would be evaluated in a drug trial would be the absolute T-helper lymphocyte number.[40] This has been shown to be useful in epidemiological studies, but whether improvement or stabilization in this parameter is the best predictor of chemotherapeutic efficacy is still an open question. Several virologic parameters may be epidemiologically useful as well, but further study is required as to their usefulness as prognostic markers after individuals undergo antiretroviral chemotherapy. Patients who have positive cultures for HIV or who have been shown to have HIV antigen in their serum (patients may be antigenemic and not viremic) tend to be more likely to become clinically ill over short periods of time.[41, 42] However, the reversal of antigenemia or the inability to culture virus after an individual has been treated with a drug may not ipso facto mean that the drug is highly effective. These parameters are undergoing careful study and will increasingly become useful in characterizing stages of HIV infection, but the highly individualized responses to infection with the retrovirus mean that it is still very hard to establish a typology that would allow clinicians to give short trials of therapeutic agents and utilize surrogate markers as a means for proving drug efficacy. In summary, in the short run there will be no quick answers as to which drugs are the most effective; rather, ongoing studies of natural history will be necessary, unless novel agents are developed which prove to be highly effective in altering or reversing the HIV-induced immunodeficiency and its sequelae.

The need for long-term, prospective, careful studies of individuals, utilizing placebos and careful controls, is clear-cut. Yet, given the magnitude of human suffering engendered by HIV infection, many clinicians feel that an academic approach is unacceptable. Some individuals have felt that historical controls can be used to establish baseline rates of progression in the natural history of HIV infection and that these can be compared to individuals who are treated with specific regimens. The problem with using historical controls is that as the epidemic evolves, there are changes in the natural history of HIV infection which have been unanticipated. Thus, comparisons of people who were infected with HIV several years ago with those who are undergoing therapeutic regimens now may lead to skewed interpretations. For example, at the outset of the epidemic, almost one-third of individuals who were initially diagnosed using the CDC definition of AIDS had Kaposi's sarcoma, whereas at the present time less than one-fifth of the new cases carry this diagnosis. It is unknown whether the decreased incidence of Kaposi's sarcoma reflects changes in behavior, changes in certain biological cofactors (such as the use of volatile nitrites, or "poppers"), or decreased transmission of another viral cofactor.

The vagaries of the natural history of HIV have complicated the need for expeditious clinical trials, and appropriate clinical concerns have been perceived by some segments of the population as an insensitivity. This has led to the burgeoning of the therapeutic underground and to an increased alienation from clinical investigators among some HIV-infected persons. Occasionally, individuals who have participated in randomized trials have gone so far as to utilize drug-analysis laboratories in order to assess whether they are receiving a placebo, and have either dropped out of trials or have supplemented their regimens with nonprotocol drugs because of their sense of urgency regarding treatment. These anecdotes reflect the exceptions rather than the rule, but they underscore the highly charged environment that is evolving in this time of uncertainty. Individual self-medication has the potential to create serious therapeutic problems, since if every individual who were HIV-infected were to experiment with different types of drugs, the results that might be obtained in specific clinical trials would be difficult to interpret. But many seropositive persons are uncomfortable not knowing whether they have received a placebo. The increased availability of AZT and the lack of a standard, accepted criterion by all clinicians in prescribing the drug create the potential to exacerbate this situation further. At the present time, it is known only that individuals who have had one episode of *Pneumocystis carinii* pneumonia or who have constitutional symptoms and other ARC-like manifestations have had their lives extended by taking AZT. However, many HIV-infected individuals who have either minor opportunistic infections, such as thrush or zoster, or asymptomatic depressions in their T-helper lymphocyte count, or both, are electing to take AZT. In the absence of clear-cut data and through the process of extrapolating from the clinical trials of sicker individuals, they prefer risking the potential toxicities of AZT to waiting until it is clearly shown that taking the drug at earlier stages of infection is useful. Blanket statements saying that individuals must either be in clinical trials or not take medication are not realistic in the current climate. On the other hand, if everybody did exactly as they pleased, utilizing any available drugs through the black market, further knowledge about the efficacy of antriretroviral therapy could be critically delayed or limited. There are no easy or glib answers. An ongoing dialogue among researchers, clinical providers, and the communities at risk for HIV infection must continue, in order to address these highly urgent human needs in a responsible fashion. Yet an adequate level of scientific rigor must also be maintained so that these crucial questions can be answered as rapidly as possible.

Up until now, clinical trials have tended to look for the magic bullet, that is, a single drug that will attenuate the effects of HIV infection. However, many researchers feel that this approach may be simplistic, since the individual with HIV infection faces two types of problems. Because the virus is immunosuppressive, the individual must have his or her immune system restored if the onset of opportunistic infections or malignancy is to be avoided. At the same time, the retrovirus itself must be inhibited from replicating in order to prevent the extension of the infection and subsequent further immunosuppression.[43, 44] Some of the first drugs to treat HIV infection were stimulators of the immune system, such as interferon and interleukin-2.[45] Whereas they tended to increase the numbers of lymphocytes which could potentially fight infection, they also tended to enhance the ability of HIV to replicate, thus abetting infection, and were ultimately not successful by themselves. Drugs like AZT inhibit specific enzymes of the virus and prevent it from multiplying, but do not restore the immune system by themselves. Thus, the possibility exists that combined chemotherapy with an immunostimulatory drug and a drug that acts specifically against the virus could be a major answer in treating individuals with HIV infection and preventing further immunologic compromise.[46] However, in order to assess adequately the potential toxicities of individual agents, such trials would have to be performed serially; in other words, the effects of either drug by itself would first have to be assessed, and only then could the drugs be studied in combination. Thus, some approaches offer much promise, but even more time may be required to study them in a responsible fashion, thus further straining the patience of individuals who are at risk for immunologic compromise. Some feel that although serial trials of these drugs represent a scientifically worthwhile approach, so many individuals could clinically deteriorate before definite data were collected that combination studies should begin in a more expeditious fashion. Previous medical experience shows, however, that when two drugs are given together, unexpected synergistic toxicities supervene instead of synergistic therapeutic effects. Dual therapy may result in lessened therapeutic efficacy of either drug alone (antagonism) in vivo even if in vitro data look promising. Thus, the dialogue between the affected individuals and the research community must take each side into account. The old dictum, Primum non noce (First do no harm), must be balanced against the problem that can result from too much delay in initiating a promising therapeutic regimen. The only answer is constant questioning and dialogue in order to expedite the process of making useful combination treatments available, without rushing to judgment in such a way that more individuals are harmed because of inadequate antecedent study.

Care-Related Issues

The AIDS epidemic raises many issues regarding the optimal delivery of services to individuals infected with HIV who subsequently develop problems related to immunocompromise. Although persons with AIDS have a markedly shortened life expectancy, they can respond well to specific treatment regimens, particularly after their first episodes of opportunistic infection. The initial approach toward the management of patients with HIV infection tended to be technologically intensive, and led to patients being hospitalized for longer periods of time. The model developed in San Francisco is one that optimally utilizes outpatient resources and maximizes home care and treatment in the ambulatory setting. Unfortunately, the ways in which health care is financed in many areas tend to create disincentives for early discharge and the provision of comprehensive outpatient services. This will become increasingly penny-wise and pound-foolish, given the availability of prophylactic regimens that require some level of medical expertise, such as the administration of aerosolized Pentamidine in order to prevent the recurrence of *Pneumocystis carinii* pneumonia. Health care planners and policymakers will need to continually talk to clinicians, patients, and advocacy groups for individuals at high risk for HIV infection in order to create the most satisfactory approaches to caring for individuals in community settings, which may provide a less depressing environment and which certainly provide a less costly one. In order for these novel programs to be successful, there must be a comprehensive set of supports which includes a wide range of health care providers, including home health aides, nursing assistants, physical and occupational rehabilitation specialists, nutritionists, and mental-health-care workers, so that the deinstitutionalized patients do not return to tertiary institutions with more complicated medical problems that could have been anticipated had the appropriate interventions been instituted earlier. Health care providers such as physicians and nurses need to increasingly become aware that many of the individuals at highest risk for HIV infection do not come from "traditional" social environments. The effectiveness of the health care team can only be enhanced if providers recognize the validity of same-sex spouses, nonnuclear family units, and nonmedical resources in communities that comprise sexual, cultural, and racial minorities. Since so much of HIV infection relates to behavioral issues, providers must educate themselves about alternative lifestyles and must understand how critical it is that they relate to clients as nonjudgmental care givers and educators.

HIV infection results in problems that involve the whole patient, who is the sum total of many parts greater than individual subspeciality concerns. Therefore, patients who are infected with the retrovirus need to be approached clinically by a multidisciplinary team of health care providers. This team must include subspecialists in areas of expertise such as infectious diseases, hematology, oncology, pulmonary diseases, gastroenterology, and often a host of other subspecialities. However, these patients have a great need to have their care integrated; thus, there will be a continuing need for primary care generalists to serve as their gateway to the health care system. In some university hospital settings, infectious disease specialists tend to be the primary providers of care for individuals with symptomatic HIV infection, but in others, general internists and family practitioners have done a fine job and have tended to be the health care providers who oversee the series of consultations that may be necessary in the course of HIV infection for any given individual. The health care team can be greatly enhanced by the inclusion of nurse practitioners and physicians' assistants who have developed specific skills around AIDS and HIV infection, since individuals with these problems may need a great deal of education, moral support, and clinical monitoring that do not necessitate the constant involvement of the subspecialist. In addition, the ongoing involvement of mental health professionals ranging from neurologists to social workers can greatly enhance the ability of individuals with HIV infection to function well in society. Not every individual with HIV infection will invariably need to see the psychiatrist or the gastroenterologist, but it is important to develop a referral network that will allow for a rational pattern of integrated health care for each individual who is diagnosed with HIV infection and its attendant clinical sequelae.

Infection Control

The last major policy issue regarding HIV infection relates to infection control. As with so many other aspects of the AIDS epidemic, the public dialogue on this issue has tended to careen between hysteria and apathy, whereas the most appropriate course is one of prudent caution based on the well-documented epidemiology of retroviral infection. The precautions that providers need to take regarding HIV infection are virtually identical to those which are taken with respect to any bloodborne disease and have been recently well described by the Centers for Disease Control.[47] One must add the caveat that individuals who are infected with HIV may be more susceptible to certain types of infections — for example, tuberculosis — that may in and of themselves be contagious to individuals with intact immune systems. Therefore, clinicians need to respond with the appropriate thoughtful caution in the care of individuals with HIV infection. Thus, if an individual who has HIV infection has an atypical chest x-ray and is coughing, it behooves the provider to suggest that the patient be placed on respiratory isolation until the diagnosis of tuberculosis is excluded. However, irrational infection control procedures serve only to stigmatize the individual, give a false sense of security to staff members, and lead to suboptimal, alienated medical care.

Traditional practice has included the documentation in the medical record of all information that could possibly be of clinical importance, on the presumption that no clinician's memory is infallible and that others may benefit from this documentation in the future. However, antidiscrimination provisions against individuals with HIV infection are lacking in most jurisdictions, and since, particularly in small medical settings, it is very difficult to keep medical information inviolate, individuals may be at risk from external social sanction if their HIV status is documented. Therefore, many have felt that information about persons with HIV infection should never be placed in the medical record. However, where HIV-related information has been obtained in a noncoercive fashion and where knowledge of this information on the part of other members of the health care team may be important for patient management, it seems that discussion should focus not on the compromise of medical care, but on how best to protect individuals from capricious or inappropriate disclosure and subsequent discrimination. Therapeutic interventions available for HIV-infected individuals, it is hoped, will continue to increase over the next few years, and as they do, the likelihood will also grow that within the health care system more individuals will be disclosed as HIV-infected. In order to avoid further exacerbation of the patients' need for comprehensive medical care, which may necessitate documentation of their clinical status, legislation that addresses the just concerns of patients is urgently needed. Discussions among medical providers, those who make public policy, and the general public must lead to a resolution that creates an environment in which individuals will not be stigmatized in the process of seeking health care.

With more than one million HIV-infected persons in the United States, any actions that potentiate alienation from the health care system and impede education around risk reduction are inappropriate. In the midst of this distressing epidemic, all of us — researchers, providers, patients, and the public — face the great challenge of having to rapidly assimilate new technical information while remodeling the anachronistic social systems that tend to increase the underlying anxieties. Until we have definitive therapeutics and chemoprophylaxis, these anxieties will persist.

Notes

1. Centers for Disease Control: Pneumocystis pneumonia: Los Angeles. *Morbidity and Mortality Weekly Report* 30:250, 1981.
2. Centers for Disease Control: Kaposi's sarcoma, pneumocystis pneumonia among homosexual men: New York City and California. *Morbidity and Mortality Weekly Report* 30:305–308, 1981.
3. F. Barre-Sinousi, J. C. Chermann, F. Rey, et al.: Isolation of a T-lymphotropic retrovirus from a patient at risk for acquired immunodeficiency syndrome (AIDS). *Science* 220:868–870, 1983.
4. M. Popovic, M. G. Sarngadharan, E. Read, and R. C. Gallo: Detection, isolation, and continuous production of cytopathic retroviruses (HTLV-III) from patients with AIDS and pre-AIDS. *Science* 224:497–500, 1984.
5. R. C. Gallo, S. Z. Salahuddin, M. Popovic, et al.: Frequent detection and isolation of cytopathic retroviruses (HTLV-III) from patients with AIDS and at risk for AIDS. *Science* 224:500–503, 1984.
6. A. S. Fauci, A. M. Macher, D. L. Longo, et al.: Acquired immunodeficiency syndrome: Epidemiologic, clinical, immunologic, and therapeutic considerations. *Annals of Internal Medicine* 100:92–106, 1984.
7. Centers for Disease Control: Update on acquired immunodeficiency syndrome (AIDS) — United States. *Morbidity and Mortality Weekly Report* 31:507–508, 513–514, 1982.
8. T. A. Peterman, D. P. Drotman, J. W. Curran: Epidemiology of the acquired immunodeficiency syndrome (AIDS). In: *Epidemiologic Reviews*, vol. 7, ed. M. Szklo, L. Gordis, M. B. Gregg, and M. M. Levine, Johns Hopkins University School of Hygiene and Public Health, Baltimore, Md., pp. 1–21, 1986.

9. J. W. Curran, Morgan W. Meade, A. M. Hardy, H. W. Jaffe, W. W. Darrow, W. R. Dowdle: The epidemiology of AIDS: Current status and future prospects. *Science* 229:1352–1357, 1985.

10. New York City Department of Health and Surveillance: The AIDS epidemic in New York City, 1981–1984. *American Journal of Epidemiology* 123:1013–1025, 1986.

11. N. Hessal, G. Rutherford, P. M. O'Malley, L. S. Doll, W. W. Darrow, and H. W. Jaffe: The natural history of HIV in a cohort of homosexual and bisexual men: A 7-year prospective study. Abstract of the Third International Conference on AIDS, Washington, D. C., June 1–5, 1987.

12. W. M. Morgan, J. W. Curran: Acquired immunodeficiency syndrome: Current and future trends. *Public Health Reports* 101:459–465, 1986.

13. G. Seage, K. Mayer, A. Hardy, J. Groopman, A. Barry, L. Weymouth, R. Ferriani, G. Lamb, H. Jaffe: Correlation of HIV non-transmission between homosexual men with virological, immunological, and behavioral factors. Abstract of the Twenty-seventh International Conference on Antimicrobial Agents and Chemotherapy, New York City, October 1–4, 1987.

14. J. J. Goedert, S. H. Landesman, M. E. Eyster, R. J. Biggar: AIDS incidence in pregnant women, their babies, homosexual men and hemophiliacs. Abstract of the Third International Conference on AIDS, Washington, D.C., June 1–5, 1987.

15. J. W. Ward, D. Deppe, H. Perkins, S. Kleinman, P. Holland, J. Allen: Risk of disease in recipients of blood from donors later to be found infected with human immunodeficiency virus (HIV). Abstract of the Third International Conference on AIDS, Washington, D.C., June 1–5, 1987.

16. P. A. Selwyn, E. E. Schoenbaum, A. R. Feingold, M. Mayers, K. Davenny, M. Rogers, et al.: Perinatal transmission of HIV in intravenous drug abusers (IVDAs). Abstract of the Third International Conference on AIDS, Washington D.C., June 1–5, 1987.

17. D. A. Cooper, J. Gold, P. Maclean, B. Donovan, R. Finlayson, T. G. Barnes, et al.: Acute AIDS retrovirus infection: Definition of a clinical illness associated with seroconversion. *Lancet* 1:537–540, 1985.

18. D. D. Ho, M. G. Sarngadharan, L. Resnick, et al.: Primary human T-lymphotropic virus type III infection. *Annals of Internal Medicine* 103:880–883, 1985.

19. CDC classification system for HIV infections: *Morbidity and Mortality Weekly Report* 35:334–339, (May 23, 1986).

20. D. I. Abrams, T. P. Hess, P. Volberding: Lymphadenopathy: Update of a 40-month prospective study. Abstract of the International Conference on AIDS, Atlanta, Ga., April 15, 1985.

21. U. Mathur-Wagh, R. W. Enlow, I. Spigland, et al.: Longitudinal study of persistent generalized lymphadenopathy in homosexual men: Relation to the acquired immunodeficiency syndrome. *Lancet* 1:1033–1038, 1984.

22. D. P. Francis, H. W. Jaffe, P. N. Fultz, J. P. Getchell, J. S. McDougal, P. M. Feorino: The natural history of infection with the lymphadenopathy-associated virus human T-lymphotropic virus type III. *Annals of Internal Medicine* 103:719–722, 1985.

23. G. V. Quinnan, Jr., H. Masur, A. H. Rook, et al.: Herpesvirus infections in the acquired immune deficiency syndrome. *Journal of the American Medical Association* 252:72–77, 1984.

24. J. Laurence: AIDS Report: CMV infections in AIDS patients. *Infections in Surgery* 603–610, October 1986.

25. W. D. Snider, D. M. Simpson, G. Nielson, J. W. M. Gold, C. Metroka, J. B. Posner: Neurologic complications of acquired immunodeficiency syndrome: Analysis of 50 patients. *Annals of Neurology* 14:403–418, 1983.

26. B. A. Navia, E. S. Cho, C. K. Petito, R. W. Price: The AIDS dementia complex: II. Neuropathology. *Annals of Neurology* 19:525–535, 1986.

27. L. G. Epstein, L. R. Sharer, V. V. Joshi, M. M. Fojas, M. R. Koenigsberger, J. M. Oleske: Progressive encephalopathy in children with acquired immunodeficiency syndrome. *Annals of Neurology* 17:488–496, 1985.

28. T. J. Thornton, ed.: Nation's hospitals awakening to increasing AIDS caseload. *AIDS Alert* 1:117–120, 1986.

29. R. W. Marion, A. A. Wiznia, G. Hutcheon, A. Rubenstein: Human T-cell lymphotropic virus type III (HTLV-III/LAV) embryopathy: A new dysmorphic syndrome associated with intrauterine HTLV-III infection. *American Journal of Diseases of Children* 140:638–640, 1986.

30. W. P. Parks, G.B. Scott: An overview of pediatric AIDS: Approaches to diagnosis and outcome assessment. Background paper. Washington, D.C.: Committee on a National Strategy for AIDS, 1987.

31. P. P. Mortimer, J. V. Parry, J. Y. Mortimer: Which anti-HTLV-III/LAV assays for screening and confirmatory testing? *Lancet* 2:873–877, 1985.

32. P. D. Cleary, M. J. Barry, K. H. Mayer, A. M. Brandt, L. Gostin, H. V. Fineberg: Compulsory premarital screening for the human immunodeficiency virus: Technical and public health considerations. *Journal of the American Medical Association* 258:1757–1762, 1987.

33. K. B. Meyer, S. G. Pauker: Screening for HIV: Can we afford the false positive rate? *New England Journal of Medicine* 317:238–241, 1987.

34. M. A. Fischl, D. D. Richman, M. H. Grieco, M. S. Gottlieb, P. A. Volberding, O. L. Laskin, J. M. Leedom, et al.: The efficacy of Azidothymidine (AZT) in the treatment of patients with AIDS and AIDS-related complex. *New England Journal of Medicine* 317:185–191, 1987.

35. J. McCusker, J. G. Zapka, A. M. Stoddard, K. H. Mayer, J. S. Avrunin, S. P. Saltzman, C. S. Morrison: HIV antibody test disclosure and subsequent behavior. *American Journal of Public Health* (in press).

36. J. B. McCormick, J. W. Mitchell, J. P. Getchell, D. R. Hicks: Ribavirin suppresses replication of lymphadenopathy-associated virus in culture of human lymphocytes. *Lancet* 2:1367–1369, 1984.

37. E. G. Sandstrom, J. C. Kaplan, R. E. Byington, M. S. Hirsch: Inhibition of human T-cell lymphotropic virus type III in vitro by Phosphonoformate. *Lancet* 1:1480–1482, 1985.

38. M. H. Grieco, M. M. Reddy, D. Manvar, K. K. Ahuja, M. L. Moriarty: In-vivo immunomodulation by Isoprinosine in patients with acquired immunodeficiency syndrome and related complexes. *Annals of Internal Medicine* 101:206–207, 1984.

39. R. S. Klein, C. A. Harris, C. B. Small, B. Moll, M. Lesser, G. H. Friedland: Oral candidiasis in high risk patients as the initial manifestation of acquired immunodeficiency syndrome. *New England Journal of Medicine* 311:354–358, 1984.

40. M. S. Gottlieb, J. L. Fahey: The clinical laboratory in the diagnosis and management of AIDS and HTLV-III/LAV infections. Plenary Session II of the Program and Abstracts of the Second International Conference on AIDS, Paris, June 23–25, 1986.

41. J. M. A. Lange, R. A. Coutinho, W. J. A. Krone, L. F. Verdonck, S. A. Danner, J. van der Noordaa, et al.: Distinct IgG recognition patterns during progression of subclinical and clinical infection with LAV/HTLV-III. *British Medical Journal* 292:228–230, 1985.

42. K. H. Mayer, L. A. Falk, D. A. Paul, G. J. Dawson, A. M. Stoddard, J. McCusker, J. S. Saltzman, M. W. Moon, R. Ferriani, J. E. Groopman: Correlation of enzyme-linked immunosorbent assays for serum human immunodeficiency virus (HIV) antigen and antibodies to recombinant viral proteins with subsequent clinical outcomes in a cohort of asymptomatic homosexual males. *American Journal of Medicine* 83:208–212, 1987.

43. D. L. Bowen, H. C. Lane, A. J. Fauci: Immunopathogenesis of the acquired immunodeficiency syndrome. *Annals of Internal Medicine* 103:704–709, 1985.

44. A. S. Fauci, H. C. Lane: Therapeutic approaches to the underlying immune defect in patients with AIDS. Abstract of the Second International Conference on AIDS, Paris, June 23–25, 1986.

45. D. Ho, K. L. Hartshorn, T. R. Rota, C. A. Andrews, J. C. Kaplan, R. T. Schooley, et al.: Recombinant human interferon alfa-A suppresses HTLV-III replication in-vitro. *Lancet* 1:602–604, 1985.

46. H. C. Lane, A. S. Fauci: Immunologic reconstitution in the acquired immunodeficiency syndrome. *Annals of Internal Medicine* 103:714–718, 1985.

47. Centers for Disease Control: Recommendations for prevention of HIV transmission in health-care settings. *Morbidity and Mortality Weekly Report* 36:3S–18S, 1987.

Glossary continued from page 36

Immunocompromise. Alterations in immune function which are suggestive of a decreased ability to fight off infections and the development of malignancies.

Immunoregulation. The processes by which the body is able to prevent immunocompromise.

Immunostimulation. The process by which substances turn on specific parts of the immune system.

In vitro. Experiments that occur in artificial laboratory environments outside the living body.

In vivo. Experiments that occur in the living organism, either using animal models or clinical studies that take place in humans.

Maculopapular. A rash that is reddened, with some irregular raised surfaces.

Neurological syndrome. Any process that results in an alteration of the nervous system. This can result in confusion, coma, muscle weakness, strange sensations, or any combination of these.

Neuropathy. Any process that impairs the functioning of specific nerves.

Opportunistic infections/ neoplasms. Infectious diseases or tumors that develop because of a weakening of the immune system, so that processes which are usually quite innocuous take advantage of the resultant immunocompromised state.

Persistent generalized lymphadenopathy (PGL). Swollen glands in more than one noncontiguous site throughout the body which stay enlarged for at least three months.

Synergism. Any combination that results in a multiplicative effect rather than an additive effect.

T-helper lymphocyte. A type of white blood cell that is responsible for orchestrating many of the interactions of different, other blood cells in the immune system. This is one of the cell types that become particularly affected by HIV, and the T-helper lymphocyte count can be a useful marker in following the progress of HIV infection in specific individuals.

Thrush. A yeast infection of the tongue.

Zoster. Reactivation of the chicken pox virus, also known as shingles. This usually results in a painful band either on the trunk or on the face, with painful blisters.

"I don't consider myself a person who's dying from AIDS. I certainly consider myself a person who's been living with AIDS. I don't consider myself an AIDS victim, and I really wish people in the media would stop using that terminology. I think that's one of the most damning things that you can say about a person, is that they're just a victim, and I think that part of the way I've come to look at this is that I'm a person who's still in control of my life and I refuse to be victimized by AIDS or anyone who's connected with this disease in any way. I maintain control."

Candida esophagitis.	Yeastlike fungus infection of the esophagus.
Hepatitis B.	Viral infection whereby a small virus attacks the liver, often producing jaundice.
Hyperallergenic subjects.	People who have heightened allergic responses.
Persistent generalized lymphadenopathy (PGL).	Persistent inflammation of the lymph nodes, particularly the axilla and groin, in response to an infection.
Transplacental or placental spread.	Transmission of the virus from the bloodstream of the mother to the blood of the unborn baby.

Epidemiology and Health Policy Imperatives for AIDS

Katherine Hill Chavigny, Ph.D., FACE
Sarah L. Turner, R.N., M.P.H., Ph.D.
Anne K. Kibrick, Ph.D.

The purpose of this article is to describe the statistics and epidemiological facts about the most virulent epidemic of our age, acquired immunodeficiency syndrome (AIDS). The discussion argues for broadened public policy to promote the surveillance of communities in order to enhance the effectiveness of data gathering for epidemiological reasoning, analysis, and control measures. To accomplish these goals, the essential characteristics of epidemiology are defined. The use of deductive and inductive reasoning is applied to describe and analyze known facts concerning the AIDS epidemic. Hypotheses are suggested from current amorphous and continually changing information to assist in further explanations of the epidemic and in the evaluation of methods of prevention and control. Current policies for sexually transmitted diseases are reviewed briefly to identify epidemiological concerns, with the aim of assisting policymakers. Implications for public policy are discussed in the context of seeking epidemiological information for the ultimate protection of the public good.

Epidemiology is logical thinking applied to health problems that threaten the public. A more generally accepted definition of epidemiology is the study of patterns of diseases and their precursors in communities; however, the essential elements of the epidemiological perspective are inductive and deductive processes of logical thought applied to problems of sickness and health in groups. Many health professionals use the concepts, processes, and results of epidemiological investigations to accomplish their goals. Epidemiology crosses the conceptual delineations of disciplines concerned with health; it seeks to identify health hazards to communities and evaluate the results of interventions, including the effects of public policy on health matters. Its main purposes are to provide information to achieve the goals of public health; to prevent and control sickness as well as disease precursors in communities, and to promote community health.

Katherine Hill Chavigny is director of the Office of Related Health Professions and Nursing Affairs at the American Medical Association in Chicago. Sarah L. Turner, an epidemiologist by training, teaches public-health nursing at Lander College in Greenwood, South Carolina. Anne K. Kibrick is dean of the School of Nursing at the University of Massachusetts at Boston.

In the new federalism that is now in vogue, the states have assumed increased fiscal responsibilities. Reduction in federal support affects administrative and government decisions at the state level.[1] Policies are codified and funds are allocated for state initiatives that are influenced by many factors besides scientific logic. In regard to human immunodeficiency virus (HIV) infections, Massachusetts has enacted laws requiring written, informed consent prior to testing for HIV antibody by physicians and health care facilities. These statutes address confidentiality, insurance, and informed consent.[2] The laws define AIDS as a handicap and invoke legal sanctions against discrimination toward persons with AIDS; also, the disclosure of test results to any person except the patient is prohibited by law. Informed consent of a person is required in written form before a test may be obtained. These state statutes protect the rights of the individual in respect to the group or community. State regulations must relate to and coordinate with national imperatives to effectively control epidemics.

At the federal and international levels, goals have been formulated, as follows, to coordinate state activities to control sexually transmitted diseases (STDs):[3]

1. To minimize disease exposure by reducing sexual intercourse with persons who have a high probability of infection.

2. To prevent infection by increasing the use of condoms or other prophylactic barriers.

3. To detect and cure disease by implementing screening programs, providing effective diagnostic and treatment facilities, and promoting health-seeking behaviors.

4. To limit complications of infections by providing early treatment to symptomatic and asymptomatic infected individuals.

5. To limit disease transmission within the community through the above efforts.

These objectives affect current policy for all sexually transmitted diseases in the United States, including the reporting and control of AIDS.

The syndrome known as AIDS is characterized by two inescapable but, it is hoped, not immutable facts that demand special policy approaches: (1) it is an infection with extended periods of infectivity (the harboring of an infective agent), and (2) eventually, the disease is fatal. It is crucial to recognize that the virus is carried and harbored by infected persons long before symptoms of acute illness occur. Owing to the longevity and fatality of HIV infection, the public requires policies for protection against a protracted, virulent, and, often, sequestered hazard. But AIDS is also a social disease; its major risk groups are associated with lifestyle behaviors such as homosexuality and illegal intravenous (IV) drug use, about which the larger society has moral and ethical preconceptions. Public policy, therefore, has to weigh civil liberties against the healthy survival of society.

Policymakers require facts to understand the risk of HIV infections, to ascertain the spread of the epidemic, and to assign resources. Basic scientific information is required to make convincing arguments for change which can be justified as objective, unprejudiced, and realistic. Epidemiology provides a comprehensive resource of scientific information about group problems for the use of administrators and legislators. All medical, social, and basic sciences are marshaled and integrated in order to apply epidemiology to the purpose of solving problems regarding the health of the community.

Policy for AIDS which meets the needs of each state requires reliable, valid, quantified information for assisting policymakers in protecting the public and the individual. National policy is based on the coordination and analysis of quantified data from state surveillance systems. Access to accurate information is a basic prerequisite for solving problems associated with community hazard. It is epidemiological practice to constantly monitor communities and collect information. Each state has a surveillance system, integrated on a national basis, to provide facts for scientific analysis. The civil concern to protect homosexual and racial rights are real and are an irrevocable constitutional mandate; however, protection of the group is an effective method of protecting individuals within the community. Statutes and policies guard the individual by expressing group decisions for mutual advantage of all people.

Methods used to determine the public good are all too frequently debatable issues. Epidemiology attempts to provide a logical basis for assessing public hazards and the effectiveness of communal solutions to protect the greatest good for all the people. Its special contribution is that it provides a rational, objective groundwork on which to base policy decisions. Facts are important to political arguments for opinion leaders, policymakers, and administrators. Valid information affords a means of allaying fear, provoking concern, and setting priorities. Assessment of risk and assessment of effectiveness of methods for the optimal protection of the people are prerequisite to setting cogent injunctions.

The public health system was slow to respond to the AIDS epidemic; too little was known about a slowly evolving but complex crisis that at first was not recognized as an infectious disease. As a result, policies that govern infectious disease surveillance were activated sluggishly. Partly because of this delay, there is a notable lack of reliable and valid information to guide epidemiologists in their quest for group parameters to assist policymakers. Measurement of community events are necessary to provide a scientific basis for policies that are well-reasoned and just.

Issues in the Analysis of Epidemiological Information

Epidemiology quantifies the incidence of disease in communities. Epidemiological surveillance provides objective data that allow comparisons between communities for decision making. But the mere collection of facts is never enough; to be meaningful, these facts require analysis and interpretation. Epidemiology as a discipline provides the scientific methods to analyze and optimize information through hypothesizing the cause of monitored problems in communities and identifying the most effective methods of prevention and control. These methods yield data to guide administrators and policymakers at all levels of government.

Hypothesizing the cause of public health problems is the central theme in epidemiology. Postulating the cause of health problems guides various strategies in analyzing observations and planning intervention in epidemic circumstances. In the interest of economy and effectiveness, it is important to choose a hypothesis that has the greatest power to produce the true associations. This is no small task, and it depends on analysis of facts that can be gleaned from the problem at issue, using hypothetical reasoning. The strength of the postulated association between potential causes and effects can be tested through inductive and deductive methods.

Scientific method is traditionally inductive, collecting observed facts to test a postulated cause. Epidemiology utilizes this approach and claims the distinction of being a science for public health. According to Karl Popper, all hypothetical reasoning is deductive, rather than inductive.[4] In other words, a causal relationship is made first and then facts are collected in support of the postulation. Popper also claims that refuting a hypothesis is more powerful than verifying the postulated relationship; the process of refutation leads to creative thinking and the selection of the most useful hypotheses. When refutation through the application of present information to test the hypothesis fails, then the hypothesis is worth testing through vigorous scientific research. Both approaches are available to yield answers to the difficult, unsolved problems concerning HIV infections; however, both methods of scientific inquiry require a body of known facts collected from the population in order to be innovative as well as effective.

The formulation of causal hypotheses as applied to populations demands special methods not always used in the strictly experimental sciences. Epidemiology uses the terminology of exposure for cause and effect for illness. There are several methods of assessing the merits of any hypothesis. Critical challenges to hypothetical association between exposure and effect include questions concerning (1) time order, (2) specificity, (3) consistency, and (4) coherence. Time order requires the exposure to precede the effect (illness) for the hypothetical association to be logical. Although it is known that some exposures can cause more than one disease, specificity is the precision of the exposure to predict illness and only that illness. Consistency is the ability of the hypothesized association to persist regardless of time, place, and person; and lastly, coherence demands the biological and clinical plausibility of the association.[5] In order to apply these (and other) logical challenges and hypothesize productively and economically, the availability of facts about the cases and their frequency is mandatory. Without facts — without the knowledge of where and when the cases of AIDS and the incidence of seroconversion (infection) are occurring — hypothesized solutions for public policy are constrained and impaired.

Issues in Measurement of the Epidemic

The need to have valid and representative information to identify an emerging epidemic and to hypothesize cause is demonstrated through the history of the emergence of the epidemic. The first necessity that arose regarding the syndrome called AIDS was to establish that a problem existed and to describe its characteristics and distribution. Although the first case of the disease syndrome was reported in 1978, it was not until 1981 that a cluster of several cases emerged indicating a possible problem.[6] Several outbreaks of *Pneumocystis carinii* pneumonia and Kaposi's sarcoma, a rare form of cancer, were reported to the Centers for Disease Control (CDC), the division of the U.S. Public Health Service which is responsible for monitoring infectious diseases in the United States. Examination of this cluster of diseases disclosed that the problem appeared to be confined to previously healthy, young, homosexual males. These differing diseases all showed the common phenomena of the evidence of immunosuppression, depleting the ability of patients to regulate and overcome infection.

Uniform case identification is crucial to any form of epidemiological investigation, whether it is descriptive or etiologic. The designation of an AIDS case was particularly difficult: not only does the disease syndrome present in several ways, but patients can have recurrent episodes and different causes of death. For instance, according to the report of the Committee for a National Strategy for AIDS, the major causes of death for HIV infection through 1986 were *Pneumocystis carinii* (64 percent), Kaposi's sarcoma (23 percent), and candida esophagitis (7 percent).[7] More recent information from the CDC indicates that the proportion of deaths due to Kaposi's sarcoma is decreasing to 11 percent relative to opportunistic infections such as candida esophagitis.[8] As with most mortality data, preexisting diagnoses are not shown. Reports usually indicate the frequency of cases and the proportions of diagnoses relative to all cases. The number of cases do not express the risk of AIDS and therefore do not relate to the community or group risk. More important, many diagnoses associated with HIV infection, such as AIDS dementia, are not systematically reported, although they are used within the new definitions for diagnosing HIV infection.[9] The methodic, consistent categorizing of persons with AIDS and the reporting of pre-mortality diagnoses are important for identifying hypotheses that will yield salient knowledge for scientists, administrators, and government leaders.

Because of the several diagnoses that accompany HIV infection as a result of reduced immunity, it became clear that a collection of signs and symptoms, a syndrome, furnished a preferred method of diagnosing the "cases" in the epidemic. In about 1982, the CDC differentiated AIDS from AIDS-related complex (ARC) and persistent generalized lymphadenopathy (PGL) in order to designate different stages of the disease. At that time, it was hypothesized that there was a linear progression from PGL to ARC to AIDS and so at least fifty thousand ARC cases were not reported to the Centers for Disease Control for inclusion in the epidemic.[10] The coherence of this postulate was soon shattered by the observation that ARC patients died without progressing to AIDS; also, PGL was not necessarily the first stage of what has subsequently been recognized as HIV infection. The CDC surveillance system, based on state reports, has not included ARC or PGL as cases of HIV infection in routine collection and reporting of epidemic data. The revised definitions of 1987 do not include the denotations ARC or PGL; however, the same syndromes are used for diagnosing the all-inclusive term of HIV infection or AIDS. Until the new diagnostic criteria are applied consistently and until enough time has passed to compile new rates rather than count cases, the extent of the epidemic remains equivocal.

The need for consistent, complete, valid information that is based on a comprehensive, consistent case definition is aptly illustrated by the fact that the true extent of the epidemic of all cases of HIV infection has not yet been detailed and made available to policymakers. Importantly, the most recent definitions may improve case finding in the future, but it will compromise any comparisons that may be made with information collected before September 1987, when the revised case definitions went into effect. The loss of comparable baseline statistics will create difficulties for policymakers who wish to have evidence of the effectiveness of regulations in slowing or deterring the spread of the epidemic.

Other epidemiological approaches are used to identify cases of infectious diseases. Any test that can measure antibodies to a specific infectious agent or a generalized response to infection is called a biological, epidemiological marker. The rationale for the use of the marker is not only to assist in diagnosis of cases but also to screen populations in order to identify the number of people who are infected in a community or in a subgroup of the general population. Epidemiological markers provide serologic evidence of present or cells suspended in a yellow fluid called serum. Antibodies to HIV and other infectious agents are found in sera that provide the serologic evidence to substantiate the presence of infection. When the tests are administered to a large group, the level of infection within the community or the proportion of those remaining susceptible to an infection can be estimated.

In many cases of infection with diseases other than AIDS, the evidence of invasion of the microbe is followed within a period of time, called the incubation period, by obvious signs and symptoms of illness. In most infections, the incubation period is short and the serum of the blood shows antibodies, a response to infection, almost at the same time that illness occurs. In some diagnoses, such as syphilis or herpes hominis II, the symptoms occur but may be too subtle to force an immediate consultation with a physician. After invasion of the body with HIV, signs and symptoms of illness may be delayed indefinitely; the only indication that the person is infected with the virus may be a positive blood test, also called a positive serology. This means that an apparently healthy person is infected with the virus and that it may be passed to others. The person is infected but has no diagnosed disease and may be unaware that he or she may be a danger to others.

The enzyme-linked immunosorbent assay, the ELISA test, made available in 1985, is an epidemiological marker for measuring the presence of antibodies to the human immunodeficiency virus in the serum of the blood. A second test to corroborate a positive serology is always required to verify the first measure, and the Western blot test is used when the ELISA suggests the presence of HIV antibody. In HIV infection, the use of the tests makes it possible to define infected populations who are without signs and symptoms of acute illness. Tests are also used to verify the diagnosis of AIDS when illness has already occurred.

In 1987, the International Nomenclature Committee and others advised that the formerly used diagnostic term (AIDS) be discarded in favor of the global term HIV infection.[11] Almost simultaneously, diagnostic criteria for HIV infection were revised, and signs and symptoms were regrouped.[12] These measures will assist in increasing the effectiveness of quantifying cases for entry into the numerator of the rate, the basic statistic of public health. Rates are important in epidemiology. The numerator is the frequency of diagnosed cases; but it can also be restricted to the number of infected, asymptomatic persons, such as those with positive blood (serology) tests. The denominator is the population at risk of exposure to the hazard at the local, state, or national level. Accuracy of rates depends on precise case identification and the size of the community where cases occur. It is also heavily dependent on the identification and reporting of cases and infected persons. Rational policy depends on access to valid rates to enhance the assessment of public problems associated with diseases that threaten the well-being of the community. Frequency of cases, the counting of the numerator of the rate, is often regarded as a questionable measure of the progress of an epidemic when the incubation period is lengthy, as in HIV infection. Lack of methods of case identification that included all HIV infections in the past has compromised the estimates of the extent of the epidemic and the hazard to the public. In the same way, lack of reporting of persons with positive serology is a serious barrier to accurate assessments of group risk; it also makes any claims that the epidemic is slowing down open to question.[13]

Describing and Analyzing the Epidemic

The use of available facts to formulate hypotheses in epidemiology is illustrated by a selective review of the evolution of the problem of AIDS. One of the first hypotheses concerning the cause of the epidemic was based on the observation that the syndrome occurred in male homosexual populations.[14] Several exposures common to this group were examined. A reasonable association from early studies was thought to be the exposure to sniffing amyl and butyl nitrite, drugs used to enhance orgasm. The amyl nitrites are commonly used to relieve anginal pain. The causal association between the use of these drugs and AIDS seemed to be refuted in later studies, mainly because the design had not included a heterosexual control group; the sample was too restrictive.[15] Subsequently, it became clear that the hypothesis did not meet the demand of criteria for establishing a causal relationship, such as time order, specificity, and consistency, although the use of these drugs may be a cofactor. The occurrence of AIDS was not always preceded by use of the nitrites; the taking of the drugs by homosexuals did not always predict AIDS, nor did this association persist in groups such as hemophiliacs.

Other hypotheses were advanced. The autoimmune reaction is depleted when exposed to spermatozoa that are forced into the bloodstream. It was thought that this antigenic response was the cause of AIDS. This postulated association was thought to be biologically plausible (coherent), because immunosuppression and the increased occurrence of tumors had been noted in primates who had had vasectomies. Although this hypothesis has not yet been clearly refuted, it lost precedence when other information emerged from increased surveillance and reporting.

Further analysis of available information showed similar patterns to hepatitis B virus infection.[16] Rates of hepatitis B are highest in those who practice illegal intravenous drug use and in persons with a history of venereal disease. Hepatitis B is spread through blood, blood products, and sexual contact. The agent is a virus. Comparison between the group pattern of hepatitis B and emerging facts about AIDS led to the hypothesis that AIDS, too, is an infectious disease, a postulate that has now been verified and that meets all logical, critical challenges.

The identification of what is now known as the human immunodeficiency virus, a retrovirus with lentivirus characteristics, was a result of the work of a group of scientists including Barne-Sinoussi,[17] Gallo,[18] and Levy[19] in 1983. As discussed earlier, the ELISA test became available in 1985 — a direct result of identifying the causal agent. This epidemiological marker traces the extent of the infection in the population; it is a screening method for detecting the presence of asymptomatic infection as well as a diagnostic tool for confirming cases. Lack of systematic screening policies has made the estimates of the extent of the asymptomatic infection in the population unreliable. It was thought that there might be between 1.5 million and 2 million seropositive people in the United States, but this was a crude guess made in the absence of evidence. The reporting of seropositivity is crucial to making the estimates valid, but policies to ensure the accurate collection of these facts are still in debate. It is not surprising that the reported estimate was recently revised and is thought to be much less, about 470,000,[20] although evidence is still sparse to support this figure. The scope of the infected but submerged reservoir of infected people is particularly troubling because the exact relationship of seroconversion to extant illness is still not clear. The occurrence of AIDS after conversion to a positive ELISA test used to be quoted as 1:5, or 20 percent. It is now thought that 50 percent of people with positive serology may develop the disease.[21]

The description of the epidemic which was derived from analysis of collected observations showed that by the end of 1986, over 24,500 cases of AIDS had been reported to the CDC.[22] It is thought that over 50,000 ARC cases had occurred during the same time period.[23] By May 1987, the total had increased to 35,318 cases of AIDS. Of the total 35,318 cases, 92.6 percent occurred in males and 7.4 percent in females; 498 cases, or 1.4 percent, were under the age of thirteen.[24]

The profile or pattern of the disease has now taken shape. Male homosexuality and male bisexuality account for 71 percent of the 35,318 cases, illegal intravenous drug use 14 percent, and male homosexuality with illegal intravenous drug use another 8 percent.[25] Illegal drug use is the major means of HIV transmission in females, followed by heterosexual activity. When the mode of transmission of HIV infection is compared to white/non-Hispanic, black/non-Hispanic, and Hispanic ethnic classifications, male homosexual/bisexual activity was a major factor in white/non-Hispanic cases. Among blacks and Hispanics, intravenous drug use was the main channel of transmission of the virus, and heterosexual transmission of HIV was highest in blacks.[26]

Few mandatory testing/screening programs for asymptomatic but infected people are in place; however, the armed forces require ELISA screening for new applicants. Information from this form of surveillance shows interesting epidemiological patterns.[27] From a total of over three-quarters of a million applicants for military service, there were fewer than two cases per thousand, or about a total of fifteen hundred persons with asymptomatic infections. Anecdotal accounts of these data suggest that many of the seropositive applicants assert they had no knowledge of their exposure to infected sources.[28] Also shown in this report are the higher rates of seroconversion in blacks and Hispanics, confirming other observations that rates of diagnosed AIDS in these minority groups are almost double the rates of overt disease in the Caucasian/non-Hispanic group.[29]

Facts describing the present status of the epidemic which may indicate intervention methods for prevention and control include the following: Among female cases, 50 percent are attributable to transmission by illegal intravenous drug use, 29 percent by heterosexual spread, and 10 percent by blood or blood components.[30] Although females form a small percentage of all reported cases, AIDS is associated with intravenous drug use twice as much in women as in men; also in females, AIDS is associated with heterosexual activity fourteen times more than in males.[31] In the larger male groups, homosexual activity and drug use, in that order, are the major forms of transmission.

The extent of the epidemic of HIV infection in women from 1981 through 1986 describes 1,819 cases, using the case definition that excluded cases of ARC[32] occurring during this time period. For this reason, these figures should be regarded as very conservative estimates. Little is known about female homosexual transmission of the virus between infected women. Usually, epidemiologists consider that compared to the male homosexual/bisexual group, there is no equivalent risk group for females.[33] The predominant method of transmission of HIV infection to women is illegal use of intravenous drugs, followed by heterosexual contact with a person at risk for AIDS. Because women have the possibility of sexual contact with groups at high risk of HIV infection, such as bisexual males, they are viewed as the interface between male homosexual/bisexual groups and the heterosexual population, where seepage of the infection to non-high-risk groups may take place. Following the progress of the epidemic through analysis of the frequency of cases in women may be a method of categorizing the spread of the infection into the heterosexual population. For instance, the proportion of cases in women which is ascribed to heterosexual transmission increased from 12 to 26 percent between 1982 and the end of 1986. It is also obvious that infected women are the source of the transplacental transmission that takes place from mother to infant, increasing the threat of AIDS to the unborn.[34] Statistics in August 1987 indicated that, under the "old" CDC case definition, 40,051 cases had been reported to the CDC from fifty states in the Union. Fifty-eight percent of these patients had died.[35] By mid-December, the total number of cases was 48,574.[36]

Methods of Transmission of HIV Infection

The transmission of an infective agent requires a reservoir that harbors the infective source; a route of transmission or vehicle for spreading the organism; a susceptible host; a portal of exit from the infected reservoir; and a portal of entry into the susceptible host. The greater the knowledge about transmission of infectious disease, the more likely that methods of prevention and control will be effective. Administrative and legislative initiatives utilize epidemiological information to break the chain of transmission, to plan services, and to allocate resources.

The mode of transmission of HIV is similar to that of the virus of hepatitis B that spreads through blood, blood products, and sexual intercourse. The transmission of the hepatitis B virus differs from HIV because chronic carriers of the hepatitis B virus are few, about 10 percent, and the incubation period is not longer than six months. It is also a recognized occupational hazard to health care workers.[37] Hepatitis B is a reportable communicable disease that is under constant surveillance by public health authorities. It is epidemic in proportions and has epidemiological tests or markers to screen high-risk populations, a practice recommended by the Immunization Practice Advisory Committee. A vaccine is available for primary prevention.[38]

The reservoirs for HIV are infected asymptomatic and symptomatic persons. Once the infection has taken place, the person remains infected and becomes a source of the virus. High levels of infectivity are found in groups whose lifestyle, such as illegal IV drug use or male homosexuality, places them at high risk. The chief vehicles through which the disease is spread are blood, blood products, and semen. Portals of entry for infected semen to enter the body of a susceptible person are provided, probably, through trauma to mucous membranes and through skin abrasions or open lesions. Another portal of entry is provided through the direct injection of the virus into the bloodstream.[39] Methods of spread are through sexual activities that may injure tissues and afford entry into the bloodstream and (perhaps) through multiple sexual contacts in a short period of time.[40] Other routes of transmission are through illegal intravenous drug use, particularly the use of shared needles, and through infected blood transfusions and blood products.

Portals of exit for infected secretions are provided through blood outlets such as bleeding gums, accidental hemorrhage, and the emission of semen from infected persons. All secretions for seropositive people have the potential to be infectious, including saliva and vaginal secretions, possibly because the virus has been retrieved from the secretions;[41] however, transmission through these means is highly unlikely, because epidemiological evidence indicates that casual social contact does not spread the disease. Direct contact with an infected person or susceptible host with appropriate portals of entry seems the necessary prerequisite for developing infection and subsequent AIDS.

Transmission of HIV infection between high- and low-risk populations is of great concern and requires further epidemiological studies to define accurately. The populations with high and low rates interface through illegal drug use, bisexual behaviors, prostitution, blood transfusions, artificial insemination, and organ transplantation.

The risk of HIV infection for health care workers who deliver direct services is low, but examination of information about the spread of disease to health workers illustrates the need to protect portals of entry, such as skin abrasions, from accidental transmission. A 1986 study by the CDC showed that out of 750 physicians and nurses exposed to body fluids of infected patients, only 3 workers, after complaining of needle sticks, were found to have converted to positive antibody tests.[42] These professionals admitted to other risk factors such as male homosexuality. In a larger study of 20,000 health care workers, 4 percent were seropositive; but it is thought that all workers with seroconversions had other risk factors besides contact with HIV-infected patients.[43]

It may be true that transmission occurs in health care workers without the presence of any high-risk factors, but such transmission seems rare. Nine cases reported to the CDC during 1987 did not admit to any high-risk lifestyles.[44] Anecdotal evidence implied that seroconversion occurred from contact with infected fluid in the presence of injured skin.[45] Four of the cases had suffered needle-stick exposures; two others had had extensive contact with infected body fluids but had failed to observe the recommended barrier precautions to wear gloves. The remaining three cases illustrate the need to provide a portal of entry for the virus to invade the body. A female worker with chapped hands applied pressure to a bleeding arterial site to prevent hemorrhage during an emergency episode; subsequently the worker had a positive ELISA test. In another case, the top of a 10 ml vacuum blood collection tube flew off, and infected blood was splattered over the faces and in the mouths of two workers, one of whom suffered from acne. The latter developed a positive serology for HIV but the other worker remains seronegative. In another incident, a major blood spill covered the gloved hands and forearms of a health care worker. She had dermatitis in one ear and may have touched the ear during the incident; subsequently she became seropositive.[46] Needle-stick injuries and exposure of mucous membranes to secretion and blood infected with the virus do not appear inevitably to result in seroconversion; however, the precise risk of transmission has not yet been defined. In spite of the general low occupational risk, it seems that the possibility of transmission will increase as the number of infected patients increases.[47]

Studies of hemophiliacs with AIDS/ARC substantiate that social contact with family and friends does not spread the disease. In a study of the family contacts of fifty children and adults with diagnosed hemophilia, sexual contact between spouses was the only mode of transmission of the disease.[48] Social interaction between friends and nonspouses with antibody-positive, asymptomatic hemophiliacs did not spread the disease. The findings in this study also showed that in comparison to the immune response in the social contacts of the antibody-negative (uninfected) group of hemophiliacs, the immune response in the social but nonsexual contacts of infected hemophiliacs was diminished. This suggests hypotheses that perhaps nonsexual social exposure results in physiological responses of the immune system, which may give some indications for research on an effective vaccine. See figure 1.

The study by Jason and McDougal which was used as the source for figure 1 was small. More recent studies substantiate that changes in the blood lymphocytes do not predict clinical change.[49] Studies of the hemophiliac group establish that transmission of the virus requires sexual contact or exposure to infected blood through a portal of entry that gives access to the bloodstream.[50]

Figure 1

Diagnosis and HIV Antibody Status of Household Contacts of Persons with Hemophilia

Health Status of Hemophiliacs	Hemophiliacs	Incidence Rate of AIDS in Family Contacts
AIDS (with signs and symptoms)	12	1 Spouse Out of 15 Contacts
ARC (with signs and symptoms)	5	1 Spouse Out of 18 Contacts
Antibody-Positive (infected but no signs or symptoms)	17	0 Cases Out of 29 Contacts (Including 7 Spouses)
Antibody-Negative (noninfected)	9	0 Cases Out of 21 Contacts
	43	83

Rate of disease in sexual partners of AIDS/ARC hemophiliacs = 14% (2/14)

Rate of disease in sexual partners of antibody-positive hemophiliacs = 0% (0/7)

Significantly lower lymphocytes in social contacts with hemophiliacs with AIDS, ARC, and antibody-positive serology than in contacts with antibody-negative hemophiliacs.

Source: Janine M. Jason, J. Steven McDougal, Gloria Dixon, et al. "HTLV-III/LAV Antibody and Immune Status of Household Contacts and Sexual Partners of Persons with Haemophilia." *Journal of the American Medical Association* 255 (1986): 212–215.

Choice of sexual behavior in heterosexuals may influence transmission of HIV infection, given that one of the partners is a reservoir for the virus. A hypothesis that anal intercourse may transmit the virus has been postulated from observations of the higher frequency of AIDS in the receptive homosexual partner. This suggests that anal intercourse may be a high-risk activity for females with an infected partner. The results of an ongoing study of females exposed to seropositive partners indicate that there is increased risk of AIDS to support this hypothesis.[51] Specialists in obstetrics and gynecology advocate tactful and sensitive inquiry into their patients' histories to obtain information on frequency of anal intercourse in order to guide counseling. It is estimated from some preliminary studies that 25 percent of American women engage in occasional anal intercourse and that 10 percent of women practice anal intercourse regularly.[52, 53] These rates are based on limited observations. Bolling and Voeller confirmed that information on frequency of anal sex in women is sparse.[54] They estimate that the frequency of anal intercourse is greater in cultural groups that use it as a method of contraception and preservation of virginity; nonetheless, it is thought that there is still a lower frequency of anal intercourse in women than in homosexual men.

Heterosexual transmission is documented,[55] but the direction of transmission from female to male was questioned. There is evidence that infected females practicing prostitution infect male heterosexuals.[56] This may be associated with the increased drug use in this group. Though the risk appears small, it is expected that by 1991 heterosexual transmission will account for perhaps 10 percent of all HIV infections.[57]

Another mode of transmission between low- and high-risk groups is transplacental spread to children born to infected mothers. A study in 1985 showed that of twenty-two babies diagnosed with HIV infection who were born to sixteen mothers, fifteen were asymptomatic at the time of birth of their first child with AIDS. Four of the mothers admitted to high-risk activities such as IV drug use and prostitution.[58] Other, more recent studies indicate that the risk of transmission of the infection to the child seems to be 1:5, or 20 percent.[59, 60, 61]

Methods of Prevention and Control

Decisions regarding the most effective methods of prevention and control require reliable evidence of modes of transmission; valid estimates of the risk of exposure to the virus; and knowledge of the virulence of the disease. Disease virulence (the serious consequences of an infection) affects policy decisions regarding prioritization of goals, assignments of funds, and allocation of resources. The virulence of a disease is measured by the case fatality rate, which is the number of deaths occurring in diagnosed cases. At present, the seven-year case fatality rate for AIDS is about 58 percent; in other words, more than half the AIDS cases reported to the CDC between 1981 and 1987 have died.[62] Perhaps of greater concern is that no diagnosed case of AIDS (or ARC) has recovered.[63] It is clear that infection is extremely virulent, and this lends great urgency to the need to seek methods to control the spread of the epidemic.

Prevention and control methods block the invasion and transmission of the virus. One of the most effective methods of preventing any infectious disease is through the immunization of populations. This primary prevention technique protects against common infectious diseases before infection takes place. For the immediate future, the availability of a generalized effective vaccine for HIV infection seems remote.[64] Effective vaccines against retrovirus infections have yet to be discovered. HIV has been described as a lentivirus that has the characteristic of antigenic variation generated during replication of the virus. The development of a vaccine that gives broadly effective immunity is quite difficult, on account of genomic diversity, or changes in the basic proteins in the chromosomes. The existence of different strains of HIV creates a major obstacle for the generation of a single, effective vaccine. This means that antibodies manufactured in response to the antigens are not effective against successive generations of the virus. Should a vaccine become available, such social concerns as how to evaluate its efficacy in populations will have to be addressed. It is important to recognize that the effectiveness of vaccination would have to be measured against baseline information that has already been collected concerning rates of infection or seropositivity, and these rates are often questionable or unavailable.

Public information and education, at present, are the most important means of primary intervention to prevent the occurrence of the disease. Education for safer sexual practices includes the use of the condom as a barrier to transmission of the virus during intercourse. Determining the efficacy of these measures to change behavior and maintain behavioral change will require reliable information. This information will be used to show decline in the rate of increase of infection. It will also require information on the distribution and characteristics associated with sexual practices and mores in several subgroups, such as the minorities. Several disciplines devoted to the study of behavioral phenomena need to research these questions. A multidisciplinary approach crossing all professional boundaries is required to develop the most effective methods of control of HIV infection.[65]

Primary prevention — intervention in the transmission of disease before the disease occurs — is the sine qua non of methods of preserving the health of the public. It is economical; it is effective; it is the most humane approach to protecting the group and the individuals within the group. Special kinds of scientific and epidemiological facts are essential to the implementation of primary prevention. For instance, a hypothesis concerning an effective vaccine must be scientifically plausible, and risk of acquiring the disease after exposure must be verified so that vaccination can be timely. This information is also important for conserving a safe blood supply.

It seems that the period between an exposure to an infected person and seroconversion varies. The Institute of Medicine in late 1986 stated that seroconversion could occur as early as six to eight weeks after exposure; however, the period is highly variable and may extend as long as eight months.[66] More recently, it has been suggested that seroconversion may occur up to twelve months after exposure.[67] The incubation period — the time between invasion and the occurrence of signs and symptoms of disease — is an important epidemiological variable and is even more uncertain. Estimations made from infected blood transfusions indicate an incubation period of about five years.[68] For adult cases not associated with transfusions, the mean incubation period may be fifteen years.[69] These analyses are compromised by limited data.

Reasons for the difficulty in identifying the incubation period are several. Establishing the date of exposure is problematic, especially without established surveillance systems denoting infected but asymptomatic persons. The incubation period may vary according to mode of transmission, the age of the patient, and the initial concentration of the virus in the infected substrate. Other strains of human immunodeficiency virus are appearing which may lack the virulence of the microbe most frequently infecting the population. Male-to-female, female-to-male transmission may be less effective than male-to-male transmission.[70] Repeated exposure to the infected person may be necessary before the susceptible partner contracts the virus, obfuscating the time of exposure. These factors and others reflect the uncertainties of the discussion on the incubation period. They also underscore the need for reliable documentation of infected persons to keep pace with the ever changing state of the art concerning AIDS.

Secondary intervention is the early detection of infected people in the population. ELISA and Western blot tests provide screening tools to identify the infected, asymptomatic pool in the population, besides verifying the diagnosis in those with illness. Once identified, those who are infected remain in the community as reservoirs for the virus for a considerable length of time. Antiviral medication does not eliminate the virus; cure for the infection is not yet within reach. For these reasons, HIV infection is called a chronic disease. Moreover, because of the variability between seroconversion and overt illness, the infected population does not always seek medical intervention; some may be unaware that they have been exposed to those with high-risk lifestyles.

Infected populations fall into two groups: the asymptomatic, who feel well; and those in whom symptoms are emerging or full-blown. Screening of populations would assist in identifying infected patients, particularly those in whom infection is not suspected. The greatest hazard to the community is the undetected infection. It has been long known in infection control in hospitals that the greatest risk to hospitalized patients and staff is from the "hidden," or undiagnosed, infected person.

Screening is part of surveillance activities that include testing of high-risk groups attending venereal disease clinics, hospital emergency rooms, and jails. Testing for more than one infection is possible and, often, routine. From the information obtained from these tests, epidemiologists provide information for the community. Administrators learn the degree of need in their locale and are able to plan resources to meet these needs. Local communities are provided with evidence of the threat that exists in their cities and neighborhoods and can organize programs to enhance education of the public. Politicians obtain facts with which they can justify acquiring funds to focus on the greatest area of concern and to encourage the promulgation of regulations to protect the public and the individual. Surveillance also documents the spread or the lack of spread of epidemics into low-risk groups; with a virulent disease such as AIDS, confirming a low prevalence of infection can allay fears and offer reassurance to concerned citizens.

Many feel that the case yield (identified cases of infection) from screening of populations is necessary only where the group may have high levels of infected persons. The danger of false positives is quoted as a reason to reduce screening activities. These arguments have merit from a statistical point of view; however, the tests have over 98 percent sensitivity and specificity — an excellent epidemiological marker to denote true cases and true noncases. In populations of low prevalence, these figures deteriorate and the problem of false positives increases. But the fact is that no test of positive serology is ever performed without a repeat test. Even in situations where prevalence of HIV infection is low, repeat testing increases the likelihood of accurate results. However, routine testing and mandated testing must be differentiated in considering policy. Routine testing consists of usual procedures of public health surveillance. Mandatory testing is supported by law. Statutes requiring written permission for testing for AIDS — the Massachusetts law is an example — create barriers to routine and confidential testing in clinics for sexually transmitted diseases. This is important, because patients in these clinics constitute a high-risk population for HIV infection.[71]

The information gained from programs identifying infected populations is a powerful tool for controlling spread of the infection among the public. Infected women can use the information to make decisions about pregnancies. Infected partners can be taught to prevent the further spread of the infection. In HIV infections, screening for seropositivity before the signs and symptoms occur identifies a group that may be willing to assist researchers in obtaining knowledge to obviate the development of the disease; this screening also identifies those in need of the latest discoveries for treating the infection.

Surveillance information can also be used to plan tertiary prevention and the optimizing of life for the chronically ill and the dying. Resources for meeting the needs of the afflicted and for tending to the dying are needed not only for reasons of humanitarianism, but also to assure the best methods of controlling accidental transmission of the disease during critically ill periods at home and in the hospital, when direct access to infected blood of the patients may occur.

Other facts are required to formulate hypotheses that justify further research, which in turn provides answers that eventually lead to intervention. Several hypotheses for epidemiological research require immediate development,[72] not the least of which is the spread of the disease into groups defined as low risk. Screening reveals populations where rates of infection are low; the armed forces, a population with mandated testing, has low rates of seroconversion; however, the spread of the infection at the interface of high- and low-risk groups may be increasing.[73] The risk of developing symptoms when a person has a positive serology may be 50 percent, but this figure remains tentative,[74] with some even projecting that, except for dying from competing causes before the symptoms of AIDS manifest, eventual occurrence of the disease is inevitable.[75]

Hypotheses are legion. It is possible that a segment of the population is immune to the virus; if this is so, it promotes areas of research with vast potential for prevention and control. Minority groups, including mothers and babies, seem to die faster from HIV infection than nonminority groups, but why this occurs is a challenging question.[76] Central nervous system AIDS may be an autoimmune reaction that afflicts only hyperallergenic subjects; if this is not the case, then other reasons for its apparently selective occurrence must be sought. AIDS in Europe and Africa is primarily a heterosexual disease, for reasons that remain obscure.[77] HIV infection is a chronic illness that suppresses the immune reaction to other infectious diseases; it is reasonable to predict a rise in other infectious diseases such as tuberculosis and mononucleosis.[78] Hepatitis B, owing to similar modes of transmission, may rise concomitantly with the HIV epidemic.[79] Increased surveillance of all infectious diseases is necessitated by the AIDS epidemic, and support for the public health system that is already in place for public protection becomes an imperative.

The questions are compelling and the problem is critical. Surveillance information that is salient, focused, and informative is urgently needed to enhance the contribution of epidemiological research so that prevention and control methods can be determined. Problems must be solved creatively so that a variety of methods of prevention can be identified through deductive and inductive reasoning; however, facts must be available from which the most plausible and coherent hypotheses can be formulated. Assignment of public and private funds may then be applied to the most productive research to assist in solving the problem of HIV infection.

Discussion

Epidemiology, a public health science, is also called social medicine. The role of epidemiology is to describe the health problems afflicting a society, seek the cause of hazards, provide logical solutions, and evaluate interventions. Because epidemiology deals with communities and provides information to protect social systems, it inevitably impacts public policy. The origins of epidemiology lie deep in the history of infectious diseases that have long plagued the human race. Its methods — which are designed to evaluate and weigh evidence, test hypotheses, and provide answers that are derived from the group experience — have established its success over time. Answers are shared with politicians, administrators, and leaders, and, because of its application to public problems, epidemiological research is often funded from public coffers. Where necessary, laws are made, on the basis of scientific inquiry, with the goal of promoting realistic and defensible regulations that are barriers to the spread of disease and that protect the rights of both the sick and the well. But the degree to which any individual requires the protection of the statutory system must be weighed and balanced against the degree of threat to the total community, if only because individual safety often depends upon protective legislation that applies to all. Objective, scientific observations of the spread of AIDS must be available to policymakers so that individual rights can be considered within the context of the public good.

Compared to many infectious disease hazards that have occurred in the past, the HIV epidemic has evolved slowly. Evidence has accumulated less quickly about a disease that causes death and is unusual in its complexity. It has not been possible to marshal the facts that were necessary to assuage fear and misconceptions that have spread within the community. The public health system was hampered by the lack of epidemiological markers such as the ELISA test until the epidemic had been acknowledged for some time. This has contributed to the delay in the customary public health methods of reporting, surveillance, and routine testing. The complexity of adequate case definition has added to the problems of activating public health reporting and surveillance systems for epidemiological purposes. Accurate information gathered from the population is still needed to allay fears, to document the lack of infection as well as its presence, and to establish the limits of spread of HIV across the boundaries of high- and low-risk groups. Policy and regulation need facts from adequate surveillance, accurate reporting, and scientific documentation of AIDS in order to support public health methods rather than obstruct the system.

Many precedents for public policy to control socially linked infections have already been set. Syphilis has long been a disease that afflicted adults, that infected mothers, and that spread to unborn infants. There was a time when it was incurable, inexorable, and misunderstood. In the past, screening for antibodies to syphilis was mandated by law for entry into the United States. Even today, testing for syphilis remains a statutory requirement in two states for obtaining marriage licenses. Costs of testing for syphilis are borne by the applicants. As with any sexually transmitted disease, persons with positive serology for syphilis require contact tracing. Social discrimination, confidentiality, and invasion of privacy remain issues that cannot be avoided. The rights to confidentiality and privacy are recognized and respected by the public health community.

Arguments against routine testing for HIV infection include prohibitive expense and the lack of vaccine or treatment for contacts. Clearly, costs are a matter of administrative and political priorities. Prevention methods for AIDS are only palliative, it is true; however, it is hoped that this will change. Not only can contact tracing yield information for the common good; it can also identify people in jeopardy of contracting AIDS and other communicable diseases such as tuberculosis and hepatitis B. Those who are infected or in need may be willing to become engaged in decisions to assist themselves and others as part of prevention activities. Contact tracing will also provide a cadre of people who require immediate treatment when the discovery of effective therapy is disclosed. Hepatitis B, a disease associated with illegal IV drug use, was subject to all the usual public health approaches of surveillance, screening, and reporting, despite the problems of contact tracing and confidentiality, even before a vaccine became available.

The American Medical Association promotes ethical standards for the practice of medicine. In 1986, partly in response to the AIDS epidemic,[80] these standards were updated and emphasized. When a physician provides treatment to a patient, confidentiality is the hallmark of professional practice. Also, the physician may not refuse to properly inform the patient of the diagnosis and treatment. The patient's consent is a prerequisite for the sharing of information with any other person, and where statistical information is shared, any personal identification must be deleted. These principles of medical ethics represent ideal standards that can be overridden only in a court of law. Physicians are the gatekeepers for patients' rights, especially for communicable diseases. With respect to HIV testing, therefore, it is difficult to justify statutes that may enable a person to bypass physician intervention and care.

Physicians safeguard the confidentiality of the patient and counsel patients about treatment in order to ensure informed consent. Nowhere is this more important than with social disease. Public health and preventive medicine have developed methods of contact tracing which are committed to the ethos of respecting individual privacy while protecting group concerns. Contacts are informed only with patient consent. Similarly, all epidemiologists are obligated to respect confidentiality. Group information for analysis is filed under conditions of strictest privacy, without any identifying information. The AMA has recently reemphasized these high precepts for the guidance and direction of ethical conduct of medical practitioners.

Anonymity is preserved through universal mandates. In other words, when testing is required routinely or by statute for groups such as prisoners, members of the armed forces, persons seeking marriage, or patients attending clinics for sexually transmitted diseases, no one is at risk of discrimination, because all must experience the same test in obedience to the law. The results of the tests are group results — they are population-based, and they supply a constant source of data for epidemiologists, who use them to further the goals of prevention and control community health hazards. These ideals should be sought and upheld by those who make public policy.

The public health community seeks to minimize disease through early detection and treatment. These are accomplished through implementing screening programs, providing effective diagnostic and treatment facilities, and promoting health-seeking behaviors. Prevention and control include limiting the complications of infection by providing early treatment to symptomatic and asymptomatic infected individuals and by limiting disease transmission within the community. These efforts are communal and require dependable surveillance systems that are accurate, reliable, and comprehensive. Enlightened public policy is required to marshal the human and technical resources of the community to protect individuals by protecting the public good.

Conclusions

Ongoing surveillance of virulent epidemics is an activity that is a national imperative. To date, information on the size and extent of the epidemic is obscure, owing to a lack of consistent, stable definitions of cases of illness for HIV infection and statutes that obstruct routine tests of high-risk populations. We now have a method of identifying the asymptomatic but infected populations — the hidden and sinister reservoir of a virulent virus. The seropositive populations can be identified through screening activities that are part of ongoing monitoring activities. Surveillance needs the support of political leadership. The interface of high-risk and so-called low-risk groups is real. All estimates of risk of spread of disease to groups with low-risk lifestyles are guesswork, based on inadequate and incomplete data. In order to secure valid information for effective decision making, influential leaders must create policy that ensures the accuracy of statistics. Only then can epidemiologists apply scientific principles for identifying the extent of the disease, the risk to the unborn, and the effectiveness of methods of prevention and control. HIV infection is a national hazard and is the concern of all the people. The challenge for policymakers is to assure protection for every human being while protecting the total community.

Notes

1. John Shannon, "De Facto New Federalism: Phase II?" *New England Journal of Public Policy* (Winter–Spring 1986): 26–36.
2. American Medical Association, Division of Legislative Activities, "AIDS State Legislative Activities" (June 1987), Chicago. Specifically, "An Act for the Confidentiality of HTLV-III Tests." Massachusetts Regular Session. Chapter 241, Laws 1986, House Bill No. 5491, approved July 15, 1986. Effective October 13, 1986.
3. American Medical Association, Board of Trustees Report YY, "Prevention and Control of AIDS: An Intermediate Report" (June 1987), p. 182, Chicago. Reports to the Board of Trustees of the American Medical Association are prepared and reviewed by medical scientists who are on the Council of Scientific Affairs. The reports are subjected to intense internal and external peer review before being submitted to the Board of Trustees. After careful scrutiny, revision, and, if necessary, further review, the reports are submitted to the House of Delegates. When they are accepted by the House, the reports enter the public domain.
4. Karl Popper, *The Philosophy of Scientific Reasoning,* 6th Impression. Revised, London, Hutchinson (1972), chapter 2.
5. Mervyn Susser, "The Logic of Sir Karl Popper and the Practice of Epidemiology." *American Journal of Epidemiology* 124, no. 5 (1986): 711–719.
6. U.S. Public Health Service (USPHS), Centers for Disease Control, "Kaposi's Sarcoma and Pneumocystis Carinii Among Homosexual Men, New York City and California." *Morbidity and Mortality Weekly Report* 30, no. 26 (1981b): 305–308.
7. National Academy of Sciences, Institute of Medicine, *Confronting AIDS: Directions for Public Health, Health Care, and Research.* National Academy Press, Washington, D.C. (1986). Cited information from the Centers for Disease Control, *1986c Acquired Immunodeficiency Syndrome (AIDS) AIDS Weekly Surveillance Report* United States Cases Reported to CDC* (September 9, 1986): 72, 73. (Hereafter in these notes, this CDC report will be referred to simply as the *AIDS Weekly Surveillance Report — United States.)*
8. Centers for Disease Control, *AIDS Weekly Surveillance Report — United States* (December 19, 1987). This report includes a comprehensive review of cases (not rates) by high risk, racial categories, and age, as well as some diagnostic classifications.
9. Centers for Disease Control, "Revision of the Centers for Disease Control Surveillance Case Definition for Acquired Immunodeficiency Syndrome." *Morbidity and Mortality Weekly Report* (September 1987) 36, supplement no. 15: 5s, A7.
10. Note 7, p. 70.
11. Kenneth H. Mayer, Steven M. Opal, "Therapeutic Approaches to AIDS." *Rhode Island Medical Journal* 70, no. 1 (January 1987): 27–33.
12. Note 8.
13. *USA Today,* December 7, 1987, 13A: interview with James Mason, director of the Centers for Disease Control, quotes the report of the USPHS interim report to President Reagan on AIDS which says that AIDS has stabilized for white homosexual males. Also *Chicago Tribune,* December 3, 1987, reporter John Crewdon quotes the same interim report to President Reagan as claiming that the general rate of new AIDS infection may have declined somewhat from the rates that prevailed in the early 1980s. The same Chicago paper (December 10, vol. 30, page 1), in an article entitled "A little good news about AIDS," says that the estimate of 1 million to 1.5 million infected Americans may be too high, and other projections suggest lower totals. But AIDS is "not spreading like wildfire," according to Dr. James Mason.
14. Note 6, pp. 305–308.

15. Discussion on causal association in case control studies. University of North Carolina Alumnae Meeting (March 1986), Chapel Hill, North Carolina.

16. Centers for Disease Control, *Morbidity and Mortality Weekly Report* 34, no. 48 (1985). Published in the *Journal of the American Medical Association* 254 (1985) and in *AIDS from the Beginning,* edited by Helene M. Cole and George D. Lundberg. Special edition, American Medical Association (1986), p. 34.

17. F. Barne-Sinoussi, J. C. Chermann, et al., "Isolation of a T-Lymphotropic Retrovirus from a Patient at Risk for Acquired Immune Deficiency Syndrome (AIDS)." *Science* 220 (1983): 868–871.

18. Robert C. Gallo, Syed Z. Salahuddin, Mikulas Popovic, et al., "Frequent Detection and Isolation of Cytopathic Retroviruses (HTLV-III) from Patients with AIDS." *Science* 224 (1984): 500–505.

19. Jay A. Levy, Anthony D. Hoffman, Susan Kramer, et al., "Isolation of Lymphocytopathic Retrovirus from San Francisco Patients with AIDS." *Science* 225 (1984): 840–842.

20. Note 12, section 1.

21. Interview with Dr. Robert C. Gallo, co-discoverer of the HIV virus. *Chicago Tribune,* December 10, 1987, section 1, p. 31.

22. American Medical Association, Board of Trustee Report SS, "AIDS Status Report: Update on Epidemiology" (1987), p. 163.

23. Note 7, p. 70.

24. Note 22, p. 164.

25. Note 22, p. 164.

26. Note 22, p. 165.

27. Centers for Disease Control, "Trends in HIV infection Among Civilian Applicants for Military Service. U.S. Oct. 1985–Dec. 1986," *Morbidity and Mortality Weekly Report* 36, no. 18 (May 15, 1987): 275.

28. Personal communication, Centers for Disease Control, Task Force on AIDS (September 1987).

29. Note 27, p. 276.

30. Note 22, p. 163.

31. Note 22, p. 164.

32. Mary E. Guinan, Ann Hardy, "Epidemiology of AIDS in Women in the United States, 1981 through 1986." *Journal of the American Medical Association* 257, no. 5 (April 17, 1987): 2039–2043.

33. Note 32, p. 2039.

34. Note 32, pp. 2040, 2041.

35. Centers for Disease Control, "Update: Acquired Immunodeficiency Syndrome," *Morbidity and Mortality Weekly Report* 36, no. 31: 522; and CDC *AIDS Weekly Surveillance Report — United States,* note 7.

36. Centers for Disease Control, *AIDS Weekly Surveillance Report — United States* (December 17, 1987).

37. "Agents for Active and Passive Immunity," chapter 67, 1125. Table 6, "Expected Hepatitis B Virus (HBV) Prevalence in Various Population Groups." *Drug Evaluations* (6th ed., September 1986, pp. 1124,1125). Prepared by the American Medical Association Department of Drugs and Technology in cooperation with the American Society for Clinical Pharmacology and Therapeutics, Chicago.

38. Note 37, p. 1124.

39. Note 7, p. 55.

40. Nathan Clumeck, Philippe Van De Perre, et al., "Heterosexual Promiscuity Amongst African Patients with AIDS." *New England Journal of Medicine* 313 (1985): 182.

41. Gerald H. Friedland, Robert S. Klein, "Transmission of the Human Immunodeficiency Virus." *New England Journal of Medicine* 317, no. 18 (October 29, 1987): 1124, 1125.

42. Centers for Disease Control, "Human Immunodeficiency Virus Infections in Health Care Workers Exposed to Blood of Infected Patients." *Morbidity and Mortality Weekly Report* 36, no. 16 (1987): 19.

43. Note 7, p. 63.

44. Note 42, p. 20.

45. Note 42, p. 20.

46. Note 42, p. 21.

47. Note 22, p. 164.

48. Janine M. Jason, J. Steven McDougal, Gloria Dixon, et al., "HTLV-III/LAV Antibody and Immune Status of Household Contacts and Sexual Partners of Persons with Haemophilia." *Journal of the American Medical Association* 255 (1986): 212–215.

49. M. Elaine Eyster, Mitchell H. Gail, James O. Ballard III, et al., "Natural History of Human Immunodeficiency Virus Infection in Haemophiliacs: Effects of T-cell Subsets, Platelet Counts, and Age." *Annals of Internal Medicine* 107 (1987): 1–6.

50. Margaret W. Hilgartner, "Aids and Hemophilia." *New England Journal of Medicine* 317, no. 18 (October 29, 1987): 1153, 1154. Also see note 35, p. 1125.

51. Nancy Padian, Linda Marquis, Donald P. Francis, et al., "Male to Female Transmission of Human Immunodeficiency Virus." *Journal of the American Medical Association* 258, no. 6 (August 17, 1987): 788.

52. David R. Bolling, "Prevalence, Goals and Complications of Heterosexual Intercourse in a Gynecologic Population." *Journal of Reproductive Medicine* 29 (1977): 120–124.

53. Bruce V. Voeller, "Heterosexual Anal Sex." *Mariposa Occasional Papers* 1B (1983): 1–8.

54. David R. Bolling, Bruce V. Voeller (letter to the editor), "AIDS and Heterosexual Anal Intercourse." *Journal of the American Medical Association* 258, no. 4 (July 24–31, 1987): 474.

55. Note 45, pp. 788–789; note 48, p. 474.

56. Robert R. Redfield, Paul D. Markham, Syed Z. Salahuddin, et al., "Heterosexually Acquired ARC and AIDS Epidemiologic Evidence for Female to Male Transmission." *Journal of the American Medical Association* 254 (1985): 2094–2096.

57. Note 21, p. 164.

58. Gwendolyn B. Scott, Margaret A. Fischl, Nancy G. Klimas, et al., "Mothers of Infants with AIDS: Evidence for Both Symptomatic and Asymptomatic Carriers." *Journal of the American Medical Association* 253 (1985): 363–366.

59. Robert W. Marion, Andrew A. Wiznia, Gordon Hutchinson, "Human T-cell Lymphotropic Virus Embryopathy: A New Dysmorphic Syndrome Associated with Intrauterine Infection." *American Journal of Diseases of Children* 140 (1986): 638.

60. Centers for Disease Control, "Recommendations for Assisting in the Prevention of Perinatal Transmission of Acquired Immune Deficiency Syndrome." *Morbidity and Mortality Weekly Report* 34 (1986b): 721–726, 731–732.

61. Note 34, p. 52.

62. Centers for Disease Control, *AIDS Weekly Surveillance Report — United States* (September 21, 1987).

63. Note 7, p. 46.

64. Note 7, pp. 221, 223, 225.

65. William W. Darrow (editorial), "A Framework for Preventing AIDS." *American Journal of Public Health* 77, no. 7 (1987): 778.

66. Note 7, p. 45.

67. Jay A. Levy, M.D., professor of medicine, University of California. "HIVs: Their Role in AIDS." Presentation at scientific seminar at the American Medical Association, December 14, 1987, Chicago.

68. Cited by Malcolm Rees, "Incubation Period for AIDS." *Nature* 330 (December 3, 1987): 428.

69. G. F. Medley, R. M. Anderson, et al., "Incubation Period of AIDS in Patients Infected Via Blood Transfusion." *Nature* 328, no. 20 (August 1987): 721.

70. Note 67; also note 7, p. 70.

71. Note 7, p. 162; also *Focus: A Guide to AIDS Research* 2, no. 5 (April 1987): 1–3.

72. Editor, "AIDS Epidemic: Neglected Issues." *Infectious Disease Alert* 6, no.19 (July 1987): 73–74.

73. Ibid., p. 73.

74. Note 68, p. 428.

75. Note 69, p. 721.

76. Richard Rothenburg, Mary Wodfel, Randi Stoneburner, et al., "Survival with the Acquired Immunodeficiency Syndrome." *New England Journal of Medicine* 317, no. 21 (November 19, 1987): 1297.

77. Note 7, p. 51.

78. Centers for Disease Control, "Tuberculosis and AIDS — Connecticut." *Morbidity and Mortality Weekly Report* 36, no. 9 (1987): 133–135.

79. Note 37, p. 1123.

80. American Medical Association, "Confidentiality." Section 5.05–5.09 in *Current Opinions of the Council on Ethical and Judicial Affairs of the American Medical Association* (1986), Chicago.

"*I'm really surprised I'm here. When I was originally diagnosed over two and a half years ago, my doctor told me I wouldn't be alive today, and he certainly didn't give me any indication that I would be able to live a more productive life, and my life has made a 180-degree turn since diagnosis. Before diagnosis I was an active alcoholic and drug addict and I've been clean for almost two years. And I'm real grateful for that chance.*"

The Acquired Immunodeficiency Syndrome in New England: An Epidemiological Review of the First Six Years

Laureen M. Kunches, R.N., M.P.H.
Jeanne M. Day, M.P.H.

Between 1981 and 1987—the six-year period following initial recognition of the acquired immunodeficiency syndrome (AIDS)—1,475 cases were reported among residents of the six New England states. Of nearly 40,000 cases nationwide, 3.8 percent occurred among New England residents, though the region's population represents 5.5 percent of the total United States population. The groups most affected include homosexual or bisexual men (65 percent) and intravenous drug users (20 percent). However, in the two southernmost states—Rhode Island and Connecticut—32 to 40 percent of all cases have used intravenous drugs. In these states, the male:female ratio of adult cases is 6:1, compared to 12:1 in the remainder of the region. In Massachusetts, the disease incidence rate is equivalent to that of Connecticut (144 cases per 1 million population); however, a greater proportion of cases (69 percent versus 45 percent) are homosexual and bisexual men, and the incidence rate for adult females is lower (49 versus 100 cases/million). Maine, New Hampshire, and Vermont have low cumulative incidence rates (<50 cases/million), and no cases among adult females or associated with blood transfusion. In northern New England, 2 percent of adults with AIDS became infected through heterosexual contact, compared to 10 percent in the southern half of the region. Sources of other data, resulting from serologic testing for human immunodeficiency virus (HIV), confirm the predominance of infection in southern New England. Rates of HIV seropositivity in military recruits, blood donors, and specific high-risk populations are uniformly lower in New England than in high-incidence regions.

This review is based on statistics provided by AIDS surveillance programs operated by the Departments of Public Health in the six New England states.

Surveillance for the acquired immunodeficiency syndrome (AIDS) has been under way in the six New England states since the original cases were described in the summer of 1981.[1] The Department of Public Health in each state requires that AIDS cases be reported according to a standard format developed by the Centers for Disease Control

Laureen M. Kunches is director of the AIDS Program at the Massachusetts Department of Public Health. She was formerly an epidemiologist with the Massachusetts AIDS Surveillance Program. Jeanne M. Day is an epidemiologist with the AIDS Program at the Massachusetts Department of Public Health.

(CDC) of the U.S. Public Health Service. From the beginning, special effort has been focused on this unusual illness to assure accurate and complete epidemiological information. Many states have supplemented their existing disease surveillance programs with additional staff members assigned specifically to AIDS case reporting. Validation studies, which have been performed to estimate the accuracy of current surveillance data, have confirmed that case reporting is 90 percent complete.[2]

AIDS, as defined for surveillance purposes, is characterized by a spectrum of rare opportunistic infections and malignancies that are typically life-threatening.[3] In the first four years of the epidemic, no specific laboratory test was available to identify the underlying cause of immunodeficiency which was common to all AIDS patients. Although the etiologic agent of AIDS was isolated in 1983 and 1984 by investigators in France and the United States,[4] the case definition for AIDS reporting did not begin to incorporate serologic evidence of human immunodeficiency virus (HIV) infection until 1985, following the licensure of antibody assays. Because of the high specificity of the indicator diseases included in the surveillance definition, positive HIV serology is not a requirement for most cases. At the present time, specific reporting of cases of AIDS-related complex (ARC) or positive HIV antibody test results is not required in any of the New England states; reporting of descriptive data without identifying information is encouraged in Maine, New Hampshire, and Rhode Island, but is optional.

There are five primary sources of information concerning the epidemiology of AIDS in New England. The direct measure of disease morbidity is derived from AIDS surveillance data. Results of testing for antibody to HIV can be interpreted in light of various types of sampling bias. Groups for which information is available include military recruit applicants; blood donors; persons concerned about possible HIV exposure who seek confidential or anonymous testing at state-operated sites; and study populations surveyed by researchers to ascertain HIV seroprevalence. Through analyzing the messages from each of these indicators, we will present a comprehensive view of the current regional trends in AIDS and HIV infection.

AIDS Surveillance Data

AIDS surveillance data have been the most consistently reliable measure of the scope and nature of this frightening new disease. They are the framework from which the modes of HIV transmission have been characterized, and the barometer of changing needs for health care resources. AIDS case reports, however, are limited in that they lag several years behind the original point of infection with HIV. An unusually long latency period, averaging between five and seven years, precedes the development of AIDS.[5] Trends in AIDS cases, therefore, reflect the events of high-risk behavior from years past. The high degree of specificity and accuracy found in reported AIDS cases provides a solid base of demographic and behavioral information from which to define the epidemic in New England.

Incidence Rates

The cumulative incidence of AIDS cases in New England (119/million residents) falls directly in the middle of the other eight U.S. regions (fig. 1: cumulative AIDS case rates per million population in nine regions of the United States). The burden of cases has been greatest in the Middle Atlantic and Pacific states, where (in the metropolitan areas of New York City, San Francisco, and Los Angeles) the original cases of AIDS were recognized.

Figure 1

Cumulative AIDS Case Rates per Million in Nine Regions of U.S.*

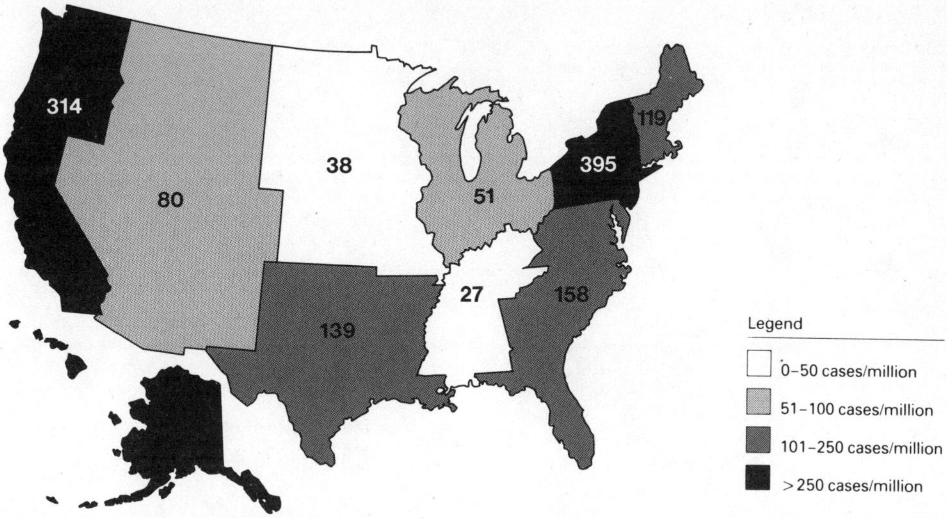

*Cumulative AIDS rates per million (1980 U.S. Census data) in New England and the Middle Atlantic, East North Central, West North Central, South Atlantic, East South Central, West South Central, Mountain, and Pacific regions. Includes 39,201 cases reported as of July 1987 from the fifty states and District of Columbia.

The six-year cumulative incidence rates in these two regions (395/million and 314/million, respectively) are approximately twice the national average (175/million), and three to four times the rate in New England.

High-incidence states like Florida and Texas (each accounting for 7 percent of the national case total) cause the cumulative rates in the South Atlantic and West South Central regions (158/million and 139/million, respectively) to exceed slightly the New England rate. Rates in the Mountain and Midwestern states range between 38 and 80 cases/million residents. The four states of the East South Central region (Kentucky, Tennessee, Alabama, and Mississippi) have reported only 400 cases, a six-year cumulative incidence rate of 27 per million.

Within the New England region, variations exist in state-specific cumulative incidence rates (fig. 2: cumulative AIDS case rates per million population in the six New England states). New Hampshire and Vermont have rates among the lowest in the nation; only four other states have reported fewer actual cases than Vermont. Rates in Rhode Island and Maine are below the national total, and these states hold ranks of thirty and forty, respectively, among the fifty states for total cases reported. Connecticut and Massachusetts are among the fifteen states reporting the most cases, and have equivalent cumulative incidence rates. Only five other states, however, have reported more pediatric cases than Massachusetts and Connecticut; fourteen children under age thirteen have developed AIDS in each of these states.

Temporal Trends

The epidemic curve in New England (fig. 3: epidemic curve of AIDS cases in New England, according to year of diagnosis) illustrates the steady slope of increasing cases over

Figure 2

Cumulative AIDS Case Rates in New England*

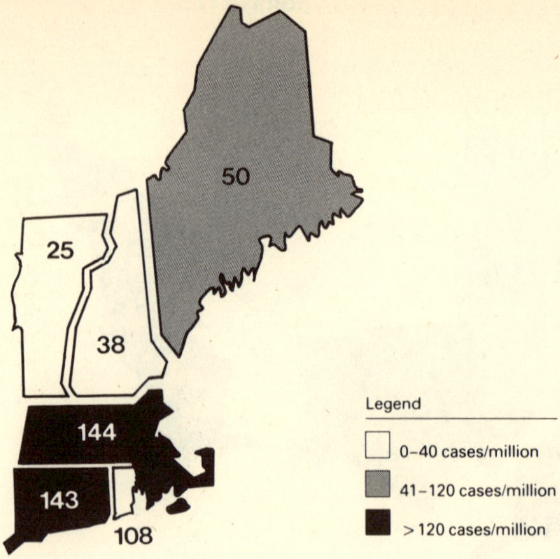

*Cumulative AIDS rates per million (1980 U.S. Census data). Includes 1,475 cases reported as of July 1987.

the period. When surveillance began in earnest in 1983, reports of 122 cases were documented for the region. Over the three subsequent years, new case reports increased by nearly 70 percent each year.

In Massachusetts, the rate of increase for new case reports has decelerated over time. The annual total for 1985 (191 cases) was 82 percent higher than the 1984 total (105 cases). During 1986, 287 additional cases were diagnosed, representing a 50 percent increase above the level of the prior year. A projection based on reports received during the first half of 1987 suggests continued slowing to a 33 percent increase over the 1986 level.

Between 1984 and 1985, Connecticut's total increased by half the margin observed in Massachusetts (41 percent). However, a 67 percent increase the following year heralded an acceleration of cases. The trend appears to have reversed in 1987, if the first six months' data are projected with allowance for delayed reports. No more than 200 total cases would be expected in 1987, representing a 10 to 20 percent increase over 1986.

Each year between 1983 and 1986, the annual case totals in Rhode Island and the three northern states combined (Vermont, New Hampshire, Maine) increased by factors of two to four. However, such small actual numbers produce unstable measures of proportional increase which are inexact and not appropriate to compare with the trends seen in Massachusetts and Connecticut. Analysis of national figures confirms the steady deceleration in the rate of new cases, although reports of new cases are not expected to reach a true plateau in the near future.[6]

Transmission Categories

After being originally described among a small number of homosexual men with unexplained immune deficiency, AIDS has continued to occur primarily among men exposed

Figure 3

Epidemic Curve of New England AIDS Cases*

(N = 1,475)

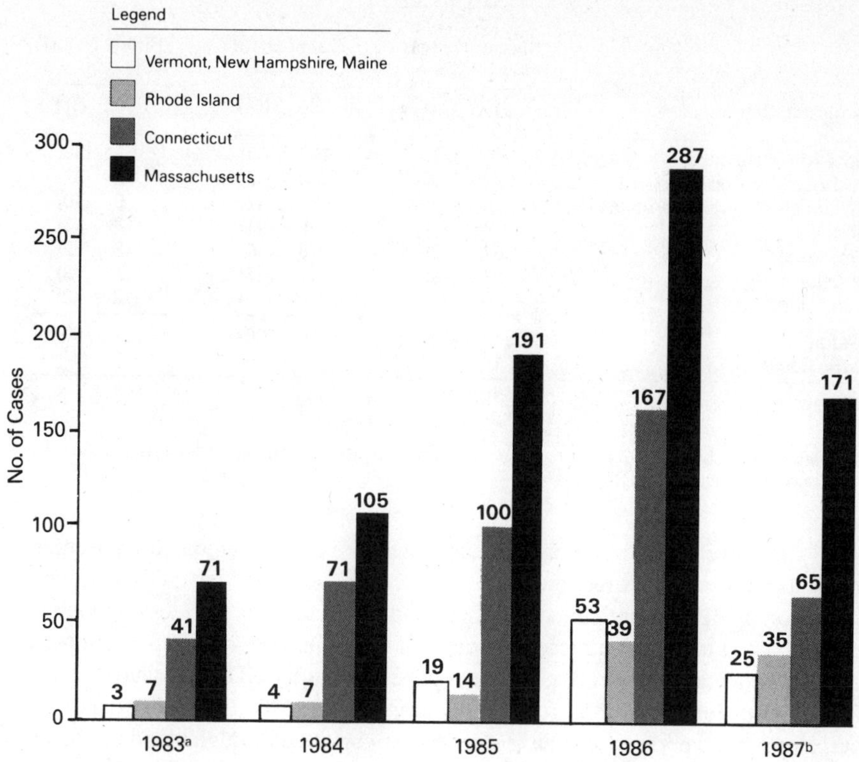

*CDC-reported AIDS cases in New England, according to year of diagnosis

[a]Includes cases diagnosed prior ro 1983.

[b]Includes cases reported as of July 1, 1987.

sexually to HIV through contact with other men. More than two-thirds of the nearly 40,000 U.S. cases reported during the first six years of the epidemic have been homosexual or bisexual men. New England AIDS cases are consistent with this trend, since 961 of the patients with AIDS (65 percent) reported homosexual contact with men, 68 of whom had the additional risk factor of prior intravenous drug use.

The relative significance of male homosexual transmission among cases reported from individual New England states is variable. For the three southern states (Massachusetts, Rhode Island, Connecticut), the male homosexual/bisexual category predominates, but accounts for fewer than half of adult cases in Connecticut, compared to nearly seven of ten cases in Massachusetts (table 1: comparison of transmission categories for southern New England AIDS cases reported as of July 1987). Rhode Island and Connecticut, perhaps because of their proximity to New York City, are more heavily affected by AIDS among intravenous drug users; this is thought to result from sharing of equipment used for injection. One-third of adults with AIDS in these states are heterosexuals who have used intravenous drugs. This heavier concentration has been persistent over the first six years but

Table 1

Comparison of Transmission Categories for Southern New England AIDS Cases Reported as of July 1987

Transmission Category	Massachusetts n = 825 No.	(%)	Connecticut n = 444 No.	(%)	Rhode Island n = 102 No.	(%)
Homosexual/bisexual	556	(69)	194	(45)	59	(58)
Intravenous (IV) drug user	107	(13)	143	(33)	33	(32)
Homosexual/bisexual IV drug user	34	(4)	31	(7)	0	(0)
Hemophilia	7	(1)	5	(1)	3	(3)
Heterosexual	64	(8)	25	(6)	2	(2)
Transfusion	23	(3)	12	(3)	3	(3)
Undetermined	20	(2)	20	(5)	2	(2)
Adult Total	811	(100)	430	(100)	102	(100)
Pediatric Cases	14		14		0	
Total Cases	825		444		102	

Source: Data provided by AIDS surveillance programs operated by the Department of Public Health in Massachusetts, Connecticut, and Rhode Island.

is expected to resolve in the future, as the accelerated rate of cases among drug users in Massachusetts moves in the direction of the Connecticut and Rhode Island experience.

Transmission of HIV through infected blood-clotting-factor concentrates (hemophilia products) and blood transfusions accounts for 53 of the adult cases of AIDS in southern New England (4 percent). Five (18 percent) of the 28 pediatric AIDS cases have been hemophiliacs or patients infected through blood transfusion. Although additional cases are anticipated among persons who have already been infected through blood products, future spread of HIV has been virtually eliminated by donor deferral and serologic screening and by inactivation steps routinely applied in product manufacturing.

In Massachusetts, the proportion of cases attributed to heterosexual transmission (8 percent) exceeds rates in neighboring states (2 to 6 percent) as well as the national average (4 percent). Such cases have occurred primarily (43 of 64 heterosexual cases) among patients who have recently entered the United States from Caribbean and central African countries, where HIV is transmitted most often heterosexually. In Zaire, Rwanda, Burundi, and Haiti, for example, AIDS cases occur with equal frequency in men and women, and rates of HIV infection are 10 to 100 times higher than in comparable age groups in the United States.[7]

Grouped together with these foreign-born heterosexual cases are patients who have had partners with high-risk behavior. The majority have had heterosexual contact with intravenous drug users, accounting for 18 cases (2 percent of adult cases) in Massachusetts and 17 (4 percent) in Connecticut. A small number of women partners of bisexual men and hemophiliacs have also developed AIDS in southern New England.

The pediatric cases are concentrated in the states of Connecticut and Massachusetts, and are primarily associated with perinatal infection due to parental drug use. Of the 28 children with AIDS in southern New England, 82 percent have parents with AIDS or with histories of high-risk drug-using or sexual behaviors; 7 percent have hemophilia; and 11 percent became infected by blood transfusion. Twenty children died of AIDS during the six-year period.

The transmission category is unknown in 2 to 5 percent of cases from these three states, a rate comparable to the national experience. Most patients listed as undetermined risk were deceased before a history of high-risk behavior could be ascertained. In a few cases, patients who have been interviewed deny homosexual contact or drug use; these patients typically report multiple heterosexual partners (including prostitute contact) and prior history of sexually transmitted diseases. Failure to clearly identify an infected partner will become more common in the future if HIV infiltrates the heterosexual population to a greater degree. Cases whose transmission category is listed as undetermined are not thought to represent new or unappreciated modes of HIV transmission; a low level of missing information is to be expected, in view of the sensitive nature of sexual and illegal drug use behavior.

In northern New England, cases have been heavily concentrated among homosexual and bisexual men (table 2: comparison of transmission categories for northern New England AIDS cases reported as of July 1987). In the tri-state area, 86 percent of the adult cases occurred among homosexual men, three of whom also used intravenous drugs. Heterosexual intravenous drug users represent 7 percent of the cases, while 2 percent of the cases are attributed to heterosexual transmission. Five persons with hemophilia have developed AIDS (5 percent); however, no transfusion-associated cases were reported in this part of the region during the period. The risk of HIV infection among hemophiliacs is consistent from region to region, because of widespread distribution of products.[8] Transfusion-associated risk, on the other hand, is related to local blood donor characteristics, and appears to vary according to the prevalence of HIV in high-risk populations and the corresponding incidence of AIDS.

Demographic Characteristics

The distribution of AIDS cases according to age illustrates the general similarities among the New England states and is comparable to the national trend (table 3: New England AIDS cases according to age, sex, and racial/ethnic characteristics). Cases occur most frequently during the third decade of life; typically, two out of three patients are between twenty and forty years old. This unusual concentration of a fatal illness in young adults at the height of their productivity further complicates the economic and social impact of AIDS.

Very few cases thus far (four in New England) have occurred among adolescents. These are most often among children with hemophilia. Given the delay between the point of HIV infection and the diagnosis of AIDS, some of the cases in the twenty- to twenty-nine-year-old age group may have been acquired through contact during adolescence.

The male:female ratio of AIDS cases nationwide is 12:1 for adults and 1:1 for children less than thirteen years old. In states where intravenous drug use accounts for one-third or more of cases, the adult male:female ratio becomes more balanced. In the two southern New England states where this is true (Connecticut and Rhode Island), male cases predominate but outnumber female cases only by a ratio of 6:1. In the three northern New England states, no AIDS cases were reported among adult women; the single female case was a child residing in New Hampshire.

The overrepresentation of racial minorities among AIDS cases in the United States is now well documented.[9] In southern New England, this appears to be true as well and may be linked to a higher incidence of intravenous drug use among urban minority populations. In Connecticut, for example, blacks account for 7 percent of the state's 3.1 million residents and 33 percent of the AIDS cases. Similarly, 16 percent of AIDS cases are Hisern New England states have low numbers of racial and ethnic minority residents, making estimates of disease distribution difficult.

In Massachusetts, age-adjusted incidence data indicate that the risk of AIDS for black men (age fifteen to forty-nine) is five times greater than for white men; Hispanic men in this age group have a fourfold excess risk compared to their white counterparts. For women, the trend is even more striking, with blacks having AIDS cases of 320/million and Hispanics of 101/million, fifteen and five times higher, respectively, than white women of the same age category.

The most common primary diagnosis among New England AIDS cases is *Pneumocystis carinii* pneumonia, reported in two-thirds of the patients. This is consistent with the national experience. Kaposi's sarcoma was reported in 20 percent of the New England cases for which data are available. Over the years, there has been a decrease in the proportion of cases with Kaposi's sarcoma which cannot be explained by a decrease in the proportion of new cases in the homosexual category. (Nearly all cases of Kaposi's sarcoma have occurred in homosexual or bisexual men with AIDS.) Epidemiologists have hypothesized that reduction of certain implicated cofactor effects, such as inhalant nitrites or other unspecified transmissible agents, may be contributing to the decline in Kaposi's sarcoma diagnoses in AIDS cases.[10] Alternatively, changes in reporting habits or other types of ascertainment bias may explain this trend; attempts to evaluate such artifactual effects have been unsuccessful.

Opportunistic infections other than *P. carinii* pneumonia have been reported in 44 percent of the cases. The most common of these infections, on the basis of Massachusetts AIDS Surveillance Program data, are esophageal candidiasis (6 percent), cytomegalovirus or cryptococcal infections (4 percent), and atypical mycobacterial infection (3 percent).

Table 2

Comparison of Transmission Categories for Northern New England AIDS Cases Reported as of July 1987

	Maine n = 56		New Hampshire n = 35		Vermont n = 13	
Transmission Category	No.	(%)	No.	(%)	No.	(%)
Homosexual/bisexual	50	(91)	26	(79)	8	(62)
Intravenous (IV) drug user	2	(4)	2	(6)	3	(23)
Homosexual/bisexual IV drug user	0	(0)	2	(6)	1	(8)
Hemophilia	3	(5)	1	(3)	1	(8)
Heterosexual	0	(0)	2	(6)	0	(0)
Transfusion	0	(0)	0	(0)	0	(0)
Undetermined	0	(0)	0	(0)	0	(0)
Adult Total	55	(100)	33	(100)	13	(100)
Pediatric Cases	1		2		0	
Total Cases	56		35		13	

Source: Data provided by AIDS surveillance programs operated by the Department of Public Health in Maine, New Hampshire, and Vermont.

Mortality Data

During the six-year period, nearly 800 AIDS deaths were documented by the New England surveillance programs. At any point in time, approximately half of all reported AIDS cases are known to have died. Nationwide in 1986, one in 27,000 deaths was due to AIDS. The high case-fatality rate and the relative youth of those affected by AIDS dramatically reduces life expectancy in certain population groups, especially in high-incidence cities. Review of national statistics on premature mortality, commonly measured in "years of potential life lost" (YPLL) before age sixty-five, indicates that 2.1 percent of YPLL in 1986 was attributable to AIDS. Although causes of YPLL usually decrease or increase slightly from year to year, AIDS moved up from the thirteenth (in 1984) to eighth (in 1986) overall, and ranks sixth for men between the ages of twenty-five and forty-four.[11] For men in this age group residing in San Francisco or Manhattan, AIDS has become the leading cause of premature mortality, accounting for more YPLL than accidents, homicides, suicides, and cancer combined.[12]

As further progress is made toward effective antiviral therapy, there is optimism that survival can be substantially prolonged. A recent New York study[13] demonstrated evidence of improvement already, particularly for patients with *P. carinii* pneumonia; in 1981, only 18 percent survived for one year after diagnosis, compared to 49 percent of cases diagnosed in 1985. The median survival period for all cases reported from New York during these five years was eleven months, with significant variability according to primary disease and demographic characteristics. For example, white men with Kaposi's sarcoma alone had twenty-seven months median survival, while black women with *P. carinii* pneumonia survived only seven months. Eleven percent of patients died at the time of diagnosis of AIDS.

Table 3

New England AIDS Cases According to Age, Sex, and Racial/Ethnic Characteristics

	Massachusetts		Rhode Island		Connecticut		New Hampshire		Vermont		Maine	
Age (years)	No.	(%)	No.	(%)	No.	(%)	No.	(%)	No.	(%)	No.	(%)
< 13	14	(2)	1	(1)	14	(3)	2	(6)	0	(0)	1	(2)
13–19	3	(0)	0	(0)	0	(0)	0	(0)	0	(0)	1	(2)
20–29	175	(21)	20	(20)	106	(24)	8	(23)	3	(23)	18	(32)
30–39	405	(49)	50	(49)	186	(42)	20	(57)	4	(31)	26	(46)
40–49	158	(19)	25	(24)	81	(18)	3	(9)	3	(23)	8	(14)
> 49	70	(8)	6	(6)	57	(13)	2	(6)	3	(23)	2	(4)
Sex												
Male	758	(92)	88	(86)	372	(84)	34	(97)	13	(100)	56	(100)
Female	67	(8)	14	(14)	72	(16)	1	(3)	0	(0)	0	(0)
Racial/Ethnic Group												
White	602	(73)	84	(82)	224	(50)			13	(100)	48	(86)
Black	155	(19)	14	(14)	149	(33)	NA*		0	(0)	2	(4)
Hispanic	63	(8)	4	(4)	69	(16)			0	(0)	1	(2)
Unknown	5	(0)	0	(0)	2	(1)			0	(0)	5	(9)

*Data not available

Source: Data provided by AIDS surveillance programs operated by the Department of Public Health in the six New England states.

Death certificate review is a commonly used method of case ascertainment, and can provide a validation tool to assess the completeness of case reporting. In Boston, a death record review of more than 2,100 certificates issued during a three-month period identified twenty deaths (1 percent of the period total) in reported AIDS cases. Three additional cases that had not been reported were identified through follow-up of deaths in young men and women which were caused by unspecified pneumonia or lymphoma. AIDS-related causes of death listed by the certifying physician, such as *P. carinii* pneumonia and Kaposi's sarcoma, were highly (80 to 100 percent) predictive of AIDS.

Projections from AIDS Cases

Using mathematical modeling, epidemiologists from the Centers for Disease Control have estimated that by 1991, 270,000 cases of AIDS will have occurred in the United States. If New England trends follow the first six years' experience, approximately 10,000 of the cases will be residents of the region. It is likely that more than 4,000 New Englanders will have died of AIDS in the ten years since the disease was recognized, and that 6,000 others will be living with AIDS and requiring specialized medical and support services.

Up to 60,000 others may have minor clinical symptoms associated with HIV infection and varying degrees of immunodeficiency, commonly referred to as ARC (AIDS-related complex). Without systematic information on the proportional relationship between AIDS cases and numbers of patients with ARC, generally accepted estimates range from 1:5 to 1:10. It is even more difficult to estimate the number of persons who are currently infected with HIV and asymptomatic. Projections for the nation, based to denominator approximations for high-prevalence population groups, suggest that between 1 million and 1.5 million Americans are already infected. If AIDS case distribution mirrors the geographic pattern of HIV in general, 35,000 to 56,000 New Englanders have been infected with HIV thus far, representing a ratio of 25 to 35 infected persons for each reported AIDS case.

Further refinement of this estimate can be achieved by focusing on the age groups likely to be infected. For adults age 20 to 39, representing 70 percent of AIDS cases, infected individuals without symptoms probably outnumber AIDS cases by a factor of fifty to one. This proportion is consistent with other population-based sources of data such as newborn screening, as well as the projected AIDS incidence data for the next five years. Using the 50:1 estimate, approximations of the number of 20- to 39-year-old adults in New England currently infected are 1 in 500 for Vermont; 1 in 156 for Maine; 1 in 215 for New Hampshire; 1 in 83 for Rhode Island; and 1 in 65 for Connecticut and Massachusetts. The likelihood of infection for males in this age group is generally twice as high as the above figures, which combine males and females. Using precise age and sex data for AIDS cases in Massachusetts and Connecticut, approximately 1 in 35 men in this age group may be infected currently. For women, rates of 1 in 200 and 1 in 400 are estimated for Connecticut and Massachusetts, respectively.

Military Recruit Applicant HIV Testing Data

The U.S. Department of Defense adopted a policy in October 1985 which required all applicants for military service to have serologic testing for HIV infection. The rationale for this policy included concern about (1) possible adverse reactions when routine immunizations (including live virus vaccines) are administered to recruits; (2) emergency blood donation requirements during battle; and (3) physical handicap or impairment of military forces. Any seropositive applicant is referred to civilian medical consultants and counselors, and is rejected from military service.

Tests of 1.1 million men and women applying to the military during the first twenty-one months of the screening program have provided valuable statistical data for HIV surveillance purposes. Since recruiting officials inform applicants that drug use and homosexual activity are grounds for exclusion from entry into military service, volunteers tested for HIV underrepresent the major HIV-infected populations (including hemophiliacs, deferred for medical considerations). The crude overall prevalence rate of 0.15 percent has remained stable during this period, with no statistically significant upward or downward trend.[14] The rate among military recruit applicants in the New England region (0.08 percent) is among the lowest in the country. In the Middle Atlantic and Pacific regions, where AIDS incidence rates are highest, the prevalence of HIV infection among military recruit applicants is two to four times higher than in New England.[15]

The prevalence of infection varies considerably from state to state and according to age, sex, and racial characteristics (table 4: comparison of military recruit applicant HIV test results in New England residents by state, according to sex and racial/ethnic characteristics). The data are consistent with AIDS incidence rates — lowest in northern New England, where only one recruit in the tri-state area was found to be seropositive. The nearly identical rates of seropositivity observed in residents of Connecticut (0.14 percent) and Massachusetts (0.12 percent) further substantiates the validity of the cumulative AIDS cases rates (144/million population for each).

The excess burden of AIDS cases among ethnic and racial minorities is reflected in military recruit data as well. Overall rates of HIV seropositivity for blacks are seven to ten times higher than for whites in the volunteers tested from Connecticut and Massachusetts. Data for other racial groups (including Hispanics, native Americans, and Asian/Pacific Islanders) come from small samples that prevent meaningful estimates of infection prevalence.

Table 4

Comparison of Military Recruit Applicant HIV Test Results in New England Residents by State, According to Sex and Racial/Ethnic Characteristics, October 1985–June 1987

Number Tested (% Seropositive) by Subgroup

	Males		Females		Black		White		Other		Total Number Seropositive	
	No.	(%)	No.	(%)	No.	(%)	No.	(%)	No.	(%)	No.	(%)
Connecticut	8,941	(.15)	1,389	(.07)	1,553	(.52)	8,200	(.05)	577	(.34)	14	(.14)
Massachusetts	16,426	(.12)	2,350	(.13)	1,536	(.52)	16,753	(.07)	487	(.41)	22	(.12)
Maine	5,515	(.00)	931	(.00)	24	(.00)	6,371	(.00)	51	(.00)	0	
New Hampshire	3,669	(.03)	587	(.00)	31	(.00)	4,190	(.02)	35	(.00)	1	(.02)
Rhode Island	3,008	(.07)	443	(.00)	214	(.47)	3,134	(.03)	103	(.00)	2	(.06)
Vermont	2,279	(.00)	370	(.00)	17	(.00)	2,620	(.00)	12	(.00)	0	
New England	39,838	(.09)	6,070	(.07)	3,375	(.50)	41,268	(.04)	1,265	(.32)	39	(.08)
United States	953,166	(.16)	151,927	(.07)	205,130	(.41)	814,316	(.08)	85,647	(.22)	1,641	(.15)

Source: Data provided by AIDS surveillance programs operated by the Department of Public Health in the six New England states.

Combined seropositivity rates for military recruit applicants in the New England region are higher for men (0.09 percent) than for women (0.07 percent). In Massachusetts, however, the prevalence of infection is uniform for male and female recruit applicants. Nationwide, the disparity between rates for men and women is more pronounced (0.16 percent vs. 0.07 percent) than in the New England region. Higher rates of seropositivity have consistently been seen among military recruit applicants age twenty-five and over, compared to those of younger ages.

Blood Donor HIV Screening

In April 1985, the first laboratory test kits for HIV antibody testing were licensed by the federal Food and Drug Administration. Since that time, more than 25 million donations of blood and plasma have been screened for HIV, in a critical step toward assuring safety of the blood supply. The nationwide trend indicates a decline in the rate of HIV seropositivity in blood donors, from 0.035 percent in 1985 to less than 0.015 percent in 1987.[16]

Data from blood donor screening have been viewed as a crude measure of the degree to which HIV is present in the so-called "general population." Since homosexual men, intravenous drug users, hemophiliacs, and their sexual partners are actively deferred from donating blood, the prevalence of HIV infection in the highly selected blood-donor population should be exceedingly low. The overall decline in the national rates of seropositivity over time is primarily the result of eliminating previously identified seropositive persons from the donor pool.

The most unbiased estimate of HIV prevalence in the segment of the population that donates blood is obtained from data on first-time donors; the cumulative statistics indicate a 0.043 percent seropositivity rate in this group. In 80 to 90 percent of donors who test positive for HIV antibody, recognized risk factors can be determined when follow-up interviews are performed.[17]

The general geographic correlation between AIDS case rates and HIV prevalence is illustrated in blood donor screening data as well. Combined data from New York (0.04 percent seropositive) and California (0.026 percent seropositive) document rates that exceed the Central and Mountain states by factors of 10 to 20. In New England, data combined for the four northern states (Massachusetts, Maine, New Hampshire, and Vermont) indicate 0.011 percent seropositivity, compared to a lower rate in Rhode Island and Connecticut (0.004 percent).[18]

Voluntary HIV Testing of Individuals with Perceived Risk

Alternative testing sites for HIV antibody testing were created to provide free and anonymous HIV antibody testing and counseling and to discourage high-risk individuals from donating blood as a way of learning their antibody status. All of the New England states have established counseling and testing sites that provide confidential or anonymous HIV antibody testing. As of June 1987, cumulative seroprevalence rates for more than three thousand persons seeking testing in the New England area have ranged from 1.8 to 6.7 percent. Overall, 2 to 3 percent of the clients tested in northern New England (Maine, New Hampshire, Vermont) were seropositive, compared with 6 to 7 percent of seropositive clients who were tested in southern New England (Massachusetts, Connecticut, Rhode Island).

In states where clients are asked to self-report their risk-group status, the seroprevalence of HIV remains highest in those risk groups — specifically, homosexual or bisexual men and intravenous drug users — which also account for the majority of AIDS cases. Eleven percent of homosexual or bisexual men are seropositive in New Hampshire, Massachusetts, and Rhode Island, while 13 percent of those tested in Connecticut are seropositive. The seroprevalence among intravenous drug users varies somewhat geographically — 21 percent of intravenous drug users in Connecticut are seropositive; 13 percent in Massachusetts; 11 percent in Rhode Island; and 3 percent in New Hampshire. Heterosexual HIV-antibody test clients who perceive themselves at risk for HIV infection have considerably lower seropositivity rates; in both Massachusetts and New Hampshire, 1.4 percent of self-identified heterosexual clients were seropositive.

Other Seroprevalence Surveys

The most meaningful measures of HIV prevalence have been drawn from studies that select a population sample according to a predetermined method that does not rely on an individual subject to volunteer for testing. Bias that is introduced when testing is voluntary can be difficult to evaluate and control. On the other hand, population-based sampling for HIV seroprevalence studies must include rigorous protocols for protection of personal identifying information, in order to assure that test results cannot be linked to individuals. To this end, samples are often batched together according to schemes that prohibit precise analysis of demographic and risk factor data. Although a ''family of seroprevalence surveys'' will be initiated nationwide sometime in 1988, preliminary information is available from New England, thanks to an innovative strategy initiated here in 1986.

Investigators at the Massachusetts Department of Public Health have developed a novel method of measuring HIV seroprevalence among childbearing women.[19] Using a filter-paper-absorbed sample of blood collected routinely on all newborn infants for metabolic screening, a mini-blot method of HIV serologic testing provides a measure of the mother's infection status. To assure absolute anonymity, specimens are batched according to characteristics of the hospital where the delivery occurred, and all identifiers are removed from the sample. By extension, the results of this survey have provided data on the true prevalence of HIV in the U.S. general population.

The overall rate of seropositivity for childbearing women in Massachusetts was estimated at 2.3 per thousand, or approximately 180 of the nearly 80,000 women who give birth each year. Half of the newborns whose mothers are infected will become infected themselves, with high probability of developing AIDS-related diseases. Within the state, seropositivity appears concentrated in inner-city hospitals serving the highest-risk women. In these areas, infection rates from the preliminary data were 7.5/1,000, although subsequent studies indicate that the rate is now 18/1,000.[20] Rates among women delivering in suburban and rural hospitals were only 1.4/1,000.

Preliminary estimates from the Centers for Disease Control indicating that nationwide seroprevalence of HIV approximates 1.9/1,000 are consistent with this population-based study, especially because other trends within Massachusetts closely reflect the combined U.S. experience. In the spring of 1988, thirty sites nationwide will embark on HIV seroprevalence studies, including long-term observation of newborn screening data as a barometer of future heterosexual spread of AIDS.

Summary

Nearly fifteen hundred AIDS cases occurring in New England during the first six years of a worldwide epidemic provide a basis for determining local resource needs and prevention strategies. The northern states of the region, having been relatively spared the severe disease burden thus far, appear to have a window of opportunity to initiate targeted intervention strategies. With low rates of seropositivity, approaches such as notification of partners of HIV-infected individuals are more feasible and potentially more effective than in other areas. Major emphasis can be placed on educating the public about sexual risk reduction and targeting patients seen in sexually transmitted disease clinics, since intravenous drug use is associated with very few of the northern New England cases.

The southern part of the region faces greater challenges to develop programs that deal with the complex interaction of HIV infection and drug use, particularly among urban minority populations. Each week that passes, four more infants are born in southern New England who are likely to develop AIDS before their second birthday. The mothers and fathers of these children face odds of developing AIDS that increase by 5 to 10 percent each year. Nearly one in four sexually active homosexual men in the urban centers has been infected already, and perhaps six thousand of them will advance to life-threatening illness by 1991. The human and economic toll of the crisis will surpass any problem of modern times.

Although New England has been only moderately affected by the AIDS epidemic compared to other areas of the United States, the task ahead is clear and ominous. With continued attention to disease trends and systematic research to monitor future spread of HIV, a reliable forecast of the region's needs and challenges can be made.

The authors gratefully acknowledge the assistance and cooperation of AIDS surveillance epidemiologists throughout New England: Julia Miller (Connecticut); David Akers (Maine); Beverly Heinze-Lacey and George Seage (Massachusetts); Joyce Cournoyer and Susan Keady (New Hampshire); Louis Dondero (Rhode Island); and Deborah Kutsko (Vermont). For the technical assistance they provided, we also thank Tim Broadbent, Mary Ann Bucci, and Heidi Hunt of the Massachusetts Department of Public Health AIDS Program.

Notes

1. Centers for Disease Control. Pneumocystis pneumonia — Los Angeles. *Morbidity and Mortality Weekly Report* 1981; 30:250–252.
2. A. M. Hardy, E. T. Starcher, W. M. Morgan, et al. Review of death certificates to assess completeness of AIDS case reporting. *Public Health Reports* 1987; 102:386–391.
3. Centers for Disease Control. Appendix A: Revision of the CDC surveillance case definition for Acquired Immunodeficiency Syndrome. *Morbidity and Mortality Weekly Report* Supplement, 14 August 1987; 36 (1S).
4. F. Barre-Sinoussi, J. C. Chermann, F. Rey, et al. Isolation of a T-lymphotropic retrovirus from a patient at risk for AIDS. *Science* 1983; 220:868–871; and R. C. Gallo, S. Z. Salahuddin, M. Popovic, et al. Frequent detection and isolation of cytopathic retroviruses (HTLV-III) from patients with AIDS and at risk for AIDS. *Science* 1984; 224:500–503.
5. G. F. Medly, R. M. Anderson, D. R. Cox, et al. Incubation period of AIDS in patients infected via blood transfusion. *Nature* 1987; 328:719.

6. Centers for Disease Control. Update: Acquired Immunodeficiency Syndrome — United States. *Morbidity and Mortality Weekly Report* 1987; 36:522–526.

7. T. C. Quinn, J. M. Mann, J. W. Curran, et al. AIDS in Africa: An epidemiologic paradigm. *Science* 1986; 234:955–963.

8. J. W. Curran, H. W. Jaffe, A. M. Hardy, et al. Epidemiology of HIV Infection and AIDS in the United States. *Science* 1988; 239:610–616.

9. Centers for Disease Control. Acquired Immunodeficiency Syndrome (AIDS) among blacks and Hispanics — United States. *Morbidity and Mortality Weekly Report* 1986; 35:655–666.

10. Centers for Disease Control. Update: Acquired Immunodeficiency Syndrome — United States. *Morbidity and Mortality Weekly Report* 1986; 35:17–21.

11. Curran, Jaffe, Hardy, et al. (note 8).

12. J. W. Curran, W. M. Morgan, A. M. Hardy, et al. The epidemiology of AIDS: Current status and future prospects. *Science* 1985; 229:1352–1357.

13. R. Rothenberg, M. Woelfel, R. Stoneburner, et al. Survival with the acquired immunodeficiency syndrome: Experience with 5833 cases in New York City. *New England Journal of Medicine* 1987; 317:1297–1302.

14. Centers for Disease Control. Trends in human immunodeficiency virus infection among civilian applicants for military service — United States, October 1986–December 1986. *Morbidity and Mortality Weekly Report* 1987; 36:273–276.

15. Centers for Disease Control. Human T-lymphotropic virus type III/lymphadenopathy-associated virus antibody prevalence in U.S. military recruit applicants. *Morbidity and Mortality Weekly Report* 1986; 35:421–424.

16. Curran, Jaffe, Hardy, et al. (note 8).

17. Centers for Disease Control. Human immunodeficiency virus infection in the United States: A review of current knowledge.

18. Centers for Disease Control (note 17).

19. R. Hoff, V. P. Berardi, B. J. Weiblen, et al. Seroprevalence of human immunodeficiency virus among childbearing women: Estimation by testing samples of blood from newborns. *New England Journal of Medicine* 1988; 318:525–529.

20. Personal communication to the authors from Donald E. Craven, M.D., City of Boston Department of Health and Hospitals.

CSF. Cerebrospinal fluid is the fluid covering the brain and spinal cord. Obtained by a lumbar puncture, this fluid may contain inflammatory cells or antibodies, or both, when there is infection in the brain.

Dysphoria. This is a negative mood such as anxiety or depression.

Endothelial and glial cells. These are nonneuronal cells found in the brain. Endothelial cells are found throughout the body; glial cells are restricted to the central nervous system.

Factor VIII. This factor is a protein that is required for the clotting of blood. People with hemophilia lack this factor and must continually take it to prevent bleeding.

Intracellular/extracellular. Viruses replicate only within cells. If the virus, or a portion thereof, remains within the cell, it is said to be intracellular. If it is liberated from the cell, generally with the death of the cell, it becomes extracellular and can be detected in various body fluids.

Monocyte. This is a cell that circulates in the blood. It may lodge in tissues and at sites of inflammation; in these loci, these cells are called macrophages.

Multinucleated, syncytial giant cells. These are large cells that have two or more nuclei. They form when cells fuse. Certain viruses, such as HIV, cause cells to fuse.

Neuromodulators. These are small proteins that are synthesized in cells of the nervous system and peripheral nerves. They are also known as neuromediator and neurotransmitter substances. They are important in transferring "information" from one nerve to another, and for movements of muscle. They also may have general, metabolic effects, and, recently, several have been found to affect the immune system.

Glossary continued on page 108

The HIV Seropositive State and Progression to AIDS: An Overview of Factors Promoting Progression

Paul H. Black, M.D.
Elinor M. Levy, Ph.D.

We have considered factors that predispose to infection by the human immunodeficiency virus as well as the clinical consequences of infection. We have also reviewed what is known about the virological status of the asymptomatic carrier, particularly the female, and the fact that pregnancy may be a cofactor for progression of HIV disease in seropositive women. Additionally, we have discussed several other cofactors that may promote the progression of HIV infection. These include intercurrent infection, excessive use of recreational drugs and alcohol, malnutrition, and stress. With respect to stress, we have reviewed evidence indicating that certain personality factors, by buffering the effects of stress, may play a role in determining the outcome of HIV disease. Possible neuromodulators that may mediate the effect(s) of stress on the immune system are considered. Also discussed is the potentially complicating role of HIV infection of the brain of asymptomatic carriers on psychosocial studies, as well as the possible dysregulation of neuromodulator levels which might result from such infection. The possibility that HIV infection of the brain may act to enhance progression of HIV infection is proposed.

One of the major issues concerning AIDS is knowledge of the virological state and infectivity of the person who has seroconverted to HIV and remains healthy — the so-called asymptomatic carrier. Equally important is the subject of cofactors — those factors which may enhance or promote the asymptomatic carrier's progression to AIDS. In this article, we shall present an overview of these topics and some implications for seropositive women who become pregnant.

Infection by the Human Immunodeficiency Virus

Upon exposure to HIV, the virus that causes AIDS, a person may develop an acute infectious mononucleosis-like syndrome with or without meningitis. Generally, these infections subside, an immune response occurs in relationship to the disease, and the patient

Dr. Paul H. Black is professor of microbiology and chairman of the Department of Microbiology at the Boston University School of Medicine. Dr. Elinor M. Levy is associate professor of microbiology at the Boston University School of Medicine.

becomes seropositive (Group I, see table 1).[1] Other people who are exposed to the virus may not develop signs or symptoms of illness, and seroconversion may take weeks to months to occur (Group II, table 1). Little is known about the factors that determine whether an acute infectious disease occurs or whether a person seroconverts asymptomatically. Moreover, relatively little is known regarding the extent of exposure necessary for seroconversion.[2] In some studies, 50 to 60 percent of male homosexual partners of infected persons become infected, as judged by antibody testing;[3] approximately the same figure applies to male-to-female transmission from HIV-infected intravenous drug users or male bisexuals.[4] Female-to-male transmission appears to be much lower, probably owing to the lower infectivity by this route.[5] Other studies reveal that four out of eight women who were artificially inseminated from an infected donor seroconverted,[6] and 50 percent of hemophiliac patients who received a contaminated Factor VIII preparation seroconverted.[7] Thus it is likely that about half of the people exposed to infectious individuals and materials will seroconvert. Factors such as the amount of virus in the infectious fluid, route of infection, or host factors, or a combination of these, must certainly be operative in determining whether seroconversion occurs after exposure to HIV.

Once an individual is infected with HIV and seroconverts, he or she is potentially infectious for the rest of his or her life. We know that the genetic material of the virus (RNA) is able to make DNA and that this DNA becomes associated with the cell's genes. This integrated proviral DNA becomes a cellular gene and, as long as the cell lives, will be a permanent part of its genetic endowment. Approximately 70 to 80 percent of asymptomatic, seropositive carriers, in whom the infectious virus cannot be found, will have the latent viral genes activated from their blood cells by various cocultivation and activation techniques. This finding indicates that most asymptomatic carriers have the capacity to synthesize the infectious virus but that it is still present in most cells in a latent state. Little is known as to the actual levels of infectious virus produced by asymptomatic carriers; however, most evidence suggests that only small amounts of infectious virus are present. Despite this, a large amount of evidence indicates that a seropositive person, symptomatic or asymptomatic, is infectious and can transmit the virus.[8]

Asymptomatic individuals can transmit the virus by means of genital secretions or blood or through transmission to the fetus. The virus is certainly in the blood cells in a latent state. Data are very sparse as to whether the virus in the genital secretions, for example, the ejaculate of males and the cervical secretions of women, is contained within cells or is free in bodily fluids in the asymptomatic individual. Some evidence indicates that the virus resides intracellularly in a latent state in cervical secretions.[9] Transmission to the fetus by the asymptomatic carrier presumably occurs through the blood, although in certain unusual circumstances newborns appear to have become infected through nursing.[10]

Asymptomatic Female Carrier

Although the virus has been recovered from the cervical secretions of asymptomatic female carriers by means of cocultivation techniques throughout the menstrual cycle, little is known about the relative levels of virus in the cervical secretions of women during various phases of the menstrual cycle or during pregnancy.[11, 12] Retroviruses in mice can be activated by certain female sex steroids.[13] This discovery raises a question as to whether female sex hormones activate virus replication in cells in the cervical secretions which harbor the virus, such as lymphocytes and macrophages and, if so, which are the activating hormones. We know very little about these phenomena in humans, but they are important, since the type and level of sex steroid vary during different phases of the menstrual

Table 1

Summary of Classification System for HIV

Group I. Acute infection
Group II. Asymptomatic infection
Group III. Persistent generalized lymphadenopathy
Group IV. Other disease
- Subgroup A. Constitutional disease
- Subgroup B. Neurological disease
- Subgroup C. Secondary infectious disease
  - Category C-1. Specified secondary infectious diseases listed in the CDC surveillance definition for AIDS
  - Category C-2. Other specified secondary infectious diseases
- Subgroup D. Secondary cancers
- Subgroup E. Other conditions

Category C-1 and Subgroup D include those patients whose clinical presentation fulfills the definition of AIDS used by the Centers for Disease Control for national reporting.

cycle and these factors may be operative in regulating the amount of virus present as well as its intracellular or extracellular location in urogenital secretions. This possibility is of obvious importance with respect to heterosexual transmission, since it is the infectious virus in cervical secretions which passes from the female to the male and transmits the disease. Many of these questions can be addressed by utilization of various techniques that have been shown to activate or stimulate virus production in vitro. For example, one could treat infected lymphocytes or macrophages, or both, with various sex steroids and measure the production of infectious HIV.

Pregnancy and the Asymptomatic Female Carrier

Of the fetuses born from women who are infected with HIV prior to pregnancy, approximately 50 percent are infected with HIV. For subsequent pregnancies, the percentage is even higher. Current evidence indicates that virus is generally passed from mother to fetus during the intrauterine residence of the fetus rather than perinatally.[14] This evidence stems from the fact that Caesarean section does not protect the fetus from infection.[15] Moreover, the virus can be recovered from the fetal compartment in cases of elective Caesarean section at twenty and thirty-six weeks.[16] Thus, most evidence indicates that the virus passes from mother to fetus transplacentally. There are reported cases, however, in which virus has been passed to the neonate via the milk.[17]

That pregnant positive women may pass the virus to the fetus in approximately 50 percent of pregnancies and that pregnancy may influence the course and progression of the disease in infected women raise many issues regarding testing for HIV positivity and counseling women who are found to be seropositive.

One important question concerns the progression of disease during pregnancy. Does pregnancy enhance the progression of disease in a healthy female carrier? There is evidence at present to suggest that HIV-infected women who have already given birth to an infected child have an increased risk of developing AIDS during the subsequent pregnancy or soon thereafter.[18] It is possible that exposure to paternal antigens of the fetus triggers an immune response that is likely to activate latently infected immune cells. Viral replication is more likely to take place in such stimulated cells. It has been suggested that these events have a cumulative effect, since the risk of AIDS does not seem to increase in the first pregnancy of an HIV-infected woman in some studies.[19] In still other studies, progression was evident in women during the first pregnancy.[20] Obviously, studies must be carried out to resolve this important issue, but it seems clear that pregnancy can be a cofactor for progression, which poses the question as to whether such progression is due to enhanced viral activation or to the immunosuppressed state that accompanies pregnancy. This subject will be discussed below.

Infection of the Brain

At what point the brain, which is affected in 85 to 95 percent of AIDS cases, is seeded with virus is not known at the present time.[21] It is entirely possible that the brain may be seeded with virus at the time of initial infection. This is what occurs with visna, a disease in sheep caused by a subgroup of retroviruses, the lentiviruses, a group to which HIV belongs. In visna infection, the virus is brought to the brain in a monocyte; presumably this happens with HIV infection, since the virus infects monocytes, and monocytes are the cells most frequently infected in the brains of AIDS patients. These monocytes may appear as multinucleated, syncytial giant cells, and viral replication has been documented in these cells. Evidence indicates that the brain is seeded with HIV in healthy, asymptomatic, seropositive individuals.[22] These conclusions are based on studies carried out with the cerebrospinal fluid (CSF). If antibody to a virus is present in the CSF, it is extremely likely that virus is replicating in the brain. In most chronic virus infections of the brain, such as measles and visna, replication of virus in the brain evokes antibody production in the brain, and the antibody subsequently appears in the CSF. Other tests can be carried out to detect viral antigen in the CSF, which is also indicative of brain infection. That the brain is seeded by the virus, possibly very early, is important, since the brain may act as a reservoir for virus replication. The brain frequently harbors chronic, subacute, and latent virus infections. Why various virus infections persist in the brain is not known. It is known that the brain is an immunologically privileged site, probably owing, in no small part, to the blood brain barrier and the lack of lymphatic supply to the brain. The fact that HIV persists in the brain will make eradication of the infection very difficult indeed, since most drugs pass the blood brain barrier poorly, if at all.

In the preceding sections, we have considered the likelihood of becoming infected with HIV as well as the consequences of infection with respect to the development of acute disease or seroconversion without clinical disease. We have also considered the viral status and infectivity of the asymptomatic carrier, particularly the woman. Pregnancy as a factor promoting progression of disease and the possible mechanisms implicated in maternal to fetal spread were also discussed. The likelihood of invasion of the central nervous system by CNS HIV was considered. The HIV carrier may feel completely well for many years, or he or she may experience progression of the disease. We will now consider the factor(s) that may influence the outcome of HIV infection.

Progression to AIDS

In table 1, a summary of the new Centers for Disease Control (CDC) classification system for HIV is presented. We define progression as the development of disease in asymptomatic individuals (Group II), which may be minor (persistent generalized lymphadenopathy [PGL], Group III) or severe (Group IV). It should be noted that in the CDC classification, several distinct symptomatic presentations of HIV infection are now included. Within Subgroup A of Group IV, for example, fall cases formerly termed AIDS-related complex, or ARC.

What, then, is the likelihood of progression? Various studies indicate that at least 50 percent of seropositive individuals will experience progression of HIV infection to a disease included in Group IV. The likelihood that progression will occur is strongly related to the length of the HIV infection.[23] Several studies suggest that the incidence of progression of persons in Group III, or PGL, is similar to that of persons in Group II.[24] What percentage of asymptomatic carriers will remain so, without progression clinically or immunologically, is not known for certain. These individuals must, of course, be followed for longer periods.

The question of whether the persistently asymptomatic state reflects containment of the replication of HIV by means of certain unspecified factors or through specific immune mechanisms, or both, remains unanswered. Although it is not known for certain, it is likely that a slower rate of progression in some individuals reflects a relative lack of cofactors; put another way, it is likely that cofactors enhance progression. We postulate that the cofactors act by increasing viral replication or by altering the capacity of the immune system to contain the infection, or by doing both. This proposed mechanism of progression is untested at present and likely will remain so for years. Nevertheless, we would assume that anything that activates viral replication or that diminishes the immune response would favor progression.

The likelihood that cofactors influence the development of AIDS is of paramount importance. We have already pointed out that pregnancy may increase the risk of developing AIDS in an asymptomatic carrier. There is much current feeling that other cofactors such as intercurrent infection, malnutrition, excessive use of recreational drugs and alcohol, and stress may all play a role in the development of disease in people infected with the HIV agent. We will discuss these factors after briefly reviewing the question of genetic predisposition.

Genetic Influence

Susceptibility to HIV infection as well as rates of disease progression may depend on genetic characteristics, for example, a predisposition for acquisition of the disease; the evidence for this, however, is very preliminary. Some data have been presented linking HIV infection with a certain genetic phenotype (group specific component [Gc]) in homosexual men.[25] Yet, in a series of seropositive hemophiliac patients, no significant difference was found between patient and control populations with respect to this genetic marker.[26]

Other studies, mainly from New York, indicate that the HLA-DR5 antigen is positively associated with Kaposi's sarcoma as a manifestation of AIDS.[27] The significance of these preliminary studies is unknown, and more studies must be done. However, the notion that there may be a genetic influence on susceptibility to, or progression of, HIV infection remains a fascinating one.

Intercurrent Infection

A large body of evidence indicates that replication of HIV may occur only in an activated cell. The infectious viral cycle generally does not proceed to virus production, but proceeds only to proviral DNA synthesis and integration in a resting lymphocyte. Upon lymphocyte activation, viral replication occurs and progeny virus is produced.[28] In a latently infected cell as well, virus synthesis may occur only after cell activation with varying agents that stimulate lymphocytes to divide, such as various antigens or infectious agents.[29] Elegant molecular biological studies have identified a factor produced by activated T-cells, a subset of lymphocytes, which enhances the expression and replication of HIV.[30] This factor is a protein that binds to the regions of the viral genome which enhance the expression of viral genes. Such studies indicate that stimulation of lymphocytes associated with another infection can activate HIV virus replication both during an acute infection and in a latently infected cell.

Infectious processes, by activating HIV replication, may promote the infection of a greater number of target cells and cause their ultimate destruction. Through this amplification, the threshold for clinical disease might then be reached. Tuberculosis and generalized viral infections have been thought to act as cofactors for HIV progression in this way.[31] There is, however, much more evidence that intercurrent sexually transmitted infections such as gonorrhea, syphilis, primary herpes simplex, hepatitis B, and nonspecific urethritis acquired after HIV infection are strongly associated with the development of symptomatic disease in two separate cohort studies.[32, 33] It has been suggested that intercurrent sexually transmitted disease may also act to promote seroconversion in the following way:[34] HIV may have infected relatively few T-lymphocytes and/or macrophages (the cells of the immune system most susceptible to HIV infection) at the site of entry of the virus, and thus may not have provided sufficient viral antigens to illicit an immune response. Such latently infected cells, when activated as part of a local, or systemic, response to infection, may then release sufficient viral particles to induce a primary specific immune response. Pinching further speculates that this phase of required HIV replication may explain the relatively long latency period between exposure and seroconversion (generally six weeks to three months; however, lag periods of up to twelve months have been reported), longer than with most other infections or immunizations.[35] One would want to have more data as to how often seroconversion is triggered by intercurrent infections, although this information might be difficult to obtain. Whether or not this hypothesis can be substantiated, the epidemiological evidence of the association of intercurrent infection and progression of HIV disease suggests that intercurrent infections are an important cofactor. Moreover, other studies indicate that the presence of lesions in the genital area which are associated with sexually transmitted diseases may be a risk factor for HIV infection, since such lesions may provide a portal of entry for the virus.[36]

Malnutrition

Many studies have indicated that severe protein calorie malnutrition and a variety of single nutrient deficiencies are causes of defective-cell-mediated immunity and of other defective immune functions.[37] Stated another way, deficiencies in calories in general as well as specific vitamins or minerals can lead to deficiencies in immune function. Malnutrition as a result of persistent diarrhea and malabsorption may contribute to further impairment of immunity and the progression of AIDS. Some evidence indicates that nutritional status decreases as the severity of HIV-related illness increases from an asymptomatic seropositive state to AIDS.[38] It is likely that malnutrition plays an important role in the progression of HIV infections in central Africa.

Recreational Drugs and Alcohol

The excessive use of alcohol or recreational drugs, or both, can cause immunosuppression.[39, 40] The contribution of alcohol and drug use to HIV-related disease is uncertain at this time, however, as recent studies were unable to demonstrate that the use of these substances contributes significantly to disease progression.[41, 42] Chronic use of alcohol, which may result in cirrhosis of the liver and diminished host resistance, could certainly act as a cofactor for disease progression.

Stress

A growing literature suggests that mental attitudes and emotions may influence the progression of infectious diseases, including those associated with HIV. Such studies, together with those dealing with psychosocial aspects as predictors of which infected individuals will progress to AIDS, are attempting to determine the relationship between mental processes and the immune system. This is a new field of study, which has been called psychoneuroimmunology.[43] Such studies are extremely important, since they may reveal mechanisms that will aid in determining whether and how stress and associated dysphoria may be cofactors in the progression of HIV infection to AIDS.

If distress is such a cofactor, it becomes important to determine the personality factors and interventions that may be instrumental in buffering the effects of stress. A number of reports have indicated that hardiness is associated with less illness in highly stressed individuals.[44] Hardy individuals are defined as those who make commitments, welcome challenge and change, and tend to feel that they can exercise control over their lives. Psychological tests to measure hardiness have found that men who are "most hardy" on the control subscale have a greater longevity following diagnosis of *Pneumocystis carinii* pneumonia.[45]

Another study has indicated that patients with Kaposi's sarcoma who are following a macrobiotic regimen have survived with their disease for as long as three to five years.[46] These patients have shown some improvement in their immunologic profile without medical therapy. Survival patterns such as these in patients with Kaposi's sarcoma are not frequently encountered. As the choice to practice a macrobiotic way of life and the ability to continue with it involve many changes and require a strong commitment, one would predict that the individuals in the study are quite hardy. In addition, an important component of the practice of a macrobiotic regimen is the belief that health can be controlled by diet. This belief presumably reduces the sense of hopelessness associated with AIDS. In animal studies, helplessness and hopelessness are associated with immune suppression. The extent to which the clinical improvement is due to the macrobiotic diet per se or the psychological involvement in the macrobiotic way of life or the particular "mind set" of those who choose an alternative therapy is not completely understood at present.

The aforementioned studies suggest that certain personality characteristics indicative of "psychological health" and a feeling of involvement and commitment may influence the course of HIV infection. It would not seem unlikely that stress and dysphoria influence progression of disease in HIV-infected persons. Numerous studies have revealed that the immune function can be diminished by many of the chemicals released from the brain or nerves, which are called neuromediators, neurohormones, and neurotransmitters and which mediate the effects of stress.[47] Furthermore, the psychological depression experienced by many people who have seroconverted to HIV may itself be immunosuppressive.[48] Although it is likely that any progression of HIV infection which is caused by stress is brought on by the immunosuppressive effect(s) associated with stress, it is also possible that the virus is directly activated in cells by certain of the neuromediators just referred to. HIV production is, for example, stimulated by corticosteroids. Activation of other viruses by several of these substances has been demonstrated in animal cells in vitro as well as in vivo.[49] In humans, certain neurohormones can also activate viruses; for example, epinephrine can activate latent herpes simplex virus infection in the rabbit eye.[50]

The effect(s) that the mind has on the HIV disease process are complicated by the possibility of the presence of HIV in the brain of asymptomatic carriers. As we have mentioned, the time when the brain is seeded with HIV is not known. It is evident that central nervous system seeding occurs eventually in most patients who progress, since the vast majority (85 to 95 percent) of patients with AIDS have pathological evidence of AIDS encephalopathy at autopsy.[51] Indeed, evidence indicates that of those diagnosed with AIDS, 20 percent may initially present with a psychiatric or neurological syndrome. Therefore, psychological or psychosocial studies on asymptomatic carriers may be complicated by the presence of HIV in the brain of an asymptomatic carrier. It is known, however, that the brain may contain HIV without psychiatric or neurological signs or symptomatology.[52] Thus, infection of the CNS may remain asymptomatic. One can determine whether the brain is seeded with HIV by examination of the CSF for HIV antigen or antibody to HIV (see above), but performance of such studies may be difficult to justify because of the risk associated with spinal tap. Recently, neuropsychological testing has been developed to identify subjects with "likely early" or "early" AIDS-related dementia.[53] This finding should allow researchers in this area to analyze their data for a possible confounding effect of organically induced alterations in mood and personality.

Although few studies have been carried out so far, it is possible that production and levels of neurotransmitter substances are altered in an HIV-infected individual who has seeded the brain. At present, there is no evidence that neurons are infected by HIV. However, the cells in the brain known to be infected by HIV (monocytes, endothelial cells, and certain glial cells)[54] elaborate substances that have been shown to affect certain neurotransmitter substances in neurons.[55] Similarly, monocytes and T-lymphocytes can also secrete factors that influence brain function. Altered neurotransmitter substances in the CNS may, in turn, affect immune function.[56] Thus, a complex interaction exists whereby products of cells of the immune system or other cells capable of secreting similar products influence the levels of neuromediators in the brain.[57] Whether HIV infection alters the function of CNS cells with respect to production of, or response to, neurotransmitter or immunomodulatory substances, respectively, is currently unknown. We speculate that because of these alterations, progression may occur more rapidly in an asymptomatic person who has HIV infection of the brain. Much work must be done to delineate further the relationship between the central nervous and immune systems, the ways in which emotions affect the immune system, and whether and how HIV infection in general, and of the brain in particular, alters these interactions. Such studies may help determine whether and how stress may be a cofactor in either the development or the progression of AIDS.

Summary

We have attempted to present an overview of the factors that may play a role in determining whether progression occurs in the HIV-positive asymptomatic person. Pregnancy, intercurrent infection, malnutrition, excessive use of recreational drugs and alcohol, and stress, as well as certain genetic factors, may influence the progression of disease. It will be important to determine whether progression occurs more rapidly in a seropositive individual with CNS infection by HIV.

Although our knowledge about the factors predisposing to the progression of HIV infection is not extensive, it is extremely likely that cofactors play an important, if not a determining, role. Thus, modifying behavior could presumably influence the outcome of an HIV infection. Present data suggest that by avoiding the use of recreational drugs and alcohol, and reducing stress or buffering its effects, one would be maximizing the host potential to combat infection. Since there is no cure for HIV infection at present, a better understanding of the psychological, biological, and behaviorial influences that act as cofactors is of great importance. Research is urgently needed in these areas, so that accurate information can be used as a basis for devising more effective treatment strategies, setting public policy, and educating persons at risk. More specific knowledge could thus be used to develop adjunctive intervention directed at cofactors rather than at the virus itself.

Notes

1. Classification system for HIV infections. *Morbidity and Mortality Weekly Report* 35(20):334–339, 1986.
2. A. J. Pinching. The spectrum of Human Immunodeficiency Virus (HIV) Infection: Routes of infection, natural history, prevention, and treatment. *Clinics in Immunology and Allergy* 6:467–488, 1986.
3. J. H. Weber, A. McCreaver, E. Berrie, et al. Factors affecting seropositivity to HTLV-III/LAV and progression of disease in sexual partners of patients with AIDS. *Genitourinary Medicine* 62:177–180, 1986.
4. Pinching. The spectrum of Human Immunodeficiency Virus (HIV) Infection.
5. J. L. Fox. AIDS: The public health–public policy crisis. *American Society for Microbiology News* 53:426–430, 1987.
6. G. J. Stewart, J. P. P. Tyler, A. L. Cunningham, et al. Transmission of human T-cell lymphotropic virus type III (HTLV III) by artificial insemination by donor. *Lancet* 2:581–585, 1985.
7. C. Ludlam, J. Tucker, and C. M. Steel. Human T lymphotropic virus Type III (HTLV III) infection in seronegative haemophiliacs after transfusion of factor VIII. *Lancet* 2:233–236, 1985.
8. D. D. Ho, R. J. Pomerantz, and J. C. Kaplan. Pathogenesis of infection with human immunodeficiency virus. *New England Journal of Medicine* 317:278–286, 1987.
9. Ibid.
10. P. Lepage, P. Van de Perre, M. Carael, et al. Postnatal transmission of HIV from mother to child. *Lancet* 2:400, 1987.
11. M. W. Vogt, D. J. Witt, D. E. Craven, et al. Isolation of HTLV III/LAV from cervical secretions of women at risk for AIDS. *Lancet* 1:525–527, 1986.
12. M. V. Vogt, D. J. Witt, D. E. Craven, et al. Isolation patterns of the human immunodeficiency virus from cervical secretions during the menstrual cycle of women at risk for the acquired immunodeficiency syndrome. *Annals of Internal Medicine* 106:380–382, 1987.
13. M. S. Hirsch and P. H. Black. Activation of mammalian leukemia viruses. In *Advances in Virus Research,* vol. 19, Academic Press, New York, pp. 265–313, 1974.
14. A. E. Semprini, A. Vucetich, and G. Pardi. HIV infection and AIDS in newborn babies of mothers positive for HIV antibody. *British Medical Journal* 294:610, 1987.
15. Ibid.
16. N. Lapointe, M. J. Pekovic, J. P. Chausseau, et al. Transplacental transmission of HTLV III virus. *New England Journal of Medicine* 312:1325–1326, 1985.

17. Lepage, Van de Perre, Carael, et al. Postnatal transmission of HIV from mother to child.

18. Pinching. The spectrum of Human Immunodeficiency Virus (HIV) Infection.

19. Ibid.

20. C. S. Peckham, Y. S. Senturia, and A. E. Ades. Obstetric and perinatal consequences of human immunodeficiency virus (HIV) infection: A review. *British Journal of Obstetrics and Gynecology* 94:403–407, l987.

21. P. H. Black. HTLV-III, AIDS, and the brain. *New England Journal of Medicine* 313:1538–1540, 1985.

22. I. Elovaara, M. Iivanainen, S. L. Valle, et al. CSF protein and cellular profiles in various stages of HIV infection related to neurological manifestations. *Journal of Neurological Sciences* 78:331–342, 1987.

23. Fox. AIDS: The public health–public policy crisis.

24. B. F. Polk, R. Fox, R. Brookmeyer, et al. Predictors of the acquired immunodeficiency syndrome developing in a cohort of seropositive homosexual men. *New England Journal of Medicine* 316:61–66, 1987.

25. L. Eales, K. E. Nye, J. M. Parkin, et al. Association of different allelic forms of group-specific component with susceptibility to and clinical manifestation of human immunodeficiency virus infection. *Lancet* 1:999–1002, 1987.

26. D. F. Nixon, R. P. Eglin, S. A. Westwood, et al. Group-specific component and HIV infection. *Lancet* 2:39–40,1987.

27. A. E. Friedman-Kien, L. J. Laubenstein, and P. Rubinstein. Disseminated Kaposi's sarcoma in homosexual men. *Annals of Internal Medicine* 96:693–700, 1982.

28. Ho, Pomerantz, and Kaplan. Pathogenesis of infection with human immunodeficiency virus.

29. A. S. Fauci. AIDS — Pathogenic mechanisms and research strategies. *American Society for Microbiology News* 53:263–266, 1987.

30. G. Nabel and D. Baltimore. An inducible transcription factor activates expression of human immunodeficiency virus in T cells. *Nature* 326:711–713, 1987.

31. Pinching. The spectrum of Human Immunodeficiency Virus (HIV) Infection.

32. Weber, McCreaver, Berrie, et al. Factors affecting seropositivity to HTLV-III/LAV.

33. J. H. Weber, J. Wadsworth, L. A. Rogers, et al. Three-year prospective study of HTLV III/LAV infection in homosexual men. *Lancet* 1:1179–1182, 1986.

34. Pinching. The spectrum of Human Immunodeficiency Virus (HIV) Infection.

35. Ibid.

36. Ibid.

37. R. K. Chandra. Nutrition and immune responses. *Canadian Journal of Physiological Pharmacology* 61:290–294, 1983.

38. N. Colman and F. Grossman. Nutritional factors in epidemic Kaposi's sarcoma. *Seminars in Oncology* 14 (Suppl. 3):54–62, 1987.

39. R. R. MacGregor. Alcohol and immune defense. *Journal of the American Medical Association* 256:1474–1479, 1986.

40. D. Blanchard, C. Newton, T. Klein, et al. In vitro and in vivo suppressive effects of delta-9-tetrahydrocannabinol on interferon production by murine spleen cells. *International Journal of Immunopharmacology* 8:819–824, 1986.

41. A. Roland, D. W. Feigal, D. Abrams, et al. Recreational drug use does not cause AIDS progression. USCF AIDS registry group. Third International Conference on AIDS Abstract:173, 1987.

42. C. E. Stevens, P. E. Taylor, S. Rodriguez, et al. Recreational drugs and HIV infection: Relationship to risk of infection and immune deficiency. Third International Conference on AIDS Abstract:179, 1987.

43. *Psychoneuroimmunology.* Ed. by R. Ader. Academic Press, New York, 1981, p. 661.

44. S. C. Kobasa, S. R. Maddi, and M. C. Paccetti. Personality and exercise as buffers in the stress-illness relationship. *Journal of Behavioral Medicine* 5:391–404, 1982.

45. G. F. Solomon, L. Temoshok, A. O'Leary, and J. Zich. An intensive psychoimmunologic study of long-surviving persons with AIDS. *Annals of the New York Academy of Sciences* 496:647–655, 1987.

46. E. M. Levy, L. H. Kushi, M. C. Cottrell, and P. H. Black. The natural history of Kaposi's sarcoma in men following a macrobiotic regimen. Submitted to *AIDS.*

47. N. R. Hall and A. L. Goldstein. Neurotransmitters and the immune system. In *Psychoneuroimmunology,* pp. 521–543.

48. E. M. Levy and R. Krueger. Depression and the immune system. *Directions in Psychiatry* 5:1–7, 1985.

49. Hirsch and Black. Activation of mammalian leukemia viruses.

50. P. R. Laibson and S. Kibrick. Reactivation of herpetic keratitis by epinephrine in rabbit eye. *Archives of Ophthalmology* 75:254–260, 1966.

51. B. A. Navia, E. S. Cho, C. K. Petito, et al. The AIDS dementia complex. II, Neuropathology. *Annals of Neurology* 19:525–535, 1986.

52. P. H. Black. HTLV-III, AIDS, and the brain.

53. D. Ornitz, H. Amitai, and J. J. Sidtis. Scales for the neurological examination and history in the AIDS dementia complex. Third International Conference on AIDS Abstract:153, 1987.

54. F. Gyorkey, J. L. Melnick, and P. Gyorkey. Human immunodeficiency virus in brain biopsies of patients with AIDS and progressive encephalopathy. *Journal of Infectious Diseases* 155:870–876, 1987.

55. H. Besedovsky. The immune response evokes changes in brain noradrenergic neurons. *Science* 221:564–565, 1983.

56. N. R. Hall and A. L. Goldstein. Neurotransmitters and the immune system. In *Psychoneuroimmunology,* pp. 521–543.

57. H. Besedovsky, A. E. DelRey, and E. Sorkin. Immune-neuroendocrine interactions. *Journal of Immunology* 135:750–754, 1985.

Glossary continued from page 96

Provirus. This is DNA made from an RNA template (of an RNA virus) by the enzyme reverse transcriptase, and it is required for replication of the virus. This DNA becomes permanently associated with the DNA of the cell and, as long as the cell lives, will remain associated with the cell's genes.

Seroconversion. The development of antibody to an infectious agent is termed seroconversion. This occurs during acute infectious diseases. It may also occur without obvious clinical disease or symptoms. In the latter case, the seroconversion may be termed silent or asymptomatic. Most infections and seroconversions with HIV are of the asymptomatic variety.

T-lymphocytes. Lymphocytes are a class of white blood cells responsible for specific immunity. T-lymphocytes are a subclass of lymphocytes and include cells that can kill virally infected cells.

"I have no immune system. You people are much more likely to give me something than I am ever likely to give you something. And I don't think very many people think in those terms, that we're the ones at risk. Just being in a room, people coughing and sneezing, could put me in the hospital, and you have virtually nothing to fear from me, so I mean, that reversal of roles has to be brought home."

Glossary

Ataxia. A loss of the power of muscular coordination.

Autonomic neuropathy. A disorder of the autonomic nervous system which manifests in abnormalities of functions governed by the autonomic nervous system, such as temperature regulation and maintenance of blood pressure.

Cat scan. Computerized axial tomography, a special radiographic examination consisting of a series of x-rays.

Cortical atrophy. A shrinkage of the outer tissues of the brain (known as the cortex of the brain).

Histopathology. The science or study dealing with the cytologic and histologic structure of abnormal or diseased tissue.

Hyperreflexia. A condition in which the deep tendon reflexes are exaggerated.

Methylphenidate. A medication that acts as a stimulant on the central nervous system.

Neuroleptic. An antipsychotic medication.

Nonfocal encephalopathy. Diffuse disease of the brain.

Obtundation. A diminished state of alertness.

Postural hypotension. A form of low blood pressure which occurs when the subject stands.

Subacute encephalitis. Inflammation of the brain which progresses at a moderate rate.

Neuropsychiatric Complications of HIV Infection: Public Policy Implications

Alexandra Beckett, M.D.
Theo Manschreck, M.D.

The human immunodeficiency virus (HIV) infects the central nervous system (CNS), causing symptoms in most persons with AIDS-related complex (ARC) and AIDS, and in a significant proportion of those classified as asymptomatic seropositive. The most common clinical syndrome secondary to CNS infection is known as HIV encephalopathy. When sufficiently disabling, HIV encephalopathy is known as AIDS dementia, and must be reported to the Centers for Disease Control as a case of AIDS.

AIDS dementia is a complex of cognitive, affective, behavioral, and motor symptoms which varies widely in its presentation. In some persons, cognitive impairment predominates, manifesting in a loss of intellectual capacities such as short-term memory, information processing, and abstract thinking. When mood disturbance predominates, it may present as irritability, anxiety, depression, or mania. Behavioral complications are most often due to confusion or psychosis, and may render the patient difficult for caretakers to manage. Motor impairments include slowing, gait abnormalities, incontinence, and paralysis.

AIDS dementia presents a significant challenge to the public health system. Physicians, other health providers, and policymakers must be educated so that they may tackle the problems of diagnosis, acute and chronic care, and public safety which are related to this illness.

AIDS is one of a spectrum of disorders resulting from infection by the human immunodeficiency virus (HIV). In addition to AIDS, there exists a number of syndromes of immune dysfunction, such as AIDS-related complex (ARC). Furthermore, it has been established that HIV causes serious neurological dysfunction in most AIDS patients, in a significant number of persons with ARC,[1] in some otherwise asymptomatic seropositives, and occasionally in persons with a false-negative serologic test.[2, 3]

Dr. Alexandra Beckett is a fellow in psychiatry at Massachusetts General Hospital, in Boston, and is an instructor in psychiatry at Harvard Medical School. Dr. Theo Manschreck is associate professor of psychiatry at Massachusetts General Hospital and is clinical director of the Erich Lindemann Mental Health Center/Harbor Area, in Boston.

Neurological Disorders: Phenomenology

Substantial evidence indicates that HIV infects the nervous system. HIV has been recovered from brain, cerebrospinal fluid, spinal cord, and peripheral nerve of patients with HIV infection and neurological disease. Over 90 percent of autopsied AIDS cases have histopathological changes in the brain.[4]

Sixty-three percent of AIDS patients have neurological symptoms during the course of their illness, and in 20 percent, these symptoms are the initial chief complaint leading to the AIDS diagnosis.[5] All levels of the nervous system may be affected, but cerebral involvement is the most common. Many factors may adversely affect neurological function in persons with an HIV infection, including prior neuropsychiatric disorders, concurrent drug treatment, systemic illness, malignancies (both primary and metastatic to the central nervous system), and opportunistic infections.

Infections afflicting immunocompromised hosts include bacterial, fungal, and viral types. The infectious agent most likely to impair nervous system function in an HIV-infected host is HIV itself. Many HIV-induced disorders, affecting each level of the nervous system, have been described.[6] In the peripheral nervous system, nerve palsies may produce painful sensory disturbance or motor weakness, or both. Autonomic neuropathy resulting in postural hypotension, with symptoms such as dizziness, is also frequently present. Damage to the spinal cord occurs in as many as 30 percent of AIDS patients, with consequent gait problems and urinary incontinence.[7]

The most common HIV-related disorder in the nervous system is known variously as nonfocal encephalopathy, subacute encephalitis, or AIDS dementia complex.[8] It is sufficiently prevalent that the Centers for Disease Control (CDC) recorded cases of AIDS dementia among its AIDS statistics as of September 1, 1987. Notably, the dementia may occur in the absence of concomitant immune disease; that is, in otherwise relatively symptom-free HIV-infected persons.

AIDS dementia is a complex of cognitive, affective, behavioral, and motor abnormalities. It usually begins with subtle alterations in mental status, such as poor concentration and mild, short-term memory loss. Patients may complain of forgetfulness, confusion, and mental slowing. Owing to attentional lapses, they may lose the train of a conversation or be unable to follow an entire television program or read a book.

Affective symptoms often include anxiety and severe depression, with loss of energy, diminished appetite, and sleep disturbance. Patients with these symptoms may be apathetic, socially withdrawn, mildly irritable, or inappropriate in their behavior. At times, behavioral changes may be more dramatic, marked by acute psychosis with agitation, hallucinations, paranoid ideation, and even mania.

Motor impairments are common and may include lower extremity weakness, ataxia, tremors, and difficulty with articulation. Patients may notice unsteadiness when walking, deterioration in handwriting, or slightly slurred speech.

The course of AIDS dementia is variable. In some individuals, it is indolent and slowly progressive. Concentration and memory may worsen, but individuals continue to work and live independently. In others, the course of AIDS dementia is rapid and catastrophic, progressing in a matter of weeks or months to severe intellectual deterioration, marked psychomotor slowing, and mutism. Hyperreflexia, urinary and fecal incontinence, and, occasionally, seizures may occur.

Because the HIV-infected individual is vulnerable to numerous influences that can manifest in a disturbance of mental functioning, the advent of a change in mental status in such a patient mandates a thorough evaluation to identify treatable causes such as tumors, opportunistic infections, drug toxicity, or metabolic imbalances. Once these have been ruled out, one is left with a diagnosis of AIDS dementia. There is no test that confirms the diagnosis, making it a diagnosis of exclusion.

As mentioned, the CDC now solicits reports of HIV encephalopathy/dementia, defined as follows: "clinical findings of disabling cognitive and/or motor dysfunction interfering with occupation or activities of daily living, or loss of behavioral developmental milestones affecting a child, progressing over weeks to months, in the absence of a concurrent illness or condition other than HIV infection that could explain the findings."[9] The appearance of this syndrome in an HIV-infected individual is now AIDS-defining; that is, its occurrence makes it a reportable case of AIDS.

The definition is necessarily vague, because the syndrome itself may have diverse manifestations, appearing singly or concurrently. In any one patient, motor, cognitive, affective, or behavioral features may predominate. Without a unique and predictable course, current knowledge prohibits the making of precise prognoses.

AIDS Dementia Complex: Epidemiology

We do not know the incidence of AIDS dementia. It is well known that most AIDS patients are grossly demented at the time of death; often, this mental decline declares itself dramatically in the last days or weeks of life. Less well known is the extent to which these same patients were functionally impaired prior to detection. This pattern is particularly apt to occur when more acute medical complications dominate the clinical picture.

Careful neuropsychological assessments of seropositives and persons with AIDS-related complex have revealed a high incidence of subclinical cognitive dysfunction. Despite the initial subclinical nature of the impairment, these individuals are coping with progressive intellectual decline that may ultimately undermine their capacity for work and social interaction.

Grant found a 44 percent incidence of neuropsychological impairment in otherwise asymptomatic seropositives, 54 percent in persons diagnosed with ARC, and 87 percent in persons with AIDS.[10] As the AIDS dementia complex becomes more widely recognized, early, subtler signs of intellectual impairment which have previously gone unnoticed or which have been understood as "functional," that is, as a psychological reaction to the diagnosis rather than organic in nature, will prompt earlier and more accurate diagnosis.

Clinical Vignette: *Mr. A., a forty-one-year-old single man, was referred to the psychiatry clinic for treatment of depression. Formerly employed as a public administrator, he had lost his job because of poor performance. Mr. A. had been in treatment for a year with a psychotherapist who was addressing issues of low self-esteem and social isolation.*

On evaluation, Mr. A. was a slovenly, mildly obese man with a slow and somewhat clumsy gait. His speech, though coherent and logical, was stuttering. Tearfully, Mr. A. described a persistent depressed mood and thoughts that others were out to get him because of past homosexual encounters. He admitted to intermittent suicidal ideation. He reported increased appetite, with a forty-pound weight gain over a year, and excessive sleep of up to fifteen hours a day, despite which he was chronically fatigued.

Mr. A. was admitted to a psychiatric hospital, where treatment with antidepressant medication was initiated. Routine psychological testing raised the question of cognitive impairment. More comprehensive testing confirmed the presence of multiple intellectual deficits.

His medical evaluation included a CAT scan, which demonstrated cortical atrophy and a white blood count that was well below the normal range. An HIV antibody test was positive, and a diagnosis of AIDS dementia was made.

Mr. A. continued to suffer mental deterioration. He was unable to care for himself and was placed in a chronic care hospital, where he died some months later from pneumonia.

What features of this case might alert the clinician to a possibility of AIDS dementia? Once the possibility of this diagnosis has been raised, what type of evaluation is indicated? How can one now help the patient?

AIDS dementia should be considered when any patient presents with a new psychiatric condition that is accompanied by cognitive deficits or neurological impairments, or both. One must ascertain risk for HIV infection, and document its presence, if the patient consents. A medical evaluation must include CAT scan or magnetic resonance imaging (MRI), followed by lumbar puncture for analysis of cerebrospinal fluid (CSF).

The purpose of this evaluation is twofold: identification of treatable illness, such as cryptococcal meningitis and toxoplasmosis, and confirmation of the diagnosis of AIDS dementia. Making the diagnosis enables the physician to counsel the patient about his or her infectiousness and intellectual limitations; facilitate the acquisition of the necessary public assistance; and refer the patient to appropriate caretakers.

As of January 18, 1988, 51,361 cases of AIDS had been identified in the United States (1,095 in Massachusetts) with 28,683 deaths. Two hundred and seventy thousand cases are anticipated by 1991, with 54,000 cases in that year alone.[11] Given an average period of four years from infection to disease manifestation, this number of AIDS cases would occur by 1991 even if no new transmissions of HIV were to take place. The incidence of ARC is thought to be two to four times that of AIDS, and the number of infected persons in the United States totals at least 1.5 million.[12] In view of the incidence of neuropsychological impairment found by Grant and others, we must confront the likelihood that thousands of persons are afflicted with AIDS dementia.

AIDS Dementia Complex Treatment

Unfortunately, there is no cure for this disorder. Early experience with Azidothymidine (AZT) in AIDS patients suggests that the drug may retard or even reverse impairments in some individuals. Controlled trials are under way to determine whether these preliminary findings are significant.

Since the virus is known to reside and replicate in the central nervous system (CNS), any effective antiviral drug must cross the blood-brain barrier and achieve sufficient levels to eradicate virus. In the absence of such penetration, the CNS could serve as a sanctuary for HIV despite its eradication elsewhere in the body. The establishment of such a sanctuary introduces additional risks to the patient and raises a series of policy-related issues. The risks are the potential for the virus to break out of its sanctuary and affect other organs; to increase damage to the central nervous system, and thereby to cognitive abilities; and to go unnoticed or undiagnosed.

The policy implications of the sanctuary problem include at least the efficacy of new treatments or vaccines and the potential for occupational impairment and consequent threats to public safety, owing to cognitive problems.

Meanwhile, such therapies as do exist are palliative, that is, they provide some symptomatic relief and enhance functioning but do not alter the course of the disease. They consist of drugs already used for patients with medical and psychiatric disorders, and include psychostimulants, antidepressants, and antipsychotics.

Given the limitations of our pharmacopoeia, appropriate therapy must include accurate appraisal of cognitive and functional capacity and assistance in adapting to individual limitations. Because of the progressive nature of the dementia complex, patients require close follow-up. Good medical care requires a multispecialty approach that may include infectious disease, neurology, psychiatry, neuropsychology, and social service expertise.

Public Health Issues

Education

Updated training and increased awareness concerning the neuropsychiatric consequences of HIV are essential for an adequate response to the epidemic. The field of knowledge is growing rapidly. Efforts to inform health professionals are especially important. Many physicians who were trained before the AIDS epidemic feel particularly uneasy tending to AIDS patients and may choose to refer them to persons they regard as AIDS "experts." It will not be possible for such specialists to provide all care. Every physician must attain a working knowledge of AIDS, making him or her prepared to provide basic care and ready to refer to other practitioners when such referrals are appropriate.

State planning committees, as well as involvement from the private sector, labor, and other social organizations, will be necessary to increase understanding and enroll support for legislative and other governmental and private solutions to the needs of these patients.

Early Diagnosis

The hallmark of successful control of disease is diagnostic sophistication. In this disease, the early manifestations may be subtle and are often in the neuropsychiatric sphere. Most health professionals have limited familiarity with the clinical and laboratory assessments of such impairments. The psychiatric specialty within medicine can respond to this diagnostic challenge but must be ready itself to accept the challenge and the central role of psychiatry in the treatment of HIV patients.

Any change in mental status in an HIV-infected individual necessitates immediate evaluation to identify treatable causes. As mentioned earlier, there are multiple possible causes for such a change, some of which are medical emergencies requiring acute intervention. A proper diagnostic workup may include CAT scan, lumbar puncture, and electroencephalogram (EEG).

Increased Demands for Care

Several problems present major challenges. First, the complexities of diagnosis, infectious and neuropsychiatric, require technical know-how from several specialties that are not organized to function together in health care settings.

Second, the kinds of clinical problems that patients have after diagnosis require medical and psychiatric input for successful management. Currently, many HIV patients are difficult to manage on a general medical ward, owing to their agitation or psychosis, or both; because their symptoms fall into the psychiatric range, there is pressure to refer them to a psychiatric facility. Unfortunately, neither public nor private psychiatric hospitals are equipped to diagnose and treat emergent medical conditions in HIV patients.

Third, HIV patients referred to public inpatient and outpatient facilities because of neuropsychiatric disturbances could create excessive demands on these services, which are already pressed by growing numbers of chronically ill and homeless mentally ill patients.

Fourth, the range of clinical presentations calls for a range of services. Some individuals are only mildly impaired, with ongoing needs for medical and psychiatric follow-up, while others are functionally incapacitated, unable to work or adequately care for themselves. HIV-infected patients have died from undiagnosed, treatable illnesses while in psychiatric facilities, underscoring the need for appropriate sites for evaluation and treatment of such patients with neuropsychiatric symptoms. Specialized treatment centers, home care support, and outpatient programming for individual, group, and rehabilitative therapy represent other services that need to be part of the solution to these problems.

Clinical Vignette: *Mr. D., a twenty-six-year-old man who had been diagnosed with AIDS four months earlier, was brought to his internist's office by three friends after he disrobed in a public park. Mr. D. was extremely agitated, talking rapidly and pacing. He admitted to auditory hallucinations and believed that God and Satan were warring within him. He refused to cooperate with a physical examination and threatened to strike anyone who came near him. The patient was brought to the emergency room by hospital security, where he was placed in a locked room.*

Mr. D.'s internist instructed emergency room physicians to refer Mr. D. to a psychiatric hospital for treatment of manic psychosis. The hospital's psychiatric unit refused Mr. D. admission, citing the unmanageability of his agitation and the potential for violence in an unlocked psychiatric facility. Mr. D. was refused admission to other general hospital and private psychiatric units.

Mr. D. was sent to a state mental hospital, where he was placed in seclusion and treated with neuroleptic medications. Twenty-four hours after admission, he developed a temperature of 104 degrees Fahrenheit, a stiff neck, and severe obtundation. He was transferred to the general hospital, where medical evaluation revealed cryptococcal meningitis. Mr. D. was admitted to the medical floor, where antibiotic therapy was initiated.

This case illustrates the dangers of preemptive diagnosis — in this instance, of "functional" psychiatric illness. When an HIV-infected patient presents with psychiatric symptoms, serious medical illness may well be present. The patient becomes a diagnostic and treatment dilemma. No one hospital or facility is prepared to meet the challenge of caring for the patient, and, all too often, the patient is transferred from one facility to another without proper and thorough evaluation.

Limited Support for Individual Patients

HIV patients are often less likely to have family involvement in their care than, for instance, Alzheimer's patients. The stigma of the illness entity contributes to this alienation, but many of those with the illness are already socially alienated, for example, many intravenous drug users and homosexual males. Lacking supports such as family increases the morbidity (suffering) of the disease. The inability to qualify for health or life insurance because of positive antibody test results is an additional obstacle to obtaining adequate support.

The issue of disability income is also a major concern. It is not currently known to what extent otherwise asymptomatic seropositives and ARC patients may develop disabling cognitive impairment. Some are partially incapacitated, while others are completely unable to work or to adequately care for themselves.

Because our current programs do not allow for distinctions between partial and full disability, patients may be forced either to (1) conceal or deny deficits until the condition becomes so advanced that such efforts are no longer possible, at which time patients must quit or lose a job and turn to the public welfare system, or (2) go on complete disability upon receiving an AIDS-related diagnosis, even though they are capable of continuing to work at the same or at a reduced level.

Because the system fails to make allowance for the subtle distinctions among HIV-infected individuals, it is often impossible for persons to continue working at a reduced capacity. Income from part-time work often causes discontinuation of disability payments, even though full-time employment is not possible.

Safety

Public safety is a policy issue, because impaired individuals may hold positions wherein their neuropsychiatric impairment may jeopardize the welfare of others. Should such individuals be restricted in their work? Should patients with impairments be allowed to drive? Currently, the answers to these and related questions are unclear; yet, the safety issue remains.

Clinical Vignette: *Mr. X., a thirty-two-year-old respiratory therapist, was diagnosed with ARC after a year of low-grade temperatures, enlarged lymph nodes, and recurrent oral thrush. Although he felt chronically ill, he was able to continue working full-time as a respiratory technician. Formerly married, he had two young children whom he supported in cooperation with his ex-wife, who worked part-time as a typist. Mr. X. was without life or disability insurance at the time of his diagnosis. He applied for both but feared that any investigation into prior conditions would disqualify him.*

Mr. X. was referred for evaluation of increasing difficulties with attention, concentration, and short-term memory. He reported "spacing-out" at work, and on one occasion mistakenly administered a medication in a dose ten times greater than ordered, not aware of the error until reviewing his paperwork from the previous day. Mr. X. felt that his cognitive difficulties reflected his anxiety and depression over his medical condition as well as his preoccupation with his financial situation.

Neuropsychological testing revealed moderate short-term memory deficits, psychomotor slowing, and difficulty with abstract reasoning. A CAT scan of the brain was consistent with a loss of brain tissue. Analysis of cerebrospinal fluid was unremarkable. A diagnosis of HIV-related encephalopathy was made. Treatment with methylphenidate, a stimulant medication, enhanced mental alertness and improved mood, but neuropsychological test results were unchanged three months later.

Mr. X. joined an ARC support group and began weekly psychotherapy with a psychiatrist. He experienced recurrent depression with suicidal ideation, and after several months stopped responding to methylphenidate. Trials of several antidepressant medications were discontinued, owing to intolerable side effects. Mr. X. was advised repeatedly that he should work at a less demanding job, but he continued to work for one year, at which time he developed AIDS. He is currently unemployed and on disability.

This case raises complex treatment and public health issues. Is this patient competent to continue working at his present job? Who is mandated to make that decision? If he is not competent to continue working, should he be considered completely disabled? What will be the course of his illness? What type of follow-up is indicated for him? What are the psychological consequences when such an individual stops working yet remains relatively well for months or years? And what are the consequences for his family and for society?

The problem of intellectually compromised persons in positions of responsibility is not a new one; substance abuse in the workplace has been of sufficient public concern that drug testing has been instituted in a number of settings. Unfortunately, there is no simple diagnostic test for AIDS dementia. Widespread HIV antibody testing would offer no answer to intellectual functioning; cognitive state can be measured only with neuropsychological testing, a time-consuming and costly endeavor. Furthermore, the results of such tests must be interpreted in view of the specific demands of the individual's work.

Psychologically, it can be devastating to a productive, self-supporting individual to be removed from the work force. Many persons on disability become profoundly depressed. Careful thought must go into developing methods for assessing the intellectual capacity of infected individuals. Rational, nondiscriminatory policies must evolve to protect the individual and society from the untoward effects of cognitive impairment.

Ongoing Psychiatric Care

HIV patients, particularly those with cognitive impairment, are at great risk for psychiatric disorders. Common diagnoses in this population include adjustment disorder; major depression; anxiety; panic disorder; organic affective, delusional, anxiety, and personality disorder; and dementia.

Individual and group psychotherapy have both been shown to be valuable in the care of these patients. Furthermore, when appropriate psychiatric services are available, utilization of other medical services may decrease.

Clinicians from a variety of disciplines (including social work, psychology, and nursing) have been working effectively with this population. However, they must always be closely allied with a psychiatrist who can recognize organic syndromes, prescribe medication, and refer for neuropsychiatric evaluation when such a referral is appropriate.

Housing

Many patients with dementia lose their housing. Financial depletion may be part of the cause, but the dementia itself may render these patients unable to live safely without supervision. Such persons would do well in a structured home setting. Currently, there is a dearth of such placements.

Persons with advanced dementia are often no longer able to perform basic activities of daily living, such as hygiene and eating. Motor impairments such as paralysis and urinary incontinence may necessitate intensive nursing care. Such patients will require a total care facility, such as a hospice, a chronic care hospital, or a nursing home.

Conclusion

We have indicated that a serious feature of HIV infection is its manifold effects on neurological, cognitive, and psychiatric functioning. These effects are frequent in this population and represent a major source of the suffering and disability associated with AIDS.

We may be encouraged that the rate of new HIV infections has slowed in certain populations; yet, at the same time, we need to soberly recognize the magnitude of the needs of persons already infected. We now diagnose and treat at an earlier point opportunistic infections and malignancies, thereby increasing life expectancy, and, with it, the incidence of clinical neuropsychiatric disorders. It is essential that we prepare ourselves to optimally care for this patient population.

We cannot rely on the medical and public health systems as they stand today; they are inadequate for the task of caring for persons who are already ill. Through education and careful planning, we must prepare ourselves for the increased demands to come.

Notes

1. D. D. Ho, T. R. Rota, R. T. Schooley, et al. Isolation of HIV from cerebrospinal fluid and neural tissues of patients with neurologic syndromes related to the acquired immunodeficiency syndrome. *New England Journal of Medicine* 1985;315:1493–1497.
2. M. C. Bach, J. A. Boothby. Dementia associated with human immunodeficiency virus with a negative ELISA. *New England Journal of Medicine* 1986;315:891–892.
3. A. Beckett, P. Summergrad, T. Manschreck. Symptomatic HIV infection of the CNS in a patient without clinical evidence of immune deficiency. *American Journal of Psychiatry* 1987;144:1342–1344.
4. B. A. Navia, E. S. Cho, M. L. Rosenblum. The AIDS dementia complex: II. neuropathology. *Annals of Neurology* 1986;19:525–535.
5. J. Berger. Neurologic complications of human immunodeficiency virus infection. *Journal of Postgraduate Medicine* 1987;87:72–79.
6. D. H. Gabuzda, M. S. Hirsch. Neurologic manifestations of infection with human immunodeficiency virus: Clinical features and pathogenesis. *Annals of Internal Medicine* 1987;107:383–391.
7. C. Petito et al. Vacuolar myelopathy pathologically resembling subacute combined degeneration in patients with the acquired immunodeficiency syndrome. *New England Journal of Medicine* 1985;312:874–879.
8. B. A. Navia, B. D. Jordan, R. W. Price. The AIDS dementia complex: I. clinical features. *Annals of Neurology* 1986;19:517–524.
9. Centers for Disease Control. Revision of the CDC surveillance case definition for acquired immunodeficiency syndrome. *Morbidity and Mortality Weekly Report,* August 14, 1987;36(15).
10. I. Grant. Neuropsychology and MRI in HIV infected groups. *New Research Abstracts of American Psychiatric Association Annual Meeting 1987,* p. 58.
11. Committee on a National Strategy for AIDS. *Confronting AIDS: Directions for public health, health care, and research.* National Academy Press 1986, Washington, D.C.
12. Laurie Kunches, Massachusetts Department of Public Health, at a meeting of the Massachusetts Governor's Task Force on AIDS.

Chemotherapeutic ablation.	Immune deficiency that is secondary to drugs given to treat an underlying disorder.
Cytomegalovirus.	A distinct virus, but a member of the herpes family of DNA viruses.
Embryopathy.	A morbid condition in the embryo or in a fetus which may become apparent after birth.
Hepato-splenomegaly.	Enlargement of the liver and spleen.
Histology.	The science that deals with the minute structure of cells, tissues, and organs in relation to their function.
Intravenous immunoglobulin.	A processed blood product with known antibody activity, given directly into the vein of an individual.
Lymphadenopathy.	Swollen glands that can be located anywhere in the body.
Lymphoid interstitial pneumonitis.	A particular lung disease that is commonly seen in children with AIDS. The exact etiology of this condition is not clear at present.
Mucocutaneous candidiasis.	Yeast infection of the mucous membranes; commonly known as thrush.
Parotitis.	Inflammation and swelling of the salivary glands.
Pathogen.	Any virus, bacteria, parasite, or other microorganism or other substance that causes disease.
Pneumonitis.	An infection of the lung which causes a diffuse change on a chest x-ray.
Sepsis.	An infection of the blood which can be carried to internal organs via the bloodstream.

AIDS in Children: An Overview of the Medical, Epidemiological, and Public Health Problems

Ellen R. Cooper, M.D.

Cases of AIDS in children under thirteen years of age have been described since 1982. Diagnosis is more difficult in children than in adults, owing to the more varied clinical presentation and the difficulty in interpretation of laboratory tests. Current diagnostic criteria of HIV infection are reviewed, as well as symptomatology, natural history, and controversies surrounding management and therapy. Without a full appreciation of the transmissibility of HIV, issues including school and day-care attendance and foster family placement remain emotionally charged. Conflicting public policies contribute to fears on the part of the general public. Because of the unique implications for the entire family when a child is found to have HIV infection, the health care profession has been obliged to confront complex psychosocial issues unparalleled in modern medicine. The medical community may provide one safe environment for the family, and so the burden of providing support falls to a profession only variably trained and equipped for this task. In the absence of a vaccine or a cure, public education directed at primary prevention and reduction of stigmatization are the keys to true control of the epidemic.

The acquired immunodeficiency syndrome (AIDS) was first described in homosexual males and intravenous drug users. It was recognized subsequently in recipients of infected blood products and in heterosexual partners of infected individuals. More recently, AIDS has been described in the population of infants born to infected mothers. In 1982, the first descriptions of this illness in children were reported. Retrospectively, however, cases can be diagnosed since 1979 in this young population. The total number of pediatric cases of AIDS reported to the Centers for Disease Control (CDC) was 820 as of February 8, 1988, but by 1991 this number is expected to reach over 3,000.[1]

The CDC has established strict criteria for the case definition of AIDS. Although these criteria continue to be revised, it must be underscored that many cases of symptomatic HIV infection may be excluded from the CDC count. Current studies of seroprevalence in newborns indicate that in the inner city of Boston, 1 in 55 babies may be HIV-positive at birth.[2] This approaches the highest rate of seroprevalence among newborns in New York City.[3] Many, but not all, of these children will go on to develop symptomatology. The true

Dr. Ellen R. Cooper is assistant professor of pediatrics in the Division of Infectious Diseases at the Boston University School of Medicine, and is director of the Pediatric AIDS Program at Boston City Hospital.

impact of this statistic with respect to pediatric AIDS will be addressed later in this article.

Widespread recognition of pediatric AIDS as a specific disease entity was delayed for several reasons. It was difficult to differentiate AIDS from other, already described causes of congenital immunodeficiency syndromes. This differentiation required an elaborate combination of epidemiological observations, pathological studies, and specific laboratory testing.

The clinical picture of AIDS in children remains quite distinct from that in adults. In general, there is a greater heterogeneity in the clinical presentation of pediatric AIDS. Although the well-known opportunistic infections seen in adult AIDS are also seen in some pediatric cases, other infectious agents are common. In contrast to adult cases, the types of pediatric infections first noted were bacterial, usually presenting as sepsis or meningitis. Primary viral infections with herpes virus or cytomegalovirus were also documented, but it remained difficult to prove the causal association with the now well-known retrovirus without more specific testing. Because of this and the relatively small number of cases, it was difficult to establish epidemiological associations early in the epidemic. There is also a greater severity of clinical disease in infants with AIDS, especially when those without opportunistic infections are compared to adults. Death often occurs early, sometimes before criteria are met to definitively establish the diagnosis of AIDS, thereby further complicating epidemiological surveys and investigations. These factors undoubtedly contributed to difficulties in accepting early reports of AIDS in infants, and continue to cloud efforts to define AIDS in pediatric patients.

In order to help with the appropriate diagnosis of what was a newly described disease, the Centers for Disease Control established specific case definition criteria for pediatric AIDS in 1984. These criteria required modification a year later, as it became more and more clear that the disease differed from AIDS in adults. In 1987, the CDC again revised its definition. It developed a definition of AIDS in children under thirteen years of age, as well as a classification schema for other forms of HIV infection in these children. The system was designed to aid epidemiological studies, disease surveillance, prevention programs, and health care planning and policy. So established, it is useful primarily in the establishment of public health guidelines. It is less useful clinically, and individual patients must be considered separately with regard to management and prognosis.

Current Diagnosis

Ideally, HIV infection in children is identified by the actual presence of the virus in blood or tissues. This may be confirmed by culture or antigen detection methods. Since these techniques are not standardized tests as of yet, they are not readily available in most centers. In most areas, physicians must rely on the presence of antibody in the serum as evidence of HIV exposure. This creates a particularly confusing situation when the infant is born to an infected mother. It is currently believed that the maternal antibody passively acquired by the infant from the mother while the infant is in utero may persist for up to fifteen months. If the child demonstrates persistence of HIV antibody for longer than fifteen months, he or she is considered to be truly infected, regardless of whether symptoms are present at that time. The problem arises in the child under fifteen months of age who is seropositive. Seropositivity in the asymptomatic infant cannot be used to definitively establish HIV infection. It is, however, an important marker, since it can certainly identify the infant at highest risk. If actual virus cannot be demonstrated in the blood or tissue by antigen or culture techniques, the child may be considered infected only if there is evidence of cellular and humoral immune deficiency as well as clinical symptomatology. These symptoms may include progressive neurological disease, specified secondary infectious diseases, secondary malignancies, or lymphoid interstitial pneumonitis. This last entity is a histologically unique condition that causes a chronic and debilitating lung disease in many children. As noted earlier, the definition of childhood AIDS remains extremely restrictive as to the type and severity of symptoms; thus, there is an underreporting of this disease in the United States. The new classification schema, it is hoped, will permit the identification of all children with AIDS as well as other forms of severe HIV infection. It is also hoped that the new schema will ensure that all children with HIV infection will be eligible for needed services and that these services will not be limited by statutory or regulatory definitions of AIDS.

Natural History of Disease

The natural history of disease after HIV seroconversion in the pediatric age group is not completely clear at this time.

The incubation period in the congenitally infected infant seems to be four to six months, but it can be longer than five years in the transfusion-infected child. Most cases of pediatric AIDS occur in very young children, with 50 percent of pediatric AIDS diagnosed during the first year of life and 82 percent by the age of three years.[4]

Although the clinical picture of congenital infection can and does vary significantly, a profile has been suggested. Common features include failure to thrive, lymphadenopathy, hepato-splenomegaly, chronic diarrhea, mucocutaneous candidiasis, and parotitis. Other hallmarks are recurrent fevers and bacterial and viral infections as well as interstitial pneumonitis. Children with lymphoid interstitial pneumonitis tend to become symptomatic later and have a better prognosis. Follow-up has not been extensive enough to provide true estimates of mortality, but CDC figures show that over 61 percent of children reported with AIDS are known to have died.[5]

Transmission

Since HIV infection in infants and children in this country is a relatively recent occurrence, a clear understanding of the modes of transmission is still evolving. It is well known that in adults the major routes for HIV infection are close sexual contact, particularly male homosexual contact; the sharing of needles and syringes in intravenous drug users; and the receipt of blood or blood products.

In the older child, HIV can be associated with these same established routes of infection. The number of AIDS patients identified during adolescence remains very low; this may be explained by the long latency period of the virus. Behaviors commonly accepted as high-risk may be initiated during these years, but symptoms of the disease may not become evident until young adulthood. Adolescents should therefore be considered a target population for education, counseling, and testing. Like adults, children have been exposed to HIV during blood transfusions; these cases currently represent 13 percent of all cases of AIDS in childhood. Another 5 percent of childhood AIDS cases can be attributed to blood products received as treatment for coagulation disorders.[6] There have also been a few reports of HIV transmission to children occurring as the result of sexual abuse.

Most children with AIDS, however, are born to mothers who themselves carry the virus. This perinatal exposure accounts for 80 percent of the children with AIDS.[7] Such mothers may have a history of intravenous drug use, prostitution, or multiple sexual partners. They may practice no high-risk behaviors but simply originate from particular geographic regions where heterosexual transmission is thought to play a major role. Here in New England we see a great number of patients from Haiti and central Africa, both of which are considered endemic areas at this time. At the time of their pregnancy, these mothers may be symptomatic, have AIDS or ARC, or be totally asymptomatic. Many are unaware of their HIV antibody status, thus increasing the difficulty in recognition of children at risk for congenitally acquired HIV infection.

The proof of transplacental transmission of HIV includes the suggestion by some investigators that HIV-infected infants have characteristic facial features. This would imply an embryopathy secondary to fetal infection. This suggestion remains controversial, and more children will need to be evaluated before it can be substantiated. The virus has been isolated from the tissues of fetuses as well as from umbilical cord blood, and this stands to indicate the presence of viral transmission from mother to infant. Transmission has been documented in infants who have been born by Caesarean section and so have had no exposure to vaginal secretions during the birthing process. In addition, infants have been found to be seropositive, and later symptomatic, even in instances when there has been no postnatal contact with the biological mother.

The incidence and the efficiency of HIV transmission in utero have not yet been well defined. It does seem clear at this point, however, that transmission of the virus to the fetus, while common, is not inevitable. With regard to twins, cases have been reported in which only one infant was infected. By most conservative estimates, however, approximately 60 percent of infants born to mothers who are themselves seropositive are infected with HIV.[8] There are no data to suggest that Caesarean section would lower the incidence of HIV transmission from mothers to infants, but this is certainly a question that has been raised in the medical community. Many studies are being conducted around the world in order to obtain better answers to this very important question. In Boston alone, several studies are trying to investigate the efficiency of transmission, the presence or possible importance of other cofactors that may impact on that transmission, and the effect that pregnancy itself may have on the progression of the disease in a seropositive woman.

Other types of perinatal transmission of HIV must be considered, although they probably do not play as major a role as transplacental passage of virus. These include passage of the virus via infected breast milk. In support of this as a potential risk, there has been a report of a child born by Caesarean section to a mother who received blood contaminated with HIV after the delivery of the infant. This child seroconverted, with the only identifiable exposure being breast milk.[9]

Although actual infective virus seems to be transmitted in approximately 60 percent of cases, there is a passive transfer of maternal antibody in virtually 100 percent of infants born to mothers who are themselves seropositive. This raises all sorts of social, political, and medical dilemmas, since currently we are unable to identify those infants who are most likely to become symptomatic. In those infants who are not truly infected, maternal antibody seems to decrease over months, until finally the babies become seronegative. Because this may take up to fifteen months, decisions regarding day care, immunizations, and treatment modalities often become an issue before the question of true infectivity can be resolved satisfactorily.

The actual incidence of HIV infection in infants will depend on several factors. These include the number of children born to HIV-infected women as well as the prevalence of seropositivity in the population of women who are of childbearing age. The prevalence of

HIV has been clearly shown to be dependent on the subpopulation group and the geographic area studied. For example, 59 percent of intravenous drug users in New York City are seropositive, while only 20 to 25 percent of intravenous drug users in Boston seem to be seropositive.[10] In Worcester, this percentage was even lower but has recently been found to be increasing rapidly.[11] As the number of infected women continues to rise, we can expect the incidence of HIV-infected infants to increase enormously.

The possibility of transmission of virus to family members and household contacts has been a particularly sensitive issue. To date, in spite of exhaustive studies, there has been no evidence to support the horizontal transmission of HIV with casual or usual household contact. In one family study, a mother who cared for her transfusion-infected child did seroconvert, but this was after very heavy and unusual exposure to blood, secretions, and excreta without proper hand washing or the use of gloves.[12] In another study, a brother of an HIV-infected child did become seropositive.[13] The only unusual exposure that was documented was a bite from the infected child. The causal relationship has not been positively determined in this case. Although HIV has been cultured from both tears and saliva, these are considered to be fluids with a very low titer of virus, and to date there have been no reports of transmission via exposure to these secretions.

A question has been raised as to the susceptibility of the infant and the young child to HIV. Although more investigation is needed before a clear understanding can be acquired, it seems that increased susceptibility may indeed be a factor, as evidenced by several epidemiological studies. In a study of transfusion-related AIDS, infants accounted for 10 percent of cases even though they had received only 2 percent of the total number of blood transfusions. There also seemed to be a shorter latency period between exposure to virus and onset of symptoms. This may be attributed to the relative size of transfusion, and therefore the load of virus.

Controversial Management Modalities

The mainstay of the management of the child with HIV infection has been largely a supportive one. Prompt recognition and treatment of all infections are of the utmost importance, as is the maintenance of good nutritional status. However, a few issues have prompted debate among the health care professionals who are caring for these children.

The utilization of immunizations has been controversial in the population of children infected with HIV. The potential hazards of the vaccines themselves must be weighed against the risk from the diseases they are designed to prevent. It has been suggested that the stimulation from the vaccine itself may cause a deterioration in the clinical status of an infected child.

The risk of live virus vaccines such as MMR (measles/mumps/rubella) and oral polio vaccine has been specifically debated. In general, children who are immunocompromised by other deficiencies or by chemotherapeutic ablation are at risk for acquiring the disease from a vaccine of this type. These vaccines are therefore not recommended for this population. With regard to HIV-infected children specifically, several retrospective studies have investigated the outcome when seropositive children were inadvertently given oral polio vaccine. Because no ill effects have been reported, and because not all seropositive infants are truly HIV-infected, current recommendations from the CDC suggest that if the child is asymptomatic it may be safe to administer routine immunization. Specific recommendations of the national Immunization Practices Advisory Committee in regard to the immunization of HIV-seropositive children have been published, but differences of opinion still exist.[14] Some feel that the theoretical risk is quite substantial and that until a large number of children have been studied, it may be wise to be conservative. At Boston City Hospital, we recommend the use of inactivated polio vaccine in all seropositive children, whether symptomatic or not. We feel more comfortable with this practice not only with respect to the infant's safety, but also because these children often have infected caretakers. Polio virus is shed in the stool for weeks to months after oral vaccine is given, and this would put infected guardians at some risk as well. We remain consistent in our view of the risk associated with live virus vaccine and thus withhold measles/mumps/rubella immunizations from seropositive children as well, although this represents no risk to other family contacts.

Inactivated polio vaccine is often difficult to obtain; when it is available, it is more costly than oral, live vaccine. In areas where immunization practices are being debated, the theoretical risk of the oral vaccine must be weighed against the relative accessibility of the inactivated form. Other routine vaccinations of childhood should be given, although some data suggest that the vaccine may not result in the production of functional antibody. When exposure to chicken pox occurs, these children should also be given passive immunization, although efficacy has not yet been determined.

The biggest problem in the management of the child with HIV infection is control of the recurrent infections that may progress to sepsis, pneumonia, and meningitis. Optimal strategies to prevent this have not yet been established. Many centers have recommended the use of prophylactic antibiotics, but these carry with them the risk of side effects, poor compliance, and the emergence of resistant bacterial strains.

Given the predisposition of children with HIV infection to develop recurrent bacterial infections, the use of prophylactic intravenous immunoglobulin (IVIG) has been suggested. A few studies have been reported, but no firm data that are based on controlled clinical trials are available. Because of a lack of other effective therapies, these early, subjective reports resulted in fairly widespread use of this preparation. Now, with the number of HIV-infected children climbing rapidly and the average cost per child of monthly IVIG totaling approximately $30,000 per year, there is pressure to demonstrate efficacy. In addition, some feel that monthly visits to the hospital for intravenous therapy may represent undue exposure to other infectious agents. Currently, a multicenter study funded by the National Institutes of Health is executing a double-blind placebo-controlled trial to address this issue rapidly and accurately. The Boston University School of Medicine is actively participating in this trial.

Special Antiviral Therapies: Choices and Dilemmas

The devastating and frequently occurring central nervous system disease in children with HIV infection has to be taken into consideration when a specific antiviral agent is chosen for study. Any antiviral drug that does not penetrate the blood brain barrier may be of little benefit in the pediatric age group.

As new antiviral agents become available for study in children with HIV infection, it will be important to have modes of comparison already established. In this way, all children will be able to receive therapy already proven to have some efficacy, either in control of symptoms or in activity against the retrovirus. The ultimate goal of therapy for HIV infection would be to control or ablate the infection altogether, and also restore the individual's ability to reconstitute normal immune function.

Although there are many potential targets for antiviral drugs, most recent efforts have been aimed at inhibiting the DNA polymerase that is unique to the retrovirus. Of the candidate antiviral agents for testing in children, the most publicized has been Azidothymidine (AZT). Preliminary trials have already begun in several centers so that optimal dosage regimens can be established. Although AZT has been shown to be efficacious in adults with AIDS and has been licensed for clinical use, it is not without problems. It is quite toxic, and most patients taking it have developed anemia severe enough to necessitate blood transfusion. Other cell lines of the bone marrow may also be affected. In addition, there may be other side effects, such as nausea, vomiting, and central nervous system disturbances. Although HIV antigen has been demonstrated to decrease during AZT therapy, it returns with cessation of treatment. AZT must therefore be considered lifelong therapy. It is not known how children will respond to this drug.

Severe opportunistic infections with viral, bacterial, and parasitic pathogens have spawned active research in the area of new therapies for these specific pathogens as well. New drugs have been developed and tested for cytomegalovirus, herpes, and *Pneumocystis carinii* infections. While these therapies may have no effect on HIV per se, they have had a great impact on the care of the infected patient.

Many AIDS patients, both adult and children, have received new therapies of one sort or another on experimental protocols after informed consent has been obtained. This has created a legal dilemma, especially in regard to the pediatric patient. Many of these children are in foster care families, with legal custody being in the hands of the state social services department. This brings up many legal questions of risk and liability on the part of the governmental agency that grants permission for participation in experimental protocols.

Of course, this problem is unique to pediatrics, since the patient is a minor and is therefore unable to give informed consent on his or her own behalf. Traditionally, it has been difficult to obtain permission in circumstances such as these. However, as more and more protocols become available, and as the number of children with devastating disease increases, these "experimental" therapies will become standard of care. The legal questions regarding liability will need to be weighed against the ethical issue of withholding possible effective therapy from children with otherwise fatal disease.

Public Health and Policy Issues

Education and day care of children with HIV infection is an emotionally charged topic, because of the severity of disease and the fear on the part of the general public. Pressure on those who make public policy has prompted hasty and sometimes overly conservative decisions. It is important to underscore again that there has been no documentation of HIV transmission in the school, at day care, or in any other casual setting.

Current guidelines from the Centers for Disease Control confirm that school-age children who have evidence of HIV infection can be comfortably included in the classroom setting. Certain unusual circumstances, however, do require special consideration in this regard. For example, children who have oozing lesions or recurrent bleeding or who lack control of their bodily secretions may pose a greater risk to their classmates. Moreover, children who may not be developmentally appropriate and who may therefore exhibit abnormal behavior, such as excessive biting, may need to be excluded from the general classroom. Although it is still unclear whether even these children truly represent a significant risk to their classmates, the Massachusetts Governor's Task Force on AIDS has upheld the CDC guidelines.

Currently, the true responsibility for creating guidelines to deal with this sensitive issue falls to local authorities. The guidelines are much more restrictive in some states than in others. Still other states have avoided the issue when possible. These discrepancies further fuel apprehensive parent and political groups, by underscoring the uncertainty on the part of policymakers as to the real danger that might exist. The *Report of the Surgeon General's Workshop on Children with HIV Infection and Their Families*, published in July 1987, suggests that the decision about whether to attend school is best left to the individual's physician.[15] This decision should be based on the general health of the individual and on a judgment as to whether school attendance would indeed pose a risk to the patient by way of excessive exposure to infectious agents. The report states that under ideal circumstances, an individual at the school should be aware of the diagnosis; however, the need for confidentiality gives children the right to have the information withheld from the school. The report emphasizes that realistic guidelines based on best current knowledge should be considered by school boards, principals, and physicians. Resources should be developed for dissemination and implementation of new information as it becomes available. The report also deals with the issue of day care for the preschooler or the developmentally delayed older child. It suggests that these toddlers be allowed to attend day care unless scientific evidence suggests that exposure of this sort could place at risk the other, uninfected children. So far, investigators have been unable to collect this evidence, and for this reason these children should not be excluded from day care arrangements.

In Massachusetts, conservative guidelines exclude children under three years of age with evidence of HIV infection from attending a group day care setting. This raises issues of ethical, political, and economic importance. While health care workers try to encourage HIV testing in high-risk populations, the day care guideline represents yet another negative incentive to families. With no alternative to day care, one or both parents may be forced out of the workplace to stay at home with the child. Coupled with the fact that one adult may be symptomatic from HIV infection, this adds yet another burden to an already stressful situation. Because the guidelines pertain to those infants who merely have evidence of maternal antibody (since it may not be possible to distinguish these children from those with true infection), the problem is aggravated still further. Counselors and health care workers are often faced with a difficult dilemma. Reporting to day care organizers may represent a breach of confidentiality, and so infringements of state regulations may go uncorrected anyway. The question of legal obligation in these circumstances is a most difficult one, and ultimately may have to be resolved by the judicial system.

Another area where lack of federal guidelines has forced local authorities to make difficult decisions is foster care. Because legal custody is in the hands of a government agency when a child is placed in foster care, the question of informed consent for HIV testing is a sensitive one. Physicians can obtain approval for testing from most social service agencies, but confidentiality guidelines vary. In some cases, foster families are not informed of the test results. This raises obvious questions of liability, since precautions for family members and medical care for the child in question may not be adequately addressed.

Psychosocial Issues and Counseling

Aside from all of the new and unusual questions that have been raised with regard to HIV, the psychosocial issues have created new challenges to the health care system. The stigmatization of this disease has complicated the health and social care of the infected individuals. School-age children have become the focus of teachers', other pupils', and neighbors' fears. Ostracism and resultant low self-esteem have often been the outcome of this public frenzy and fear. Adolescents who have acquired this disease by engaging in "high-risk behaviors" must deal with admissions to the behaviors in addition to the disease itself. Well-publicized incidents of discrimination, accompanied at times by acts of violence, have created an environment in which the family with an infected individual has sometimes chosen to be totally anonymous rather than search for help. This reduces the possibility of psychiatric, social service, religious, or community support.

In addition, the misconceptions within different cultural, ethnic, and even community groups have further complicated the feeling of alienation on the part of the afflicted family. Some individuals have been forced out of housing, others turned away by their family or friends. In some cases, churches have been afraid to give comfort to these families, even refusing to house funeral or memorial services. In addition to the obvious psychosocial burden on the family, this places a great stress and responsibility on the medical community, since it is often only through this system that any support may be obtained. This is considered a "safer" environment in which to vent frustrations, anger, and sadness surrounding the diagnosis; but it means that the medical staff often accepts this burden alone.

Identification of a seropositive infant brings up other problems for the family. Many of these children are already the victims of drug-using families and low socioeconomic status. When a mother is told that her infant is seropositive, she must also be told of the likelihood that she herself is infected with HIV. This message must convey the serious and usually fatal nature of the illness in the infant; the likelihood of infection and potential for illness and death in the parents; the need for changes in sexual expression in order to prevent subsequent transmission; and the possibility of avoidance of future pregnancies. Fear, guilt, and sadness further complicate an already complicated scenario. An older, uninfected sibling must face the possibility of losing not only a sibling, but both parents as well. This type of "family disease" has not been described or paralleled in modern medicine.

Any discussion of the psychosocial issues regarding HIV infection must include the medical team and other support services through which care is provided for the child. Because of the problems just discussed, caring for these patients can be a draining experience for the pediatricians, who usually see patients improve under their care. Even for physicians and others who care for chronically and terminally ill children, the family nature of this disease can be overwhelming. The social problems are far-reaching, and the feeling of impotence on the part of the medical team can reach a point of desperation. A large number of people are needed to care for a particular child, owing to the multidisciplinary nature of the required services, and this can lead to miscommunications. We have found that regularly scheduled discussion and support groups are necessary for dealing with this situation, especially as a particular child becomes more symptomatic and hospitalizations become more frequent and prolonged. As the number of infected children increases, we will have to look to other techniques to reduce burnout and depression among health care workers.

A Comprehensive Approach to the Problem

Owing to the unique problems presented to the medical community by the child with HIV infection, new approaches to the organization and execution of care have been attempted.

The Boston Comprehensive Pediatrics AIDS Program is the residential unit for infants and toddlers with HIV infection who cannot be cared for at home. The program functions within the Boston City Hospital grounds, with support from the Massachusetts Department of Public Health and the Boston Department of Health and Hospitals. It is set up as a home for these children until their parents are able to care for them or until other parenting arrangements can be made. It currently has a four-bed capacity, and, almost since the program opened in February 1987, there has been a waiting list for these beds. Respite workers provide direct child care on a twenty-four-hour basis. The philosophy of the program supports and facilitates the creation of a warm, caring environment. Through the combined efforts of a program coordinator, a social worker, a registered nurse, eight child health care workers, and volunteers, this program offers each child a specialized program for promoting maximum wellness. When it is appropriate, families are included in activities. Overnight visits, which allow the parents to learn to care for their child's special needs, may facilitate preparations for eventual discharge. This residential unit was developed for children who are medically stable and who need only "home medical care." When a child has an acute problem for which she or he needs ongoing medical care, transfer to an inpatient ward is arranged. This separation allows for a normalization of life for children while they are in the residential facility.

Also at Boston City Hospital is housed Boston's only outpatient medical clinic designed to deliver multidisciplinary care to pediatric patients with HIV infection. Care is provided through a team approach, and staffing consists of infectious disease specialists as well as other subspecialty physicians. All children are followed with nutritional and developmental assessments. Social service and educational counseling are available to all patients as well. Communication with primary care physicians who have referred patients is maintained, and the program works in close association with the Boston City Hospital Adult AIDS Program, further establishing a family-based treatment program. The same team follows the patient and helps direct decision making when the child is admitted to the hospital, thus providing care of these families. In addition, all appropriate treatment protocols are made available to these patients and their families.

Control of the Epidemic

Currently, very exhaustive attempts are being made to develop a vaccine that will prevent HIV infection in individuals who have not yet been exposed. Numerous problems exist, making the search for an effective vaccine a very difficult one. The effort is complicated by the diversity of subtypes of the virus and by the lack of knowledge regarding the actual role of antibodies and cell-mediated immunity in the defense against HIV.

The objective of most investigators working on candidate vaccines is to develop a vaccine that will induce neutralizing antibody. It has been shown, however, that most patients with HIV infection have neutralizing antibody that is not effective in preventing AIDS. Direct cell-to-cell spread of virus may exist in conjunction with virus latency to "protect" HIV from the immune system. At the present time, it is not known how vaccination will effect either seronegative or seropositive donors. Animal testing is hampered by a shortage of chimpanzees; therefore, it will probably be necessary to test most vaccines in HIV-seronegative human volunteers.

We are a long way from being able to rely on a vaccine to control this epidemic, so other avenues must be explored.

Although universal blood screening of blood and blood products for HIV has not eliminated the risk of transfusion-associated acquisition of HIV, it was an important step in decreasing the number of new cases. Because of the long latency period of the virus, however, new transfusion-related cases will continue to be diagnosed for some time.

Prevention of perinatally acquired disease will depend on the number of births to HIV-infected women. Efforts to identify and educate infected women who can transmit HIV to their children must be aggressive. Women who are at high risk must be counseled to undergo voluntary screening, and they must be educated about the risks associated with pregnancy in the seropositive mother. Of course, education must also focus on behavioral modification, including avoidance of high-risk sexual activities and of intravenous drug use.

Clearly, populations that are already at high risk must be counseled and educated. But the true spread of the AIDS epidemic will not be controlled until the general public is made aware of the risks. Containment of this disease will rest on our ability to effect changes in behavior and lifestyle so that the chain of transmission can be broken. The mass media, which often emphasize the sensational aspects of the AIDS epidemic, must educate the public so that fear does not spawn drastic policy measures that are unwarranted in terms of what is known about the actual risk.

Significant portions of the population, including intravenous drug users, adolescents, and persons with language barriers, are not being reached with the educational message conveyed through traditional media. The techniques of marketing research should be used to identify the most effective means of communicating with all segments of the population. Alternative communication resources should be explored. Only in this way can the stigmatization be reduced, thus allowing affected individuals to openly be counseled, tested, and provided with care. Without these measures, the number of HIV-infected adults, children, and infants will continue to grow to even more tragic proportions.

Notes

1. Personal communication from the AIDS Program, Center for Infectious Diseases, Centers for Disease Control, Atlanta, Georgia.

2. Personal communication from the Boston Department of Health and Hospitals, Boston, Massachusetts.

3. Bruce Lambert, "One in 61 Babies in New York City Has AIDS Antibodies, Study Says," *New York Times,* January 13, 1988, A1.

4. S. D. Barbour. Acquired immunodeficiency syndrome of childhood. *Pediatric Clinics of North America* 34, no. 1 (February 1987): 247–268.

5. *Report of the Surgeon General's Workshop on Children with HIV Infection and Their Families.* Office of Maternal and Child Health, U.S. Department of Health and Human Services, July 1987. Single copies available from the National Maternal and Child Clearinghouse, 38th and R Streets N.W., Washington, DC 20057; (202) 625–8410.

6. M. F. Rogers. AIDS in children: A review of the clinical epidemiological and public health aspects. *Journal of Pediatric Infectious Disease* 4 (1985): 230–236.

7. Ibid.

8. A. Rubinstein, M. Sicklick, et al. Acquired immunodeficiency with reversed T4/T8 ratios in infants born to promiscuous and drug addicted mothers. *Journal of the American Medical Association* 249 (1983): 2350–2356.

9. Centers for Disease Control. Recommendations for assisting in the prevention of perinatal transmission of human T-lymphotropic virus type III/lymphadenopathy-associated virus and AIDS. *Morbidity and Mortality Weekly Report* 34 (1985): 721–732.
10. Personal communication from the Massachusetts Department of Public Health.
11. Ibid.
12. Centers for Disease Control. Apparent transmission of human T-lymphotropic virus type III/lymphadenopathy-associated virus from child to mother providing health care. *Morbidity and Mortality Weekly Report* 35 (1986): 75–79.
13. V. Wahn et al. Horizontal transmission of HIV infection between two siblings. *Lancet* 2 (1986): 694.
14. Centers for Disease Control. Immunization of children infected with human T-lymphotropic virus type III/lymphadenopathy-associated virus. *Morbidity and Mortality Weekly Report* 35 (1986): 595–606.
15. *Report of the Surgeon General's Workshop on Children with HIV Infection and Their Families.*

References

A. J. Ammann, W. J. Cowan, et al. Acquired immunodeficiency in an infant: Possible transmission by means of blood products. *Lancet* 1 (1983): 956–958.

American Academy of Pediatrics. Committee on Infectious Diseases. School attendance of children and adolescents with human T-lymphotropic virus III/lymphadenopathy-associated virus infection. *Pediatrics* 77 (1986): 430–432.

S. D. Barbour. Acquired immunodeficiency syndrome of childhood. *Pediatric Clinics of North America* 34, no. 1 (February 1987): 247–268.

T. A. Calvelli, A. Rubinstein. Intravenous gamma-globulin in infant AIDS. *Journal of Pediatric Infectious Disease* 5 (1986): S207–210.

Centers for Disease Control. Classification system for human immunodeficiency virus infection in children under 13 years of age. *Morbidity and Mortality Weekly Report* 36 (1987): 225–236.

———. Education and foster care of children infected with human T-lymphotropic virus III/lymphadenopathy-associated virus. *Morbidity and Mortality Weekly Report* 34 (1985): 517–521.

———. Immunization of children infected with human T-lymphotropic virus III/lymphadenopathy-associated virus. *Morbidity and Mortality Weekly Report* 35 (1986): 595–606.

———. Recommendations for assisting in the prevention of perinatal transmission of human T-lymphotropic virus III/lymphadenopathy-associated virus and AIDS. *Morbidity and Mortality Weekly Report* 34 (1985): 721–732.

J. W. Curran, W. M. Morgan, et al. The epidemiology of AIDS: Current status and future prospects. *Science* 229 (1985): 1352–1357.

G. H. Friedland, B. R. Saltzman. Lack of transmission of HTLV-III/LAV infection to household contacts of patients with AIDS or AIDS-related complex with oral candidiasis. *New England Journal of Medicine* 314 (1986): 344–349.

H. L. Grierson, D. T. Purtilo. New developments in AIDS. *Infectious Disease Clinics of North America* 1, no. 3 (September 1987): 547–558.

J. E. Kaplan, J. M. Oleske, et al. Evidence against transmission of human T-lymphotropic virus III/lymphadenopathy-associated virus in families of children with the acquired immunodeficiency syndrome. *Journal of Pediatric Infectious Disease* 5 (1985): 468–471.

R. W. Marion, A. A. Wiznia, et al. Human T-cell lymphotropic virus type III embryopathy. A new dysmorphic syndrome associated with intrauterine HTLV-III infection. *American Journal of Diseases of Children* 140 (1986): 638–640.

K. Martin, B. Z. Katz, G. Miller. AIDS and antibodies to HIV in children and their families. *Journal of Infectious Disease* 155 (1987): 54–63.

Massachusetts Department of Public Health. Governor's Task Force on AIDS. Policies and Recommendations (January 1987).

M. F. Rogers. AIDS in children: A review of the clinical epidemiological and public health aspects. *Journal of Pediatric Infectious Disease* 4 (1985): 230–236.

A. Rubinstein, M. Sicklick, et al. Acquired immunodeficiency with reverse T4/T8 ratios in infants born to promiscuous and drug addicted mothers. *Journal of the American Medical Association* 249 (1983): 2350–2356.

Report of the Surgeon General's Workshop on Children with HIV Infection and Their Families. Office of Maternal and Child Health, U.S. Department of Health and Human Services, July 1987. Single copies available from the National Maternal and Child Clearinghouse, 38th and R Streets N.W., Washington, DC 20057; (202) 625–8410.

Glossary

ADCC.	Antibody-dependent cell-mediated cytotoxicity.
Adjuvants.	Materials used with vaccines to enhance the activity of a vaccine.
Cytotoxic (killer) T-cells.	A component of the immune response involving a subgroup of lymphocytes that kill virus-infected cells.
Lymphokines.	Chemicals produced by lymphocytes to communicate with other lymphocytes.
Transmucosally.	Across mucous membranes such as those lining the vagina and rectum.
Virion.	A single virus particle.

The Quest for an AIDS Vaccine

Robert T. Schooley, M.D.

More than fifty thousand cases of AIDS have been reported in the United States since the disease was first described in 1981. Many times this number of people are infected with human immunodeficiency virus (HIV), which has been identified as the agent responsible for the illness. The seriousness of the disease, coupled with the relatively rapid spread of HIV, has fueled the effort for development of an effective vaccine.

Much is now known about the life cycle of the virus, and about its structural components. This information, and information about methods of transmission of the virus, form the basis for a rational vaccine development program. A successful program depends both on technological advances and on the political will to create a climate in which interpretable vaccine trials can be undertaken. This review will focus on some of the impediments to rapid development and licensure of an AIDS vaccine.

Since the initial description of AIDS in 1981, and the initial definition of the human immunodeficiency virus (HIV) as the etiologic agent for the syndrome, much progress has been made in understanding the cell and molecular biology of HIV, and in defining the components of thc immune response to the agent. In parallel with the growth in basic understanding of HIV, the agent has spread rapidly in the United States and worldwide, primarily through sexual, blood-borne, and perinatal exposure. It has been estimated that between 1 million and 3 million residents of the United States are currently infected with HIV, and that at least as many individuals are infected in other parts of the world. This relatively rapid spread of HIV, despite educational efforts aimed at interdicting spread of the agent, underscores the urgent need for development of an effective AIDS vaccine. This article will outline current prospects for development of an AIDS vaccine, and will delineate the steps required for the proof of efficacy in clinical trials.

Initial Infection and Spread of HIV

HIV gains access to the body either transmucosally (across mucous membranes) in sexual

Dr. Robert T. Schooley is associate professor of medicine at the Harvard Medical School and is a member of the Infectious Disease Unit at the Massachusetts General Hospital.

transmission, or directly into the bloodstream or soft tissues with blood-borne (needle stick or transfusion) exposures (figure 1). In that the virus lives primarily within cells, it is not clear whether spread involves free virus or virus transmitted within cells. Once within the new host, the virus enters susceptible cells. The genetic material of the virus is acted upon by an enzyme known as reverse transcriptase, which is brought into the cell by the virus. The genetic material of the virus is then integrated into the host cell DNA. The virus may remain latent and be transmitted to any progeny of the infected host cell, or it may begin to reproduce and be transmitted to previously uninfected, susceptible cells. Although it is possible that a vaccine might slow secondary transmission of virus to uninfected cells, the primary goal in most vaccination programs involves prevention of establishment of the initial infection.

In the case of HIV, this initial interception of virus by the immune response might be complicated by the ability of the virus to spread directly from infected to uninfected lymphocytes through cell-to-cell spread, and by the possibility that the initial infection of host cells might occur at mucosal surfaces such as vaginal and rectal linings. Initial infection at these sites might significantly limit the effectiveness of immune response induced by traditional vaccines.

Figure 1

HIV Pathogenesis

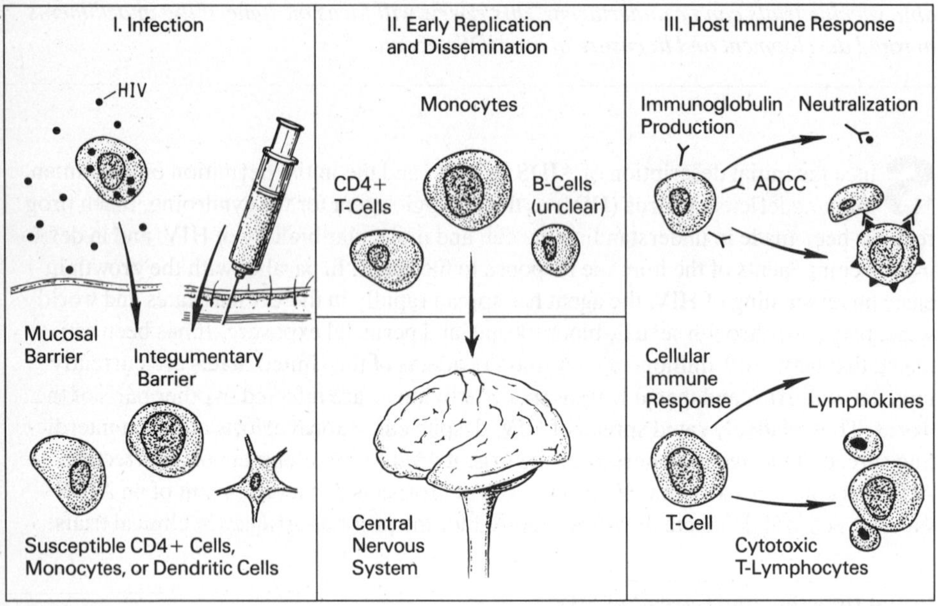

The figure describes interaction between HIV and the infected individual. The virus gains entry to the body through mucous membranes with sexual exposure, or more directly through blood-borne exposure. After entry, the virus infects certain cells of the immune system and the brain. The immune response that is evoked by the virus is multifaceted and probably slows the rate at which the virus causes illness. Greater knowledge about the characteristics of this immune response will be useful in vaccine development.

Host Immune Response to HIV

Once the virus is within an individual, replication of HIV proceeds at a rate that may be dependent on a number of factors, including the state of activation of host cells; the HIV-specific host immune response; and, possibly, virus-specific strain differences. As the initial cycles of viral replication proceed, a vigorous antibody and cellular immune response to the virus is developed. The antibody response to HIV is directed to a number of viral components. These antibodies are useful diagnostically in the identification of HIV-infected individuals, but, more important, they provide insight into the components of the virus recognized by the host as being foreign.

Antibody activity can be measured in functional assays that measure biologic effects of the antibodies. The functional assay that has been most extensively studied for the purpose of vaccine strategy is the neutralization assay. In this assay, dilutions of sera to be tested are mixed with a known amount of virus. After exposure of the virus to serum for a defined length of time, the ability of the serum-exposed virus to infect susceptible cells is tested. If protection of susceptible cells by a given dilution of serum is demonstrated, the serum is said to contain neutralizing activity at that dilution. Neutralizing activity appears within the serum of most HIV-infected individuals within the first several months following infection. These assays are useful in planning vaccine approaches because they permit investigators to determine which parts of the virus are able to elicit antibodies that cripple its ability to infect host cells. In the case of HIV-1 (the most common AIDS virus type in the United States), this neutralizing activity is most easily demonstrated in antibodies that react with the envelope (surface) of the virus.

Although one can demonstrate neutralizing activity specific for the envelope of HIV-1, such knowledge is far from sufficient for providing an effective vaccine. As noted above, such antibodies must be present at the site of initial infection, such as the rectal or vaginal mucosa. Furthermore, HIV possesses an envelope that varies significantly from strain to strain. In addition to the two currently known types of HIV, within each type there are many, many strains. Thus, an antibody that is able to neutralize one strain of virus may be less able to neutralize other strains of virus, or may be incapable of doing so. In addition, with the description of a second type of HIV, now termed HIV-2, which was initially isolated in west Africa, vaccine development is faced with the need to deal with at least two types of HIV.

Although the antibody response to HIV is the aspect of the immune response which has been most intensively studied, it is clear that neutralizing antibodies represent only one component of a multifaceted response. In addition to antibodies that neutralize the virus, cytotoxic (killer) T-cells are induced by HIV infection. These cells are capable of seeking out and killing HIV-infected cells. They, thus, form a second impediment to uncontrolled replication of the virus, and may play an important role in slowing the rate at which HIV causes symptoms in infected individuals. These cytotoxic T-cells are directed at the envelope of HIV, but, in addition, cells with activity against other components of HIV are present. The other components of HIV tend to vary less from strain to strain and thus are more conserved. These observations are of importance in AIDS vaccine development in that inclusion of more strictly conserved components might allow development of vaccines that have activity against a wider variety of strains.

Because of the relentless progress of infection in most individuals, the effectiveness of the HIV-specific immune response that can be detected within the first several months of infection has been called into question. Despite this consideration, it should be noted that individuals, once infected with one strain of virus, are rarely, if ever, infected by other strains, even when repeated exposure to other strains occurs frequently. This suggests that although the naturally occurring immune response might fail to prevent onset of disease following infection, it is at least capable of preventing infection with additional strains of virus. Thus, if an immune response that closely mimics the response following natural infection can be elicited by an AIDS vaccine, subsequent infection with live virus might well be preventable.

Steps in the Development of an AIDS Vaccine

As basic understanding of the HIV-specific immune response is developed, application of this information to the technical aspects of vaccine development will be increasingly effective. Induction of an effective immune response requires delivery of an appropriate stimulus (termed *antigen*) to the immune system prior to exposure to the natural agent. Antigen delivery may be achieved through the use of either living or nonliving material (table 1). One of the oldest approaches to vaccines has involved growing the agent itself in the laboratory, then purifying and killing it by chemical means. The purified, killed material is then injected into the individual being vaccinated and, thus, is presented to the immune response. The magnitude of the immune response is highly dependent on how a vaccine is delivered (that is, whether it is injected or given by other routes) and on carrier or other materials (termed *adjuvants*) that may be added to the killed virus. Killed virus approaches have the advantage that they are technologically straightforward, but the disadvantage that most of the material injected consists of portions of the infectious agent that are irrelevant to the immune response in developing protective immunity. Thus, the theoretical possibility exists that undesired vaccine side effects may be induced by the presence of unnecessary vaccine components. Finally, there is the unlikely possibility that the inactivation procedure may be incomplete. If the vaccine preparation steps do not completely kill the virus, infection with the agent for which the vaccine is intended in the first place could occur. In addition, there has been at least one instance in which killed vaccine was contaminated with a virus of a different type (in the case of an early lot of polio vaccine) which was not killed by the inactivation procedure. Although these two latter possibilities are increasingly unlikely with modern technology, they are not totally outside the realm of possibility.

Table 1

Antigen Delivery Systems

A. Nonliving antigen delivery systems
   1. Killed whole virus
   2. Viral components
      a. Purified from whole virus
      b. Prepared by recombinant DNA technology

B. Live antigen delivery systems
   1. Attenuated virus
   2. Viral components carried by a nonpathogenic (or minimally pathogenic) unrelated virus

A second approach to vaccine preparation using nonliving material involves use of viral components, termed *subunits*. These subunits can be purified from whole, killed virus, or they can be prepared with DNA technology. This approach involves introduction of a selected portion of the viral genetic information into the genetic material of another living organism, such as a bacterium or a yeast. The material normally encoded by the viral gene selected is then made by the new host. When the new host is grown in the laboratory, large amounts of the HIV component are also produced. This material can then be purified and utilized as a vaccine. The advantage of this approach is that it has the potential to produce well-characterized portions of the virus at great purity. By selecting a portion of the viral genetic material which encodes for portions of the virus which appear to be targets of the protective component(s) of the immune response, one can avoid introduction of deleterious or irrelevant viral components. Thus, one could include only selected portions of the viral envelope or other components. Recombinant DNA technology has the disadvantage, however, of producing material that might be more likely to induce an immune response that is specific only for the strain (or closely related strains) from which the initial genetic information was procured. Recombinant DNA technology also runs the risk of producing material that will be slightly different from the material encoded by the native gene, owing to events that occur within cells following initial protein production. These events relate mainly to the way in which the proteins are folded after production, and to the addition of sugar molecules. Newer developments in molecular biology have circumvented some, but not all, of these problems.

Live virus approaches have several potential advantages over those utilizing nonliving material. These include the fact that vaccine delivery may be achieved without injection (for example, through oral or aerosol routes). It has also been said that live agent approaches may be more likely to stimulate a more global immune response, both in terms of the viral components recognized and in terms of the development of immunity at likely sites of infection, such as mucosal surfaces. The live virus approach that is used most frequently involves the introduction of changes (termed *attenuation markers*) in the normal viral genetic material which make the agent less likely to cause disease. A virus that has been modified by addition of these attenuation markers is termed an *attenuated virus*. Once the host has dealt with the attenuated virus, the immune response developed during this interaction is capable of preventing infection with the natural (wild) virus. This approach is the one that was used in the production of the Sabin vaccine for polio.

The final potential advantage of live agent vaccines is that they might spread to unvaccinated contacts of the persons initially vaccinated. Thus, vaccinating one individual might lead to the protection of others, who become secondary vaccinees. Secondary vaccination may be good for the population, but the potential for harm exists, as well, if the attenuated agent is introduced into individuals whose immune responses are incapable of preventing morbidity even from the attenuated strain of virus used in the vaccination. The biggest drawback concerning the use of attenuated viruses as vaccines relates to uncertainty as to whether the changes introduced to include attenuation are stable. If these attenuation markers revert to the wild state after replication begins to occur in an individual receiving the vaccine, the deleterious effects are obvious.

An alternative to using attenuated virus involves the insertion of a portion of the viral genetic material important for induction of immunity into an agent that does not normally cause illness. As the agent of low pathogenicity replicates, the host immune response is also presented with the immunologically relevant portion(s) of the agent being vaccinated against. The resulting immune response then, in theory, prevents infection with the wild agent if it is subsequently encountered. Although this approach shares many of the advantages of the attenuated virus approach, the possibility of inadvertently introducing wild virus is eliminated. One of the potential hazards, however, relates to concerns that while the carrier virus chosen might be unable to cause disease in individuals with intact immune responses, it might be capable of causing severe disease in individuals with immune dysfunction. In the case of the most intensively studied carrier virus (vaccinia), such concerns would exist in vaccination plans in which individuals who were already HIV-infected might be inadvertently vaccinated. This concern would include either direct or secondary vaccination, as discussed above.

Current Status of HIV Vaccine Research

At the time of this writing (March 1988), a large number of academic and industrial investigators have focused attention on AIDS vaccine research and production. Most of the scientific attention has centered on approaches that utilize the viral envelope or portions of the envelope as the primary component of candidate vaccines. Live and killed virus approaches have succeeded in producing immunogenes (vaccines) that induce neutralizing antibodies in laboratory animals ranging from mice to nonhuman primates. To date, most, if not all, of the animals vaccinated have produced antibodies that will neutralize only the strain or type of the virus from which the candidate vaccine was derived. Thus, attempts to produce a vaccine that might offer broad protection against a wide variety of strains or types have been unsuccessful. Vaccines useful in the United States may have limited utility in parts of the world where other viral strains are prevalent.

Only a handful of studies have progressed to the point that chimpanzees have been vaccinated with a candidate vaccine and then have been challenged with live virus. Most of these studies have not yet been reported in peer-reviewed scientific literature. In these studies, in general, although neutralizing antibodies have been elicited by the candidate vaccines, animals subsequently inoculated with live virus, even of the vaccine strains, have become infected. This failure to prevent infection might stem from any one of a number of factors. These include the inadequacy of the candidate vaccine and the probability that the live virus inoculation studies have used an excess amount of virus. In the chimpanzee challenge studies performed to date, most animals are challenged intravenously with many thousands of infectious virions. In human infection, it is clear that most sexual exposures do not result in transmission of virus. Those exposures which result in infection may do so because slightly more virus is present, or because of defects in the rectal or vaginal surfaces. Thus, in order for the chimpanzee challenges to accurately reflect human infection, it would be necessary to develop a model whereby animals were inoculated with much smaller amounts of virus, preferably administered to mucosal surfaces. In such inoculations, most animals would not become infected. In order to demonstrate protection, it would be necessary to vaccinate a large number of chimpanzees, and to then inoculate them with a small enough amount of virus that most of them would not become infected, even if unvaccinated. In such a study, one might immunize 100 animals with a test vaccine and another 100 with a sham (or fake) vaccine. One would then inoculate each animal with an amount of virus just in excess of what might infect a minority of unvaccinated animals. At the end of a study like this, a successful vaccine might reduce the number of infected animals from 8 of the 100 in the sham-vaccinated group to 2 of the 100 in the group receiving the active vaccine. Such studies would require tens to hundreds of chimpanzees per vaccine candidate. Given the short supply of chimpanzees, and the cost of each animal (currently approximately $70,000), it is unlikely that such studies are feasible.

Thus, at this point, a number of vaccine candidates have been developed. Many produce neutralizing antibodies in vaccinated animals. None has yet been demonstrated to protect animals from live virus challenge. Even if a vaccine demonstrated protection from infection in the chimpanzee model, it would not necessarily imply protection of humans in the real world setting. Therefore, even with all the knowledge theoretically available from animal studies, human vaccine studies will be required prior to licensure of an AIDS vaccine.

Human Studies with Candidate AIDS Vaccines

The human studies that must be undertaken in the evaluation process for AIDS vaccines will be patterned after such studies with other vaccines in the past. A logical sequence of studies progressing from simple dose-finding studies to larger-scale clinical trials will assure the most timely evolution of AIDS vaccine and will minimize the inherent risks to study subjects which are encountered with evaluation of any vaccine or drug product.

The process that is generally followed involves Phase I studies, in which the candidate vaccine is administered to a small group of healthy human volunteers who are at minimal risk for acquiring the agent being vaccinated against. In these studies, the primary goal is to determine whether any toxicities not anticipated from animal studies might be manifest in human subjects. In addition, through the use of several laboratory assays, these studies seek to measure the magnitude of the immune response induced by the vaccine. This endeavor will not necessarily identify adverse effects that might occur at a low frequency or that might occur in populations not included in the preliminary testing. The immunologic changes that are measured will be useful only in that they will indicate whether the immunologic impact of the vaccine in humans is similar to that experienced by animals in the prior studies.

The Phase I studies might involve several different vaccination schedules or doses of vaccine, and might compare the magnitude of the response encountered when the vaccine is given with various adjuvants (immune-enhancing materials). In some vaccine development programs, the Phase I studies are performed in several stages, in which adverse and immunologic effects are measured in a very small group of volunteers (five to ten persons) before they are repeated or modified for application to a larger number of volunteers.

After Phase I testing has been completed, information should be in hand about optimal dosing schedules and adverse effects of a vaccine. The next phase of the studies focuses on whether a vaccine actually prevents infection in the field. In such studies, members of a group or groups at risk for acquiring the agent are recruited and invited to participate in a placebo-controlled trial. In these studies, subjects are randomly allotted to one of two or three groups who will either receive the vaccine candidate or an identical-appearing placebo. Subjects are allotted by chance to these groups; neither the subject nor the investigator knows who receives the theoretically active material. Subjects are then followed to determine whether the group or groups receiving the vaccine are infected at a lower rate over time than those who receive the placebo. Only after such evidence is in hand is a vaccine considered safe and effective and is it offered for general use. Such information is mandatory, because premature licensure and use of an ineffective vaccine would give the public a false sense of security and would encourage behavior that would increase the rate of infection. In general, most effective vaccines offer a significant degree of protection, but not complete protection. The speed with which a trial can demonstrate the effectiveness of a vaccine is directly related to the rate at which the study population acquires the agent being studied, and to the proportion of vaccinated individuals who are protected from infection by virtue of being vaccinated.

Although the need for such studies seems self-evident, in the case of AIDS vaccine studies practical and ethical concerns will make them extremely difficult to design. In the initial studies, it will be critically important to be certain that individuals who are already infected with HIV, or who are likely to become so in the ensuing several months, are excluded. This is important, since one would not wish to put a potentially useful vaccine at risk of being prematurely discarded because clinical manifestations of HIV infection are mistaken for untoward effects of the vaccine. In most vaccine studies in the past, these concerns have caused investigators to move totally out of "at risk" groups for the very early studies. Politically, this might prove to be difficult with respect to an AIDS vaccine, since individuals at risk for HIV infection have expressed a strong desire to be an integral part of any vaccine studies, from even the earliest phase through the finish. This consideration has caused some investigators to consider offering enrollment to HIV-seronegative homosexual men who have been abstinent for three months and who will guarantee abstinence during the period of the vaccine trial.

In the placebo-controlled trial, in which participants will be at risk of HIV infection, other ethical considerations are operative. Subjects must understand the study design in terms of the placebo inclusion. They must be told that even if they receive active material, the vaccine may not work. Finally, participants must be counseled about modes of infection and must be advised not to put themselves at risk of infection. To the extent that the counseling is effective, it will be increasingly difficult to demonstrate a protective effect of the vaccine. This is related to the fact that in order for a vaccine to demonstrate protection from infection, vaccine recipients and control subjects need to have a significant exposure rate. If trial members receive vaccine or placebo, and then are never exposed to the virus, it will not be possible to determine whether the vaccine is protective. An additional consideration relates to the need to protect the confidentiality of study subjects. This extends beyond usual concerns for such studies, because vaccinees will likely be designated HIV-seropositive by the standard HIV serologic screening tests. To the extent that widespread mandatory testing is employed or appears to be on the horizon, potential vaccine study participants will have a strong disincentive to take part in such vitally important trials. It has been proposed that vaccine trial participants be given certificates indicating participation in HIV vaccine trials in order to indemnify them from retribution from insurance companies and others. These certificates might or might not be useful to

Table 2

Attributes of an Ideal AIDS Vaccine

1. Effective against a wide variety of HIV strains and types
2. Lacking immunopathogenic or other untoward effects
3. Effective against genital, blood-borne, or percutaneous exposure
4. Inexpensive to prepare
5. Easy to administer
6. Stable upon storage

participants, and would certainly expose them to a loss of confidentiality in terms of risk group behavior if they were utilized.

A final consideration relates to the fact that successful completion of placebo-controlled vaccine studies in one risk group will not assure protection to persons in other risk groups. In the case of sexual exposure, it is likely that less virus is presented than with intravenous exposure with intravenous drug use and in transfusion-associated HIV transmission. In addition, in that intravenous drug users and hemophiliacs not infected by HIV are frequently immunosuppressed by drugs and clotting factors, respectively, the immunologic response to a candidate vaccine might be less vigorous than that in healthy homosexual men. Thus, it will be necessary to carry out vaccine trials in several different risk group populations (for example, homosexual men, intravenous drug users, heterosexuals, and hemophiliacs).

The Ideal Vaccine

The ideal AIDS vaccine must satisfy several requirements (table 2). Development of such a vaccine requires a thorough understanding of the modes of transmission of HIV, of the mechanisms by which the virus causes illness and death, and of strain variability among HIV isolates. The ideal vaccine must be safe; effective against a variety of HIV isolates; protective against either sexual or blood-borne exposure through needle sticks; inexpensive to produce; easy to administer; and stable in storage for prolonged periods. Technological progress in basic vaccine design over the past decade makes it likely that such a vaccine will ultimately be produced. However, the impediments to development of such a vaccine are substantial and are unlikely to be overcome in the near future. Although any timetable must be viewed as highly speculative, a possible one is presented in table 3. The vaccine development process is already well under way, having begun with the initial description of the syndrome in 1981. As outlined in the table, vaccine development should be viewed as an orderly process that consists of a series of temporally overlapping but discrete phases. At the present time, limited dose-finding studies have begun. These studies seek to determine whether vaccine preparations are safe to administer, and what dosing schedule induces the most potent immune response. Once an optimal dosing regimen has been established, larger, more elaborate trials will be required to determine whether the vaccine or vaccines actually prevent infection. Following this demonstration in several risk groups, the vaccine will be made available for commercial production. Although it is extremely difficult to make such predictions with precision, it seems unlikely to this author that AIDS vaccines will be widely available until at least 1994 or 1995.

Table 3

Timetable, Past and Potential, in the Development of an AIDS Vaccine

1981	Clinical recognition of acquired immunodeficiency syndrome
1983–84	Identification of HIV as etiologic agent for AIDS
1984–87	Delineation of components of HIV recognized by host immune response
1987–88	Phase I human studies (safety and dose finding)
1989–93	Phase II and Phase III human studies (controlled larger-scale clinical trials with vaccine candidates)
1994–95	AIDS vaccine licensure

Conclusion

In summary, much is now known about the immune response to HIV. This basic knowledge has formed the framework for initial plans for developing AIDS vaccines. AIDS vaccine studies have progressed to the point that portions of the virus have been identified which are capable of generating neutralizing activity in animals. To date, however, no vaccine preparation has been shown to prevent infection with live HIV following a challenge with the pathogenic virus. Human studies are in the earliest phase at this writing, but are both technically and ethically highly complex. It is likely that a vaccine or vaccines that offer a degree of protection, if not full protection, will be developed. It is the opinion of this investigator that such a development is at least five years away.

Other Journeys

Phillip Dross

Phillip Dross was a writer. He was forty-three years of age when he died of AIDS in January 1987. Four years earlier, he had come to Newburyport, Massachusetts, to live and to face hard realities about himself— the legacy of a painful, confusing childhood in Florida, where he grew up, bouts with alcoholism, and his own shortcomings as a writer, for although he drove his friends to distraction talking about writing, he could not endure long hours alone, especially at the typewriter.

He made progress — the slow, plodding progress that characterizes the struggle within oneself that can be resolved only within oneself. And then, the diagnosis of HIV infection brought him face to face with new realities and the final confrontation with self.

Ironically, his writing was never better. Stripped both of the need for and the diversion of pretense, of the excesses that often mar the work of writers who seduce themselves with the sheer abundance of their own talents, he developed clarity, economy, and a pristine, almost fastidious, sense of the sufficient.

The disease spread rapidly. Months before the end he could no longer hold a pen or use a typewriter, and finally he lost the ability to speak.

But, of course, he still speaks . . .

---

21 September 1985

I would call this the first day of winter. Yesterday had the signs that today promised. A subtle quality I felt, certain summer was over. I only recognized two seasons, warm and cold. Fall is wonderful, crisp, clear, gloriously colorful, and cold. The air is dry, smelling of apples and manure, wildflowers and pine.

This clumsy drivel is without meaning.

Ever so slowly I become cognizant of what I'm supposed to be doing, aware gradually of just how I'm going to beat this disease. . . . The task looms larger every day and my faith in myself stays just ahead of the doubt. The magnitude of the change required daunts me, but the changes are long-time heart's desires. It's how I have wanted to change myself and couldn't figure a way. It is, in other words, a welcome challenge in many ways. I

These extracts from Phillip Dross's diary were compiled by his friend David Polando.

could have continued, would not have discovered, would not have learned, had the shock not been mortal.

I have AIDS. Can you imagine! I would have told you that I could imagine it once, but the reality has a quality beyond imagination. I guess nothing in recent history has so stirred the imagination as this disease has. The reaction in the general public seems to reach beyond reason in dark primal areas of fear. Suddenly one cannot avoid the subject. On television, radio, in newspapers and magazines, it is omnipresent. It took me about two months to absorb, to really fully comprehend, that they were talking to me when they said AIDS victim. I have developed a slurring in my speech which only now diminishes slightly, recurring when I am tired or speaking about it. I am still unable to write, my hand shakes uncontrollably. At the social security office I sat for an hour refusing to believe I couldn't fill out the forms, could not write my name! Relieved and rescued by a kind woman, or I might still be there utterly bewildered.

27 September 1985

Okay. I'm 42 years old. I have AIDS. I have no job. I do get $300.00 a month from social security and the state. I will soon receive $64.00 a month in food stamps. I am severely depressed. I cannot imagine how I will acquire even a part-time job off the books so as not to endanger my disability status. I cannot live on $300.00 a month. After $120.00 a month for rent and $120.00 a month for therapy, I am left with $60.00 for food and vitamins and other doctors and maybe acupuncture treatments and my share of the utilities and oil and wood for heat. I'm sure I've forgotten several expenses like a movie once in a while and newspaper or a book.

All this doesn't include my worry about the disease. I find that I tire easily, so a job is a mixed desire. My car is not very dependable either. It seems as if I am trapped in a dilemma, largely of my own making, from which I see no escape. I have determined that this writing down in black and white of my situation must at least lump it all together and provide perhaps a clue to the solution — there must be a solution — mustn't there?

I am still alive. Is it too late to reconstruct my life? How can I still live if I can't manage to afford life?

I wake up every day facing these things — trying to maintain the positive outlook I must have if I am to surmount this illness.

I never planned on this scenario.

I am rapidly running out of food, of vitamins, of money, of ideas, of hope.

3 October 1985

Today is schizophrenic, or rather I am schizo today, up one minute — way down the next. This phenomenon does give one the impression that there is movement, and that is some comfort. This morning I couldn't think why I should go on living and tonight I feel confident that I shall. Even the eleven o'clock news about AIDS doesn't get to me. The incessant coverage is a major trial to bear, but life has become all trial, with little or no recess. If checking out were easy — if one could lightly reject the quality of one's life — determining that it was insufficient, I would have done it weeks ago. It is not, however, easy. I still cannot figure out how to do it, so I suppose I'm not ready after all.

8 October 1985

Can't figure out why it's so hard to write. It was a shock to discover I hadn't written in all this time. How sad to waste the days like this. It's not like I have days to waste. I don't seem to get depressed in the same way lately, or maybe I'm simply getting used to being depressed. I wake up dreading the days. They stretch before me empty and lonely, without meaning. The flavor is gone.

26 December 1985

Wan sunlight and slightly blue sky dress this bitterly cold day. This present approach to the typewriter has been even more fraught with dread than before, preceded by weeks of thought, anticipated with unspeakable fear and trembling. Events here evolve with unabated pace, though I can't fault their character.

On the physical front, I continue to feel rather good. The last blood tests were much improved. The cancer grows only slowly. Saturday I see my acupuncturist's teacher from England, reputed to be preeminent in the field. I continue to seek after a job, with some leads but no action.

My mental condition has improved somewhat, only more slowly than I had hoped.

January 1986

I am a pacifist at war with myself, a world at war, a man spending his life in self-destruction, a dog snarling at his own image on the surface of the water.

10 June 1986

Understanding what's happening is not easy. I have AIDS, the word terminal is associated with this condition, and not getting better is a new experience. When you have a cold you get better, a toothache, you have it attended to, this is a singularly different experience. The levels of my acceptance continue, and the closer I come to a real acceptance, the better it feels. There is a peacefulness associated with the simplicity imposed by the physical realities of the disease. I can't work anymore, so I'm home a lot, and alone, and free to contemplate the whole situation — not always a pleasant experience.

Last week I said to myself, "well as soon as I feel less tired, I'll write some of this down." The next day I realized I may not feel less tired, what then?

I go to a gym three times or four times a week. I've never done drugs in my life, and the man that I thought was sitting home being as nice as I was was obviously doing other things, and he infected me. I went through a lot of things before they diagnosed me. I went through six months of biopsies, and I got cut up, and sliced up, and I got spinal taps 'cause I wasn't in the so-called high-risk category and that's something that I think is really important. They have to stop going on about high risk and low risk because I wouldn't have gotten sliced up and cut up and put to sleep and put in the hospital over and over again like I did had they just said, "These are your symptoms; this is what you might have, even though you're a white, middle-class female."

AIDS: Prophecy and Present Reality

Victor De Gruttola, D.Sc.
William Ira Bennett, M.D.

Mathematical modeling of the AIDS epidemic can be useful for policymakers even though precise projections are not possible at this time. Models are useful in establishing ranges for current and future prevalence of HIV infection and incidence of AIDS, as well as in predicting the effect of a given intervention strategy. Most decision makers are using models implicitly when they use epidemiological information as a basis for policy; formulating a model explicitly permits examination of the underlying assumptions. By creating and testing a variety of models, an investigator can determine whether the models reflect more the underlying assumptions or the available data. Modeling is a process that helps the policymaker test and refine his or her own beliefs about the future of the epidemic and the effect of behavioral intervention. In this report, the process is examined in relation to five policy problems posed by the AIDS epidemic.

Because AIDS is, in many respects, an utterly novel disease, formulation of policy has proved difficult. In the normal course of events, policymakers rely on experience — often, to be sure, quantified experience — to reach decisions. The duration of the world's experience with AIDS amounts, for all intents and purposes, to half a decade. If sound policy is to be developed soon enough to be of any value in protecting public health, ways must be found to maximize the amount and accuracy of information that can be extracted from such a brief history.

In this instance, the strategy for wringing wisdom from brief experience has two major components.

First, people well versed in several different analytic strategies must collaborate to create models of the disease. Such models can be used as a basis for investigating policy options. ("Policy" in this case includes not only such obvious elements as legislative or police action to interdict transmission, but targeting and content of educational and screening programs, as well as the design of research projects.) A wide variety of models

Dr. Victor De Gruttola is assistant professor of biostatistics at the Harvard School of Public Health. Dr. William Ira Bennett is editor of the Harvard Medical School Health Letter *and is lecturer on medicine at the Harvard Medical School.*

based on very different assumptions must be available for this approach to be useful. If a certain strategy is optimal in most models, for all reasonable assumptions used to construct them, then the strategy may be regarded as "robust" to the choice of model. If a strategy makes sense only for models with very specific and untestable assumptions, then the strategy is open to serious question.

Second, models must be repeatedly tested against new data from the epidemic itself to see how close they come to being true. If models are constructed, tested, and revised in a reasonably formal, iterative fashion, many errors can be corrected before they become misleading.

Like it or not, this is the only procedure available for guiding us through the epidemic, and everyone in a position to make decisions about AIDS policy uses it, though most of the time in tacit or informal ways. The hazard of informality is that people will behave as though solutions were easier than they are, or alternatively, that they will respond to the complexity of the task with inaction.

In this article, we wish to discuss the features that make models of AIDS useful and the limitations of such models which must be explicitly recognized. We will also discuss the different types of models that may be developed; some models require complex assumptions about sexual behavior and biological characteristics of HIV infection, while others may be more strictly mathematical.

Further, we will consider five policy problems and the type of information that must be obtained to approach them: (1) whether to close sites for anonymous sex, such as bathhouses; (2) whether to promote use of condoms and "safer sex" behaviors, or, as a variant of this question, whether to concentrate resources on increasing condom use or reducing needle-sharing behavior; (3) how to use AIDS tests for screening; (4) how to budget and allocate resources for the future growth of the epidemic; and (5) what information to collect to improve the accuracy of predictions about the disease and therefore the value of interventions.

The "Reality" of the Model

Suppose that we are interested in estimating the rate of growth of the epidemic by different regions and by different routes of infection throughout the United States. In other words, we want information sufficiently fine-grained to provide an estimate of the difference between rates of growth among heterosexuals living on the West Coast and heterosexuals in New York. Two factors will determine the accuracy of the estimates.

The first is bias. Our estimate may have to be based, at least partly, on the experience of a population that does not accurately represent the population in which we are most interested. For example, the information on rate of growth of the epidemic among heterosexuals in New York may or may not be of any use in estimating the rate of growth among heterosexuals on the West Coast or among intravenous drug users in New York. If it is not, then using such information in estimating rates for other populations may give biased results.

The second factor is variance. The variance of an estimate refers to the range of values in which the estimate is likely to lie; if the range is small, then the estimate is known precisely. For example, if we are interested in rate of growth of heterosexually acquired AIDS on the West Coast, we could simply report the observed annual increase in number of cases. Such observed rates of growth are likely to be very unstable estimates of the real rate because of the small number of people who have acquired AIDS from heterosexual contact on the West Coast. Our estimate is unbiased (provided that reporting is accurate), because it is based exclusively on the population of interest; yet, it is not precise. There are so few of these cases that minor, random fluctuations in the epidemic or in reporting would have a large effect on estimates of growth rate; the variance is very high. Thus, the effect of splitting the data into fine categories is to generate values with minimal bias but high variance.

It is a fundamental limitation of model-based estimates, however, that they do not work equally well to minimize bias and to estimate variance.

An alternative approach to "splitting" is "lumping" — combining data on heterosexuals in all regions, for example, or combining data on all risk groups from one region. The number of cases is now larger, so variance is decreased. But your estimate for the specific group of interest (West Coast heterosexuals) may be highly biased if the epidemic is growing at different rates in different regions or as a function of the route of exposure to the AIDS virus.

The basic choice between lumping or splitting is itself a form of modeling. You believe either that all regions of the country are alike or that they are so different that there's nothing to be learned on the West Coast from the experience of the East Coast. Both models take extreme positions. One minimizes bias while forgetting variance; the other does the opposite. The best approach may be to construct an intermediate model that makes some trade-off between bias and variance.[1] The drawback is that this procedure requires more thought.

To estimate growth rate among West Coast heterosexuals, you could devise a weighted average combining the observed rate of growth in that specific category with an expected value of this rate based on the observed rates in other, more broadly defined categories. The weights depend on the amount of data in each category. When there are a lot of data, they are heavily weighted. But when data are sparse, more weight is given to estimates derived from related cells with larger numbers (such as all American heterosexuals or all people on the West Coast, regardless of the route of exposure to the AIDS virus). Technically, the weights are inversely related to the relative sizes of the variance estimates for the two approaches to estimation. This procedure takes advantage of the similarities between the coasts and the various groups at risk, while acknowledging that there may be important differences. The less sure we are about the differences, the more we depend on similarities to draw inference.

The point of this example is to illustrate that a model may be made more complex by having it allow for smaller and smaller effects, or by making finer divisions in region or category of risk. In general, this procedure reduces the amount of bias, but it can also reduce precision of an estimate applied to a particular region or risk group of interest, because finer distinctions necessarily reduce the number of cases in any given category.

To the extent that the obligation for AIDS planning and policy falls on states and local jurisdictions, it becomes important to recognize the perils of projecting trends in specific categories (drug users in Baltimore, heterosexuals in San Francisco) and to be aware of the techniques appropriate for attempting such projections. In particular, the trade-off between minimizing bias and minimizing variance must be kept in mind.

It is important not only to get a precise estimate of the average value of a given parameter, such as the rate of new partner acquisition, but also to estimate the variability in that rate. Even if we had an accurate estimate of the average number of new partners acquired by sexually active people but did not know the variability in this number, our models might be very misleading. There is good theoretical reason to believe that the growth of the AIDS epidemic, at least in its early phases, was driven by a small group of very promiscuous gay men. The ratio of the variance in acquisition of new partners to the mean for the gay male population at large appears, from one important study, to have been the driving factor that determined the rate of growth of AIDS.[2] This hypothesis, if true, has important implications for strategies to control the epidemic. As long as the hypothesis remains viable, it implies that collecting information about the range of behaviors is as important as getting an accurate estimate of the average number.

The point of our examples is this: The type of model you choose for analyzing any given situation is a matter of style, emphasis, and purpose. Models are designed to answer specific questions, not to reproduce reality. At the end of the 1980s, what we want from a model of AIDS is to know the small number of major factors that determine the answer to a given policy question. We want to be able to distinguish between these crucial factors and the remaining details. Nevertheless, when there is insufficient information to make a clear distinction, you may ask a simple question and still get a complex answer.

Toward a Model of AIDS

A useful model of the evolving AIDS epidemic requires many inputs and a complex sampling procedure. Models of the AIDS epidemic may be constructed for a variety of purposes. One of the most difficult challenges is to estimate the future number of AIDS cases for a given population. Currently among the most important goals of modeling is testing the potential effect of a strategy for intervention. Models can also be useful for learning what information needs to be collected, and with what precision. For example, simple modeling of the heterosexual epidemic reveals that there is little point in gathering very detailed information about heterosexual behavior unless more information about the time course of infectiousness is also gained.

The utility of models should not, however, be seen as just a slightly more quantitative way of guessing about the future than inspecting the entrails of dead birds. Models can be used to answer questions about the validity of contemporary observations (What is the evidence that behavior is really changing? Can the epidemic be propagated by heterosexual transmission? When will the epidemic peak in San Francisco?)

Information required to model some aspect of the AIDS epidemic is likely to include one or more of the following:

- the rate at which the virus is transmitted from one person to another, according to sex of partner, along with each of the potential routes of contagion (sexual activity, type of blood-borne contact, and so forth)
- how this rate changes over the course of infection
- a measure of how transmission is influenced by the presence of cofactors, such as other diseases and use of drugs
- the rate at which susceptible partners (sexual, drug using) are acquired
- the frequency and type of sexual contact between such partners

- the average duration of the relationship during which the relevant activities occur

- the extent to which the relationships and activities occur within relatively closed networks, as opposed to extending throughout the population

- the elapsed time between becoming infected and becoming ill (really the distribution of times, now known to range from a few months to more than seven years)

Because, in practice, the whole epidemic cannot be modeled, not all of these items may be needed in any one model. The point is to choose the specific question about a specific population which is to be answered, then choose the model that is appropriate for that purpose and find or estimate the value of parameters needed to construct it.

Policymakers may, and frequently do, base their decisions on their predictions of political consequences and on certain prior commitments — to values, to a constituency. These elements have weighed heavily in many policy decisions with respect to AIDS. It ought to be possible, nevertheless, to agree that the highest priority should be given to the question of effectiveness. Whether or not a particular measure violates the beliefs or behavioral preferences of various social groups, its potential effectiveness in stopping spread of the disease should weigh most heavily in judging it. Given our ignorance not only about AIDS as a disease but about the behaviors that transmit it, modeling becomes a crucial way to predict the effect of an intervention.

The following examples will illustrate aspects of this process.

Closing the Baths

Closing down places where homosexual men go for anonymous sex is one of the simpler measures that could have been taken to try to control spread of AIDS. However, the effect of such a measure depends on a rather complex interplay of factors. In this case, the effort to construct a model is itself instructive, though it may not yield an unambiguous answer about the preferable course of action (or inaction).

Closing these places may alter certain key parameters in the transmission of the AIDS virus. The rate of transmission per sexual act between an infected and an uninfected individual would probably not be affected, but the average rate of acquiring new partners might be, as would the variability in this rate, and so would the degree of mixing between infected and uninfected people.

Closing the baths could reduce the variability in the rate of new partner acquisition by making very high levels of promiscuity more difficult. However, closing centralized facilities with a certain relatively well defined clientele could have the paradoxical effect of increasing dispersal of infected people within a region. That is, it might induce former patrons to find other, less centralized outlets and thus to have a correspondingly higher chance of encountering uninfected people (who were not habitual bath-goers). On the other hand, by eliminating bathhouses as sites of sexual tourism, this measure could reduce the free mixing of people from different cities and thus slow the rate at which the disease spreads from one region to another.

A crucial parameter in any model of the effect of this action is the infectiousness of an infected person — that is, an estimate of how easily that person transmits the virus to others as a function of time since infection as well as other cofactors. How closing the baths affects the whole epidemic is influenced by the biology of AIDS and is not only a result of the effect of the measure on sexual behavior. If, for example, infectiousness is highly concentrated in a few individuals, then preventing them from having high rates of contact with susceptible people might have a major impact on the epidemic. If most infected people are infectious, but have only a low risk of infecting a partner, then closing the baths might make less difference.

For an illustration of this effect, imagine 1,000 gun owners, each of whom possesses 1,000 bullets — 999 blanks and a real one. It won't matter whether each of these people fires all 1,000 bullets at one target or at many; in any case, only one of each person's targets can wind up with a hole. Next imagine that a few gun owners have a higher proportion of real bullets, and the remainder have none. Now it makes a big difference whether the gun owners always fire at the same target or fire at many. In the second case, limiting the number of targets anyone can shoot at has a much bigger effect than in the first.

Until more information is available both about the biology of AIDS and on sexual behavior, it will be difficult to assess the effect of any intervention, such as closing the baths, aimed at limiting choice and availability of sexual partners. Any model of this effect must therefore be tested with extreme estimates of both maximal and minimal value of the parameters that are consistent with available data. "Sensitivity analysis" of this type will give a range for the likely effect of an intervention.

Of course, closing the baths, which are a social institution as well as a location for sexual activity, may have consequences that extend beyond the purely demographic. Harder to model, but nonetheless real, is the behavioral reaction of the clientele to loss of an accustomed place of sexual activity. A potential cost of closing the baths is the disappearance of a site for intensive education and behavior modification of a group that is at high behavioral risk. Alternatively, such a vivid message might be sent in the act of closing these places that behavior would be favorably influenced ipso facto.

Making Sex Safer

The object of any campaign to encourage safer sex is to alter only one parameter in the list of those causing the epidemic to grow — the infectivity per sexual act.

If the intervention being evaluated is promotion of condom use, two pieces of information are needed: the reduction in rates of transmission from wearing a condom, and the frequency of condom use.

The extent to which reducing infectivity per sexual act (as by wearing a condom) will limit growth of the epidemic depends a good deal on the variance of another parameter — promiscuity. If there is a great deal of variability in the number of partners acquired over any period of time, as appears to be the case, then targeting the most promiscuous group in the population for maximum education and intervention may have the highest yield. Even if the number of partners is not reduced, the net effect of reducing the infectiousness of behaviors among the most promiscuous may be appreciable.

It is important to bear in mind here that there is a crucial distinction between protecting a population and protecting the individual. Promoting use of condoms may prove quite effective for diminishing the rate of growth of the AIDS epidemic, especially if relatively promiscuous people use them most. But the level of protection that condom use offers any individual may, over the long run, not be very high if some of that person's partners are infected. And this is for the simple reason that risk accumulates with each repetition of an act. What may seem to be good odds on a single occasion (say, 1 in 1,000) may come to look rather poor after 10 or 50 repetitions. Thus if a program is to be judged in terms of how many participants have truly reduced their personal risk of AIDS, it must be judged by how many have really eliminated their risky behavior completely. It can be demonstrated that for a given background prevalence of infection (that is, the prevalence for the population from which partners are being selected), reducing the number of partners or using condoms does not much lower personal risk unless the number of partners is reduced nearly to one or the condoms are used nearly 100 percent of the time.[3]

On the other hand, if a program is to be judged by its overall impact on public health — how it affects growth of the epidemic — then another standard must be used. Reduction in risk that does not necessarily provide much protection for the individual might have significant effect on the epidemic as a whole.

The reason for this is that an intervention may significantly lower the basic reproductive rate of the epidemic even though it is a measure that does not assure the individual of protection. The basic reproductive rate is simply the average number of people who would be infected by an infectious person if he or she were exposed to a large group of susceptibles. This rate must be above 1 for the epidemic to propagate. If, in a given population, the rate is only slightly above 1, occasional condom use might bring it below 1. Thus, even though occasional condom use does not much alter the risk to an individual who is selecting partners from a population with a given prevalence of infection, the background prevalence itself might well be lowered if most members of the population occasionally used condoms. In any real-life situation, a model is needed to predict the magnitude of the effect.

For a simple heterosexual epidemic model in which the population is homogeneous, the basic reproductive rate can be calculated as the square root of the product of the average annual number of women infected by men (r_w) and the average annual number of men infected by women (r_m), times the duration of infectiousness (d).[4] This is expressed as $(r_w\ r_m)^{1/2}d$. If this number were close to 1, and were brought below that value by occasional condom use, then the epidemic could not propagate in that population by heterosexual contact. For example, suppose that the duration of infectiousness is 5 years, and that r_m is .1 and r_w is 1 for populations that do not use condoms and that r_m is .05 and r_w is .6 for those which do. Condom use would reduce the basic reproductive rate from about 1.6 to about .9 even though the individual using a condom with an infected partner might still be at high risk.

With respect to male homosexual practices, the impression has grown — on the basis of research reports — that anal intercourse is the most hazardous sexual practice and that oral intercourse is much less hazardous. Indeed, there is only one reported case of AIDS unambiguously attributable to oral sexual exposure.[5] However, it should be borne in mind that the power of available epidemiological methods to detect or measure the level of risk from oral exposure is exceedingly low. The value of efforts intended to shift erotic focus from one behavior to another depends on the real difference in risk between the two behaviors.

From even this short discussion, it should be clear that the value of safer sex campaigns, while undoubtedly real, should continue to be analyzed. Population-wide campaigns may be less valuable than highly targeted ones, and in any case there is an ethical obligation to distinguish between benefits that may come to the population as a whole and a level of protection that any one person may find inadequate for himself or herself.

Designing Screening Programs

There's an obvious reason for wanting to screen the population for exposure to the AIDS virus: one wants to know the total number of people infected and to know the prevalence of infection in specific subgroups of the population.

However, because of the intrinsic properties of any screening program, results are likely to be misleading for a population of very low prevalence (or, for that matter, for a group in which infection is highly prevalent). At one extreme, a large proportion of positive results is bound to be false, and at the other extreme, a sizable number of negative results will be false. For example, suppose that the test only rarely yields a false positive (say, 1 per 1,000 tests). If the test is used in a population in which infection is even more rare (say, 1 infection per 10,000 people), then a large majority (over 90 percent) of the positive test results will be false. This creates something of a paradox: you want a prior estimate of the prevalence of infection before you begin screening any particular population.

The reason for this is that you want to know how to screen to get the best estimate of overall prevalence (you don't want to concentrate your effort in areas of low prevalence). In addition, screening tells you only about specific groups like army recruits or mothers giving birth. Even if you do population-based surveys, you only find out about people who are sufficiently compliant to participate in the study. Thus, an independent estimate of prevalence is desirable, and one way to obtain such an estimate is from model-based approaches.

One such model can be constructed from data on the number of cases of AIDS in the population and the distribution of latencies (that is, the rate at which disease develops after infection, expressed not as an average but as the number of people in every interval). For another type of model, a small group is intensely studied, then its experience is projected to the whole population, making allowances for whatever is atypical about the group under study — necessarily an imprecise procedure.

In either case, modeling can help you decide whom to screen and can help in the interpretation of screening data after you get them. If, for example, your model of heterosexual transmission told you that a self-propagating epidemic among heterosexuals was impossible, then you would know that the rare cases of infection that you observed from low-prevalence areas would be more likely to have resulted from atypical behavior than from the start of a heterosexually transmitted epidemic.

Planning for the Future

There are at present reasonably good data, though far from perfect, on the growth of AIDS in the United States from the beginning of this decade. Not known — and undiscoverable from this information — is what the future growth of the curve will be.

What would make projection more precise is the shape of the curve of infection to date, but this is not known. It is not possible at present to reject either of two hypotheses: that rate of growth has been linear (increasing in a straight line) or that it has been sigmoidal (building to a peak rate of growth, then tapering off in a symmetrical fashion). The two shapes would result from different types of epidemics. If the epidemic is being spread mainly by a small number of highly infectious or promiscuous people, we may expect a linear shape, whereas if the epidemic is propagated by most of the already infected people with fairly homogeneous behavior, the sigmoidal curve may result. Existing data are consistent with either the sigmoidal or the linear model. Depending on which you believed, however, you could get estimates that ranged between 400,000 and 2 million cases of HIV infection in the United States, and projections for the future depend heavily on this estimate.[6]

It is crucial to recognize that a single model cannot be "confirmed" by showing that it fits the available data. This would be like saying, "The ground looks flat, so the world must be a plane." It is necessary to see how many different theories fit all available data. At present, a lot of different curves fit the observed growth of AIDS in the United States.

The point of continuing to construct and test these models is that, sooner or later, if one model can be rejected, we will have some useful information about the factors favoring spread of AIDS, and therefore some way of evaluating the potential effectiveness or efficiency of an intervention.

What We Need to Know

Every example we have given indicates the extreme importance of knowing more about the infectiousness of people carrying the AIDS virus. The frequency with which evidence of the virus can be recovered from genital secretions (the only important route of transmission besides needle sharing) is known, but finding the virus is a far cry from telling us what rate of transmission is typical for sexual exposure to that fluid. To get any useful information about infectiousness, large and carefully designed studies of sexual partners are needed.

Two crucial groups are those infected through blood transfusion and those infected through exposure to anti-hemophilia factor. In both of these groups, it is feasible to obtain a reasonably accurate estimate of the time of exposure. Many of the infected people also have had sustained sexual relations with a partner, so that the rate at which virus is transferred from one to another for a given frequency of sexual activity can be estimated. The essential data to gather from such people include (1) the time from probable exposure to evidence of infection, and (2) an account of sexual activity, including the type and frequency of specific acts.

The opportunity to study these groups, however, is about to be lost. New exposures have been reduced to a minimum by measures to protect the blood supply. Meanwhile, many significant events in the lives of the existing group (transmitting the virus, becoming ill) have already occurred.

Even if we had perfect information on everything else, we would still need to know about infectiousness or we would be unable to rule out the possibility that there is wide variation in the probability that AIDS will be transmitted.

The essential question about models used to develop policy is how different ones are affected by that policy. If a given policy seems best for models that make very different assumptions about unknown parameters and processes, then the policy is not dependent on more advanced knowledge. If the choice of policy is highly dependent on these assumptions, then the model has revealed where research must be conducted to obtain the vital information.

For example, a relatively robust conclusion is that heterosexual transmission of AIDS will be most effectively diminished by reducing the sharing of needles by drug users. It is clear from existing data that most heterosexual transmission will be from men who have acquired the virus through sharing of needles and who then pass it to women by way of sexual intercourse. This pattern will dominate the statistics for years to come, regardless of whether an independent epidemic can be sustained by heterosexuals.[7]

On the other hand, the effect of safer sex campaigns depends heavily on the nature of infectiousness. If the epidemic is being driven mostly by a few highly infectious and promiscuous people, then the effect of strategies like reducing number of partners or promoting use of condoms is different than if infectiousness is more diffusely distributed.

Although data are not available to model the AIDS epidemic with great precision, modeling can still be useful in making policy decisions. Uses of modeling in formulating policy include the following:

- estimating the precision with which current prevalence of HIV infection and future incidence of AIDS can be known
- making explicit the assumptions on which such estimates are based
- evaluating the likely impact of behavioral intervention or vaccination strategies
- evaluating the precision with which information must be collected to make estimates as accurate (but only as accurate) as necessary

Models need not be complex to be useful. But they must be sufficiently varied to determine under what conditions a given control strategy appears effective — does it work under a broad range of reasonable assumptions about the dynamics of the epidemic or only under special conditions? That is, models should indicate the degree to which the opinions of the modelers, as opposed to the underlying data themselves, determine the results. Modeling is a mechanism that enables the policymaker to test and refine the beliefs he or she already holds.

This research was supported by Grant No. 24643 from the National Institute of Allergy and Infectious Diseases.

Notes

1. Scott Zeger, "Methods for Trend Analysis of the AIDS Epidemic," paper presented at the Johns Hopkins Conference on Statistical and Mathematical Modeling of AIDS, Baltimore, Md., November 17, 1987.
2. Robert May and Roy Anderson, "Transmission Dynamics of HIV Infection," *Nature* 326 (1987): 137–142.
3. Harvey Fineberg, "Education to Prevent AIDS: Prospects and Obstacles," *Science* (in press).
4. May and Anderson, "Transmission Dynamics of HIV Infection."
5. Victor De Gruttola and Kenneth H. Mayer, "Human Immunodeficiency Virus and Oral Intercourse," *Annals of Internal Medicine* 107 (1987): 428–429.
6. Victor De Gruttola and Stephen Lagakos, "The Value of Doubling Time in Assessing the Course of the AIDS Epidemic," Technical Report No. 564z, 1987. Copies may be obtained from the Dana Farber Cancer Institute, Binney St., Boston, MA 02115.
7. Victor De Gruttola and Kenneth H. Mayer, "Assessing and Modeling Heterosexual Spread of HIV in the United States," *Reviews of Infectious Diseases* 10, no.1: 138–150.

Understanding the Psychological Impact of AIDS: The Other Epidemic

Marshall Forstein, M.D.

HIV has created two epidemics, one of disease, the other the consequence of the psychological response to that disease. Thus far, behavioral change is the only effective means of interrupting the transmission of HIV. The underlying psychological dimensions of the societal and individual responses to AIDS are discussed, with suggestions for how both rational thinking and irrational fears and anxiety contribute to the development of public policy. Examples are given of how short-term solutions to reduce anxiety may actually create long-term problems, potentially increasing the risk of transmission of HIV. Specific psychological mechanisms that contribute to the epidemic of fear are explained. Understanding the fears and incorporating them into a coherent plan for addressing behavioral change are essential if the epidemic is to be contained. Public figures have a responsibility to resist short-term solutions in response to public anxiety.

Historical reflection upon the impact of AIDS will eventually document the development of two epidemics, one involving the biophysiological and medical response to a viral illness, the other a psychosocial phenomenon affecting every social, religious, educational, financial, political, and cultural institution within American society and throughout the world. Ultimately, the way in which we as individuals, societies, and nations respond to the psychological effects of this viral, sexually transmitted, blood-borne disease will be as significant as the way in which we respond to the virus itself, with respect to the extent of the epidemic's impact on society.

This article will explore the psychological dimension of the epidemic of fear and anxiety which compounds the disease itself. AIDS has undeniably elucidated many of the problems, deficits, and failures of our society which have been inadequately addressed for some time, such as unequal access to health care, substance abuse, sexually transmitted disease, homophobia, and unequal protection of civil rights. If we are to sufficiently contain the epidemic and minimize the devastation to individuals and social institutions, choices will be required of us individually and collectively which will be made at the

Dr. Marshall Forstein is codirector of the Outpatient Psychiatry Department at the Cambridge Hospital in Cambridge, Massachusetts, and is an instructor in psychiatry at the Harvard Medical School. He is a member of the American Psychiatric Association's Committee on AIDS and is secretary of the board of directors of the AIDS Action Committee of Massachusetts, in Boston.

intersection of public health policies, societal values, scientific technology, and an economic reality that includes increasing world needs and decreasing resources. While it is unlikely that all of society's problems will be solved as a means of stopping the epidemic, addressing those problems is essential if appropriate interventions are to be realized. Complicating the societal issues are the complex psychological factors of human sexual behavior, substance abuse and addiction, and varying capacities of individuals to manage fear and anxiety.

AIDS requires, for example, that we take the most difficult, most emotionally charged concerns of our civilization and within the extremes of existing values, morals, social structures, and economics cut through to the essential tasks involved in halting a sexually transmitted disease. Of all the infectious agents in the biosphere for which we do not have a vaccine, HIV is among those we best know how to avoid getting or transmitting. The epidemiology and routes of transmission are clear, although for various reasons there is a curious denial of those data, allowing people to believe what they want to about the disease. Because the virus is transmitted almost always by willful, consensual behavior, the containment of the epidemic is dependent on people knowing what behaviors and risk factors facilitate the transmission from one person to another. This requires education as to the facts, and strategies for helping people integrate psychologically the behavioral changes that will protect them from transmitting or receiving the virus.

So the essential question is, Given what we know, why aren't we doing what we know we can do to stop the transmission of this virus? What is getting in the way of our taking the appropriate steps, of committing our resources to putting an end to the transmission of this virus? Despite the amount of information we have regarding the mode of transmission and the behaviors that put one at risk, many people believe that scientists are wrong, that doctors cannot guarantee complete safety from all risk, and that taking actions to protect oneself, even if they are irrational and in violation of others' basic rights, is warranted.

In the novel *The Plague,* Albert Camus poetically lays out the essential conflict, and resolution, of the task before us through the observations of Dr. Rieux, who begins to fathom the deepest psychological implications of the task of containing the plague:

> Only the sea, murmurous behind the dingy checkerboard of houses, told of the unrest, the precariousness, of all things in this world. And, gazing in the direction of the bay, Dr. Rieux called to mind the plague — fires of which Lucretius tells, which the Athenians kindled on the seashore. The dead were brought there after nightfall, but there was not room enough, and the living fought one another with torches for a space where to lay those who had been dear to them; for they had rather engage in bloody conflicts than abandon their dead to the waves. A picture rose before him of the red glow of the pyres mirrored on a wine-dark, slumbrous sea, battling torches whirling sparks across the darkness, and thick fetid smoke rising toward the watchful sky. Yes, it was not beyond the bounds of possibility. . . .
>
> But these extravagant forebodings dwindled in the light of reason. True, the word "plague" had been uttered; true, at this very moment one or two victims were being seized and laid low by the disease. Still, that could stop, or be stopped. It was only a matter of lucidly recognizing what had to be recognized; of dispelling extraneous shadows and doing what needed to be done. Then the plague would come to an end, because it was unthinkable, or, rather, because one thought of it on misleading lines. If, as was most likely, it died out, all would be well. If not, one would know it anyhow for what it was and what steps should be taken for coping with and finally overcoming it.
>
> The doctor opened the window, and at once the noises of the town grew louder. The brief, intermittent sibilance of a machine-saw came from a nearby workshop. Rieux

> pulled himself together. There lay certitude; there, in the daily round. All the rest hung on mere threads and trivial contingencies; you couldn't waste your time on it. The thing was to do your job as it should be done.[1]

The job to be done is to contain the spread of the virus. This means finding a cure or adequate treatment for those infected, a vaccine for those not yet infected, and/or a method for behaviorally containing the spread of the virus. These attempts to curtail the devastation of this virus in society call upon the most sophisticated technological and biomedical techniques, and upon complex ways of changing individuals' drug usage and sexual behavior. What lies at the heart of the psychological difficulties facing individuals and social institutions is that currently the containment of the spread of HIV infection is almost exclusively dependent on changing at-risk behaviors. The fear that the AIDS virus is out of control parallels long-standing fears in our society that sexual and addictive behaviors are also out of control.

Psychological Responses: The Limbic/Cortical Partnership

An essential characteristic of the human mind helps to explain the psychological dimensions of the epidemic of fear and anxiety. The most ancient part of the human brain, evolved over millions of years, continues to share structure and function with the brains of lesser animals, such as reptiles. These structures collectively constitute the limbic system, the repository of human emotions such as fear and anxiety, and visceral drives such as hunger, thirst, and sexual desire. This might be called our reptilian legacy. What distinguishes humans from other species is a much more recent, evolutionarily speaking, part of the brain called the neocortex. The human cortex allows for the development of language, of logical and deductive reasoning, of rational thought. Further, it allows human beings, perhaps alone among all species, to contemplate their own existence, to know and perceive the passage of time, and to foretell their own mortality.

As a species, we are still on a journey to make the most of this exquisite partnership of limbic and cortical capacities. Neither capacity alone is capable of sustaining human life, but either one alone is capable of destroying it. Emotional, irrational responses that are based on fear can prevent us from making reasoned, albeit difficult, choices needed to contain crises that threaten us. Purely rational responses that ignore emotional impact may seem logical yet be impossible to implement. Each challenge to our species, such as the AIDS epidemic, requires further maturation of the delicate balance between cortical and limbic systems; paying attention to the limbic system allows us to understand and experience our fears, while attention to the cortical system allows us to manage those fears in a way that leads to effective control and appropriate changes.

Given this schematic representation of the human psyche, three potential modes for approaching the presence of HIV in our society can be described. One mode is confined to limbic arousal and response, such as the fight-or-flight reflex. This is the need to do something immediately to quiet the anxiety and fear of AIDS. Decisions that are based exclusively on limbic arousal lead to the perception that the fear is allayed, while not addressing the immediate and long-term effects of such responses. The second mode involves a strictly cortical response. It assumes that the whole of human behavior and motivation, and the AIDS virus itself, can be managed with a totally rational approach. Relying only on logic, cause-and-effect argument, and quantification of the problems associated with the HIV epidemic obviates the need to acknowledge and treat the fear and anxiety.

The essential problem with an exclusively rational approach is that it precludes the concern for the psychological consequences of any decisions. Denying that even rational decisions engender emotional responses simplifies the situation greatly, but does not provide for the emotional consequences.

The third mode, which is in fact the only really viable one, derives from understanding and utilizing both the limbic arousal and the cortical capacities to formulate an integrated response to any human dilemma or crisis. This requires respect for the complexity of human behavior and emotional conflict which must inform intellectual decisions. It allows us to know the fears for what they are, and enables us to contain them when reason suggests they may be out of control and harmful to the long-term prospects of societal survival.

Two psychologically important capacities have an impact on human sexual and addictive behavior, and on those social structures which are intended to protect people from the unpredictability of the world. These are the capacity to contain ambiguity and uncertainty, and the capacity to act on the basis of the relative risks or benefits of any particular activity.

The necessary balance between the cortical and limbic structures depends on the capacity to understand and contain ambiguity and uncertainty. This capacity develops as a complex psychological response to a world in which a person perceives, feels, and believes in the tenuousness and mystery of life while at the same time believing that he or she has some ability to affect, perhaps even to manage, the vicissitudes of life. In an existential way, the capacity to contain ambiguity and uncertainty correlates with the capacity to contain anxiety about the very nature of human existence. Fear and anxiety increase the desire for answers and action, even if the long-term effects of such are undesirable. Short-term solutions to ameliorate anxiety are often more acceptable than tolerating that anxiety and delaying the gratifying, more long-term solution. When the fear and anxiety become overwhelming, irrational choices and decisions may be employed to attempt to decrease the painful feelings. The desire to reduce pain, physical or emotional, is a basic drive, and the basis of much human behavior. At times, addictive behavior, whether with drugs or sex, may be the only available level of adaptation which can even momentarily alleviate the psychic pain.

The psychological capacity to manage fear and anxiety results from a very complex evolution of personal character, experience in the world, native intelligence (cognitive ability), and basic beliefs and tenets about the human condition. Within any society confronting something as frightening as the AIDS epidemic, there is inevitably a great range of ability to conceptualize, contain, and manage the emotional impact of the reality. Like the individual brain, the societal mind must understand its components, validate and acknowledge the emotional issues, but not allow fear to preclude reasoned choices that take into account the human response to any particular decision.

The ability to make decisions on the basis of a perception of the relative risk of certain activities compared to that of others is evoked in the extreme when feelings of uncertainty, fear, and vulnerability collide. Mothers, for example, who don't think twice about sending a child to school on a bus will take the child out of school for fear of infection because a child with AIDS is attending, although the risk of the child dying in a bus accident is greater by a thousand-fold. The unwillingness of some, even after the epidemiological data are presented, to change that attitude and behavior (of withdrawing their child from school) may be a representation of the irrational distortion of the relative risks involved. In a way, AIDS allows parents to do something to protect their children. But the attempt to protect their children from the dangers of living in this world gets particularly exacerbated with respect to AIDS precisely because parents are so terrified of the very activities that are associated with the transmission of the virus: sexual activity and drug use. Now, more than ever, it is impossible to deny that those very activities which challenge the control parents have over their children are associated with death itself.

The lack of faith and belief in their own parenting capacities leads to the refusal to acknowledge the nearly zero risk of their child getting infected by attending school with a child with HIV positivity or with AIDS. Parents irrationally try to control the situation in the present, when the fears are those which extend into their future sense of how much control they will have over their children, perhaps even over their own lives.

Politicians and policymakers, for example, may try to quiet the popular anxiety, and their own, by formulating immediately acceptable policies, even though the long-term effects of such policies may be counterproductive. For scientists, especially physicians, having an immediately available test result, for example, may decrease uncertainty in the short term without necessarily achieving the long-term goals.

Examining in detail the history and use of HIV antibody testing will highlight these essential psychological issues as they pertain to the policy and educational decision making whose stated goal is to stop the transmission of HIV.

HIV Antibody Testing: The Psychological Dimensions

The development of the antibody test began with the expressed desire to make the blood supply safe from contaminated blood donors. As a laboratory test, the HIV ELISA is exquisitely sensitive, capturing in its net almost all of the contaminated blood donated. "Almost all" will always be the best that any test can do when it comes to screening blood for anything. In the case of HIV, donors who are infected but have not yet produced antibodies will not be captured by the present tests. Even an antigen test, which will presumably not have the same window of incubation before antibodies are identifiable, will suffer from the statistical latitude of error that is inevitable in any laboratory test situation. Thus, at the very best, blood recipients can expect an extremely safe blood supply, but not a perfectly safe one. This means that we must all accept a certain level of risk and make informed judgments about the use of blood transfusions. In a positive way, AIDS has probably done more to reduce the inappropriate use of blood products than all of the medical education doctors get about the risks and benefits of transfusions.

The public, however, finds it difficult to tolerate any level of risk when it comes to the blood supply. At the basis of this is perhaps more than the question of quantifiable relative risk. The individual's subjective perception of that risk may be fundamental. The same people who clamor for a perfectly safe blood supply, and who become outraged when science cannot deliver it, are likely to take significantly greater risks with their lives every day, such as driving a car, flying, and so on. In comparison, the risk of dying from AIDS as a result of a blood transfusion after March 1985, when antibody screening of blood began, is less than one in one hundred thousand. A white male who lives in an urban area in the United States has a one in one hundred and thirty chance of being killed by a gun. For a black male, that chance increases to one in five.

How are we to understand why some risks are tolerable even if they are statistically so much greater than others? Why does the person who rails against the imperfect blood supply not become enraged by the lack of gun control? How do we come to expect medicine and doctors to be perfect in the pursuit of saving lives while at the same time accepting the potential perpetration of violence by one human on another? Do anti–gun control enthusiasts, perhaps, manifest the magical belief that guns provide a certainty of safety and control in an essentially uncontrollable world?

Perhaps the underlying fear manifested by the blood transfusion issue has also to do with the fear of being hurt in an accident, and having others — medical personnel — make decisions of life and death in a moment of complete vulnerability. All of us can imagine daily events in which car accidents may precipitate crises. As horrible as that possibility is, the thought of it is manageable with some denial that it will actually occur. When it comes to the issue of dying at the hand of a gunman, the horror is too much to handle, and more complete denial becomes the psychological device for managing the basic fear of losing one's life. In reality, although having a gun may make a person more potentially lethal to others, it does not make one less vulnerable to another gun.

We associate blood transfusions with crises we consider manageable, and therefore don't totally deny — thereby increasing, perhaps unreasonably — our expectations of safety; we associate gun control with crises that aren't manageable, leading us to totally deny the relative risk, or creating the illusion of total safety by having a gun.

Some fears, to be managed at all, require different levels of repression, leading to different types and degrees of emotional expression. The same psychological mechanisms of defense may be operative with the threat of nuclear disaster.

No one would argue about the rationale for continuing to screen blood for HIV antibodies. No one would argue that increasingly better laboratory tests should be pursued to increase the level of safety. Problems arise, however, when the rational use of HIV antibody testing to screen blood becomes the basis of public health policy that establishes programs for screening large populations of people, with the assumption that doing so will necessarily lead to a reduction in the spread of HIV.

As evidence of how short-term solutions may be sought to allay anxiety, one might examine the U.S. immigration policy, which now requires that persons applying for U.S. residence be HIV antibody tested. Ostensibly, this requirement is put forth as a way of preventing the spread of disease and overloading of the U.S. medical establishment, which already feels the strain of the HIV epidemic. Asymptomatic individuals who are HIV-positive are prevented from immigrating, yet people with other sorts of chronic illness, such as diabetes, arthritis, and cardiovascular disease, are not denied entrance even though they are as likely to utilize U.S. medical resources. While in the short run this policy may seem to contribute to protecting the U.S. population, the long-term implications have never been fully addressed.

For example, what if other nations follow the example of the United States in barring immigrants who test positive? One can imagine that nations, then fearing each other, might begin requiring all tourists and people traveling on business to be certified HIV-free. Soon countries might have standing policies based on the paranoid fantasy that anyone could be carrying the virus and on the unstated acknowledgment that people may have consensual sexual relations. The policies would also arise out of the fear that infected individuals would seek the best level of care possible, burdening nations that had the greatest access to medical care.

Should the notion of testing to protect national boundaries become more acceptable, the consequences might be felt within the United States. The Commonwealth of Massachusetts (well known for its medical establishment and already the mecca for persons suffering from rare or difficult medical problems) might begin to think it should protect its medical system from ruin by refusing to let neighboring states, which have fewer medical resources, refer all their HIV cases to Massachusetts. At first, Massachusetts hospitals might refuse to treat persons from out of state, but as people found ways to circumvent the rules in order to obtain the best possible AIDS care, state borders might begin to be enforced, with persons being required to produce certification that they had recently tested negative before being allowed to cross state lines.

Although such paranoid fantasies may seem "beyond the bounds of possibility," the statements of public figures suggest otherwise. Some have called for all HIV-positive people to be distinctively marked so that others might avoid contact with them; others have recommended that all people in high-risk groups, essentially all gay men and intravenous drug users, be contained in some sort of protected "camp"; and some fanatical religious leaders have even called for the outright eradication of homosexual people.[2]

Even reasonable people, when confronted with the rising statistics on those infected and on the estimated cost of treating and caring for the ill, begin to contemplate irrational means of trying to control the epidemic — for instance, by attempting to control other people's lives. Implementing large-scale mandatory testing with this goal in mind may appear to be rational until one looks at the long-term implications and the cost of implementation.

Let's assume, for instance, that everyone applying for a job or currently employed or entering school or presenting at a hospital or clinic were to be mandatorily tested for HIV. Perhaps as many as 100 million tests would have to be performed, at a cost of at least $3 for each ELISA and approximately $60 to $100 for each confirmatory test. All those who tested negative would have to be routinely tested on a regular basis, since the test might not catch HIV-positive people who were without antibodies at the time of testing, or persons who became infected between tests. It could well require several hundred million dollars every several months just to do large-scale screening.

Aside from the cost in dollars, moreover, would be the cost to the well-being of persons who were positive but for whom at this time nothing could be done. Additionally, since in large-scale testing of low-incidence populations there would be an equal number of true and false positives, half the people identified as positive, but who in fact were not, would suffer the psychological damage and stigma of being identified as HIV-positive. The cost to society in terms of productivity would be immeasurable.

Most significantly, the intended goal of such large-scale screening, to reduce the spread of HIV, might actually be negatively affected. There is no evidence, scientifically, that knowing one's HIV serological status in any way correlates with the ability to manage risk-taking behavior. Once the meaning of the test is clear, people react in many ways to obtaining the results of the test, whether positive or negative. Studies[3] done in several cities, such as Chicago and New York, do not support the position of the Centers for Disease Control (CDC), which advocates that people at high risk be HIV tested. The CDC's position is based on its belief that knowing one's antibody status leads to appropriate behavioral modification. In fact, the research to date[4] suggests that individuals who find out their antibody status may differ significantly in their responses. Preliminary research has indicated that people who perceived themselves to be at high risk and who had not made appropriate behavior changes were not likely to do so because of the results of the test. Both for those who were positive and those who were negative, the capacity to behave safely was not affected by the test itself. In some cases, it becomes even more difficult to change at-risk behavior after finding out test results, whether positive or negative.

Psychologically, several possible inferences, supported by clinical experience across the United States, can be made from these findings. Individuals who test negative may begin to feel that they are immune, assuming that if they haven't been infected already they must be invulnerable to the virus. Others develop severe forms of survivor's guilt, not unlike what is seen in Holocaust survivors. Many of these individuals have lost intimate friends and sexual partners to AIDS, and begin to wonder why they have been spared. For some, there is actually an increase in unsafe practices, almost in defiance of their luck to date and in support of their denial about their own mortality.

Individuals who test positive may respond in a number of ways upon learning their antibody status. For some, the fact that they are already infected and the perception that they will die from AIDS engenders a nihilistic, self-destructive attitude. Occasionally, the thought of "taking others with you" becomes revenge for the anger and betrayal they feel on account of contracting AIDS. This derives partly from the stimulation of self-hate in the infected individual, in turn often resulting from internalized homophobia for gay and bisexual men, and from self-loathing in intravenous drug users, who may feel morally corrupt and guilty for their addiction. In addition, the very behavior that places an individual at risk, whether it be addictive use of drugs or compulsive sexual activity (or both), becomes the most available means of decreasing the underlying anxiety.

The growing consideration of the impact of testing on an individual's ability to manage at-risk behaviors has led most public health officials not to support the idea of mandatory testing or of contact tracing. But officials who might be able to manage their own anxiety about not being able to control the epidemic immediately face the fear and demands of some who insist that restrictive policies be enacted to protect society.

Camus again warns of the danger from irrational responses to anxiety-provoking and fearful situations:

> All I maintain is that on this earth there are pestilences and there are victims, and it's up to us, so far as possible, not to join forces with the pestilences.[5]

Educating people and providing access to information and social and psychological supports in order to curtail activities that may transmit HIV are the only available methods of rationally addressing the epidemic. Even with the most powerful, all-encompassing efforts, it is certain that there will be casualties: that certain people, for whatever reasons, will continue to engage in activities that put themselves and others at risk. The mere fact that something so small as a virus is transmitted by something so powerful and universal as sexuality, and that it can have such devastating effects on the individual and such enormous consequences for the entire society, upsets our basic sense of security.

AIDS and the Social Environment: The Psychological Implications

The context in which AIDS developed in the United States is inextricably linked to the psychological difficulties both of infected people and of people responding in any number of ways to the epidemic. Although scientific data and epidemiological studies throughout the world have linked the spread of the virus to blood-to-blood transmission and to sexual activity in which the virus is transmitted (independent of sexual orientation), the fear and anxiety propelling irrational responses are clearly related to what drug use and sex symbolize and mean in our culture. That homosexuality initially was causally associated in both the scientific and the lay mind with the spread of HIV only exacerbated the problem.

If the first U.S. cases had not been described in sexually active gay men and in intravenous drug users, but in the white, heterosexual sons of congressional leaders, for instance, the emotional response and mobilization of resources would have been substantially different from what they were. The prolonged silence of the U.S. government, its public policies, and the political ramifications of AIDS arose from the fear of addressing the fundamental issues of homosexuality and drug addiction in the United States. The silence of those in responsible leadership positions allowed the worst attitudes and prejudices to intensify. Imagine, for instance, if soon after the epidemic was under way, the president of the United States had held a press conference, perhaps while sitting on the bed of a man with AIDS, and said: "My fellow Americans, I want you to know that your government is fully committed to dedicating whatever resources we have toward finding a cure and a treatment for those afflicted, and to educating us all about the transmission of this virus. I furthermore implore you not to punish or ostracize people who are sick or who are drug-addicted because of your fear of AIDS." Hearing and watching the president model a posture that deplores homophobia, racism, and irrational acts would provide many Americans with some psychological supports for containing their fear.

The ability of a U.S. president to take such a stance would depend on the public being able to deal with basic issues around sexuality (particularly homosexuality) and drug addiction. From the point of view of persons infected early on — drug addicts and gay men — the position of outcast was already extant. After all, how does a society begin to address the medical and psychological needs of homosexually oriented people who are intentionally invisible within the fabric of American life, and whose basic civil rights are not clearly guaranteed by the Constitution? Furthermore, the very sexual activity that is associated with the transmission of the disease is considered criminal behavior in most of the United States.

Underlying the response by the public and its leaders is the long-standing fear that sexuality and pleasure-seeking behavior, if left unchecked, threaten to tear apart the fabric of society. Those social, legal, and religious institutions which are designed to contain the worst impulses of the species become the deterrents to the use of reasonable strategies for containing this particular epidemic.

How does a government that is purportedly based on the constitutionally determined separation of church and state deal with the teachings of particular religions and the changing social morality, and the need to contain a sexually transmitted disease? What will it take for the condom to be seen as an instrument of death prevention rather than birth control?

When will the debate about whether teenagers should or should not be having sex before marriage or adulthood give way to the reality that the sex lives of pre-adults are not within the control either of institutions or of individuals other than those engaging in sex?

Statistically, about 10 percent of all AIDS cases in the United States are in the age group twenty to twenty-four.[6] Given the latency period of perhaps two to seven years, there can be no doubt that teenagers are being infected. While teens become infected and the reservoir of HIV-positive people increases, the debate continues as to whether the government can support with public funds the kinds of printed materials that graphically speak to the issues of safer sex and condom use. If parents are to feel that they are realistically preparing their children to protect themselves, they must confront their own anxiety about discussing sex with their children, perhaps even their own anxiety about sex itself, and about the inevitable necessity of giving up control of their children.

Many of the fears that operate within each person become institutionalized in public policy. Thus, several psychological issues contribute to the particular way in which AIDS has become an epidemic of fear arising out of personal experience, or as part of a cultural legacy. The fear of people who are different, such as in racism or homophobia, may be an internalized, acceptable aspect of a particular culture, institutionalized in spite of legal or stated social positions. Take, for example, the Catholic church's position on homosexuality. The church asks us to love the person but deplore the sexual activity. It further supports the denial of homosexuals' basic civil rights, under the guise that these rights are already guaranteed by the Constitution, a position that interpretations of the Supreme Court do not support. The conflict within such powerful institutions as the church becomes incorporated psychologically into the fear and anxiety of the individual who sees homosexuality, perhaps even all of sex, instead of the virus, as the cause of AIDS. Homophobia, the irrational dread of being confronted by homosexuality, becomes the basis for what is publicly put forth in the name of protecting the public health.

A comparison of the AIDS virus with a virus that caused an epidemic of lesser proportions, such as Legionnaires' disease, may be instructional. After all, even though Legionnaires' disease was spread through respiratory contact, breathing did not become a disgraceful, shameful activity. There is something quite different about sex than almost any other human activity which psychologically makes our culture respond regressively and often punitively. The association of sex and death, now profoundly etched in our consciousness, and the basic fears of intimacy and sexual expression which have always been part of our society have created special barriers to the development of coherent, reasonable approaches to this disease. In other nations, where sexuality has traditionally been more easily addressed, the response of the governments has been more decisive, swifter, and less tinged with moral consternation. In Great Britain, for example, where consensual homosexuality is not criminalized, the debate about teaching safer sex is not whether to, but how to.

Similarly, in the United States drug addiction is treated both as a criminal act and as a medical illness. This conflict represents an underlying psychological ambivalence about whether an individual is to blame for his or her addiction or whether, in fact, it is a disease. The arbitrary distinctions between the use and abuse of alcohol and the use and abuse of other substances illustrates the difficulty in addressing AIDS in the drug-addicted population. Rationally, the best way to curb the spread of HIV is to provide sufficient access to treatment for persons who are addicted, and to legalize and control access to substances that individuals choose to use, separating out the use of the substance from the mechanism of transmission of HIV, that is, sharing contaminated needles. To develop such an approach would require changing institutionalized attitudes and myths about people who become drug-addicted.

Public Policy: The Psychological Context and Constraints

The success of any long-term program in decreasing the transmission of HIV will ultimately depend on the provision of support and impetus for people to change the behaviors that put them at risk. While the society at large debates the morals and merits of homosexuality, the gay male community has taken charge of itself and has redefined its sexual mores, so that acceptable behavior is now safer behavior. It appears to be more difficult for people who are already sexually active to change their sexual habits than it is to help people just coming out and becoming sexual to incorporate the safer sex behaviors into their lives.

A proactive, "sex positive" message depends on the presence of a visible gay and lesbian community, with resources to provide persons seeking intimacy with alternative ways of obtaining affirmation of their sexual identity. In rural, isolated areas, such support may be lacking, and the very anxiety of being "out" in some areas may in fact impel gay men to seek out unsafe sexual practices as a way of quelling the anxiety about being homosexual. Public policies, therefore, that are intended to stop the spread of AIDS have got to support the basic protection and civil rights of homosexual people in the United States. Forced underground, considered less valuable in the eyes of society, gay men and lesbians internalize the hatred within that they experience and feel from others who are validated in the world. Public policy can protect the rights of human beings without condoning or encouraging any particular behavior. That is the essential principle behind freedom of choice. Likewise, public policies must take into account the long-term effects of "sex negative" messages that are "rationally intended" to stop AIDS but that ignore the emotional and psychological impact on human beings, who need intimacy and sex in their lives to form the kinds of relationships that make society compassionate and caring. What will our nation look like twenty years from now if a generation of children grow up terrified of sex, more homophobic, more racist, and more addictophobic?

Stopping the spread of HIV in the addicted community requires that sufficient resources be allocated to provide treatment for the underlying disease that leads to the transmission of HIV. The debates about clean needle exchange and what type of drug treatment is best point to the ambivalence the medical profession and society have about treating drug addiction as an illness. We feel morally bound to treat people who are ill, and in fact usually offer a range of treatments for any single medical problem. By criminalizing drug addiction, we absolve ourselves of the responsibility of treating behavior that is self-destructive and potentially dangerous to others. Those who make public policy must be educated about the complex meaning of sharing needles within the IV drug subculture, and what economic opportunities, incentives, and social changes will be required in order to preclude the need for such rituals within the IV community.

If the necessary changes in human behavior are to occur which can minimize the spread of this virus, attention must be paid to the important interface of the psychological, medical, and public policy issues. The inherent bias against psychological understanding, perhaps even a fear of psychological thinking, is evident at even the most sophisticated levels of discussion. The International Conference on AIDS,[7] attended by scientists and policymakers from all over the world, has had virtually no representation from the psychiatric or psychological profession, even though, when asked, everyone admits that changing behavior is the only available, effective means of stopping the transmission. That scientists meeting with the stated purpose of halting the transmission of AIDS could create an international conference at which psychological professionals are conspicuously absent — even from the planning committee — speaks to the difficulty of addressing the complex psychological aspects of HIV infection. Dealing with such important issues as sexual behavior change and addiction treatment has not heretofore been acceptable within the province of medical science. Yet the achievement of substantial progress in reducing the spread of AIDS is dependent on effectively dealing with those anxiety-provoking issues. How is the general public to begin to deal with the fear and anxiety if professionals themselves set out to deal with AIDS without adequately addressing the psychological issues? Even after three years of such a conference, and with complaints by members of both the psychiatric and psychological professions, the conference planning committee has chosen to neglect psychological and psychosocial input in favor of what is considered "hard science." The reality is that scientists are no better prepared to deal with the difficult issues of sex, drugs, and death than the lay population.

The resistance to spending time and energy on the complex psychological dynamics of addiction and sexual behavior is based partly on the way in which that very psychological understanding would force a different approach to public policy and decision making. Human psychology complicates any simple answer to problems that involve changing deeply imbedded values and habits. Not addressing these issues allows for seemingly straightforward answers and simple solutions, such as testing people premaritally for HIV. Addressing these issues points out the inconsistencies and long-term problems associated with simplistic policies.

Public policy that develops to stop the spread of AIDS must be divided into short-term and long-term plans. Short-term plans require crisis-oriented activities, considered, it is hoped, in terms of the potential long-term ramifications. Strategies that decrease anxiety immediately, or that give a false sense of security and discount the psychological ramifications, may in fact contribute to, rather than stop, the spread of AIDS. Long-term plans must evolve on the basis of what is known about human learning, and behavioral patterns and change. Sex and drug education must begin with the very young, allowing children to grow up without much of the anxiety adults now have about even discussing such subjects. Current community values and doctrines must be challenged so that education that allows for informed, reasoned choices becomes the standard throughout the nation. Critical changes must be made in terms of how sexuality, particularly homosexuality, is dealt with socially and legally. Civil-rights legislation must be seen not as condoning any particular lifestyle, but as essential to guarantee freedom of choice, access to medical care, and protection from punitive public policies. The long-term benefits of allowing younger people who are homosexual to grow up in a society that does not treat them as lepers, criminals, or satanic beings must be understood in terms of how sexual behaviors are used to survive and affirm an identity in a hostile world. Allowing homosexually oriented people to develop healthy self-concepts, to be freed of the anxiety that drives many toward unsafe sex, must inform the change in civil-rights protection.

Drug addiction must be seen as an illness, just like alcoholism. Drugs must be decriminalized, even regulated and administered perhaps in much the same way alcohol is. That would mean confronting the economic implications of the drug traffic in this country and providing access to treatment and rehabilitation. The cost to do so is staggering.

To truly respond to the psychological aspects of AIDS will cost this government and society both dollars and existing public policies and laws. The education of the young will need to be re-prioritized, so that children are coherently educated from the beginning to understand and believe in both the risks to life and the possibilities for decreasing those risks. The separation of church and state will have to be complete, permitting the church to disagree but not regulate education or public policy, which will protect the people through reasonable and appropriate programs.

Finally, public officials and scientists must acknowledge the importance of understanding the anxiety we share as human beings about our mortality, and our attempts to mitigate our fears of it. Public policy must derive from a comprehensive view of human life, with its fears and phobias, inconsistencies and incongruities. Society must be seen as a complex organism, neither wholly rational nor wholly irrational. That individuals sometimes do not act the way others might want, or even the way they might want to act themselves, is part of the human condition. A species as complex as ours requires a complex set of public policies and multiple levels of strategies. No single plan or program will be enough. The makers of public policy carry the significant responsibility of not responding reflexively, but rather leading society into a future that acknowledges the psychological aspect of human beings and pays attention to it in the development of all strategies that attempt to control the spread of this virus or any future threat.

Notes

1. Albert Camus, *The Plague* (New York: Vintage Books, 1948), 39.
2. The author has personally heard this view set forth twice by public figures, one a leading member of the Moral Majority, the other a representative of a pro-family, "anti-AIDS" group from New York City who stated the position during a panel discussion on AIDS in which the author participated and which was aired on the *Dave Finnegan Show,* on Boston's WNEV-TV, Channel 7.
3. HIV Negative Test Often Prompts High Risk Behavior, *AIDS Record* 1:3, March 15, 1987.
4. Personal communication from David Ostrow, M.D., Ph.D., University of Michigan.
5. Camus, *The Plague,* 236.
6. *AIDS Weekly Surveillance Report — United States,* AIDS Program, Center for Infectious Diseases, Centers for Disease Control, February 1988.
7. Third International Conference on AIDS, Washington, D.C., June 1987, and Fourth International Conference on AIDS, Stockholm, Sweden, to be held in June 1988.

I'm of the Jewish faith. Both of my parents were in concentration camps and my father made a comment to me when he first found out what was wrong with me: "Now you know how I felt when I was twenty-two years old and I could die at any minute," and when he said that, that just . . . that did it, I just decided you can live or die with this, and I chose to live with it. He survived the Holocaust and I'll survive this."

HIV Antibody Screening: An Ethical Framework for Evaluating Proposed Programs

Ronald Bayer, Ph.D.
Carol Levine, M.A.
Susan M. Wolf, J.D.

Introductory Note

In May 1985, the Food and Drug Administration (FDA) licensed the first test kits to detect antibodies to the human immunodeficiency virus (HIV), then known as HTLV-III. The test kits were developed to screen donated blood in order to detect contaminated units so that they could be discarded. Only a small percentage of AIDS cases had been traced to transfusions; however, federal officials assigned a high priority to developing a method of identifying contaminated blood because of immense public concern about the safety of the blood supply. Moreover, the means of preventing transmission in this way — unlike changes in sexual or needle-sharing behaviors — was amenable to technological intervention.

The introduction of the test kits — formally known as ELISAs, or enzyme-linked immunosorbent assays — for this purpose (still the only FDA-approved one) led almost immediately to a variety of other proposed uses. Some of these appeared to be valid on grounds of public health and ethics; others were suspect on both counts.

Staff at the Hastings Center had begun to consider the ethical ramifications of AIDS as early as 1983, and the result of the first project on AIDS was a set of guidelines on confidentiality in research, published in *IRB: A Review of Human Subjects Research* (November–December 1984). The Hastings Center research group then turned its attention to a range of other problems and quickly agreed that the uses of the HIV antibody test were of paramount concern. The result of a series of meetings involving public health officials, philosophers, lawyers, gay rights advocates, and others was the article printed here — an attempt to lay out an ethical framework for considering proposed uses of the test. Although the authors alone are responsible for the views set forth in it, the article represents the consensus view that had emerged: opposition to widespread mandatory testing and support for expanded voluntary testing, with appropriate counseling and confidentiality and antidiscrimination protections.

Dr. Ronald Bayer is associate for policy studies at the Hastings Center. Carol Levine is executive director of the Citizens Commission on AIDS for New York City and Northern New Jersey. She was formerly codirector of the Hastings Center's projects on AIDS. Susan M. Wolf is associate for law at the Hastings Center.

That was the view overwhelmingly endorsed at a conference called by the Centers for Disease Control (CDC) in February 1987. What the CDC had planned as a small, informal discussion turned into a media event attended by over eight hundred public health officials, civil rights advocates, and others. Many criticized the CDC for even the decision to place mandatory testing on the agenda. The conclusions reached at the conference are expressed in a CDC document entitled "Recommended Additional Guidelines for HIV Antibody Counseling and Testing in the Prevention of HIV Infection and AIDS" (dated April 30, 1987). The participants favored "the increased use of voluntary confidential HIV antibody counseling and testing as an adjunct measure in the prevention and control of AIDS." They also concluded that "mandatory testing other than for screening donated blood and plasma was not useful, nor should it be required for the prevention and control of HIV infection and AIDS." Surgeon General C. Everett Koop advocated a similar approach.

At the same time, however, Secretary of Education William J. Bennett took the political lead in calling for increased "routine" testing of individuals in certain age groups and on specific occasions, such as admission to a hospital or application for a marriage license. Rep. William E. Dannemeyer (R–Calif.) promoted the same idea but was more open in calling it "mandatory" testing. At a dinner the night before the opening of the Third International Conference on AIDS in Washington, D.C., President Reagan, speaking out for the first time on AIDS, also called for "routine" testing of several groups. A Gallup Poll taken in July 1987 found that 52 percent of Americans favored testing all Americans, and as many as 90 percent of those polled favored testing of selected groups, such as immigrants.

At the time the original version of the article printed here was published, the Department of Defense was already screening military recruits and rejecting those who were seropositive, and screening active duty personnel and reassigning those who were seropositive. The federal government has moved toward expanding the screening net to include Foreign Service applicants and active personnel; applicants for the Department of Labor's Job Corps; federal prisoners; immigrants; and undocumented aliens seeking to regularize their status under the amnesty program.

States have also moved to institute mandatory screening programs. Two states — Louisiana and Illinois — have mandated premarital screening, although the provisions in each state are somewhat different. Other states are considering a range of settings for screening. Some hospitals have announced policies of screening all admissions; many others are screening selected patients surreptitiously. Insurance companies vigorously defend their right to test applicants for life insurance and even health insurance and to deny coverage to those who are infected. Most employers are not screening job applicants or employees; a few, however, do so.

New concerns have been raised about the accuracy of the current screening tests when applied to populations in which there is a low reservoir of infection — such as marriage license applicants and hospital admissions. A study published in the *Journal of the American Medical Association* (October 2, 1987) concluded that universal premarital screening in the United States "currently would detect fewer than one tenth of 1% of HIV-infected individuals at a cost of substantially more than $100 million. More than 100 infected individuals would be told that they were probably not infected, and there would likely be more than 350 false-positive results." A report in the *Lancet* (September 12, 1987) warned that the latency period between infection and the development of antibodies might be as long as fourteen months, rather than the six months previously thought to represent the outer limit. And, as experience with testing accumulates, more reports show that even positive results confirmed by Western blot may occasionally be false positives. Pregnant women, for example, may be in this category because of cross-reactivity to the father's antigens.

Public health officials are caught between the public pressures to test and professional concerns about the wisdom and cost-effectiveness of widespread testing of populations unlikely to be infected. The New Jersey Department of Health's policy on testing, issued in September 1987, is as much a refutation of mandatory testing as it is a proposal for expanded voluntary and routine testing (with informed consent) in state-funded clinics for prenatal care, family planning, and sexually transmitted diseases.

Without a vaccine, without a cure, and with only the beginnings of effective treatment, AIDS will continue to present a challenge to those who make public policy. Faced with a new and lethal disease, the public demands action, any kind of action. The HIV antibody test is a valuable tool, but not a solution. The principles outlined in the following article, I believe, still constitute an ethical approach to the use of the test, but they may not withstand the political pressures.

— Carol Levine

The acquired immunodeficiency syndrome (AIDS) poses a compelling ethical challenge to medicine, science, public health, the legal system, and our political democracy. This report focuses on one aspect of that challenge: the use of blood tests to identify individuals who have been infected with the retrovirus human immunodeficiency virus (HIV). In this article, we follow the terminology recently proposed by the International Committee on the Taxonomy of Viruses; that is, we use the term *human immunodeficiency virus*. This replaces the more cumbersome dual terminology of human T-cell lymphotropic virus type III/lymphadenopathy-associated virus (HTLV-III/LAV).

The issue is urgent: the tests are already in use and plans to implement them much more broadly are being proposed.[1] The issue is also complex: at stake is a potential conflict between the community's interests in stopping the spread of a devastating disease and in preserving important values of individual liberty and equal rights.

Screening may seem to be a minor intrusion in the face of a deadly disease; yet even such an ostensibly limited intervention can have dramatic and deleterious consequences for individuals. Such intrusions must, therefore, be warranted by the potential public health benefits.

It is important to reaffirm our society's commitment to promoting the health of its citizens, but public health efforts undertaken with a beneficent intent have sometimes had the opposite effect. An example is mandatory screening for sickle cell trait among blacks in the 1970s, which resulted in misinformation, stigmatization, and discrimination.[2]

This report is addressed to all those considering the introduction of screening and testing programs, including employers, public health officials, legislators, health care providers, and insurers, as well as those who would be screened and whose interests would be affected. We have adopted prevailing usage and define *screening* as the application of the HIV antibody tests to populations and *testing* as the application of that procedure to individuals on a case-by-case basis.[3] Using this distinction, blood donations tested for HIV antibodies are screened; people who go to an alternative test site for the same procedure are tested.

We believe that in each situation in which screening is considered, the proposed program should be subjected to ethical analysis. This report provides a framework for that task. Ethical evaluation is necessary but not sufficient for decision making; it should be performed in conjunction with other types of evaluation, such as legal and economic analyses, before screening is instituted.[4] In addition, those who consider screening should consult with members of affected populations, since these individuals are best able to identify the potential hazards of proposed programs.

This document argues at various points in favor of moral obligations without advocating legal coercion. In a society that recognizes individual privacy and liberty, law and ethics are often distinct spheres. Not all moral obligations should be translated into law.

Screening for HIV Antibodies

The test now being used to detect the presence of antibodies elicited by HIV viral antigens is an enzyme-linked immunosorbent assay — the ELISA (or EIA) test. Because the ELISA test was developed to protect the blood supply, the cutoff between reactive and nonreactive values was set very low to capture all true positives. The price of such sensitivity is a loss of specificity. In high-risk populations, there will be comparatively few false positives. In low-risk populations, however, as many as 90 percent of the small number of initially reactive results will be false positives. To distinguish true positives, it is necessary to repeat the ELISA and to use an independent, supplemental test such as the Western blot.[5]

In addition to the false positives, there may be false negatives; that is, the tests may fail to detect antibodies, or there may be none even though the person is infected. The problem of false negatives is only partly a characteristic of the test; it also reflects the latency period (on rare occasions as long as six months) between infection with HIV and the development of antibodies.

Despite these problems, the ELISA test has satisfactorily served its initial purpose — screening blood donations. The antibody test also enables clinicians to monitor the infection status of their patients. It may be useful in establishing risk to the patient when immunosuppressive therapy is contemplated. It may provide epidemiologists with baseline data for the conduct of longitudinal studies of the natural history of AIDS. Finally, it may provide many individuals with data that are useful in supporting their voluntary modification of sexual, drug-using, and reproductive behavior.

The current screening method (a repeated ELISA plus a supplemental test) compares favorably, in terms of accuracy, to other screening methods used in medical practice, all of which have some limitations. Concern about the possible misuses of test results must not be confused with challenges to the accuracy of the tests.

Principles and Prerequisites for Evaluating a Screening Program

To evaluate the ethical acceptability of a proposed screening program, we recommend an analysis that is based on seven prerequisites. The prerequisites are based on the principle of respect for persons and the principles of harm, beneficence, and justice. These four widely accepted ethical principles are derived from secular, religious, and constitutional traditions and are commonly applied to medicine, research, and public health.[6, 7] A brief discussion of each of the four principles follows.

1. *Respect for persons* requires that individuals be treated as autonomous agents who have the right to control their own destinies. It requires that persons be given the opportunity to decide what will or will not happen to them. The right to privacy and the requirement of informed consent flow from this principle. A corollary — requiring that persons with diminished autonomy be given special protections — may also apply to some populations, such as children and prisoners.

2. *The harm principle* permits limitations to be placed on an individual's liberty to pursue personal goals and choices when others would be harmed by those activities.

3. *Beneficence* requires that we act on behalf of the interests and welfare of others. The obligations of beneficence apply to actions affecting both individuals and the community. Potential risks must be weighed against potential benefits, followed by adoption of the actions with the most favorable risk-to-benefit ratio. The justification for public-health authority derives from both the harm principle and the beneficence principle.

4. *Justice* requires that the benefits and burdens of particular actions be distributed fairly. It also prohibits invidious discrimination.

These ethical principles may sometimes conflict. For example, the principle of beneficence and the harm principle may outweigh the need to obtain consent in some situations, but they never outweigh the obligation to treat persons with respect for their intrinsic worth and dignity.

The following seven prerequisites are based on the preceding principles. These prerequisites constitute the threshold requirements for ethical acceptability, but they do not cover all the ethical problems that may arise, as we will see later.

1. *The purpose of the screening must be ethically acceptable.* There is at present one acceptable purpose for screening: to stop the spread of AIDS. This purpose draws on the principle of beneficence — the duty to protect the welfare of those who might become infected with HIV. The use of medical tests and of the public health power of the state is justifiable to protect the health of the community. However, use of these resources merely to express social disapproval of sexual orientation or of drug use violates the principles of justice and respect for persons. If a therapy or vaccine becomes available, screening may be justified to benefit those at risk.

2. *The means to be used in the screening program and the intended use of the information must be appropriate for accomplishing the purpose.* If a screening program is intended to stop the spread of HIV infection but is designed in a way that precludes achieving that end, it is unjustifiable, since it would involve an invasion of privacy without any public health benefit. For example, screening all food handlers is not justifiable, since there is no evidence that the disease is spread through food.

3. *High-quality laboratory services must be used.* Given the importance of interpreting not just one but a series of tests to arrive at a confirmed positive result, the availability of highly qualified technicians and laboratory services is essential. Beneficence requires that persons not be subjected to any risk — whether social, psychological, or medical — if the information about them to be generated in screening does not meet the current standard levels of accuracy. The need for confirmatory testing applies both to low- and high-risk populations.

4. *Individuals must be notified that screening will take place.* Respect for persons requires that individuals be notified that they are or may be the subjects of screening. In some cases, individuals may choose not to participate in the activity for which screening is required (for example, they may choose not to donate blood or semen). In other cases, they may not have that option, but they should, nevertheless, be notified to protect their autonomy; they should also be made aware that highly sensitive data about them will be generated, with the associated psychological burdens and risks of breaches of confidentiality. Physicians who contemplate testing an individual on the basis of membership in a risk group should notify the person and should seek consent. This prerequisite does not preclude the use, without notification, of blood or other samples unlinked to personal identifiers in research approved by institutional review boards (IRBs).

5. *Individuals who are screened have a right to be informed about the results.* There is no ethical justification for withholding test results. Certainly that information may be profoundly disturbing — not just to the individual but to the health care provider who has to convey it — but the principles of respect for persons and beneficence support notification.

The converse — that individuals have a "right not to know" — is in dispute. We believe that persons who are screened and whose seropositivity is confirmed have a moral obligation to learn that information; that is, we reject the right not to know in this case.[8]

The most important potential benefit of the knowledge of a positive test result is the motivation for an individual to change behavior that puts others at risk. A person at low risk (for example, a blood donor who has no knowledge of a sexual partner's drug use) has no reason to suspect that he or she is infected and, therefore, has no reason to change behavior. To protect others, that person must know the fact of potential infectiousness.

This conclusion is generally accepted; the major controversy concerns the right of individuals at high risk not to know. The claim is made that as long as such an individual acts as though he or she were seropositive and avoids high-risk behavior, there is no need for knowledge of seropositivity. Moreover, the argument continues, such information may be so psychologically devastating that the individual will suffer greatly without any benefits to himself or herself or additional benefits to others.

We acknowledge the potential burden of such information. We also recognize that there is insufficient evidence to determine whether notification will in fact motivate behavioral change or whether it will lead to enormous distress with no compensating benefits. However, there are two problems with the arguments in favor of a right not to know. First, they underestimate the power of denial and the difficulty of sustaining behavioral change in the absence of specific information. Second, there is no way to discern in advance which of the infected people will modify their behavior without notification and which will not, much less which ones will be consistent in these changes.

Therefore, we conclude that given the disastrous consequences of HIV infection and the imperative of the harm principle, those who are infected have an obligation to know their antibody status, to inform their sexual partners, and to modify their behavior. We urge immediate research into both the positive and negative consequences of notification.

6. *Sensitive and supportive counseling programs must be available before and after screening to interpret the results, whether they are positive or negative.* Individuals should be counseled about the test before screening; should be told the significance of both positive and negative results; and should be informed about the availability of future counseling. A confirmed positive test result should not be conveyed by letter. It should be provided by personal contact in the context of, or with referral to, competent counseling services. Referral to a person's private physician may not be adequate, since many physicians in general practice, particularly those in low-incidence areas, have little experience with interpreting HIV antibody test results.

7. *The confidentiality of screened individuals must be protected.* Respect for the privacy of those who undergo therapeutic and diagnostic procedures demands that the results of such procedures be kept confidential. In the case of HIV antibody testing, where the inadvertent or unwarranted disclosure of positive test results could have disastrous social consequences for individuals, preserving confidentiality is especially critical.

However, there are a few circumstances in which public health reasons could provide a justification for the breach of confidentiality. For example, if it were known that a seropositive individual had recently donated blood, notifying the blood collection agency would be appropriate on grounds of benefiting blood recipients. However, that agency would then have the obligation to protect the confidentiality of the information received.

Appropriate legislation or administrative regulations should be designed to protect the confidentiality of antibody test results. Whenever disclosure is to occur, individuals must be informed that a breach of confidentiality will take place and must be told why it is necessary. Under no circumstances should test results be used in ways that bear no relationship to legitimate public health concerns.

Mass Screening and Screening in Special Settings: Applying the Ethical Prerequisites

Using the framework we have established in the previous sections, we will now discuss the specific application of the principles and prerequisites to the current policy debates.

Should Universal Mandatory Screening Be Undertaken?

Universal mandatory screening can be justified on the basis of beneficence when a therapeutic intervention is available or when an infectious state puts others at risk merely through casual contact. However, neither is the case with AIDS. Thus, there is no demonstrable public health benefit that justifies universal mandatory screening, given the invasion of privacy involved.

Representing the extreme position, advocates of universal mandatory screening suggest it be a prelude to isolation.[9] This would entail a sweeping deprivation of civil and human rights — the segregation of a million or more people for life on the assumption that they will behave in ways that spread disease. Such a drastic measure cannot be justified, particularly when less intrusive measures are available. Isolation would probably increase the incidence of disease, because those who were segregated would become a closed community, with the prospect of repeated reinfection.

Others justify mandatory screening less drastically. They see it as a way of making each individual learn his or her antibody status, hoping that this will prompt behavioral change. However, long-term behavioral modification is a complex process that is less likely to be achieved under circumstances of coercion, where long-term follow-up and support are nearly impossible to provide on a mass scale. Even in this case, universal mandatory screening would require the creation of an immense and costly apparatus. Since screening would have to be repeated periodically, it would be necessary to trace each individual's whereabouts to preclude avoidance of the test. Even were such screening feasible, it would require an extraordinary and repeated intrusion into the privacy of all Americans, with little probable benefit. Therefore, on grounds of beneficence, it would be unacceptable.

Should Mandatory Screening Be Implemented in Special Settings?

In certain limited circumstances, mandatory screening is appropriate — only where it can be shown, under stringent standards of scientific evidence, to reduce certain dangers. The mandatory screening of all blood donations has aroused virtually no opposition, because everyone has an interest in a blood supply that is free of HIV. For similar reasons, there should be routine screening of semen donors for artificial insemination and of organ donations for transplant purposes, both under conditions consistent with our ethical prerequisites.[10] With respect to donations of blood, semen, or live organs, individuals can avoid screening by avoiding the activity; these activities may be desired but are not central to a person's life plans.

Screening all applicants for marriage licenses presents quite a different situation. Marriage, unlike the act of donating blood, is central to an individual's freedoms. The likelihood of detecting a significant number of true positives, a goal that might be defended on grounds of beneficence, is exceedingly small in relation to the economic costs and ethical dangers of invasions of privacy and potential curbs on individual liberties in instituting a screening program. Those at risk for contracting AIDS are not likely to be the ones applying for marriage licenses. Moreover, neither sex nor childbearing is dependent on marriage in our society.

The state has an interest in stopping the spread of AIDS, but any bar to marriage for a seropositive individual would pose serious legal and ethical problems. Seropositive heterosexuals, like gay men in long-term relationships, can practice safer sex and take their antibody status into account in making childbearing plans. Individuals who are at high risk or who are concerned about their own or their partner's antibody status may voluntarily take the test before marriage, with appropriate counseling.

General screening in the workplace is unjustifiable under our ethical prerequisites, because the usefulness of such screening for the protection of others is unsupported by epidemiological or clinical evidence.[11] In some cases, although the protection of the public health is the stated purpose for workplace screening, the underlying reason is the desire to avoid the economic burden of providing health care benefits for people who might become ill with AIDS. The economic costs of AIDS are a matter of serious concern and ought to be addressed directly, so that equitable mechanisms for sharing the burden can be developed. However, to disguise these concerns as matters of public health serves neither purpose well.

But are there circumstances that fall between the extremes of blood screening and general employment screening where mandatory screening might be ethically acceptable? A range of settings must be considered.

Employment settings. Since casual contact is not a route of transmission of HIV, the only employment settings in which mandatory screening might be justified are, first, health care involving the open wounds of others and, second, prostitution. Careful investigation of the potential of HIV transmission from infected workers and professionals to patients indicates no evidence of such transmission when standard infection control precautions are taken.[12] Since the risks are, therefore, only theoretical, no grounds currently exist for instituting routine screening of health care workers, including dentists. Prudence, however, dictates that health care personnel who are themselves at high risk for AIDS, whether or not they know their antibody status, take all precautions when they enter a situation in which contact might pose a hazard to others.

A strong public health argument can be made for screening prostitutes. First, male and female prostitutes may have significant rates of seropositivity, either because of drug use; because of a greater risk of infection, owing to their large numbers of sexual contacts; or because of high-risk sexual practices in which they may engage. Second, seropositive prostitutes can potentially infect large numbers of people. Because the great majority of infected persons in this country are male, and because male-to-male transmission of HIV is most common, it is likely that male prostitutes constitute a greater threat to their clients than do female prostitutes at this time. Finally, prostitutes' motivation to practice safer sex or to stop prostitution may be questionable; even if they are so motivated, the pressures to maintain their current behavioral patterns are probably considerable.

As a practical matter, however, only where prostitutes are licensed and subject to periodic health examinations could such screening, when used in conjunction with license revocation, interrupt the transmission of HIV without creating huge problems. Nevada has recently introduced such screening.[13] Where prostitution is illegal, screening can occur only as an adjunct to arrest. Those prostitutes who are seropositive would have to be threatened with rearrest and perhaps with isolation if they continued to engage in prostitution. Effective and consistent enforcement would raise difficult logistic and legal questions.

These practical difficulties, and the moral issues raised by singling out one group for a regimen of screening, arrest, and isolation, warrant immediate attention. Although moving incrementally is morally permissible, targeting a specific population requires particular justification to prevent invidious discrimination. There is an urgent need for educating prostitutes and their clients. It is also important to examine possible ways to reduce the spread of HIV which take into account the social realities of prostitution.

Since the only ethical justification for workplace screening is derived from beneficence — reducing the risk of infection to others — the Department of Defense's routine screening of all recruits and active duty personnel is troubling. Communal living does not result in the transmission of HIV. The Department of Defense publicly justifies its policy with the claim that each member of the armed services is a potential blood donor and that in a battlefield emergency there would be no time to screen blood.[14] However, it is not at all clear that soldier-to-soldier battlefield transfusions are standard practice today. Moreover, the rejection of seropositive recruits cannot be justified on such grounds if seropositive active duty personnel are not also being discharged. Even if all seropositive individuals were discharged, one-time screening would not suffice to protect the military donor pool over time. Given the social costs associated with repeated screening, it would be more appropriate to ensure alternatives to battlefield soldier-to-soldier transfusion.

More plausible is the justification that screening identifies those whose compromised immune system might lead to adverse reactions to live-virus vaccines routinely given to recruits. But even this paternalistic justification is weak. The HIV tests are not the only way to identify these individuals.

As in general-employment screening, other factors may be concealed under the guise of public health: the military's policies against homosexuality and drug use; relations with foreign governments that are concerned about the exportation of AIDS by U.S. servicemen; and the desire to avoid the economic burden of AIDS. Here, too, we urge that these concerns be discussed directly, not masked as purported public health issues.

Clinical and residential settings. Because hepatitis B is far more infectious than HIV, it is widely accepted that those institutional precautions which are currently in place to prevent infection by hepatitis B are sufficient to protect against infection by HIV (see note 15). Since the routine screening of hospital admissions for hepatitis B is not deemed necessary, neither is the routine mandatory screening of all hospital admissions for HIV infection.

Dialysis centers are the only clinical setting in which routine hepatitis B screening occurs. Yet here the CDC has argued against routine antibody screening for HIV because of the potential breaches of confidentiality, although it does not object to dialysis on separate machines for those with clinically diagnosed AIDS.[15] Epidemiological evidence has provided no evidence thus far of transmission of HIV infection in dialysis centers. However, given the frequent occurrence of blood spills in such centers, we believe that the routine screening of dialysis patients for HIV and the adoption of especially careful precautions for those who are seropositive require further consideration. Such screening, however, should never be used to deny dialysis.

In other settings, such as mental hospitals and residential homes for retarded people, routine screening might be considered because of the possibility of sexual contacts among residents or patients. Especially in those settings where sexual segregation is practiced, homosexual contact — voluntary and involuntary — is known to occur. Given the reduced competence and diminished autonomy that characterize residents of mental hospitals and homes for retarded people, it might be appropriate to consider screening residents and patients in such settings as a way of protecting those who are uninfected from possible HIV infection. However, the need to provide extra supervision for those who are seropositive does not warrant isolation, stigmatization, or the deprivation of services.

The screening of infants born to mothers at high risk, prior to foster care or adoption placement, raises unique issues.[16] The purpose of antibody testing under these circumstances would not be to stop the spread of AIDS or to benefit the child, but to provide potential foster and adoptive parents with information that would undoubtedly play a role in their decision to care for the child. But for that purpose, the test results may be inconclusive. Some babies born to seropositive mothers may be seropositive at birth but not viremic and may lose the antibodies in the first year of life.[17]

A seropositive child may be difficult, if not impossible, to place in a foster or an adoptive home, even though the child may never develop illness. Isolation and stigmatization would almost inevitably follow. The tension is between the potential harm to such children and the interests of the prospective foster and adoptive parents in obtaining this information. These issues require further study.[18]

Finally, screening in prisons has been discussed. Since there are substantial numbers of intravenous drug users in prisons, and since homosexual activity, including instances of homosexual rape, is known to occur, proponents of screening argue that it is the obligation of the state to protect inmates from possible infection. Those who oppose such screening point out that the identification of seropositive prisoners might well place them in imminent danger of violence from other inmates. To prevent such violence, and to protect other inmates from infection, isolation has been suggested by proponents of prison screening. The logical consequence of such a proposal would be the creation of a separate prison system. The problems of logistics posed by such an effort would be staggering. Furthermore, segregating those who are seropositive without measures to educate and protect them from repeated infection would only increase the likelihood of disease.

In prison and in clinical and residential settings, a question ought to be asked of all proposals for mandatory screening: Are there alternative measures less intrusive than screening which could provide the necessary protections? If so, then screening cannot be justified.

In fact, alternatives to screening in prisons do exist. The state could reduce the risk of forcible spread of HIV infection by seeking to reduce the incidence of prison rape. The spread of HIV infection in prison would also be reduced by providing condoms and education regarding the risks of drug use and high-risk sexual behaviors.

Screening and insurance. Both health insurance and life insurance are at issue here. First, with respect to health insurance, we have determined as a society that, with the exception of the very poor and the elderly, it will be available through the private sector, largely through the workplace. The acquired immunodeficiency syndrome has provided the occasion to reexamine elements of that system, including exclusions for preexisting conditions and reliance on experience rather than community rating.[19]

The sole purpose for which screening would be instituted by health insurance carriers would be either to deny coverage or to increase sharply premiums for those who are seropositive.[20] Persons who apply for insurance as individuals, rather than as members of groups, are particularly vulnerable, but dangers exist as well for persons covered by group plans. Employers who are self-insured may seek to dismiss employees, penalize them, or refuse to hire applicants who could increase the costs of health care coverage. In any case, given the proportion of the population which would be involved, screening for group health insurance would be, in essence, universal mandatory screening, and the arguments presented against that policy apply here as well.

Although we recognize that this view is controversial, we believe that state regulatory agencies should not permit those who provide group or individual health insurance coverage to exclude persons who are at increased risk for any illness, including AIDS. A denial of health insurance would ultimately create overwhelming burdens for the public and private hospitals that would be forced to provide uncompensated care to the uninsured. From a societal perspective, the central issue is whether the cost of health care for AIDS patients and others at high risk for illness will be broadly distributed or borne by those who become sick, and by their friends and families, reducing them to dependency on the welfare system. The moral issue is one of justice.

The moral problems posed by life insurance are more difficult to evaluate, since it is not as basic a need as health insurance. The social purpose of life insurance is to provide protection for dependents in the event of death, although individuals may purchase life insurance for other purposes as well. Those who are at increased risk for a broad range of medical conditions face barriers to life insurance either through formal exclusion or prohibitive premium rates, especially when insurance is purchased individually rather than through a group.

Insurance carriers fear that those who know they are at risk for AIDS will seek large amounts of life insurance coverage, thus potentially endangering a company's solvency and its ability to pay other claims. Consequently, insurers seek to protect the interests of their other policyholders and stockholders by screening applicants in high-risk categories for HIV antibodies.

Despite such fears, there is no solid information yet on the potential impact of AIDS on insurance companies' solvency or on future premium rates. Moreover, there is a substantial risk to individuals who are screened; the information produced may be accessible to employers and others with no legitimate public health interest. Those who are denied life insurance coverage may also be denied loans, mortgages, and other forms of credit.

In determining public policy, state regulatory agencies must entertain the full range of issues beyond narrow actuarial considerations. If screening is ultimately permitted by state regulatory agencies for life insurance, these agencies should also explore innovative arrangements to provide appropriate coverage to seropositive individuals, and should mandate strict confidentiality requirements as well.

Alternatives to Screening: The Promise of Voluntarism

We believe that those who are at high risk for developing AIDS have a moral obligation to take all possible steps to prevent harm to others, including taking the antibody test. This moral obligation should not, however, be translated into legal coercion. Mandating universal screening, as we have explained, would violate norms of beneficence and respect for persons and might drive the HIV infection underground, thus subverting public health goals.

Where voluntary testing programs are instituted, they should follow the relevant ethical prerequisites set out earlier: that is, high-quality laboratory and data services must be used; individuals who are tested must be informed about the results; sensitive and supportive counseling programs must be available before and after testing to interpret the results, whether positive or negative; and the confidentiality of tested individuals must be protected. In addition, voluntary testing should involve full disclosure of risks and benefits as well as informed consent.

Some have rejected the moral obligation to take the test, arguing that all members of high-risk groups should simply act as if they were antibody-positive. These persons cite dramatic changes in sexual behavior (as measured by a reduction in sexually transmitted diseases in homosexual men in San Francisco and New York) in populations that include men who have not taken the test.

If such advice were sufficient to motivate radical alterations in sexual conduct and in childbearing plans among the diverse populations involved, it might not be necessary to encourage the use of the antibody test. No conclusive evidence exists on either side, but there is reason to doubt that advice alone provides sufficient motivation.[21] Given the risks associated with AIDS and the uncertainty about what will in fact modify high-risk behavior, there is a strong community interest in encouraging voluntary testing. Public health authorities and clinicians should encourage the use of such tests, to be taken anonymously or with strict confidentiality protections.

In addition, antibody-positive individuals have a moral obligation to notify their partners, especially when their partners have no reason to suspect that they have had contact with an individual at risk for HIV infection. Counselors have a professional duty to encourage such notification.

We recognize that sexual contact tracing by public health officials might be considered the next logical step, since some individuals may refuse to notify their sexual partners directly. This issue requires further discussion, to consider both whether this is an appropriate strategy at this time and what kinds of protection would be needed. Sexual contact tracing might be justified in low-risk and low-incidence areas, for example, but not in other settings.[22]

Women who are at high risk should be encouraged to undergo testing as they consider the prospect of childbearing.[23] In the case of positive results, pregnant women should be fully informed about the risks to themselves and their fetuses (the risks are high but not necessarily determinative) so that they can make informed decisions about whether to terminate the pregnancy. However, encouragement to undergo testing should be just that, not coercion.

Because of the uncertainty and anxiety that surround the issue of confidentiality, antibody testing has been undertaken under conditions of anonymity in many cities at alternative test sites. In these settings, individuals do not provide their names; are counseled about the test; and, if they decide to take the test, are given a number. It is up to the tested individual to request the results and to obtain further counseling. Anonymous testing thus offers the greatest protection for the confidentiality of test results. As a result, testing under such circumstances has been recommended as the single most effective way of encouraging the voluntary use of the test. However, drawbacks to such testing do exist. It may preclude appropriate counseling and follow-up and may make long-term epidemiological studies in the tested populations either difficult or impossible. In the short run, anonymous testing may be the only effective strategy for both privacy and public health reasons. Ultimately, if it were possible to construct stringent confidentiality protections, anonymous testing with its obvious limitations might be replaced.

The most serious threat to the widespread use of voluntary testing comes from proposals or already enacted regulations that require reporting to state public health officials the names of those who are antibody-positive. The arguments for such reporting resemble those which are used to justify the mandatory reporting of AIDS itself — now universally required in the United States — as well as other venereal diseases and infectious conditions. It has been asserted that epidemiological study, sexual contact tracing, and future therapeutic interventions all require mandatory reporting by private physicians and by all health care facilities.

In fact, mandatory reporting by name instead of code may deter rather than encourage voluntary testing. The knowledge that names will be given to public health authorities, even when those authorities affirm their commitment to confidentiality, is not conducive to voluntary testing. Some have even suggested that mandatory reporting may encourage anonymous sexual activity, so that individuals could not be named as sexual partners if contact tracing were implemented.

For voluntary testing to be effective, it would have to be widely available, not only in alternative test sites, but also in clinics established for the treatment of sexually transmitted diseases, in drug treatment facilities, and in prenatal clinics. Information in these settings should describe the services available in alternative test sites under conditions of anonymity as well.

Moreover, under the principle of justice, voluntary testing should be publicly funded. Many individuals at high risk, especially those who are intravenous drug users, do not have the resources to pay the cost of testing. The cost of widely available testing programs will be substantial, especially when the requisite services of counselors are considered. But to the extent that significant public health benefits might be achieved, these costs should not be a barrier to the creation of testing centers throughout the United States. Furthermore, since the primary purpose of testing is the protection of other individuals, including potential offspring, the burden of paying for testing ought to be borne by the public.

Summary

In conclusion, we believe that the greatest hope for stopping the spread of HIV infection lies in the voluntary cooperation of those at higher risk — their willingness to undergo testing and to alter their personal behavior and goals in the interests of the community. But we can expect this voluntary cooperation only if the legitimate interests of these groups and individuals in being protected from discrimination are heeded by legislators, professionals, and the public. Yet voluntary testing is not enough. We must proceed with vigorous research and educational efforts to eliminate both the scourge of AIDS and the social havoc that has accompanied it.

Permission to reprint the original version of this article was granted by the *Journal of the American Medical Association,* which published the article in its October 3, 1986, issue (vol. 256, no. 13, pp. 1768–1774; copyright 1986, American Medical Association; one edition in English only).

The Hastings Center research project on AIDS, entitled AIDS: Public Health and Civil Liberties, is funded by the American Foundation for AIDS Research, the Field Foundation, the Norman Foundation, the Pearl River Fund, and the Pettus-Crowe Foundation.

For their comments and criticisms of earlier drafts of this article, the authors wish to thank the members of the Hastings Center's AIDS research project: John D. Arras, Ph.D.; Dan Beauchamp, Ph.D.; Allan Brandt, Ph.D.; Daniel Callahan, Ph.D.; James Chin, M.D.; Robert Cohen, M.D.; Christopher J. Collins, J.D.; Irene W. Crowe, Ph.D.; Harold Edgar, LL.B.; Daniel Fox, Ph.D.; Willard Gaylin, M.D.; Lawrence Gostin, J.D.; Bruce Jennings, M.A.; Mathilde Krim, Ph.D.; Sheldon Landesman, M.D.; Jeffrey Levi; Robert J. Levine, M.D.; Ruth Macklin, Ph.D.; Deborah J. Merritt, J.D.; Alvin Novick, M.D.; Mel Rosen, C.S.W.; Stephen Schultz, M.D.; Mervyn Silverman, M.D.; Joseph Sonnabend, M.D.; Paul Starr, Ph.D.; Thomas Stoddard, J.D.; and David P. Willis, M.P.H.

Notes

1. Additional recommendations to reduce sexual and drug abuse-related transmissions of human T-lymphotropic virus type III/lymphadenopathy-associated virus. *Morbidity and Mortality Weekly Report* 1986;35:152–155.
2. R. F. Murray, Jr., M. Chamberlain, J. Fletcher, et al.: Special considerations for minority participation in prenatal diagnosis. *Journal of the American Medical Association* 1980;243:1254–1256.
3. J. M. Last: *Dictionary of Epidemiology.* New York, Oxford University Press, 1982, pp. 32–33.
4. Important to consider will be pertinent constitutional provisions, laws, and legal precedent on the federal, state, and local levels, such as the Fourteenth Amendment to the U.S. Constitution; the Federal Vocational Rehabilitation Act of 1973, 29 US 794; state statutes such as California Health and Safety Code Chapter 1.11 199.20 et seq.; city ordinances such as the San Francisco Police Code Article 38; and judicial decisions such as *Codero vs. Coughlin,* No. 84, Civ 728 (SD NY 1984); *District 27 Community School Board vs. Board of Education,* 130 Misc 2d 398, 502 NYS2d 325 (NY Sup 1986); *South Florida Blood Service, Inc., vs. Rasmussen,* 467 S2d 798 (Fla App 1985); and *La Rocca vs. Dalsheim,* 120 Misc 2d 697, 467 NYS2d 302 (NY Sup 1983). This list is by no means exhaustive, and the specifics of any screening or testing proposal will dictate the legal research required.
5. S. H. Weiss, J. J. Goedarat, M. G. Sarngadharan, et al.: Screening test for HTLV-III (AIDS agent) antibodies: Specificity, sensitivity, and applications. *Journal of the American Medical Association* 1985;253:221–225.
6. National Commission for the Protection of Human Subjects of Biomedical and Behavioral Research: The Belmont Report: Ethical Principles and Guidelines for the Protection of Human Subjects of Research, publication (OS) 78-0013. U.S. Department of Health, Education and Welfare, Washington, D.C., 1978.
7. T. L. Beauchamp, J. F. Childress: *Principles of Biomedical Ethics,* New York, Oxford University Press, 1979, pp. 97–126.
8. Provisional public health service interagency recommendations for screening donated blood and plasma for antibody to the virus causing acquired immunodeficiency syndrome. *Morbidity and Mortality Weekly Report* 1985;34:1–5.
9. J. Grutsch, A. D. Robertson: The coming of AIDS: It didn't start with homosexuals and it won't end with them. *American Spectator* 1986;19:12–15.

10. Testing donors of organs, tissues, and semen for antibody to human T-lymphotropic virus type-III/lymphadenopathy-associated virus. *Morbidity and Mortality Weekly Report* 1985;34:294.

11. Recommendations for preventing transmission of infection with human T-lymphotropic virus type III/lymphadenopathy-associated virus in the workplace. *Morbidity and Mortality Weekly Report* 1985;34:681–686, 691–695.

12. Update: Evaluation of human T-lymphotropic virus type III/lymphadenopathy-associated virus infection in health-care personnel — United States. *Morbidity and Mortality Weekly Report* 1985;34:575–578.

13. Prostitutes to undergo HTLV-III testing. *American Medical News* 1986;29:30.

14. C. Norman: Military AIDS testing offers research bonus. *Science* 1986;232:818–820.

15. M. S. Favero: Recommended precautions for patients undergoing hemodialysis who have AIDS or non-A, non-B hepatitis. *Infection Control* 1985;6:301–305.

16. Education and foster care of children infected with human T-lymphotropic virus type III/lymphadenopathy-associated virus. *Morbidity and Mortality Weekly Report* 1985;34:517–521.

17. R. W. Marion, A. A. Wiznia, R. G. Hutcheon, et al.: Human T-cell lymphotropic virus type III (HTLV-III) embryopathy: A new dysmorphic syndrome associated with intrauterine HTLV-III infections. *American Journal of Diseases of Children* 1986;140:638–640.

18. Acquired immunodeficiency syndrome in correctional facilities: A report of the National Institute of Justice and the American Correctional Association. *Morbidity and Mortality Weekly Report* 1986;35:195–199.

19. G. M. Oppenheimer, R. A. Padgug: AIDS: The risk to insurers, the threat to equity. Hastings Center Report 1986;16:18–22.

20. See a mimeograph entitled "White paper: The acquired immunodeficiency syndrome & HTLV-III antibody testing." American Council of Life Insurance, Health Insurance Association of America, February 1986.

21. C. E. Stevens, P. E. Taylor, E. A. Zang, et al.: Human T-cell lymphotropic virus type III infection in a cohort of homosexual men in New York City. *Journal of the American Medical Association* 1986;255:2167–2172.

22. M. Mills, C. B. Wofsey, J. Mills: Special report: The acquired immunodeficiency syndrome. *New England Journal of Medicine* 1986;314:931–936.

23. Recommendations for assisting in the prevention of perinatal transmission of HTLV-III/LAV and acquired immunodeficiency syndrome. *Morbidity and Mortality Weekly Report* 1985;34:721–726, 731–732.

"This is a great disease to be a drama queen with. I mean, it's really easy to fall into that 'victim role' trap and have everybody running around getting you glasses of water and doing all sorts of stuff for you. But I made a decision that first day, or possibly the second day—I was crying too much that first day—to choose life, and I've never looked back. I assume responsibility for my own life. I don't blame people. I assume responsibility for my own life. I refuse to play the victim role. I feel that I have control over my life. I have the right to lead a rich and full, rewarding life. I still play softball. I refuse to let this disease dictate my life."

HIV Antibody Testing: Performance and Counseling Issues

Michael Gross, Ph.D.

This article assesses the performance of currently used tests for exposure to human immunodeficiency virus (HIV), the infectious agent associated with acquired immunodeficiency syndrome (AIDS); suggests, in view of that information, guidelines for counseling people seeking HIV antibody testing; and evaluates the claim that because antibody test results will effect behavior change in those who are infected, all members of high-risk groups should be tested.

HIV testing is likely to yield a high proportion of false-positive results in low-risk populations and infants born to infected mothers. A negative result may not establish freedom from infection in high-risk groups or the offspring of infected mothers. Counseling should relate these generalizations to a client's motivation for and expectations from testing. In evaluating a client's risk of exposure, past and present, counseling should provide both information about and reinforcement for behavioral risk reduction.

The assertion that members of high-risk groups ought to learn their antibody status is questioned in view of concerns about test performance and even more serious questions about the psychological impact of test results — both short- and long-term — on people's adaptation to protective sex and modification of drug use patterns.

In November 1983 — not long after scientists had concluded that AIDS was caused by a transmissible agent and months before the disease was definitively associated with a new virus — the New York Academy of Medicine published a comprehensive summary of the state of knowledge about the syndrome. In the book's more than six hundred pages, containing dozens of papers about AIDS, just three index entries on blood screening refer to two short papers attempting to measure the efficacy of requesting that prospective donors who are at risk defer themselves. In current AIDS compendia, in contrast, techniques, applications, and interpretations of testing occupy whole chapters.

From a technical interest — how best to screen donations of blood and tissue for the agent associated with AIDS — testing has evolved into a major area of biomedical research and an even larger preoccupation, sometimes a battleground, of public policy.

Dr. Michael Gross coordinates support services for persons who are HIV-antibody-positive for the Massachusetts Department of Public Health. He also serves as a Support Service (hospice) volunteer with the AIDS Action Committee of Massachusetts, in Boston.

Should some or all citizens be subjected to mandatory testing? Is testing appropriate for purposes of insurance underwriting? Is testing a productive adjunct to risk-reduction education and counseling efforts? Are there any occupations for which screening is necessary to prevent transmission in the workplace? Are there valid reasons for testing institutionalized populations?

Test Methods and Performance

An important consideration in determining valid uses of testing is the performance of currently available methods. This section, therefore, examines the methods, accuracy, and efficacy of current procedures and the possible meanings of test results. The next section considers the implications of that information in an individual's decision about whether to elect for HIV testing, and in relation to his or her adherence to risk-reduction guidelines. Some of the patterns of response by individuals to their test results are then described as a context for a discussion in the following section of principles that ought to underly the adoption of testing programs.[1]

Is There a Test for AIDS?

The so-called AIDS test does not diagnose AIDS. An AIDS diagnosis requires actual illness, typically infections or cancers that indicate severe immune system damage. Even in the presence of such indicators (opportunistic infections like *Pneumocystis carinii* pneumonia or toxoplasmosis and cancers such as Kaposi's sarcoma or non-Hodgkins lymphoma), other possible causes of immune suppression must first be ruled out, including the use of immune suppressive or steroidal drugs or primary cancers that are themselves immune suppressive.[2]

Direct evidence for HIV infection would result from detecting the virus itself. Such methods, however, are used mainly for purposes of laboratory investigation.[3] Detection of an immune response to the virus, in the form of antibody to the virus, is the most widely used form of testing for such purposes as blood screening. But the mere presence of antibody to HIV does not establish an AIDS diagnosis, nor does it foretell with certainty the onset of HIV-related illness in the future; moreover, early detection of HIV does not lead to prevention of subsequent symptoms.[4]

Why Use Antibody Tests?

In general, the presence of antibody is a more consistent indicator of present *or* past infection than the presence of the disease-causing pathogen itself. Antibody will remain long after the causative agent of an infection has been cleared from the body. Before much became known about the natural history of HIV infection, it seemed possible that, like many other viruses, HIV might be eliminated by some individuals' immune response. Antibody would then be the only trace of past infection or of ongoing infection with undetectably low levels of virus. It now seems that most or all individuals infected with HIV never successfully eliminate the virus altogether. But in its latent state, the virus would be undetectable by antigen tests and possibly difficult to recover by viral isolation methods. Therefore, an antibody test is the most consistent index of HIV infection available which is practical to use on a large scale for screening purposes.

Why Use the ELISA Technique?

The most widely used screening method, employing an enzyme-linked immunosorbent assay (ELISA or EIA), is relatively inexpensive (typically, less than $5 per test for the cost of reagents and equipment), highly reproducible, and technologically adapted for processing large batches of samples with efficient, automated laboratory apparatus. In contrast, other procedures (for example, viral isolation, Western blot) have technical limitations. They usually depend on the competence, consistency, and particular recipes employed in a given laboratory[5] and are correspondingly more expensive. They may entail procedures that require special handling (for example, the radioactive reagents used in DNA probe studies and radioimmune precipitation). They also may be more difficult to interpret: for instance, both viral isolation and antigen tests frequently fail to detect virus in samples from truly infected individuals.[6]

What Are Current Procedures for Testing?

The protocol used by the Massachusetts Department of Public Health in its testing and counseling programs, and by the American Red Cross New England Region Blood Service screening program described here, is typical of testing programs across the country and internationally.[7]

Evaluation of a sample begins with an ELISA test. If the reactivity of the sample falls below a predetermined cutoff value standardized for the particular test kit being used, the result is judged negative, that is, no antibody detected. No further testing is undertaken. If the observed reactivity is above the cutoff value, the same sample is tested again using the ELISA procedure. When reactivity registers below the cutoff value on repeat testing — not an unusual occurrence for samples from low-risk individuals — the sample is interpreted as negative.

If the repeat ELISA test is also reactive or borderline, the sample is subjected to a more specific procedure that ordinarily has the capability to distinguish antibody to HIV from antibody to something else. The immunoblot, or Western blot, can show whether the antibody detected by ELISA binds to known classes of viral protein. The distinctive banding pattern that appears when the HIV antibody is present confirms a positive ELISA result. The lack of such a pattern indicates that antibody detected by ELISA was probably elicited by some agent other than HIV which happens spuriously to cross-react with biological material that was not eliminated when the test kit was prepared.

If the immunoblot pattern is ambiguous, for instance, if the observed bands are only very faintly perceptible, still another procedure may be employed: the immunofluorescence assay.[8] Cells known to be infected with HIV, along with uninfected (control) cells, are exposed to a serum sample and appropriate reagents. Infected cells will become coated with a fluorescent dye if the serum sample being tested contains HIV antibody, while uninfected control cells will show no label. Such a result is considered positive. If neither infected nor uninfected cells become labeled, the sample is considered free of HIV antibody. If both infected and uninfected cells become labeled, the meaning is ambiguous, and the outcome described as "indeterminate."[9]

How Accurate Are Antibody Test Results?

We do not know definitively. ELISA test kits from commercial manufacturers score differently on tests meant to standardize their performance. In 1986, five products ranged from 98.3 to 100 percent in sensitivity, which measures a test's ability to detect infection when it is present. They ranged from 99.2 to 99.8 percent in specificity, which indicates how well a test discriminates true infection from absence of infection.[10] These small percentage changes make a big difference in the proportion of false positives, as discussed below. The most sensitive tests are the least specific.[11] Making comparisons is difficult, because each manufacturer's tests were standardized using different test samples, and performance varies from batch to batch, even from the same manufacturer. In a study of ELISA performance in five hundred laboratories, thirty-five of approximately seven thousand positive samples were labeled negative. The laboratories, it should be noted, were voluntarily participating in these proficiency studies, and extra care may well have been taken, since the study samples were so labeled.[12]

Western blot tests are even more difficult to standardize or compare, because only one commercial test has been licensed. Most laboratories that perform Western blot testing use reagents they prepare with their own procedures, and they define the standards to be used in judging whether results for a sample are categorized as positive, indeterminate, or negative.[13] Ten of nineteen laboratories seeking U.S. Army contracts for Western blot testing were rejected because they failed a test panel at least once.[14] Using panels of ambiguous samples, the College of American Physicians found 12 to 15 percent of laboratories labeling two of three reactive samples indeterminate by Western blot.

The comparative performance of immunofluorescence assays — another form of confirmatory procedure — is even less well studied than that of Western blot tests.

Although specimens used in laboratory studies to standardize the performance of HIV tests receive optimal treatment, in the real world samples may be abused.[15] No systematic studies have been published which examine how much mistreatment of samples is permissible before antibody testing may lead to inaccurate results, or whether error would be more likely to be in the direction of false positives or false negatives.

Are There Many False Positives?

A "false positive" means that someone tests positive or shows reactivity on an antibody test even though he or she is not really infected. Even with a very low rate of false-positive test results, in a population of low-risk individuals a large proportion of those few results which are positive will falsely label as infected someone who is free of HIV.[16] These residual positive results are likely to remain positive on subsequent tests.[17] If antibody is spuriously cross-reacting with HIV, it is not likely to disappear spontaneously. Furthermore, other confirmatory tests are not likely to clarify the situation. Neither viral isolation nor antigen tests are ultimate arbiters. Failure to detect virus during viral isolation may be due to very low levels of virus, rapid death of cells harvested for culture purposes, or other sources of failure of that very exacting procedure. Failure to detect antigen may result from a latent infection in which HIV is not actively replicating, since latent virus may not be detected by antigen tests.

If I Test Positive, What Are the Chances I Am Truly Infected?

The likelihood that a positive result truly indicates infection is related both to the person's level of risk and to the accuracy of the test or, customarily, combination of tests used. The lower the risk, the more likely it is that a positive result is misleading; the greater the risk, the more likely it is that a positive result is a true indicator. For instance, a female who meets blood-donor eligibility criteria and who has tested positive has only a one in seven chance of truly being infected even when the combined accuracy of ELISA and confirmatory test is as high as 99.95 percent. If the combined accuracy of the test drops to 99.50 percent, then the likelihood of true infection is 1 out of 50.[18] Conversely, for a sexually active gay man in Los Angeles, New York, or San Francisco, or an intravenous (IV) drug user in Greater New York, chances are better than 99 out of 100 that a positive test result accurately indicates HIV infection.

These data make sense if we consider a simple example of two hypothetical populations — one low-risk, one high-risk — of 1,000 people each. A variety of studies suggest that roughly 1 of 1,000 members of the "general population" tested randomly in such procedures as military screening or studies of serum samples from routine hospital admissions will be found positive.[19] Gay men in such second-tier cities (with regard to infection rates) as Pittsburgh and Chicago have an infection rate of about 300 per 1,000. Suppose a false-positive rate of 0.1 percent, or 1 per 1,000, applied to each such group. In the first case, the chances of obtaining a true and a false-positive outcome are equal (1/1,000). Put another way, the chance that a positive test is a valid predictor of infection is 50:50.[20] In the second example, the likelihood of true infection when a sample tests positive is 300 times greater than the likelihood of a positive result arising from test error. In other words, in a high-risk population, the predictive value of such a test is much greater than in a low- or no-risk population.

How Long Does It Take for Detectable Antibody to Form After Exposure?

The U.S. Public Health Service implies that when exposure leads to infection, three months is a sufficiently long period for antibodies to develop to detectable levels.[21] But it is not that simple, and the question is difficult to study. Estimates using animal models or immune responses of humans to other viruses may be invalid.[22]

Definitive information comes from the very few known cases of seroconversion after a needle-stick accident or a blood transfusion. But these cases, involving direct inoculation of a substantial quantity of blood, may occasion a different rate of antibody development than the more typical routes of viral exposure through sexual contact or IV drug use (in which injected blood droplets are highly diluted). Also, the speed of response may be affected if IV use itself or concomitant infections have compromised the individual's immune system.

Published literature documents a few dozen instances of seroconversion within a few months after apparent sexual exposure in gay men.[23] But other examples[24] show latency periods prior to seroconversion among gay men of twenty-three,[25] thirty-four,[26] and thirty-six months.[27] Some studies of IV drug users show intervals of nine, fourteen, and eighteen months between apparent exposure and the development of detectable antibodies.[28] None of these studies bears on the likely interval for seroconversion in low-risk or very low dose exposures.[29] Also, the design and manufacture of particular test kits — for example, the amount, species, and source of HIV protein selected — may affect their sensitivity.[30]

Finally, viral infection and antibody response within the central nervous system — detectable by studying cerebrospinal fluid — may not be apparent from studies of serum antibody.[31] However, such a compartmentalization of infection and antibody response is believed to occur only rarely.

Are There Many False Negatives?

We do not know. For instance, ELISA-negative sera are not routinely screened by other procedures such as the Western blot,[32] even though when such studies are done they reveal a rate of false negatives in the neighborhood of 1 percent or higher,[33] owing solely to problems in the consistency of test performance. The value of a single negative test result in establishing freedom from infection with HIV among people with a history of high-risk behavior is questionable, since the sensitivity of the ELISA test is based on studies of low-risk individuals.[34]

In various situations, even the most sensitive test is ineffective, because the subject being studied, although infected, does not or cannot produce detectable antibody. It is not at all unusual, for instance, to find false-negative results in symptomatic HIV-infected patients.[35] In one study of "high-risk" gay men[36] (more likely to be infected than the general gay male population), four of the ninety-six patients studied harbored virus despite persistent negative results on antibody tests.[37] In another research report, two of sixty-six high-risk gay men were found to harbor virus even though their serum did not reveal antibody.[38] Because viral isolation procedures and antigen tests do not always identify true infection,[39] these results may, if anything, underestimate the rate of false negatives. In another series, 8 percent of healthy infected gay men were negative by ELISA, but their infection was detected by Western blot, which would not ordinarily be performed on ELISA-negative specimens.[40] This statistic is consistent with theoretical estimates of 7 percent based on current test accuracy and typical infection rates for a city like Boston.[41]

An example indicates why negative test results may be problematic. In one 1985 study,[42] a healthy twenty-four-year-old gay man was evaluated who had had 250 lifetime sexual partners but fewer than 10 since 1981. He had been receptive during anal intercourse only with 4 partners, and his last oral or anal exposure to ejaculate had occurred four years before the study. His only symptoms were swollen glands in his neck and recurrences of herpes. During the two years prior to the study, he had become consistent in the practice of "safer sex" and was clinically healthy. A series of antibody test results were negative. In view of the interval since his period of greatest risk, his adherence to protective sex guidelines, his current health, and the pattern of repeatedly negative antibody test results, even very cautious counsel would affirm that very probably he was not infected. However, upon further study, his serum was found to contain evidence of HIV even though no antibody was detectable.

What About Testing Newborns and Infants?

False-positive results are likely during the first year or so of life in an uninfected child born to an HIV-infected mother. False negatives are not unusual, at one to two years old, if the child was infected pre- or perinatally.

During the first year or more after an infant is born to an infected mother, her HIV antibody, which was transferred across the placenta, may remain detectable in the baby's circulation.[43] There is, during that interval, no routine way to determine whether antibody to HIV detected in such a baby's serum derives from passive transfer of maternal antibody or from an active response to HIV infection by the infant's immune system. Positive results, in short, may well be misleading.

As the baby's immune system develops and maternal antibody disappears, the child may fail to mount an antibody response to HIV if he or she has been infected since birth.[44] The baby's immune system may not react to HIV that has been present during its entire life in the same way as it reacts to a foreign substance; consequently, there may be no immune response — no HIV antibody — even though the child is infected.

Does Presence of Antibody Prove Infectiousness?

Once infected, an individual probably remains infected. But an infected individual may not be producing enough virus at all times to be able to transmit it to others. Since there is no way to know when one is highly infectious and when one is not, consistent use of risk-reduction techniques is essential for people who are HIV-positive and for anyone else who may have been exposed but who does not know his or her antibody status.

Attempts to isolate HIV from blood of antibody-positive individuals succeed about 75 percent of the time.[45] Because viral isolation is a difficult procedure, this statistic suggests that virus is present in any individual who shows HIV antibody reactivity, even though virus may not be recoverable from a particular specimen. On the other hand, antigen tests, which show the presence of active virus or viral fragments in the specimen being tested, may be positive in only a small fraction of individuals who display antibody reactivity.[46]

Another indirect source of data is epidemiological: Do individuals with positive antibody tests infect steady sexual partners when they do not follow protective sex guidelines? They do, sometimes after only a single exposure. On the other hand, about half of the steady male partners of infected men may not be infected even though the uninfected partner may have been receptive during anal intercourse with the infected partner on hundreds of occasions.[47] The same pattern occurs in heterosexual partners, with considerable variance from study to study.[48] In a recent study of heterosexual partners of people unknowingly infected by blood transfusions, 92 percent of male and 82 percent of female sexual partners — with an average, respectively, of 180 and 156 unprotected sexual contacts — escaped infection.[49] A pattern of steadily increasing risk to the uninfected partner is suggested by research on the female partners of hemophiliacs (70 to 90 percent of whom are believed to be infected as a result of having received contaminated blood product concentrates prior to the introduction of screening programs and heat-treatment processes). Studies of these women suggest that the likelihood of infection with HIV during unprotected sexual contact increases with the length of time the infected individual has carried the virus.[50] There are two possible explanations. As more contacts occur, perhaps the chances become greater that whatever combination of factors is required for transmission is present. Or, as time passes, people who carry HIV may become more infectious, perhaps because their health deteriorates to the extent that they begin to produce larger quantities of virus than their immune system can inactivate.

Counseling Issues

Counseling individuals seeking HIV antibody testing can accomplish two important objectives:[51] (1) individualized assessment of risk and delivery of tailored, specific, focused risk-reduction information; (2) assurance of fully informed consent prior to testing. Informed consent implies an assessment of whether the test can address the client's motives for testing as well as an evaluation of whether the individual feels capable of managing the test outcome, whatever it is. The question of motivation forms the starting point for the following outline of issues that ideally should be reviewed in counseling individuals seeking antibody testing.

1. Why is the individual seeking testing *now?* What triggered the decision to have the test performed?

2. How accurate is the individual's understanding of the meaning of the test in relation to his or her concerns?

3. How will test results be used? What will be the behavioral and emotional outcomes?

4. Is there a clear understanding of AIDS risk-reduction guidelines?

Why Seek Testing Now?
Much can be learned by finding out not only why an individual has concluded that testing is worthwhile, but, more specifically, what immediate concern prompted the decision. Responses to that question may reveal specifically relevant circumstances in the person's life, and ways in which the person might use test results both profitably and harmfully. Some typical triggering motives include the following:

- Coercion or insistence from a partner that one be tested. (Is the partner also seeking testing? Are there issues of guilt, responsibility, power, or moral superiority underlying this pressure? Would the person seeking the test persist in seeking it without such pressure?)

- Concern about symptoms. (Has the individual consulted a physician? Can some concerns be discounted as unrelated to HIV? Will negative results cause the condition to remain untreated? Will a positive test result lead to inappropriate self-diagnosis, failure to seek medical attention, or suicide?)

- Recent notification that one has been exposed from a past partner who has tested positive or who has received a diagnosis of AIDS or AIDS-related complex (ARC). (How does this new information change anything if the individual already follows risk-reduction guidelines? If the motivation for testing is to allay anxiety that has suddenly escalated, will a negative result accomplish that? Is testing motivated by the wish that a negative result will allay guilt on the part of the infected contact?)

- Recent sexual assault, after which the individual wants to establish a "baseline" antibody status, showing that as of the time of the assault, she or he was not infected; or a past assault, as a result of which the individual wants to be sure she or he was not infected by the attacker. (Does the assault survivor understand that a baseline negative result shortly after the assault may not be definitive [since *any* other possible exposure in the months before the assault could also account for the development of a positive result in the months after the assault]? If the test is to be used in prosecuting the attacker, has a lawyer been consulted for advice about the kind of evidence and testimony that will be required to pursue such redress? Will the testing procedure itself impede the process of counseling and recovery in the weeks and months following the assault? Is the testing procedure timed in such a way that the individual will have a strong support system should the result prove positive? How will test results affect the individual's motivation to practice safer sex?)[52]

- Pressure from a parent or a guardian. (Does the individual's behavioral history agree with the perception of those who are applying pressure for testing? Is the individual being tested able to distinguish his or her own best interests from the demands of those attempting to pressure him or her?)

- A specific news item or media report about AIDS. (Does the individual have an accurate understanding of the information and its context? [For instance, reports speculating about unusual or unproven modes of transmission need to be labeled as such.] Are there genuine risks that the individual has not recognized which should lead him or her to adopt risk-reduction guidelines?)

Does the Individual Understand the Meaning of the Test?

Prior to the advent of AIDS, the technical content involved in counseling — even in complex decisions regarding prenatal diagnostic procedures and outcomes — was relatively straightforward and unchanging, so that attention could be devoted to the ethical and psychological issues involved. With AIDS, the relevant technical information is not only complex and difficult, but also incomplete on many key points, and rapidly evolving. At a minimum, anyone contemplating HIV testing needs to understand the following:

- A positive test result does not mean that the individual has AIDS or necessarily will develop AIDS.

- By itself, a positive test result in an individual with medical symptoms does not explain the cause of these symptoms.

- A positive test result means that the individual should consider him- or herself able to transmit HIV to others sexually, through sharing injection equipment (for any purpose, not just the use of recreational drugs, and regardless of whether the skin is punctured intramuscularly or intravenously); during pregnancy; at delivery; and possibly through breast-feeding.

- A negative result does not necessarily *prove* that an individual is free of infection. Its meaning depends on how long a time has passed since the most recent possible incidence of exposure; even with the passage of well over a year since such an incidence, there remain some false negative results, particularly, it is assumed, among individuals at high risk.

- A positive result may not be an accurate indicator of infection in individuals with very little or no identifiable risk of exposure; there may be no ultimate standard or measure to which to appeal except monitoring one's medical status for possible HIV-related developments, while scrupulously following risk-reduction guidelines.

What Will Be the Impact of Test Results?

Not enough information is yet available about the specific personality profile or psychological determinants that characterize people who respond well or poorly to HIV testing.

Many, if not most, people who seek voluntary testing assume that they will test negative and are thus hoping for reassurance that they are not infected. Often they have not considered realistically the ways in which a positive result might affect them. Many people who are in ongoing counseling or psychotherapy never mention their concerns about AIDS or their interest in HIV testing to their therapist. And if they do, their counselor may have encouraged them to be tested, secure in the belief that the test would reduce the client's anxiety, without ever having examined with the client the possible impact of a positive result. Certainly, the test is specifically contraindicated by a risk of suicide, homicide, or other sociopathic behavior; risk of abandoning drug treatment; or other probable adverse outcomes.

In the absence of risk of those specific adverse outcomes, it is important to try to ascertain whether the individual's behavior will be any different if he or she tests positive than if he or she tests negative. If an individual feels that he or she may be infected, risk-reduction guidelines may be appropriate whether or not she or he is tested, and whether the test is positive or negative. Using test results to make career choices or financial plans may be inappropriate, since the test is an uncertain predictor of actual illness.

If a woman or a couple is using the test to help make a decision about becoming pregnant or terminating a pregnancy, even with a positive result the best choice is not a foregone conclusion. As with any other application of the test, results must be evaluated in relation to one's history of risk. And even if a mother is truly infected, it is by no means certain that her infant will become infected; the prevailing estimate — that about 50 percent of infants born to infected mothers are also infected — averages statistics from specific studies whose estimates range from about 20 percent to as high as 80 percent. Finally, just as women may reasonably choose to bear a child knowing that it may be born with Down's syndrome, hemophilia, or Tay-Sachs disease or that it may develop Huntington's chorea, so a parent or parents may determine that the risk is acceptable of giving birth to a child that may or may not be infected and, if infected, may or may not proceed to develop AIDS.

When a principal motive for testing is reduction of anxiety, the individual must consider whether a positive outcome would greatly exacerbate his or her anxiety and whether some uncertainty actually is preferable. For an individual at very low or no risk, a positive result is unlikely and, should it occur, may be misleading because it may well be a false positive. When the risk of obtaining a false positive is about equal to the risk of actual infection (for example, for people who were transfused with one or two units of blood in a low-risk area prior to the introduction of routine blood screening in the spring of 1985), the decision about whether to proceed with testing is a difficult judgment to make.

Experience with repeat and chronic test-takers suggests that although people may expect test results to allay anxiety, for many people they do not. Sometimes people seize (appropriately or not) on the ambiguities inherent in a negative result and seek repeat testing even though no amount of testing will finally dissipate their anxiety. Some people who test negative and appear at first to be greatly relieved that they have been spared may find, with the passage of time, that they are *less* able to maintain risk-reduction behavior. They repeatedly put themselves at risk, and chronically reappear for testing as a way to "monitor" whether they have gotten infected yet.

When people seek testing as a license to abandon risk-reduction precautions, they fail to recognize that it becomes more and more likely as time goes on that each new partner will be infected. The need will become progressively greater to adopt safer sex techniques and to be sure that if drug injection equipment is used it is sterile. Although the test may allay worries about the past, for most people the greater challenge looms in the future: developing and stabilizing habits that provide continuing protection from the possibility of infection. The apparent clarity of a positive or a negative result may obscure the daunting but necessary effort to adapt to a changing environment in which safer sex must become the norm.

Does the Individual Understand and Follow Risk-Reduction Guidelines?

Few situations illustrate better than the AIDS epidemic that individuals do not fit into simple, unitary categories. Actual behaviors are more important than self-designated identity in evaluating someone's risk of exposure and, more important, in delivering risk-reduction information. A gay man who always preferred very safe sex practices may nevertheless have had an accident or illness that required multiple blood transfusions before screening was introduced. Some men with hemophilia are gay, and some gay men with hemophilia inject recreational drugs and share needles. Loving husbands and devoted fathers may sustain long-term partnerships with other men in a similar situation without defining themselves as "gay," "homosexual," or even "bisexual." Former intravenous drug users who have been clean for months or years may continue to have sexual relationships primarily with other ex-users or current users. Lesbians sometimes want a gay male friend to father a child. Some heterosexual women like anal intercourse. Heavy drinkers who black out may forget not only what kind of sex they engaged in but also the gender of their partner. It matters when and where risky behavior occurred. For instance, unprotected heterosexual intercourse with a man with hemophilia living in Pittsburgh may be much more risky than with an IV drug user in Ottawa.

Risk-reduction recipes sound simple in principle. Needle sterilization seems as easy as rinsing out a drinking glass, and lists that assort safe, possibly safe, and unsafe sex acts appear perfectly straightforward. But when people nod their heads and say, "I understand," they may be suffering under significant misconceptions, or may be finding themselves unable to talk about how hard it is to put those simple guidelines into practice.

The phrase "exchange of bodily fluids" euphemistically avoids key particulars. Saliva, sweat, and tears are far less menacing than blood or semen. "Exchange," which sounds like a bank transaction, offers little clarification about how HIV may actually infect. When the phrase "direct blood contact" is employed to clarify "exchange," it may mislead, because the important blood cells in HIV infection are white, not red. The white blood cells that HIV attacks may be present at any site of infection and inflammation, as well as locations where blood vessels are actually ruptured or penetrated.

Since the beginning of the AIDS epidemic, "promiscuity" has recurrently been cited as a key factor in HIV transmission. But an emphasis on number of partners may belie the obvious: that a mutually monogamous, unprotected sexual relationship with an infected partner is much riskier than scrupulously safe sex with a multiplicity of strangers. Gay men in monogamous relationships seem less likely to be consistent about risk-reduction guidelines than men who have nonsteady partners.[53] For instance, an important reason why some gay men in San Francisco continued receptive anal intercourse was that they accepted a single-minded public health emphasis on the dangers of promiscuity and "anonymous partners" and believed that having fewer sexual partners would protect them.[54] But statistical analysis suggests that even in 1982 the spread of HIV in that city was such that a 50 percent reduction in the number of partners per year with no change in actual sexual practices would have reduced the likelihood of exposure by only about 10 percent.[55]

Not all sexual contacts are consensual. Even in less coercive settings than sexual assault, the obstacles to adopting protective sexual practices may not be informational, but situational: a woman with young children whose sole source of financial support is an abusive husband who has multiple sexual partners or a pattern of chronic needle sharing during IV drug use, or both; a family, religion, and culture that tell this woman that her fulfillment in life requires that she accede to her partner's demands; a man who obtains sexual release only after drinking so much that he cannot remember whom he has slept with or what kinds of sex he had; anyone who agrees that the measure of their love and devotion or the guarantor of monogamy in a relationship is their willingness to have unprotected sex; a sex worker (someone who is paid for sex) whose client will pay a much higher fee if he does not have to use a condom.

What Are the First Reactions When People Learn Their Test Results?

People usually react to the news of a negative result the way one would expect — with considerable relief. Surprisingly often, however, some respond with indifference, and occasionally, with almost a sense of letdown.[56] People who learn that their test was positive display a wider range of immediate responses, including outbursts of strong feeling, especially sorrow and anger; withdrawal; stoic acceptance; a jumble of questions and thoughts; and intellectualizing (for example, "It's what I expected," "Now I'll do whatever I have to do to keep from getting sick"). It has been suggested that for some, the definitive information that one is infected may be calming because it reduces the anxiety that results from uncertainty. I have observed this response on only a few occasions. Even in the case of persons who appear most genuinely convinced that they have been infected with HIV, a positive result dashes the optimism and hope that they seem to bring with them to the test situation.

Over Time, How Do People Deal with Being HIV-Antibody-Positive?

People who have tested positive are divided about whether they ever should have had the antibody test. Those who value it feel that it has been helpful in making decisions about matters such as medical care, health maintenance, and financial planning; in setting priorities; and in helping them to affirm the relative importance of various relationships with lovers, family, and friends. They rarely, if ever, feel that testing has significantly changed their commitment to protective sex — unless one views a change from consistently safe sex to abstinence as a significant contributor to public health.

Those who regret having learned their status experience a wide range of problems.[57] Some persons who have tested positive describe, even years after learning their antibody status, profound — sometimes omnipresent — feelings of foreboding, gloom, and impending disaster. The resulting anxiety and depression may become self-perpetuating, particularly when such feelings are interpreted as early signs of neurological damage due to the progress of an HIV infection. In a support group I co-led for seropositive gay men, the most guarded fear, which was verbalized only in the tenth week of a twelve-week program, was the fear of literally losing one's mind to HIV infection.

Often there is tremendous uncertainty about how to deal with a medical situation that is constantly changing. Optimistic news of an experimental treatment one day is juxtaposed the next with reports of a gloomy prognosis for anyone who is infected. It is easy to collect a portfolio of tales of insensitive, AIDS-phobic, homophobic, and drug-phobic providers in medicine, dentistry, mental health, and alternative healing modalities. But even warm, patient, trusted, sensitive providers have biases about the benefits and risks of specific treatments, whether conventional, experimental, or alternative. This diversity of opinion may be healthy, but it imposes a burden that many medical consumers have neither the training nor the temperament to bear. Gaining sufficient knowledge to make responsible choices may become as consuming as a full-time career, and also may leave the affected person with an overwhelming and inappropriate sense of responsibility for his or her own medical fate.

People having difficulty with the knowledge that they tested positive describe struggle and pain in their relationships. Friends sometimes withdraw, perhaps out of irrational fear of exposure or anxieties triggered about their own situation. Or they may become oppressively solicitous. The issue of disclosure may become a preoccupation. Does one tell family members? Which ones, and when? Must or should one tell one's employer, and, if so, when? Gay men liken the experience to "coming out," but without the sense of joyous celebration that often accompanies acknowledging and beginning to experience one's sexual identity.

Relationships may become problematic, especially if one's current sexual partner tests negative or does not know his or her status. Does one inform any or all past sexual partners or fellow drug users? What about the possible emotional fallout: blame, guilt, sorrow, old wounds reopened? Does one tell a prospective sexual/emotional partner? Can a relative stranger be trusted with this information after only a first encounter? What about the pain of rejection if the news is shared only when the relationship has gained in closeness and significance? If the information is conveyed after a sexual encounter, even a scrupulously safe one, how does that affect trust in the future, if the relationship survives such a disclosure? If one decides to restrict sexual relations only to those who have also tested positive, how does one meet them? If one chooses celibacy, how are needs for interpersonal warmth, intimacy, and physical closeness to be met?

Policies for Testing

Testing is now one of the most popular items in AIDS budgets. Counting becomes confused with controlling.[58] The principal reasons for this derive as much from emotion as from reason. Everyone experiences a sense of urgency to *do something*, preferably something palpable, quick, easy, universally applicable, and mechanically predictable. The uncharitable perception endures, usually with respect to groups other than those to which authors of pro-testing recommendations belong, that "they" will change behavior only if they are somehow shocked or flogged into it by the distress of a positive test result.[59] The misconception persists among many policymakers that people who test negative need be less worried about transmission that those who test positive. Testing also has the effect, desirable to some, of diverting educational dollars into fiscal support of laboratories and collection of epidemiological data. A mechanical procedure like drawing blood samples and running them through a laboratory procedure seems somehow more hard-hitting, objective, and productive than education, which seems soft — just a cozy little chat about sex.

Does Knowing One's Antibody Status Lead to Risk Reduction?

Long-term reactions to learning one's antibody status remain poorly documented and mostly anecdotal. This is important, because longitudinal studies of the factors important in maintaining safer sex do not agree with cross-sectional studies.[60] Relatively few people have known their HIV antibody status for more than a year or two. Many of those who have been studied are in individual therapy or support groups or research studies, all of which select subjects who are in certain ways nonrepresentative.[61] Some clinical interventions may select specifically for people experiencing difficulty managing this knowledge. Others may attract those who already are coping very well. Besides knowledge of antibody status, usually all subjects in such studies are receiving some form of systematic professional attention, educational interventions, and support as part of the research protocol.

What we do know is not especially encouraging. Some studies of short-term outcomes do indeed suggest that people who learn they have tested positive reduce risky behavior to a greater extent than people who have tested negative.[62] This is not as reassuring as it may sound — assuming that the negative result *is* a valid indicator of freedom from infection — since there remains the risk of future exposure. Other findings suggest that those who learn they have tested negative may be less committed to adopting safer behavior than those who do not learn their antibody status.[63] Although the U.S. Public Health Service suggests that learning one's antibody status is "an important component of prevention strategy" for individuals with a history of high-risk behavior, presumably because it will motivate them to make a concerted effort to reduce risk,[64] the most methodologically sound research studies to date suggest that, at least for gay men, other factors besides knowledge of one's antibody status weigh more heavily in the consistent, sustained practice of safer sex.[65] Of great importance to these persons is the perception that they are situated in a supportive peer community that holds shared values about the importance of safer sex. Paradoxically, persons with the greatest sense of vulnerability to AIDS — such as those who have tested positive — may have the greatest difficulty in adjusting to and maintaining safer practices.[66] Individuals already having difficulty with impulse control — who have not integrated knowledge of risk reduction with behavior — may not become more cautious upon learning they are infected with HIV.[67] This is consistent with the observation that intravenous drug users who are in the early weeks of drug treatment and who learn they are antibody-positive are more likely to drop out of such programs or return to injecting drugs, or both, than if they learn they are antibody-negative or do not learn their antibody status.[68] Anecdotally, people who have been in recovery from drug addiction for a year or more have remarked to me that they doubt they could have handled news of a positive antibody status during their first three to six drug-free months.

Should All Members of "High-Risk" Groups Be Tested?

Antibody screening has been recommended for *all* members of so-called high-risk groups and is required of any captive or disenfranchised populations available to the federal and various state governments, including immigrants seeking to become naturalized citizens; prisoners; and military, Peace Corps, Vista, and all foreign service personnel. In a pioneering analysis of HIV antibody screening programs,[69] Bayer et al. have stipulated ethical principles and have located pragmatic grounds for rejecting mass screening for hospital admissions (except perhaps in custodial institutions), marriage, prison, or the workplace (except perhaps "prostitutes").[70] Most public health officials concur, sharing concerns about the accuracy and efficacy of tests, the relative costs in comparison with other prevention interventions, and legal as well as ethical implications.[71]

But, setting aside three basic principles that they propose — "respect for persons," "beneficence," and "justice" — Bayer et al. focus on a fourth, "the harm principle," and deny that individuals at high risk should have "the right not to know" their antibody status. They argue for use of the antibody test because "there is reason to doubt that advice alone provides sufficient motivation" for "radical alterations in sexual conduct and in childbearing plans. . . . Given the risks associated with AIDS and the uncertainty about what will in fact modify high-risk behavior, there is a strong community interest in encouraging voluntary testing." The authors acknowledge, however, that "such information may be so psychologically devastating that the individual will suffer greatly without any benefits to himself or herself or additional benefits to others."[72]

I believe their position is flawed for three reasons. First, the argument poses a false dichotomy: we are not forced to choose between advice and testing. Another option must be made available for anyone — aware of their antibody status or not — having difficulty reducing high-risk behavior or in danger of relapse: sensitive, responsive, creative programs that support the process of achieving a satisfying adaptation to the requirements for sexual risk reduction.[73] Second, why assume that when "advice" does not effect behavioral change, "information" — in the form of knowledge of one's antibody status — will? This is particularly problematic, for reasons given by Bayer et al.: "There is no way to discern in advance which of the infected people will modify their behavior without notification and which will not,"[74] nor, I would add, is there a way to discern in advance which persons, given notification, will modify their behavior in harmful ways.

Third, Bayer et al. institute a revealing double standard. For health care providers performing invasive procedures, a risk of HIV transmission exists which is more than "only theoretical," for instance, if an accident exposes the open wound of a patient to blood from a health care worker. Health care personnel are advised to take "standard infection control precautions . . . whether or not they know their antibody status."[75] Such precautions are futile for accidents in which blood is drawn — for example, when a blade slips and cuts through single or double latex gloves. Why not here, too, accord priority to the harm principle and argue forcibly for submission to voluntary testing by all health personnel who perform invasive procedures? Why suppose that knowledge of one's antibody status is an indispensable motivator for sexual risk reduction but has no bearing on scrupulousness about infection control, no influence on the care taken to avoid accidents, and no relevance to the desirability of voluntary job reassignment for HIV-infected health personnel performing invasive procedures? The point here is not to argue that health care workers performing invasive procedures have no right to remain uninformed of their antibody status, but rather to suggest that there is serious inequity in denying "the right not to know" to conventionally defined high-risk groups while implicitly extending it to everyone else.[76]

How Should Testing Programs Be Evaluated?

To the ethical principles Bayer et al. propose in their analysis of screening programs, I suggest adding two criteria for the evaluation of testing proposals: (1) that they are the least intrusive way to accomplish a necessary goal, and (2) that they obey the fundamental dictum of medicine to do no harm.

As an example of the first principle, the need for epidemiological data on rates of infection can be met without testing and labeling specific individuals as infected. Blind samples, coded by source (for example, inner-city vs. rural newborn infant blood samples used in an ingenious study of childbearing women in Massachusetts[77]) can reveal a great deal about infection rates in the general population, and voluntary testing programs as well as noncoerced participation in research studies already have provided much information, not only about overall rates of infection, but about the dynamics of HIV transmission.

The second principle encapsulates the problem with widespread use of HIV testing as a means of effecting behavior change: it is a psychologically invasive procedure of unproven benefit. Although no physically invasive procedure — chemotherapy, surgery, or other medical treatment — is widely adopted without evaluating whether its anticipated benefit equals or exceeds its risk, HIV testing has not been so stringently reviewed. Yet it is sufficiently psychologically intrusive to have been the immediate precipitating factor for some suicides. And it is experimental — of uncertain benefit and of unknown risk in terms of long-term adverse psychological sequelae.

The cautious evaluation of drugs used to treat patients with AIDS models appropriate care in evaluating unproven treatments. The medical profession weighs seriously the physical harm done by a drug with dangerous side effects, even though human compassion and the danger of imminent death both dictate the most expansive availability of any promising therapeutic agent for AIDS. In contrast, advocates of testing programs may cavalierly dismiss psychological morbidity.[78] They may never even mention that an evaluation plan needs to be implemented for analyzing outcomes, and weighing their risks and benefits.[79]

Drug trials offer a valid paradigm for considering risky, unproven psychological interventions. Although Suramin was an effective antiviral agent in the test tube, it apparently did more harm than good when employed on a small sample of people with AIDS: careful, skeptical evaluation was essential to spare people from misuse of a drug that appeared at first to be promising. When Azidothymidine (AZT, or zidovudine, or Retrovir) was shown in the laboratory to be of apparent benefit in inhibiting the growth of HIV, it was distributed widely to AIDS patients only after two phases of trials: one to identify whether a dose existed that the human body could tolerate without irreversible harm, and a second to establish whether treatment conferred any benefit. In that second phase, parallel double-blind placebo-controlled studies enrolled patients from specific subgroups.[80] On the basis of such studies, AZT currently is recommended only for persons with AIDS as diagnosed by a history of *Pneumocystis carinii* pneumonia and for persons with helper T-cell counts below a specified threshold. Without sufficient evidence of benefit for other subgroups, AZT is not routinely recommended for all people with AIDS, much less all people infected with HIV.

Compare that caution and specificity with the blanket recommendation that all individuals in so-called high-risk groups seek voluntary HIV antibody testing, or with arguments for even more widespread mandatory testing (sometimes euphemistically referred to as "required" testing). We need to know how intravenous drug users react who are not in treatment, who are in methadone programs, who are now drug-free, who are in Alcoholics Anonymous, Narcotics Anonymous, or other twelve-step recovery or self-help programs, who are breadwinners for families, who are in shelters for the homeless or in community housing, who are living alone, and so on. We need to know how gay men in long-term monogamous relationships react to test results, compared to gay men who are not, compared to married bisexual men. We need to know how test results affect gay men still practicing high-risk sex with various partners, compared with gay men who are practicing high-risk sex only with long-term monogamous partners, compared with gay men who routinely are essentially safe in sexual behavior. Hardly any information exists about the specific psychological profile — in terms of such factors as locus of control, risk taking, capacity for intimacy, tolerance for ambiguity, self-esteem, and so on — of persons likely to benefit from testing. And until such research is done, it is no more ethical to prescribe antibody testing for all members of high-risk groups than it would have been to recommend AZT for everyone infected with HIV.

Public health policies that endorse widespread or "routine" testing may compound the problems already experienced by health educators who deal with AIDS. A single example may suffice. Mistrust of medical expertise already accounts for unyielding public concern about AIDS transmission via casual contact. What will be the effect on public trust and public policy of testing programs that falsely label half of those who test positive as infected carriers of a lethal virus, while erroneously reassuring thousands of infected people who test negative that they have nothing to worry about?

Notes

1. The views expressed in this article do not necessarily represent those of the Massachusetts Department of Public Health.

2. Only in the most recent modification of the Centers for Disease Control surveillance definition of AIDS has the "AIDS test" in certain circumstances become a necessary part of the differential diagnosis of AIDS. It is employed where an individual with a history suggesting possible exposure to HIV is severely ill — for instance, having lost 10 percent of body weight, with chronic diarrhea or fatigue, or dementing — and no other specific explanation can be found other than infection with HIV. "Revision of the CDC Surveillance Case Definition for Acquired Immunodeficiency Syndrome," *Morbidity and Mortality Weekly Report* (supplement) 36, no. 1S, 14 August 1987.

3. Limitations of each of the principal methods for establishing the presence of the virus restrict their usefulness for screening purposes.

   a. Microscopy: If HIV is not actively reproducing and is instead in a latent state, it will not appear under microscopic observation. Even if it is actively replicating, it still may be present in such a small proportion of cells that it will escape observation.

   b. Viral isolation: The growth of HIV from a tissue specimen or body fluid sample does prove that the virus is present. But growing sufficient virus to be detected takes time, requires skill, and often does not yield reproducible results. Thus, viral isolation may underestimate the presence of virus in a truly infected specimen.

   c. Antigen testing: If HIV is latent — incorporated in its "proviral" form into the DNA of an infected cell — there will be no reactivity on an antigen test. Because antigen tests most accurately measure active HIV infection, a principal use of antigen testing is to evaluate the effect of antiviral agents on viral replication.

   d. DNA probe (Southern blot; *in situ* hybridization): Fragments of viral DNA in the chromosome can be detected by the binding of radioactively labeled or colorimetrically detectable probes constructed of complementary DNA sequences. The proportion of chromosomal DNA in an infected cell contributed by viral genes is very small, as is the proportion of cells actually infected with HIV. Some method of amplifying the amount of viral DNA is necessary so that it can be detected. Such a method has only recently been developed for laboratory use. See Jeffrey L. Fox, "Monitoring and Diagnosis of HIV," *American Society for Microbiology News* 53 (1987): 430. The technical difficulty of handling radioactive materials makes this procedure costly and not now widely applicable.

   e. Indicator cell lines: This procedure depends on the conservation of special regulatory genes and proteins among variant strains of HIV which are not found in other viruses. It is more complicated than current antigen or antibody tests but would detect latent as well as active infection. See Barbara K. Felber and George N. Pavlakis, "A Quantitative Bioassay for HIV-1 Based on Trans-Activation," *Science* 239 (1988): 184–186.

4. Kenneth H. Mayer, "The Clinical Challenges of AIDS and HIV Infection," *Law, Medicine and Health Care* 14 (1986): 281–289.

5. Commercial Western blot reagents manufactured by DuPont have been licensed during the past year but cost more than laboratories spend preparing the equivalent materials using their own procedures. Consequently, cost savings override the possible benefits of standardization, in practice.

6. Kenneth H. Mayer et al., "Correlation of Enzyme-Linked Immunosorbent Assays for Serum Human Immunodeficiency Virus Antigen and Antibodies to Recombinant Viral Proteins with Subsequent Clinical Outcomes in a Cohort of Asymptomatic Homosexual Men," *American Journal of Medicine* 83 (1987): 208–212.

7. "Update: Serologic Testing for Antibody to Human Immunodeficiency Virus," *Morbidity and Mortality Weekly Report* 36, no. 3 (8 January 1988): 833–845.

8. F. K. Mundon et al., "Analysis of Discrepant Anti-HIV ELISA Reactives," *III International Conference on AIDS Abstracts Volume* (Washington, D.C.), 1–5 June 1987, Abstract TP. 248, p. 103.

9. In such ambiguous situations, which have occurred in less than 1 percent of samples evaluated thus far in voluntary screening programs in Massachusetts, another sample is usually requested. If the ambiguity resulted from very low levels of antibody developing in the early stages of infection, a sample drawn four to eight weeks later should be plainly reactive. If the ambiguity resulted from low levels of cross-reactive antibody first elicited by something other than HIV, the borderline or ambiguous results would persist after such a time delay (workshop presentation by Victor Berardi, Director of Virology, Massachusetts Department of Public Health, State Laboratory Institute, Jamaica Plain, Massachusetts, 4 January 1988).

10. Paul D. Cleary et al., "Compulsory Premarital Screening for the Human Immunodeficiency Virus: Technical and Public Health Considerations," *Journal of the American Medical Association* 258 (1987): 1757.

11. Ibid.

12. "Update: Serologic Testing" (note 7).

13. Klemens B. Meyer and Stephen G. Pauker, "Screening for HIV: Can We Afford the False Positive Rate?" *New England Journal of Medicine* 317 (1987): 238–241; also, "Update: Serologic Testing" (note 7).

14. Roger N. Taylor et al., "Summary of the Centers for Disease Control Human Immunodeficiency Virus (HIV) Performance Evaluation Surveys for 1985 and 1986," *American Journal of Clinical Pathology* 89 (1988): 1–13. See also Cleary et al. (note 10).

15. Long periods of time may pass before the serum used in ELISA testing is separated by centrifugation from blood cells. If the cells break down before serum is separated, some breakdown products (hemolysis) may affect the structural integrity of serum antibody. Bacterial contamination of samples, particularly if they are left unrefrigerated for several days (as may occur if samples are sent by surface mail), may also affect serum antibody.

16. Meyer and Pauker (note 13).

17. False-positive results can occur for a variety of reasons. Every individual has the potential to produce antibodies of millions of different specificities; from a lifetime of exposures to foreign antigens, we may each carry antibody of thousands of different specificities. Some people even make antibody to polystyrene, the plastic substrate used in several commercial ELISA test kits! (Confirmatory Western blotting would rule out that source of reactivity as HIV-related, however.) Antibody elicited by one sort of foreign entity and strongly reactive to it may happen to react, to a lesser degree, with other molecules as well: antibodies do not, after all, "know" with what they should and should not react. In screening thousands of individuals, it is therefore not surprising to turn up dozens who have antibody that happens to react to some portion of HIV or to materials used in test kits and who thus appear to test positive even though they have never been exposed to the virus. Such false-positive results are even likelier among those who (1) have been exposed

to unusually large amounts of diverse antigens or (2) have a disease process that results in unusually large quantities of antibody. An explanation of each category follows.

Drug injections with equipment that has not been sterilized may include such foreign materials as blood cells and plasma proteins from others. Proteins and other components of semen emitted during anal intercourse may enter the bloodstream through ruptured capillaries in the anorectal canal. Ordinary blood transfusions and the concentrated blood products used in the treatment of hemophilia contain massive quantities of foreign antigen. Although these potential sources of false-positive results bear more heavily on members of the main risk groups, the higher prevalence of infection in such groups makes it likely nevertheless that a positive test result accurately indicates HIV infection. To its pregnant mother a fetus is, immunologically, a large transplant of foreign tissue. Ordinarily, the placenta keeps the mother from rejecting the fetus but, especially at delivery, the mother's circulation may be exposed to fetal cells. This mechanism explains why women who have had many pregnancies may be somewhat likelier to test positive for HIV antibody although they have never been exposed to the virus. See Jay B. Hunter and Jay E. Menitove, "HLA Antibodies Detected by ELISA HTLV-III Antibody Kits" (letter), *Lancet* 2 (1985): 397.

Abnormally large amounts of antibody produced by patients with systemic lupus erythematosus and rheumatoid arthritis may cross-react with the antigens used in HIV tests. Injections of immune globulin may cause transient reactivity. See Paul D. Cleary et al., "Compulsory Premarital Screening for the Human Immunodeficiency Virus: Technical and Public Health Considerations," *Journal of the American Medical Association* 258 (1987): 1757. Although no such false-positive results were observed in the few samples from such patients during initial evaluations of ELISA test specificity, in studies of larger numbers of patients with no known risk of HIV exposure, some samples have been found to be reactive. Failure to clear antibody from the circulation — for instance, as a result of liver damage caused by very high levels of alcohol consumption or chronic active hepatitis — may also lead to unusually high levels of antibody. See C. J. Mendenhall et al., "False Positive Tests for HTLV-III Antibodies in Alcoholic Patients with Hepatitis," *New England Journal of Medicine* 314 (1986): 921–922, and F. R. Cockerill et al., "'False Positive' Antibodies to Human Immunodeficiency Virus (HIV) Detected by an Enzyme-Linked Immunosorbent Assay (ELISA) in Patients at Low Risk for Acquired Immune Deficiency Syndrome (AIDS)," *III International Conference on AIDS Abstracts Volume* (Washington, D.C.), 1–5 June 1987, Abstract MP.147, p. 34. Moreover, since all biological materials spontaneously degrade, those antibodies which remain longest in the circulation may have altered specificity — they may become more "sticky" — which would cause them to react with HIV test antigens. Other mechanisms are mentioned in connection with an elevated association between anti-HIV and antimalarial antibody in African subjects. See Robert J. Biggar et al., "ELISA HTLV Retrovirus Antibody Reactivity Associated with Malaria and Immune Complexes in Healthy Africans," *Lancet* 2 (1985): 520–523.

18. Meyer and Pauker (note 13).

19. Jeffrey L. Fox, "AIDS: the Public Health–Public Policy Crisis," *American Society for Microbiology News* 53 (1987): 426–430; Department of Health and Human Services, U.S. Public Health Service, "Human Immunodeficiency Virus Infections in the United States: A Review of Current Knowledge and Plans for Expansion of HIV Surveillance Activities. A Report to the Domestic Policy Council," November 30, 1987; "Human T-Lymphotropic Virus Type III/Lymphadenopathy-Associated Virus Antibody Prevalence in U.S. Military Recruit Applicants," *Morbidity and Mortality Weekly Report* 35: 421–428; and Rand L. Stoneburner et al., "Risk Factors in Military Recruits Positive for HIV Antibody" (letter), *New England Journal of Medicine* 315 (1986): 1355.

20. Cleary et al. (note 10) believe that the proportion of false-positive results may be as high as 85 percent under certain real-world testing situations.

21. "Public Health Service Guidelines for Counseling and Antibody Testing to Prevent HIV Infection and AIDS," *Morbidity and Mortality Weekly Report* 36: 510–515.

22. Humans may respond differently to HIV than primates (which do not appear to get AIDS after infection with HIV). See R. Yanagirhara et al., "Attempts to Produce a Progressive Immune Deficiency and Encephalopathy in Nonhuman Primates with the Human Immunodeficiency Viruses," *III International Conference on AIDS Abstracts Volume* (Washington, D.C.), 1–5 June 1987, Ab-

stract TP.29, p. 67. The time required for an immune response to other viruses such as hepatitis B may be misleading, because most inocula of HBV contain larger quantities of virus than inocula of HIV. Also, HBV is not a retrovirus; HIV is. That means HBV does not, like HIV, enter a latent phase during which it is inactive, incorporated into the DNA of its host's immune cells, and not immunogenic. Because infection with HBV means that large amounts of virus are available to stimulate an immune response, the time course of response to infection with HBV is likelier to be more predictable and more rapid than with HIV.

23. For instance, see Hans Gaines et al., "Antibody Response in Primary Human Immunodeficiency Virus Infection," *Lancet* 1 (1987): 1249–1253, whose subjects required two to seven weeks to seroconvert.

24. Jean-Pierre Allain et al., "Serologic Markers in Early Stages of Human Immunodeficiency Virus Infection in Haemophiliacs," *Lancet* 2 (1986): 1233–1236, observe a series of six seroconversions requiring 1, 1, 3.5, 3.5, 5, and 9 months, respectively.

25. C. M. Farber et al., "Persistent Human Immunodeficiency Virus (HIV) Detection in Seronegative Asymptomatic Carriers," *III International Conference on AIDS Abstracts Volume* (Washington, D.C.), 1–5 June 1987, Abstract MP.124, p. 30.

26. Annamari Ranki et al., "Long Latency Precedes Overt Seroconversion in Sexually Transmitted Human Immunodeficiency Virus Infection," *Lancet* 2 (1987): 589–593. Persistent HIV antigen or very low levels of core antibody were detected in seven of forty-seven gay men and in one woman who tested nonreactive on conventional ELISA tests. Three of the seven showed a defect in cell-mediated immunity, which may account for their delayed or indolent antibody response. (Both underlying cancer and immunosuppressive drugs may cause a loss of antibody reactivity on ELISA tests. See Richard G. Marlink et al., "Low Sensitivity with ELISA Testing in Early HIV Infection" (letter), *New England Journal of Medicine* 315 (1986): 1549–1550. However, false-negative results remain a concern for individuals at high risk, whether or not a state of immunocompromise lengthens the time required to seroconvert.

27. Harold A. Kessler et al., "Diagnosis of Human Immunodeficiency Virus Infection in Seronegative Homosexuals Presenting with an Acute Viral Syndrome," *Journal of the American Medical Association* 258 (1987): 1196–1199. The case report reads as follows: "Patient 3 had been in a strictly monogamous relationship for three years and practiced 'safe sex' with his partner, who was asymptomatic and negative for HIV by culture and serologic analysis for antibody and antigen. This suggests that this patient, who was also HIV culture positive, may have been asymptomatically infected for up to three years before the onset of his acute syndrome."

28. The form of antibody produced during a primary or initial immune response to HIV (IgM) is not detected by conventional antibody tests. Normally, this is not a problem, because IgM antibody typically disappears in several weeks, and is replaced by a more stable form of serum antibody (IgG) that is detected by conventional antibody tests. However, sometimes the primary-response IgM antibody species remains for many months and is not detected by conventional antibody tests for IgG even though the individual is infected during the entire period. G. Bedarida et al., "HIV IgM Antibodies in Risk Groups Who Are Seronegative on ELISA Testing," *Lancet* 2 (1986): 570–571, and "Anti-IgM Screening for HIV," ibid., p. 1456. One infected, HIV-IgM-positive subject in this series still had not developed detectable IgG antibody at 18.5 months of follow-up.

29. Kenneth H. Mayer, "The Epidemiological Investigation of AIDS," *Hastings Center Report*, August 1985, pp. 12–15. A detailed sexual and drug history and serial tests for antibody, alongside multiple tests for virus or antigen, would yield more reliable norms concerning the rate of false-negative antibody results by risk group and the time intervals between exposure, infection, and seroconversion. This has been done only in one study (see note 26), and it would require hundreds or possibly thousands of subjects as well as great expense for the battery of laboratory tests necessary to cross-verify whether subjects actually harbor HIV.

30. A test that performs with excellent sensitivity in low-risk populations may be less reliable in assaying high-risk samples. See L. Grillner et al., "False-Negative Result by the Wellcozyme Anti-HIV Assay in Testing an HIV-Positive Haemophiliac," *Lancet* 1 (1987): 1200–1201.

31. Mark S. Greenberg, "Neuropsychological Manifestations of AIDS" (lecture, Harvard University), 17 December 1987.

32. National Institutes of Health, "The Impact of Routine HTLV-III Antibody Testing on Public Health," Consensus Development Conference Statement 6, no. 5, *Journal of the American Medical Association* 256 (1986): 1778–1783.

33. Dana Gallo et al., "Comparison of Detection of Antibody to the Acquired Immune Deficiency Syndrome Virus by Enzyme Immunoassay, Immunofluorescence, and Western Blot Methods," *Journal of Clinical Microbiology* 23 (1986): 1049–1051.

34. Michael J. Barry, Paul D. Cleary, and Harvey V. Fineberg, "Screening for HIV Infection: Risks, Benefits, and the Burden of Proof," *Law, Medicine and Health Care* 14 (1986): 259–268.

35. Jerome E. Groopman, "Clinical Spectrum of HTLV-III in Humans," *Cancer Research* 45, Suppl. 9 (1985): 4649s–4651s; and James R. Carlson et al., "AIDS Serology Testing in Low- and High-Risk Groups," *Journal of the American Medical Association* 253 (1985): 3405–3408.

36. These "high-risk" gay men were selected because they were believed to be most likely to be infected although antibody-negative: they had been sexual partners of infected individuals, or had had hundreds of sexual partners, or showed laboratory signs of immune system aberration while being clinically healthy.

37. S. Zaki Salahuddin et al., "HTLV-III in Symptom-Free Seronegative Persons" (letter), *Lancet* 2 (1984): 1418–1419.

38. Kenneth H. Mayer et al., "Natural History of HTLV-III/LAV Infection in Asymptomatic Male Homosexuals in Boston" (abstract), International Conference on Acquired Immune Deficiency Syndrome, Paris, 23-25 June 1986.

39. The same research laboratory was able to detect HIV in only 43 percent of seropositive subjects. See D. D. Ho et al., "Primary Human T-Lymphotropic Virus Type III (HTLV-III) Infection," *New England Journal of Medicine* 313 (1985): 1606.

40. Groopman (note 35), p. 3405.

41. Barry et al. (note 34).

42. Kenneth H. Mayer et al., "Human T-Lymphotropic Virus Type III in High-Risk, Antibody-Negative Homosexual Men," *Annals of Internal Medicine* 104 (1986): 194–196.

43. J. Q. Mok et al., "Infants Born to Mothers Seropositive for Human Immunodeficiency Virus," *Lancet* 1 (1987): 1164–1168.

44. W. Borkowsky et al., "Human Immunodeficiency Virus Infections in Infants Negative for Anti-HIV by Enzyme-Linked Immunoassay," *Lancet* 1 (1987): 1168–1171; Kwang Ho Pyun et al., "Perinatal Infection with Human Immunodeficiency Virus," *New England Journal of Medicine* 317 (1987): 611–614; and Leonard R. Krolov et al., "Longitudinal Serologic Evaluation of an Infant with Acquired Immunodeficiency Syndrome," *Pediatric Infectious Disease Journal* 6 (1987): 1066–1067.

45. In the earliest attempts to isolate HIV (then called HTLV-III or LAV or ARV), the virus was detected in 30 to 54 percent of adult AIDS patients and in 50 to 86 percent of "pre-AIDS" (ARC) patients. Robert C. Gallo et al., "Frequent Detection and Isolation of Cytopathic Retroviruses (HTLV-III) from Patients with AIDS and at Risk for AIDS," *Science* 224 (1984): 500–502; and Jay A. Levy et al., "Isolation of Lymphocytopathic Retroviruses from San Francisco Patients with AIDS," *Science* 225 (1984): 840–842.

46. J. A. M. Lange et al., "Viral Gene Expression, Antibody Production and Immune Complex Formation in Human Immunodeficiency Virus Infection," *AIDS* 1 (1987): 15–20; and Deborah A. Paul et al., "Correlation of Serum HIV Antigen and Antibody with Clinical Status in HIV-Infected Patients," *Journal of Medical Virology* 22 (1987): 357–363.

47. Kenneth H. Mayer, "Male Homosexual Transmission of HIV Infection," Annual Meeting of the American Association for the Advancement of Science (Boston), 11–15 February 1988.

48. Gerald H. Friedland and Robert S. Klein, "Transmission of the Human Immunodeficiency Virus," *New England Journal of Medicine* 317 (1987): 1125–1135.

49. Thomas A. Peterman et al., "Risk of Human Immunodeficiency Virus Transmission from Heterosexual Adults with Transfusion-Associated Infections," *Journal of the American Medical Association* 259 (1988): 55–58.

50. James Goedert, "Natural History of HIV Infection," Annual Meeting of the American Association for the Advancement of Science (Boston), 11–15 February 1988.

51. See also for general guidelines and suggestions Gabriele Dlugosch, Marc Gold, and James Dilley, "AIDS Antibody Testing: Evaluation and Counseling" and "Diagnosis/Treatment: Disclosing AIDS Antibody Test Results," *Focus* 1, no. 8 (July 1986): 1–3; Peter Goldblum and Neil Seymour, "Whether to Take the Test: Counseling Guidelines," *Focus* 2, no. 5 (April 1987): 1–3; Stephan L. Buckingham, "The HIV Antibody Test: Psychosocial Issues," *Social Casework* (September 1987): 387–393; and Mark Gold, Neil Seymour, and Jeffrey Sahl, "Counseling HIV Seropositives," in *What to Do About AIDS,* ed. Leon McKusick (Berkeley: University of California Press, 1986), pp. 103–110.

52. These issues, which have not been much discussed in print, grew out of planning discussions and plenary and workshop sessions of a recent conference entitled AIDS and Rape (Needham, Massachusetts), 7 January 1988.

53. Leon McKusick et al., "Prevention of HIV Infection Among Gay and Bisexual Men: Two Longitudinal Studies," *III International Conference on AIDS Abstracts Volume* (Washington, D.C.), 1–5 June 1987, p. 213.

54. David G. Ostrow et al., "Sexual Behavior Change and Persistence in Homosexual Men," *International Conference on Acquired Immunodeficiency Syndrome* (Atlanta, Georgia), 14–17 April 1985 (Session 26.3), p. 71.

55. J. M. Van Druten et al., "AIDS Prevention and Intervention," *Lancet* 1 (1986): 852–853.

56. This observation is based on the author's experience with delivering antibody test results to over 1500 individuals in the greater Boston area. See also Susan D. Cochran, who concluded, from a study of 150 asymptomatic gay men, that "knowledge of a positive HTLV-III/LAV result may have negative consequences for psychosocial functioning, but a negative result does not lead to less distress than not knowing," in "Psychosomatic Distress and Depressive Symptoms Among HTLV III/LAV Seropositive, Seronegative, and Untested Homosexual Men," *III International Conference on AIDS Abstracts Volume* (Washington, D.C.), 1–5 June 1987, Abstract MP. 202, p. 43.

57. Cochran (note 56) and Dlugosch et al. (note 51).

58. This is pointed out in Barry et al. (note 34).

59. An unfortunate example was recently published by a member of the President's Commission on the HIV Epidemic: Theresa L. Crenshaw, "HIV Testing: Voluntary, Mandatory, or Routine?" *Humanist* (January–February 1988): 29–34.

60. Jill G. Joseph et al., "Magnitude and Determinants of Behavioral Risk Reduction: Longitudinal Analysis of a Cohort at Risk for AIDS," *Psychology and Health* (in press).

61. Laura Dean and J. L. Martin, "Differential Participation Rates and Epidemiologic Estimates of AIDS," *III International Conference on AIDS Abstracts Volume* (Washington, D.C.), 1–5 June 1987, Abstract THP. 79, p. 176. The authors conclude that "the highest risk individuals, the highest rates of HIV infection, and the highest rates of AIDS are to be found in the subset of individuals who never enroll or are unwilling to continue participation in behavioral and serologic AIDS studies." By extension, those most harmed by testing procedures may be least accessible to follow-up.

62. See Dlugosch et al. (note 51) and Thomas J. Coates, S. F. Morin, and Leon McKusick, "Consequences of AIDS Antibody Testing Among Homosexual Men: The AIDS Behavioral Research Project," *III International Conference on AIDS Abstracts Volume* (Washington, D.C.), 1–5 June 1987, Abstract WP. 184, p. 141.

63. Robin Fox, N. Odaka, and B. F. Polk, "Effect of Learning HTLV-III/LAV Antibody Status on Subsequent Sexual Activity," *II International Conference on AIDS Abstracts Volume* (Paris), 23–25 June 1986, Session S18d, p. 167. "Disclosure of a negative Ab test," in comparison with testing positive or not learning one's status, "did not result in a comparable reduction in sexual activity. . . . [T]he effect of informing gay men of their Ab status may be contrary to the goal of public health programs, which is to decrease the spread of HTLV-III/LAV through sexual activity."

64. "Public Health Service Guidelines" (note 21). See also Thomas J. Coates, Stephen F. Morin, and Leon McKusick, "Behavioral Consequences of AIDS Antibody Testing Among Gay Men" (letter), *Journal of the American Medical Association* 258 (1987): 1889.

65. Joseph (note 60); Karolynn Siegel et al., "Factors Distinguishing Homosexual Males Practicing Safe and Risky Sex," *III International Conference on AIDS Abstracts Volume* (Washington, D.C.), 1–5 June 1987, Abstract TP. 171, p. 91; and (in Vancouver, BC, Canada) Brian Willoughby et al., "Sexual Practices and Condom Use in a Cohort of Homosexual Men: Evidence of Differential Modification Between Seropositive and Seronegative Men," *III International Conference on AIDS Abstracts Volume* (Washington, D.C.), 1–5 June 1987, Session M.6.3, p. 5.

66. Jill G. Joseph et al., "Perceived Risk of AIDS: Assessing the Behavioral and Psychosocial Consequences in a Cohort of Gay Men," *Journal of Applied Social Psychology* (submitted), and Carol-Ann Emmons et al., "Psychosocial Predictors of Reported Behavior Change in Homosexual Men at Risk for AIDS," *Health Education Quarterly* 13 (1986): 331–345.

67. Marshall Forstein, director of outpatient psychiatry, Cambridge Hospital, and medical director, Gay and Lesbian Counseling Service, Boston, "Why HTLV-III Antibody Testing May NOT Be Best for Everyone," 1986 (Xerox), 4 pp.

68. Richard G. Marlink et al., "High Rate of HTLV-III/HIV Exposure in IVDA's from a Small-Sized City and the Failure of Specialized Methadone Maintenance to Prevent Further Drug Use," *III International Conference on AIDS Abstracts Volume* (Washington, D.C.), 1–5 June 1987, Session TH.5.1, p. 156.

69. Ronald Bayer et al., "HIV Antibody Screening: An Ethical Framework for Evaluating Proposed Programs," *New England Journal of Public Policy* 4, no. 1 (Winter–Spring 1988): 173–187. This article, in its original version, appeared in the *Journal of the American Medical Association* 256, no. 13 (October 3, 1986): 1768–1774, and permission to reprint the article was granted by the *Journal of the American Medical Association.*

70. Ibid.

71. Cleary et al. (note 10); Barry et al. (note 34); and Nan D. Hunter, "AIDS Prevention and Civil Liberties: The False Promise of Proposals for Mandatory Testing," American Civil Liberties Foundation, June 1986 (Xerox), 23 pp.

72. Bayer et al. (note 69).

73. Coates, Morin, and McKusick (note 64). Information alone is not enough: see, for instance, Jeffrey A. Kelly et al., "Relationships Between Knowledge about AIDS and Actual Risk Behavior in a Sample of Homosexual Men: Some Implications for Prevention," *III International Conference on AIDS Abstracts Volume* (Washington, D.C.), 1–5 June 1987, Abstract MP.174, p. 39. Nor is knowledge of antibody status enough to consistently motivate safer behavior: for instance (in addition to sources in note 66), see Jane McCusker et al., "Changes Over Time in Anogenital Practices in a Cohort of Homosexual/Bisexual Men," *III International Conference on AIDS Abstracts Volume* (Washington, D.C.), 1–5 June 1987, Abstract WP.172, p. 139. See, for commentary, Paul R. Gustafson, "Prevention of HTLV-III Infection" (letter), *Journal of the American Medical Association* 256 (1986): 346–347.

74. Bayer et al. (note 69).

75. Ibid.

76. This inequity is underscored by the issue of consent. Men having sex together, for instance, have been well warned of the risk of sexual exposure. Arguably, the entire population has been warned about risks of unprotected sex and failure to use sterile drug-injection equipment. In contrast, patients are not warned that on the average, 6 percent of health care workers are infected and the rate of infection among health care workers not attributable to conventional risks (for example, sexual, needle exposure) is almost twice that for the rest of the population (5 percent vs. 3 percent [data presented by Brian Saltzman, "HIV Transmission by Casual Contact and among Health Care Workers," Annual Meeting of the American Association for the Advancement of Science (Boston), 12–15 February 1988]). That is, two to three health care workers per thousand carry HIV and have no reason to suspect that they do so.

77. Charles Marwick, "HIV Antibody Prevalence Data Derived from Study of Massachusetts Infants," *Journal of the American Medical Association* 258 (1987): 171–172.

78. Crenshaw (note 59).

79. Cochran (note 56); Roger Stempel et al., "Patterns of Distress Following HIV Antibody Test Notification," *III International Conference on AIDS Abstracts Volume* (Washington, D.C.), 1–5 June 1987, Abstract WP.199, p. 143; and Calvin Pierce, "Several Suicides Follow Positive Tests, Underscore Urgency of HIV Counseling," *Clinical Psychiatry News* 15, no. 10 (October 1987): 1, 29.

80. Those subgroups included people with AIDS diagnosed by a bout of *Pneumocystis carinii* pneumonia in the previous four months; people with ARC; people with Kaposi's sarcoma but no history of *Pneumocystis carinii;* and people with severe neurological symptoms. On the basis of such studies, AZT currently is recommended only for people with AIDS as diagnosed by a history of *Pneumocystis carinii* pneumonia and for people with helper T-cell counts below a specified threshold. Still under investigation also are the effects of AZT for infants with AIDS, and the impact of AZT on progression of disease in asymptomatic seropositive patients.

"The PWA does have an integral role to play in this health crisis. But government health agencies and politicians, especially the ones in power, tend not to take PWAs too seriously. Many have never seen a PWA in their life; there may even be people in this room who have never met a PWA in their life. We tend to be a novelty act, and when that novelty wears off, the doors may not open to us anymore. I don't believe the government has ever had to deal with patients' organizations like this before and they simply don't know what to make of us, so they humor us. PWAs are not seriously consulted on decisions that affect our lives and our freedoms. PWAs are always the last to know anything about what the government is doing."

Glossary

Etiologic agent. The cause or source of a disease; in the case of AIDS, the infectious virus.

Immunosuppression. Abnormal or depressed ability to maintain immunologic integrity; especially, an inability to fight infection.

Interferon. A protein capable of limiting superinfection; produced by cells when infected with a virus.

Interleukin. A protein substance produced by white blood cells which regulates the function of other white cells and intracellular virus replication.

Seroepidemiology. The prevalence and distribution of antibodies, reflecting the degree and extent of infection of a population.

Ethical Issues in AIDS Research

Michael A. Grodin, M.D.
Paula V. Kaminow, J.D.
Raphael Sassower, Ph.D.

There is a need for carefully controlled and scientifically rigorous research studies of the acquired immunodeficiency syndrome (AIDS). The morbidity and mortality associated with AIDS patients and the public health concerns for control of this epidemic have distorted the usual process of research. The Institutional Review Board at Boston City Hospital is suggested as an appropriate mechanism for clarifying the distinctions between research and innovative therapies and for assuring the protection of this vulnerable population of research subjects. This article addresses ethical concerns relating to the time frame of research, drug and antibody testing, vaccine trials, and questions of justice in micro- or macro-allocation. The unique problems in AIDS research with informed consent and confidentiality are discussed. Finally, the need is outlined for careful balancing of individual welfare and rights and those of society.

Perhaps the least controversial point in all discussions about AIDS and AIDS-related complex (ARC) is the need for research. The need to discover the etiology, natural history, epidemiology, and treatment of AIDS is indisputable. However, ethical dilemmas surrounding the priorities, methodologies, and timing of research strategies pose unique problems for patients, researchers, clinicians, hospitals, institutional review boards (IRBs), public health workers, health care policymakers, and society at large.[1]

From the earliest case reports in late 1979 of male homosexuals with Kaposi's sarcoma, immunosuppression, and opportunistic infections, through May 1984, when the human immunodeficiency virus (HIV, formerly known as HTLV-III/LAV) was accepted as the etiologic agent of AIDS, to the present, medical scientists have been and continue to be involved in clinical, epidemiological, and basic science research into AIDS.[2] The Centers for Disease Control (CDC) has been involved in surveillance and epidemiological re-

Dr. Michael A. Grodin is director of the Program in Medical Ethics and is associate professor of pediatrics and social and behavioral sciences (ethics), Boston University Schools of Medicine and Public Health, and is chairperson of the Institutional Review Board (IRB) at Boston City Hospital. Paula V. Kaminow, J.D., was special assistant corporation counsel for the City of Boston and is an ex-officio member of the IRB. Dr. Raphael Sassower is assistant professor of philosophy at the University of Colorado and was a member of the IRB.

search, while other federal agencies, such as the National Institutes of Health and the National Cancer Institute, have sponsored and carried out other investigations. Privately funded commercial, pharmaceutical, and hospital-based research has also been initiated. The rapid mobilization of the medical research community in the face of this deadly, immensely complex, and emotionally charged public health problem has caused some wobbles in the balance that is carefully maintained between individual patient welfare and the public welfare — a balance that has always been an integral part of the ethical principles of medical research.

The Nature of AIDS Research

The primary goal of medical research is to contribute to the development of general knowledge about a particular disease or condition; the primary goal of clinical therapy, on the other hand, is to benefit the individual patient. When medical research enters the clinical therapy setting in the form of testing new drugs, vaccines, or diagnostic procedures, a blurring between these two objectives often occurs. The goal of participating in the testing of a new drug or an innovative therapy may be one thing for the patient and the clinician team, another for the research scientist, and quite another for the sponsoring agency.

The potentially competing interests of the various parties involved in human experimentation present a crucial issue in AIDS research. Additional surveillance is needed because of the wide array of unvalidated and innovative therapies being tested on AIDS patients — members of a special population with a fatal disease who may be willing to incur greater risk to themselves for the good of others. This surveillance must be undertaken by a group that represents the interests not only of the researchers and sponsoring agencies but also of the patients and the public at large.

Institutional Review Boards

IRBs are the intra-institutional committees established under regulations promulgated by the U.S. Department of Health and Human Services.[3] They are mandated to review research involving humans and to monitor the protection of human subjects in order to ensure that socially accepted ethical norms are met.[4] IRBs require that research protocols involve sound scientific design; competent methods of investigation; favorable balance of risks and benefits; adequate informed-consent mechanisms; equitable selection of subjects; justification for research on special populations; and consideration of compensation for research-induced injury. Those who comprise IRBs fall into one of two groups, broadly speaking: individuals who are affiliated with the institution or hospital, such as physicians, nurses, scientists, pharmacists, and public health workers; and unaffiliated lay members, such as philosophers, theologians, lawyers, and other community representatives. Such broad representation and mandated authority place IRBs in the pivotal position necessary to provide additional surveillance of AIDS research.

Time Frame for Research

The high morbidity and mortality of AIDS patients and the serious public health concerns regarding the etiology, natural history, and transmission of HIV have accelerated the standard medical research time frame for AIDS research. Although the pressure to speed up AIDS research is understandable, perhaps even desirable, such distortion of standard research practice implies potential dangers. Moreover, the publicity concerning AIDS research has created a public image of medical research that is quite different from reality.

Standard medical research is a slow, meticulous process. Once the safety and efficacy of proposed therapies have been established, controlled clinical tests are performed. To minimize human risk, animal studies are used when possible before human studies; competent adult patients are studied before incompetent patients; and, when applicable, healthy volunteers are studied before sick or exposed volunteers. Special protections are needed for the study of populations who are at special risk of possible coercion or duress. As a rule, indiscriminate or premature use of therapies that have not been vigorously tested and verified is discouraged.

In AIDS research, however, there has been a rapid movement from basic-science studies to clinical trials. Researchers have been quick to report the results of their work, and the publication of these results has been almost immediate through the news media. Data from such research may be quickly transferred to the clinical setting, where they are often applied without controlled clinical testing. This is understandable. Physicians want to be able to treat their AIDS patients as effectively as possible, and they also want to be able to educate their patients and the public appropriately in order to prevent the spread of AIDS. AIDS patients, searching for hope of survival, scan the medical literature and news reports for access to new drugs or therapies. Premature media coverage of research results has often been accompanied by unwarranted claims of success, thereby raising the public's expectations unfairly. When the initial studies of interferon and interleukins were released by the press, AIDS patients from all over the country flooded researchers with requests for treatment.

Public health concerns about the prevention and spread of AIDS have caused the early introduction of research data into public policy debates. Epidemiological studies are sought as a means of dealing with disease risk management. Such data are used in arguments for and against policies regarding persons with AIDS and their school attendance; the safety and appropriateness of their employment; acceptance for health and life insurance; and possible large-scale screening and quarantine.

Through the rapid publication of their data, many investigators have gained professional and personal renown as well as guarantees of future research funding. The race to cure AIDS has even spurred one research team in France to bring a legal suit against a U.S.-based research team in an argument over who really discovered the AIDS virus.[5]

The rather unorthodox methodology of AIDS research has led to several problems. Data are presented which have not been adequately tested or controlled. Reports of conflicts in data or errors in data cause alarm among clinicians and patients alike. Premature claims of certainty about results which prove to be inaccurate and the continual updating and reclarifying of results of epidemiological studies and clinical tests have confused the public and shaken its confidence in AIDS research.

Because of the urgency of AIDS research, IRBs have felt increased pressure from both researchers and the public to approve AIDS research protocols rapidly. Since it is both the function and responsibility of IRBs to protect human subjects in medical research, they must assume the crucial tasks of helping to maintain ethical and standard research procedures and of helping to develop responsible modifications in those procedures. However, IRBs cannot and should not be the sole gatekeepers safeguarding the integrity of AIDS research.

AIDS Drug Testing

The discovery of experimental antibiotics and antiviral agents that may help fight AIDS and the complicating opportunistic infections found in AIDS patients has spurred the early clinical testing of such drugs. Research protocols involving these drugs represent some of the most ethically complex situations that come before IRBs. Researchers ask IRBs for approval to bypass standard research procedures and to grant compassionate use of drugs they believe will be of particular benefit to AIDS patients. Private pharmaceutical companies are eager to introduce their new antiviral products, because sometimes the mere suggestion of the possible success of an experimental antiviral agent has caused stock in the companies producing such drugs to rise rapidly. Requests are also made for special, expedited approval for new uses of approved drugs without controlled trials or standardized testing.

An excellent example of the dilemmas associated with drug testing in AIDS patients is the case of Azidothymidine (AZT).[6] From the moment this antiviral agent was shown to have some efficacy with the AIDS virus, an emotionally charged and ethically complex series of questions arose. Should the drug go through the standard three-phase, slow medical research protocol of exhaustive testing of safety and efficacy in animals and humans? What patients should be used in human experimentation, and how should they be selected? Should a standard controlled clinical trial of the experimental agent matched against a placebo-control group be undertaken to prove clinical efficacy scientifically? How much of a role should AIDS patients, ARC patients, physicians, scientists, drug companies, and the public play in determining the research trials of AZT? If a randomized clinical trial of placebo versus AZT were undertaken, at what point should the code be broken, identifying which patients received AZT and which received placebo in such a blind study? Once a trend toward efficacy has been established in the course of clinical experimentation, when should the trials be terminated and the drug made available? Is a desperately ill, dying patient with AIDS the appropriate subject for study, or are patients with ARC or HIV-antibody-positive patients with no symptoms a more justifiable group in which to conduct clinical trials? How should one assess the relative risks and benefits in these populations? Should dying patients be included in the randomization, or should they be treated with drugs outside of clinical trials as a last glimmer of hope? Can patients who are dying give an informed consent? Even if they are competent to do so, should they be approached with new, untested drugs with no clear evidence of safety or efficacy? Who should bear the cost of the research project and of the drugs themselves? If a drug appears to be effective late in a clinical trial, can the research subject be asked to pay for the drug? After the research trials are over, can a patient who appears to have responded continue to have access to the experimental agent? As newer drugs become available, should they be tested against placebo controls or against other existing drugs, such as AZT? What control should IRBs have in the resolution of these dilemmas? And, finally, what role should such regulatory bodies as the Department of Health and Human Services or the Food and Drug Administration (FDA) play in monitoring and granting final approval for AIDS drugs?

The history of AZT, from its early synthesis as an anticancer drug through animal and human testing and then to FDA approval and marketing, represents a fair balance between the expediency of drug development and the protection of human subjects at risk. AZT was first tested for in vitro activity against HIV. When the drug's efficacy with HIV had been demonstrated, animal trials were undertaken. The first human experiments were conducted at the National Cancer Institute as an open, nonrandomized trial. Once AZT showed promise as an agent in vivo against HIV, a randomized, placebo-controlled clinical trial was carried out at several medical institutions caring for AIDS patients. Early in the controlled trials, researchers broke the code to identify patients receiving the drug when it became apparent that some patients benefited from the trial more than others.

On the basis of accumulated data from these trials, the FDA approved AZT for clinical use on March 19, 1987. After AZT was approved, the manufacturer began to charge for its use. Initially the cost of AZT was approximately $10,000 per year, but the increasing market and efficiency of production have already led the manufacturer to begin lowering this figure. However, the cost may still present an economic hardship for some. Increased production of the drug seems to have alleviated the problems of access that accompanied its emergence. Insurance coverage may vary, though it appears that access has not been limited nationally by inability to pay. In Massachusetts, all third-party payers, including Medicaid, have covered the cost of AZT. Massachusetts has also recently established a program to cover the cost of the drug for patients who have no other means to pay. AZT has thus proven to be a paradigm for a reasonable approach to drug testing in AIDS.

In June 1987, partly in response to AIDS drug testing, the FDA issued final regulations outlining procedures under which "promising, investigational new drugs could be made available to desperately ill patients before general marketing begins."[7] The regulation applies to "patients with serious and immediately life-threatening diagnoses for which no comparable or satisfactory alternative drug or other therapies exist." The FDA also defined "conditions under which drug manufacturers may charge for investigational new drug products." It remains to be seen whether such FDA regulatory changes will accomplish the goal of releasing new drugs to patients prior to marketing while at the same time protecting the scientific clinical-trials process for testing safety and efficacy and protecting the human subjects participating in research.

HIV Antibody Testing

Perhaps the clearest example of the quick transition of AIDS research from the laboratory to the clinic is the HIV antibody test. Because of the need to identify subjects carrying the HIV antibody in order to protect the blood supply from contaminated donor units, antibody testing was one of the first priorities of AIDS research. The test was also necessary for quantifying epidemiological data and for therapeutic trials and screens. Once developed, the HIV antibody test was rapidly introduced into research protocols and clinical practice, but problems of sensitivity and specificity resulted because experience with the significance and variances of the test was not complete. Beyond test reproducibility, questions about the reliability of HIV antibody positivity and the significant false-positive and false-negative rates caused concern about how quickly this test was being used for clinical screening and public policy guidelines. Extending the use of the HIV antibody test to patient care is complicated by the questions of where, when, how, and why it should be used. In using antibody testing, the distinctions between purposes of epidemiology, diagnosis, and public policy have not always been clear.

HIV Vaccine

As more is learned about the structure and function of the AIDS virus, several research groups have begun work on the development of an HIV vaccine. If and when such a vaccine becomes available, how should it be tested? Do safety and efficacy studies in animals warrant the move to human studies? Who should be used for human studies — patients who are already infected with the virus, or normal subjects with no evidence of viral infection? Is it appropriate to test the vaccine on at-risk populations when education and change in lifestyle are known to be effective preventive measures? Once the vaccine is administered, how will immunity be tested? Should such subjects be challenged with the virus or allowed or even encouraged to continue their high-risk behavior? The laboratory development of an HIV vaccine may raise the hope of universal protection through immunization, but there will be significant ethical debate about research trials and subsequent recommendations for widespread clinical use.

Justice in Micro-Allocation

The main concern of persons with AIDS is the possible avoidance of what appears to be an inevitable early death. This fact brings into focus the problem of population selection for AIDS research. It is reasonable to assume that some experimental drugs will eventually be effective in combating AIDS. Are chances of survival increased when an AIDS patient participates in many research protocols involving different experimental drugs? How are participants to be selected? Who serves as the control group for these drug trials? Should selection be based on the ability to pay, on special needs, or on special merit? Since participation in AIDS research may be viewed as a public good that may also be helpful to the individual AIDS patient, questions about distributive justice must be addressed. How should promising experimental therapies be distributed among all too many claimants in a research setting?

Distributive justice also enters into the problem of disseminating knowledge about AIDS research. Who should know about it? How should such knowledge be provided? Who should pay for it? Should the public as a whole bear the burden of learning and teaching all there is to know about AIDS? Should all the media outlets devote time to AIDS-related issues? Should all public schools devote regular sessions to AIDS-related issues? Should the public be alerted as soon as possible to all new stages of AIDS research?

Justice in Macro-Allocation

Most medical research in the United States is funded either by government agencies or by private foundations and corporations. More specifically, when the research pertains to national epidemics or to medical ailments that are of concern to a wide portion of the population, funding has been provided largely by government agencies. Because AIDS was not viewed at first as an epidemic of national concern, however, AIDS research was initially given little attention and little funding.

Several explanations can be given for this early public policy decision. First, AIDS was thought to afflict only a small minority and thus was not a national concern. Second, some viewed AIDS in theological terms and claimed that this disease was divine punishment against the immoral acts of homosexuals. Third, political pressure to do anything about AIDS was lacking. This is understandable, given the politically conservative stance of the current administration, especially toward the population at risk for developing AIDS.

Political compromises regarding AIDS became quite evident to the growing population of potential AIDS patients. The male homosexual populations of cities like Boston, New York, and San Francisco flexed their political muscles and demanded that their city governments do something about AIDS. These powerful grassroots efforts provided the popular support that city mayors needed to pressure their state legislators for funds to help with AIDS research and education programs. Finally, through pressure from local and state governments and the public at large, the federal administration began to provide funds for AIDS research through the office of the secretary of health and human services.

If only a marginal segment of the population is afflicted with a certain disease, it seems reasonable and just that only a small proportion of public funds earmarked for medical research be allocated for the study of that disease. This was the original proposition advocated in the case of AIDS on both logical and ethical grounds. But this reasoning cannot hold. Now that cases of heterosexual partners and children with AIDS have been confirmed, it remains unclear how small or large the at-risk population is. Because the potential risk to the public at large is uncertain, it is not obvious how to proceed. Should funds be provided only according to the proven proportion of the population which has already contracted the disease? Or should the potential spread of AIDS be taken into account?

Questions also arise concerning the priority of other ongoing medical research. Should federal funding for the less urgent areas of medical research be halted and those funds channeled to AIDS research? Such a suggestion could be defended if one were able to show that unless the government did just that, millions of lives would be endangered. Arguments of this sort presuppose that it is possible to establish a medical research agenda with an agreed-upon set of priorities determined by society as a whole. There are, of course, practical problems with setting such an agenda. How could all of society participate in such a discussion? Can any procedure guarantee democratic control of the setting of these priorities?

A discussion of the macro-allocation of resources for AIDS research would not be complete without considering what it is that private foundations and corporations have at stake in funding AIDS research. Are these organizations concerned with the well-being of those afflicted with AIDS? Or are they hoping to discover the cure in order to capitalize on their discovery and make huge profits? It is possible to claim that the motives for research are unimportant as long as the results are beneficial to patients and society. Moreover, whether or not profits will be secured remains an open question that has little bearing on the ability of the private sector to supplement the federal funds allocated for AIDS research. There are always potential conflicts of interest on the part of those involved in research, in terms of compromises that might be made to maximize profits.

Although IRBs should be cognizant of these issues, their concern about funding sources is limited to the ways in which financing may affect the well-being of human subjects. Is there adequate funding to assure the completion of the proposed research, so that the claimed benefits will indeed outweigh the risks the subjects are asked to incur? It should also be noted that the role of the IRBs is not to set up or implement any specified research agenda but merely to ensure the protection of the subjects who are enrolled in medical research projects.

It is impossible and would be presumptuous to provide any answers or even rules for action regarding the many questions raised so far. The main purpose of this discussion and that which follows is to illustrate the complexity of the ethical issues surrounding AIDS, both for society as a whole and for the individuals involved, and to show that these issues are intimately connected to other social and political concerns.

Informed Consent

Obtaining informed consent in any type of research is a demonstration of respect for an individual's autonomy. Informed consent has three primary components:

- the individual giving consent is mentally competent;
- the individual giving consent is presented with enough information to make rational decisions; and
- the consent is uncoerced — freely given by a nonvulnerable, autonomous individual.

AIDS research raises ethical questions about each of these components. First, when research involves a new vaccine or treatment, both the scientific community and the subjects are faced with more unknowns than knowns. Because AIDS research is so new, the range and magnitude of the unknowns are great. Researchers may believe that their ethical obligations are fulfilled by advising the subjects of the range of unknowns and asking them to weigh the potential risk/benefit ratio on that basis. However, at some point, particularly where new ideas are being rushed through the research system and virtually no information may be available, potential subjects may be placed at too great a risk. IRBs need to make this kind of assessment and, if necessary, restrict participation in such a study.

Second, some persons with AIDS show clinical signs of a central nervous system dysfunction associated with the AIDS virus. To the extent that such symptoms render them mentally incompetent, they will be unable to give informed consent. A question that arises when research is directed at central nervous system AIDS is, Who, if anyone, can or should give consent for the patient? This question arises in both clinical and research settings. Generally, substitute decision makers (for example, parent, spouse) are approached.[8] But what happens when an individual with AIDS is alienated from his or her family and has no legally recognized spouse? The individual who is closest to and who best knows the patient may not be legally recognized as such and may know of difficulties between the patient and other family members.

Third, and finally, when research involves a dying patient whose body has been ravaged by a continuous series of recurring infections and the patient is given a glimmer of relief, the consent can hardly be considered freely given by a nonvulnerable person. Or, how about the symptomatic or asymptomatic individual who feels a sense of guilt from the possibility of having infected a loved one and who is willing to undergo unusual risks to make amends? How about the intravenous (IV) drug user who may link the research with access to methadone?

What obligations do researchers have to look beyond the surface of consent and protect the individual? How paternalistic may the researcher be? Or, conversely, are members of a group uniquely infected by a virus under some obligation to society and the other members of their group to sacrifice their individuality in order to help avert further infection? IRBs are in a position to protect the rights of individuals to make autonomous and informed decisions and not be pressured either by researchers or by the population of persons with AIDS. In this sense, then, IRBs may be considered paternalistic when attempting to maintain the rights and welfare of potential research subjects.

Confidentiality

Preservation of the confidentiality of individuals with AIDS or of other participants in AIDS research is a major concern of clinicians, researchers, lawyers, ethicists, and community groups.[9] The right to privacy, as associated with individual liberty and autonomy, is an important ideal in our society. All medical clinicians and researchers are obligated to maintain confidential information acquired in the clinical and research settings. In the therapeutic environment, such ethical obligations are supported by legal rights in order to permit a free exchange of information between patient and clinician so that possible benefits of treatment will be maximized. The federal guidelines for federally funded research require that researchers provide for confidentiality of records and subject information and that IRBs consider this issue when reviewing research protocols.[10]

The complexity of AIDS research makes difficult demands on researchers with regard to confidentiality. First, in a society in which homophobia exists and AIDS phobia runs rampant, the risk of information leaks is quite high. Individuals may be stigmatized generally for being gay or drug users, or specifically for having a fatal, contagious disease. There are cases in which people either with AIDS, ARC, or HIV antibody positivity have been denied insurance benefits or have suffered the loss of their jobs. Medical providers, acting on their unsubstantiated fears of treating individuals with AIDS, may inappropriately gown or glove before entering the patient's room, may over-isolate AIDS patients, or may even refuse to treat AIDS patients altogether. Another repercussion of AIDS is a family's discovery that a family member is a homosexual or an IV drug user. Further, certain activities that contribute to the spread of AIDS, such as prostitution and IV drug use, are illegal. Knowledge of the individual's status may be followed by legal prosecution. However, in a fear-driven society, failure to release information about particular individuals with AIDS may subject all members of high-risk groups to being ostracized, denied benefits, and treated in a discriminatory fashion. Should such a societal response justify invasion of an individual's privacy and liberty?

Recognizing the importance of medical research, both the federal government and the Massachusetts legislature provide mechanisms for protecting confidentiality by limiting access to research records in certain cases. Under federal law, a researcher can apply for a confidentiality certificate when engaged in mental health research, including research on the use and effect of alcohol and psychoactive drugs, to prohibit access to information by compulsory process.[11] The Massachusetts statute similarly protects certain information from release under subpoena.[12] Laws regarding the protection of confidentiality and access to research records may vary among states.

One major dilemma for researchers who learn that an individual has AIDS, ARC, or HIV antibody positivity and may therefore be infectious is how to preserve the patient's confidentiality while at the same time protecting medical personnel from exposure to AIDS. An example from Boston City Hospital will illustrate this point. When the HIV antibody test was first developed, it was available only for research and blood bank use, not for clinical purposes. At that time, the Centers for Disease Control and the Massachusetts state health agencies felt that, in the absence of treatment for the AIDS antibody, the information would be of little clinical value and would result only in negative consequences for the patient. Since that time, the CDC has become more interested in tracing the course of the virus at earlier stages and has encouraged antibody testing in clinical settings where the information would assist clinical management.

Seroepidemiological studies of HIV with IV drug users, including a substantial number of pregnant addicts, were conducted at a drug treatment clinic operated by Boston City Hospital. The researchers in this instance had information about the clients which they could not disclose to other clinicians without proper consent. These other clinicians believed such information would be invaluable in the clients' treatment plans. The problem was further complicated for pregnant addicts, because a particular physician could be both a researcher and a clinician for them. How could the clinician advise the obstetric and pediatric staffs at the hospital where the clinician practiced, and where the clients would deliver their babies, to take precautions against blood exposure from mother and infant without disclosing the mother's HIV antibody status, learned only through research? Should all high-risk mothers and infants be considered infectious?

In AIDS research, it may be important to distinguish between confidentiality and anonymity. If the only concern is an epidemiological analysis of prevalence, then anonymity may be preferred. However, if there are good reasons — such as the ability to trace a person with AIDS in order to provide therapeutically relevant data or to alert a victim that a new therapy is available — then keeping patients' names in confidential files may be preferred. IRBs have emphasized this distinction and have challenged researchers to decide whether anonymity or confidentiality is preferable and for what reasons.

Conclusion

The ethical and societal concerns about AIDS research which are raised by the relationship between research findings, available clinical treatments, and public health policy actions call for a national assessment of medical research priorities and intermediate goals for AIDS research.[13] Assessments must then lead to directing research funds in accordance with the national research agenda in the most cost-efficient manner. Such a public policy could be cooperatively addressed by private researchers and institutions and public agencies and officials. To some extent, such forums have already been established in various states. For example, in Massachusetts the Governor's Task Force on AIDS is composed of researchers, public health officials, and community representatives. All of the New England states have established similar investigational bodies. State plans should be consistent with broader, more comprehensive national agendas.

Many ethical, legal, and public policy considerations are involved in addressing the problems associated with AIDS research. Professionals in all aspects of health care need to recognize and understand the possible alternative approaches to resolution of these practical and moral quandaries. IRBs can serve as locally based forums for the initiation of debate. Such boards have had ample experience in dealing with the substantive issues of consent, confidentiality, the balancing of risks and benefits, and the proper selection of populations for research. This experience is complemented by federally mandated guidelines that assure proper procedures for the protection of human subjects in research. Since the procedures are open to public scrutiny and since these boards have public representation, IRBs are particularly appropriate forums for public participation in addressing AIDS research.

Although the principles of biomedical ethics, such as beneficence, justice, and respect for persons, are not unique to AIDS research, the enormity and gravity of AIDS necessitate a careful application of these principles. The continuous balancing of the rights and welfare of individuals and the rights and welfare of the public is a crucial element in resolving the complex ethical issues involved in AIDS research.

This article is an adaptation of a paper entitled "Ethical Issues in AIDS Research," which originally appeared in October 1986 in the *Quality Review Bulletin* (volume 12, number 10). The article is printed by permission of the Joint Commission on Accreditation of Healthcare Organizations.

The authors would like to thank George Lamb, M.D., and Donald Craven, M.D., for their helpful comments on this manuscript, and Adrienne Dillon for secretarial assistance.

Notes

1. See generally Hastings Center (Hastings-on-Hudson, N.Y.), "AIDS: The Emerging Ethical Dilemmas," *Hastings Center Report* (special supplement) 15, no. 4 (August 1985):1–32.
2. See Anthony S. Fauci (moderator), "Acquired Immunodeficiency Syndrome: Epidemiology, Clinical, Immunologic and Therapeutic Considerations," *Annals of Internal Medicine* 100 (January 1984):92–106; Samuel Broder, Robert C. Gallo, "A Pathogenic Retrovirus (HTLV-III) Linked to AIDS," *New England Journal of Medicine* 311, no. 20 (November 15, 1984):1292–1297; Sirkka-Liisa Valle, Carl Saxinger, Annamari Ranki, Jaako Antonen, Jukka Suni, Juhan Lahdevirta, Kai Krohn, "Diversity of Clinical Spectrum of HTLV-III Infection," *Lancet* 1 (February 9, 1985):301–304; James W. Curran, W. Meade Morgan, Ann M. Harding, Harold Jaffe, William Darrow, Walter Dowdle, "The Epidemiology of AIDS: Current Status and Future Prospects," *Science* 229 (September 27, 1985):1352–1357; and Sheldon H. Landesman, Harold M. Ginzberg, Stanley H. Weiss, "The AIDS Epidemic," *New England Journal of Medicine* 312, no. 8 (February 21, 1985):521–525.
3. See Code of Federal Regulations, 45 C.F.R., 46 (1974, rev. 1981, rev. 1983).
4. See generally Tom L. Beauchamp and James F. Childress, *Principles of Biomedical Ethics* (New York: Oxford University Press, 1983) and Robert J. Levine, *Ethics and Regulation of Clinical Research* (Baltimore and Munich: Urban and Schwartzenberg, 1986).
5. See Colin Norman, "News and Comments," *Science* 231 (January 3, 1986):11–12.
6. See Ruth Macklin and Gerald Friedland, "AIDS Research: The Ethics of Clinical Trials," *Law, Medicine and Health Care* 14, no. 5–6 (December 1986):273–286.
7. See Code of Federal Regulations 21 C.F.R., 312.
8. See Robert Steinbrook, Bernard Lo, Jill Tirpack, James Dilley, Paul Volberding, "Ethical Dilemmas in Caring for Patients with the Acquired Immunodeficiency Syndrome," *Annals of Internal Medicine* 103 (November 1985):787–790; and Kevin Kelly, "AIDS and Ethics: An Overview," *General Hospital Psychiatry* 9, no. 5 (September 1987):331–340.
9. See Charles Marwick, "Confidentiality Issues May Cloud Epidemiologic Studies of AIDS," *Journal of the American Medical Association* 250, no. 15 (October 21, 1983):1945–1946.
10. See Code of Federal Regulations 45 C.F.R., 46.111, and 45 C.F.R., 46.116.
11. See ibid., 42 C.F.R., 2a; 42 U.S.C., 242(a).
12. Massachusetts General Laws Ch. 3, 2.4A.
13. American Medical Association, "Task Force Formed to Coordinate Study, Testing of AIDS Therapies," *Journal of the American Medical Association* 255, no. 10 (March 14, 1986):1233–1242; and Edward N. Brandt, "Implications of the Acquired Immunodeficiency Syndrome for Health Policy," *Annals of Internal Medicine* 103 (November 1985):771–793.

"Someone once described AIDS like being in a canoe in the middle of a hurricane. It's pretty lonely and it's pretty terrifying. But when someone is in that canoe with you it's not nearly so frightening. So it is with our coalition of PWAs. We even believe that we can bring that canoe into a safe harbor."

The AIDS Epidemic: A Prism Distorting Social and Legal Principles

Alec Gray

The AIDS epidemic is affecting American society in far-reaching and unexpected ways. It touches our institutions, our value systems, and our private lives. Social issues seem to change and become distorted by the epidemic's prismlike effect. This article examines some of the major public health issues raised by the epidemic, ranging from testing to contact tracing and quarantine. It argues that while the civil rights of individuals may have to be sacrificed to stem the spread of the disease, those rights should not be abandoned unless a clear benefit to the public health would result.

Issues of discrimination in housing, employment, insurance, and medical services are considered to determine whether additional protections are needed. Other measures for contending with the epidemic, including the use of criminal statutes, are reviewed to determine whether they could realistically be expected to have a beneficial effect.

The effect of the disease on personal, private, and religious beliefs is considered, and a legal perspective is applied to the various implications of the epidemic. The conclusion is reached that while there are no easy or simple answers, common sense must be the basis for any workable approach.

To say that AIDS is the public health issue of the century is to state the obvious. The assertion that AIDS is everyone's concern is no longer subject to challenge. The disease has caused and will continue to cause major revisions in the ways in which we live, structure our society, and define our beliefs. It attacks the human body with devastating consequences. It attacks the fabric of our society in ways that are perhaps more subtle but that have equally drastic consequences.

A basic tenet of U.S. political philosophy is that every human being has inalienable rights, including the rights to life, liberty, and the pursuit of happiness. Few things could directly challenge the existence of all three of these inalienable rights. The AIDS epidemic has that potential.

Now, for the first time in recent history, a disease threatens life through the very act of intimacy. By its fatal nature, AIDS directly challenges the right to life of all who are ex-

Alec Gray is a former assistant attorney general for the Commonwealth of Massachusetts. In his current law practice, he works in an advisory capacity with private and governmental agencies on issues surrounding the AIDS epidemic.

posed to it. The means by which the disease is transmitted affects the willingness and ability to engage in intimate sexual relations. The right to pursue happiness through loving and intimate relationships has been challenged. Even the right to liberty has come into question, as more and more political leaders call for the segregation of those who are ill and those who are infected.[1]

The central question posed by this epidemic is whether we will be able to maintain our traditional values and principles while dealing with a threat to our very existence. To maintain the health of the entire community, some individual rights may have to be sacrificed. Of particular concern in the legal community is the question of what quantum of protection will justify the lessening of personal freedoms. In this century in this country, thousands of Americans of Japanese ancestry were rounded up and forced to give up their homes, their property, their jobs, and their freedom because of the suspicion that they posed a threat to the country's safety. The action was legally challenged, and the final decision, rendered from the nation's highest tribunal, was that the governmental action was justified and proper.[2] Yet the idea that a mere suspicion is enough to cause the wholesale termination of personal freedoms is anathema to the American concept of justice and liberty.

In the public health arena, the power of health commissioners to impose quarantine is well known. When faced with a threat to the health of the public, the state, through its inherent police power, can impose burdens and lessen freedoms. Courts have traditionally upheld this prerogative when it is exercised in accordance with the sound discretion of appropriate officials. At the beginning of this century, the U.S. Supreme Court upheld the mandatory inoculation for smallpox.[3] Since then, other courts from diverse jurisdictions have upheld the exercise of the police power to meet a health emergency.[4] Some decisions have indicated that in this regard, the constitutional protections simply do not apply.[5] This body of law does not date from an ancient period of history. In 1980, the West Virginia Supreme Court of Appeals set forth the minimal due-process guarantees that were to be applied to efforts to quarantine patients with tuberculosis.[6]

In considering these cases, the "reasonableness" standard has traditionally been applied. Because its interpretation relies upon the subjective view of the public health commissioner, this standard is quite troubling. It is not for the court to second-guess the professional judgment of the executive-branch official who is entrusted by law with the power to make this type of decision.[7]

A more useful means for ascertaining the reasonableness of a mandatory public health measure is to determine whether it will afford protection to the public health as a matter of reasonable medical certainty. This requires more than the belief that the matter is necessary or efficacious; it requires that public health officials be able to offer solid medical or epidemiological evidence that the mandatory public health measure will, in fact, be able to protect the public health. If the contemplated measure will offer real protection, then the determination of reasonableness must be made by balancing the degree of intrusion into personal liberties that would result from its imposition against the degree of protection that the measure would provide to the general populace: the greater the intrusion, the greater the degree of protection that must result.

This balancing approach will be called into play as various state and city legislatures and public health departments contemplate and impose new public health measures designed to address the AIDS epidemic. Certainly, the proper authorities must be given the power to address this epidemic. But the measures that are imposed must not compromise the individual freedoms of those who are affected without a corresponding benefit to the public good.

The extent to which personal liberties may be intruded upon will depend, in part, upon existing statutory schemes. The Constitution provides certain basic guarantees, such as due process and freedom from unreasonable search and seizure. But the more immediate and applicable rights derive from state or federal legislative enactments. For example, it is unlawful for employers who receive money from the federal government to discriminate on the basis of handicap.[8] Massachusetts has a law that prohibits discrimination against the handicapped in employment but does not prevent discrimination in housing.[9] Unless there is a statute prohibiting discrimination on the basis of AIDS, a public health measure requiring an AIDS virus test may result in a loss of employment, housing, and insurance for the person being tested. Whenever mandatory public health measures are contemplated, corresponding consideration should be given to whether additional protections are needed to preserve individual civil liberties.

When the general welfare is threatened, it is appropriate for the government to take appropriate action to preserve and protect the common good.[10] Accordingly, it is not surprising that the first round of debate on the AIDS epidemic is occurring in Congress, in the state legislatures, and in public health councils around the country. These are the proper deliberative bodies to formulate policies and to devise the means by which the disease can be treated and its spread curtailed.

But government must deal with the AIDS problem in a separate context as well. It must decide how to deal with those people who have AIDS and who live in or who are confined in public institutions. How to treat persons with AIDS who are in direct state care and what to recommend for or impose on the general public with regard to AIDS should be consistent, or at least not contradictory, even though the considerations for each are somewhat different.

Governmental Response: The General Population

Mandatory Public Health Measures

Traditionally, government has had the right to take drastic and even devastating actions to control the spread of disease.[11] Quarantine,[12] segregation,[13] testing,[14] and vaccination[15] have been not uncommonly imposed on past generations to deal with epidemics. These same measures are being discussed today as potential means for fighting the spread of HIV infection.[16]

Testing. The primary focus of most current governmental discussion about mandatory health measures with respect to AIDS is the idea that certain people should be required to be tested for the AIDS virus. This idea has initial appeal. It seems to make obvious good sense to know who has the disease, to learn how widespread the infection is so that the problem can be addressed in an informed manner. The AIDS test is a relatively simple laboratory procedure performed on blood. The degree of intrusion with respect to a person's bodily integrity is relatively minor. The potential benefit seems to be considerable. But if testing is to be imposed, who should be tested and the consequences of the test result must both be determined.

Testing was first imposed for those in the armed forces and for military recruits.[17] Here, the justifications for testing are strong: The armed forces must be healthy. In case of emergency, all personnel must be available to provide blood transfusions. The armed forces are dispersed throughout the globe. It is proper for this country to take steps to prevent or at least retard the exportation of disease to other countries.[18] The same considerations have led to the mandatory testing of State Department personnel who are assigned to overseas operations.[19] The testing of military personnel for the AIDS virus is not without serious potential consequences. Soldiers have been charged with criminal conduct as a result of having sex after having tested positive.[20] A civilian band leader assigned to a foreign army base has been released from duty for having tested positive to the HIV antibody.[21]

Many jurisdictions are considering a mandatory AIDS test for all who apply for a marriage license.[22] President Reagan has advocated this idea.[23] It has a superficial appeal. Politicians who suggest premarital testing for AIDS may appear to be doing something to curb the spread of the disease. Traditionally, states have taken action to require that those who are entering the holy state of matrimony undergo venereal disease tests.[24] With respect to the AIDS virus, some hold that it would be unfair to the betrothed to enter a marriage in which the partner is infected with a life-threatening disease that could be transmitted to the spouse or to the children, or both.

However, the issue is far more complex. The HIV antibody test is about as accurate as any medical test, but it is not completely accurate. Even with a reliable confirmatory test, there are many instances of false-positive test results.[25] If the test is applied in a population with a low prevalence of viral infection, the number of false positives is appreciable. For example, if the test were to be administered to members of the general population (which is presumed to have a low seroprevalence), many true instances of infection would be discovered. But it could also be expected that many false positives would result.[26]

Applying these false-positive statistics to the notion of premarital testing, it could be anticipated that if all couples about to be married were tested, more than 380 perfectly healthy, happy persons would (incorrectly) be told that they were HIV-positive. The effect that such information would have on the marital plans can easily be imagined. Further, the testing project would cost somewhere in the vicinity of $100 million,[27] and the use of these monies for this sort of testing would mean that funds would not be available to offer testing to individuals who might well be infected and for whom the test would produce more accurate results.

The concept of the state stepping in to require full and informed consent prior to marriage is equally troubling. While it might appear to be a good idea to require potential husbands and wives to be truthful about their medical status, it would similarly be wise to require them to be truthful about their financial status and about their past criminal history.

The proposal for premarital testing should be evaluated with the same criterion that is applied to other public health measures: Is the degree of intrusion into personal liberties justified by the corresponding benefit to the public health? The degree of intrusion could be serious; marriage has long been considered to be a fundamental right,[28] and any requirement of premarital testing or disclosure would impose a significant burden on the right of individuals to marry at will, without governmental restriction. The benefit to be derived from the test would be speculative at best. Many, if not most, of those who seek to be married have presumedly already engaged in intimate sexual relations. Testing for those about to be married would not be focused on a population that is particularly at risk of infection, nor would it be imposed at a time when the knowledge derived from the test would be most useful. In this situation, the intrusion into personal liberties would not be justified by a corresponding benefit to the public health.

The president has also advocated the mandatory testing of aliens who are applying for permanent residence status.[29] This is a notion whose initial appeal readily dissipates upon even a cursory examination.

Traditionally, quarantine was used to isolate a ship coming in to port which potentially carried infected goods or people.[30] The ship was kept in the harbor, and neither anyone nor anything was allowed off the ship until proper inspection could be made to determine that it would not be dangerous to allow disembarking.[31] It is from this historic perspective that the testing of aliens derives its appeal.

The idea of denying entrance to those infected with a deadly disease may have merit, especially if the disease is not already rampant within the general population. The proposed restriction, however, does not apply merely to individuals outside the United States who are seeking admittance for the first time; it extends to individuals who are already in this country, regardless of the length of their residence. Many of those applying for permanent residence have lived here for years, as students, as temporary workers, or as visitors.[32] To assume that it is only after they gain permanent status that they will begin to engage in sexual relations or intravenous drug use is absurd. To now refuse them permanent status is simply unjust and far more serious than closing the barn door after the horse is gone. Requiring them to leave this country may amount to the mandatory exportation of the virus to other nations. This public health measure will have little, if any, effect on the spread of the disease in the United States. All that it will accomplish is to deny citizenship to individuals because of their medical condition.

While to date mandatory testing has been advocated only for the military and for State Department personnel, those seeking marriage licenses, and aliens, other populations will soon be the focus of such efforts. Prostitutes, who are apt to be intravenous drug users,[33] are at least a potential bridge between traditional high-risk groups (homosexual men and intravenous drug users) and the mainstream of society. Besides the use of prostitutes by heterosexual men, it is not unheard of for a "straight" man to employ a male prostitute. Thus, the HIV infection may pass from a prostitute (having been infected through drug use or homosexual acts) to a heterosexual man and from him to his wife, girlfriend, or next sexual partner. The concern about prostitutes has been heightened by media reports of both male and female prostitutes who have continued to work after learning that they were infected with the AIDS virus.[34] The public outrage is understandable.

Realistically, it is not clear what can be done about the prostitute-AIDS connection. Suppose a prostitute were charged and convicted and an HIV antibody test were ordered. The prostitute would obviously have to be held in custody until the test results were known. If the results came back positive, there is serious question as to whether the sentencing judge would take that medical status into consideration in imposing a sentence. If a harsher sentence were imposed because of the HIV antibody status, the prostitute would have been punished for having a disease rather than for committing a crime. This concept is antithetical to the American concept of criminal justice,[35] especially given the likelihood that the prostitute would have been ignorant of his or her medical status prior to committing the act for which the criminal charges were pressed. It might be possible to make the medical test result part of the probation or criminal record so that the information could be used the next time such charges were leveled against the prostitute. But for the test results to be used, the prostitute would have to be charged with a new crime in which he or she was clearly engaging in the act of prostitution after having been diagnosed as HIV-positive. Further, even if the new crime were enacted, the penalty would not have been pre-specified. A longer and a mandatory prison sentence could be imposed for the new crime, but it is not clear that this would have an impact on the disease, and the increased penalties might create new problems for the penal system.

Another suggestion for dealing with the AIDS-prostitute problem is to legalize prostitution and require periodic medical examinations of those who seek to work in this field. The idea is that by licensing prostitutes, some check or control could be placed on their medical status, and those who chose to use a prostitute would be able to employ someone whose health had been established. There are two essential problems with this approach. First, even if some prostitutes were working legally, there would still be those who worked without the benefit of a license and a medical certificate. Second, the current test detects antibodies to the AIDS virus, not the virus itself. It takes the body some time, estimated at three weeks to six months, to generate these antibodies after initial exposure to the virus.[36] To be sure that a person is free of the virus, it is necessary to test twice, with a six-month interval, and to ensure that during those six months the person engages in no conduct that could expose him or her to the virus. Imposing these restrictions on prostitutes would seem to be particularly unworkable. Finally, the solution is simply impracticable. A prostitute might be licensed and certified as healthy and then become infected, while carrying a certificate of health attesting to a disease-free status and presumably stating that no new test would be required for several months. In the interim, more and more clients would rely on a health certificate that was inaccurate. While the idea of legalized prostitution may be meritorious, it does not gain any support as a tool for fighting the AIDS epidemic.

There are those who take a more altruistic view of the problem concerning AIDS and prostitutes. They suggest that for prostitutes who are engaging in sex in order to finance a drug habit, the solution is to treat the drug addiction. Providing prostitutes with counseling, a chance to develop skills, and help with finding other forms of employment would be ways of doing this. Education about the dangers of drugs and the realities of AIDS might well have a beneficial impact. Clearly, all of this would require more methadone treatment centers, more counselors, more teachers, and more money. But to believe that such efforts would halt the practice of prostitution in the near future would be naive.

The prostitute's client may also be an appropriate party to educate about the dangers to which he is exposing himself and others. Mandatory education programs are now a common way of dealing with drunk drivers.[37] Perhaps a mandatory AIDS education program for those convicted of using a prostitute would be helpful. It might provide not only useful information, but also a deterrence from the use of prostitutes in general.

Another group that will likely be singled out for testing are pregnant women, who are now urged to undergo an HIV antibody test. The potential for an infected mother to transmit the disease to a child is quite high.[38] Doctors are urging women with identifiable risks for HIV infection to consider this reality in deciding whether or not to have a child.[39]

The idea of encouraging pregnant women to undergo an HIV test does not pose any risk to civil liberties. It remains for the women herself to decide whether she wants the information and to decide what to do with the test results. Civil liberties are implicated only when the concept is expanded to *require* that all pregnant women submit to such a test. The true issue is not the test, but the consequence of the test. Will there be a suggestion that infected mothers cannot give birth? If so, what other prenatal tests can be required to ensure that only the healthy procreate and only the well are born?

In this connection, it could be argued that there is a benefit to requiring testing of all pregnant women and a benefit to requiring that women who test positive for the AIDS virus not give birth. Such a requirement would certainly lessen the number of children born with this fatal and costly disease. However, the degree of intrusion into personal liberties is so total and so devastating that it could not be justified by any countervailing improvement to the public health.

Contact tracing. One public health measure that is currently under discussion is sexual contact tracing, which is a standard public health measure for dealing with venereal disease.[40] Existing statutes and regulations in most jurisdictions could be readily adapted to AIDS.

Contact tracing involves contacting those individuals who may have been exposed to the disease. It requires that when people test positive for the infection, they reveal the names and addresses of those whom they may have infected. In the AIDS context, this would mean revealing the identity of past sexual partners as well as the identity of those with whom intravenous needles were shared. The identified individuals would then be contacted by public health workers and urged to be tested for the virus. While the standard approach is to phrase the law in terms of a mandatory requirement, there is often no penalty for noncompliance or for inadequate or incomplete compliance.

These laws have generally been upheld as reasonable public health measures designed to deal with venereal disease.[41] Despite the intrusion into personal freedoms, there is an undeniable benefit to the public health. By identifying those individuals who are infected with VD, treatment can be offered which can eliminate the infection within a matter of days. This remedy is simply not available with AIDS. While the sources of infection may be identified, no treatment can be offered to eliminate the infection.

Contact tracing could have a beneficial effect in dealing with the AIDS epidemic, especially in populations with a low incidence of HIV infection. A person who has no suspicion that he or she may have been exposed to the virus is much less likely to practice behavior that will reduce the risk of spreading the disease. Informing infected persons of their HIV status may influence them to terminate conduct that could spread the disease.

Obviously, a program of mandatory contact tracing would have a great impact on the right of individuals to privacy. Whenever a governmental employee asks for the identity of past sexual partners, the potential for abuse is great. The potential for effectively curtailing the spread of the disease, however, is not assured. People can be expected to lie about their sex and drug partners. Some will be dissuaded from being tested if they know that they will be asked to reveal the identity of others. In populations such as the male homosexual communities of San Francisco and New York City, where up to 50 percent of the members of the community are already infected, the potential benefit from such a program would be marginal, as the same people would likely be identified over and over again. The rights/benefits analysis would indicate that in some communities the right of individual privacy may outweigh the unlikely benefits.

In communities with low seroprevalence, there may be a sufficient benefit to the public health to warrant the imposition of contact tracing. Even in these circumstances, every effort would have to be made to preserve the confidentiality of all concerned. If a sufficient matrix of statutory protections exists banning discrimination on the basis of HIV status, the burden on individual liberties may be lessened further, thereby justifying this public health measure.

A more workable approach might be to inform people who do test positive of the nature of the disease and to explain that they may have exposed other people who, perhaps, are in the process of exposing still others. They should be urged to contact those whom they may have infected. As an alternative, a program should be offered to them whereby trained, professional public health workers can contact those who may have been exposed in order to explain the situation in an anonymous context. Such a program would provide information to those who need it without needlessly infringing on the right of privacy.

Quarantine. A suggestion not openly discussed is quarantining those with AIDS and HIV infection. Quarantine was used earlier in this century to deal with the threat posed by tuberculosis.[42] Those who were confined in sanitaria (and only after a court determination that they were unable or unwilling to take proper precautions)[43] were nonetheless confined apart from the population and against their will.

Tuberculosis is an airborne disease.[44] A person can contract it simply by being in the same room with someone who is infected. There was an undeniable need for drastic measures to deal with tuberculosis. HIV is transmitted only through the exchange of blood or semen; some type of direct blood-blood or blood-semen contact is required. But the conduct that transmits HIV is private in nature and therefore not easily susceptible to regulation. Those who favor quarantine argue that while AIDS is not communicated as readily as TB, there is no effective way to guarantee that those who are infected will refrain from conduct that will transmit the infection.

An idea that is advanced only by the most zealous is to mark or tattoo those who are infected. The argument goes that if the potentially dangerous conduct cannot be successfully regulated, at least persons who come into contact with those who are infected should have fair warning. The idea is offered as a modern-day version of the leper's bell.

These suggestions are frightening. Few things are more devastating to personal liberty than being quarantined for life. The idea of a tattoo smacks of Nazi Germany and is particularly abhorred by the gay community, since homosexuals were tattooed in the concentration camps and were made to wear the infamous pink triangles.[45]

The first question with regard to quarantine is, Who would be removed? The answer would be, necessarily, all those who are infected. Merely quarantining those with clinical, CDC-diagnosed AIDS would not remove all those who are infected. All who are HIV-positive would have to be removed. All 2 million.[46] And, because the antibodies to the virus (which is all that the test currently detects) are not present for up to six months after initial infection,[47] the quarantine effort would have to be ongoing. Designing a plan by which the entire population would be tested routinely twice each year would be staggering. It would dwarf any military registration system that has ever been implemented.

But even if such a system could be designed and put in place, it wouldn't be successful. As noted earlier, the test is not foolproof.[48] There would be instances of false negatives. In a general population of 100,000 tested, 29 people who are in fact infected would have a false-negative test result[49] and accordingly would be allowed to remain at large, spreading the virus. Additionally, some people never develop the antibodies, so although they are infected, they would continue to test negative. The potential for abuse and subterfuge would only be increased by the consequences attendant on a positive test result. Dividing the country between the infected and the healthy would jeopardize all notions of liberty and justice. It would separate the country as decisively as the South's secession did.

Another form of segregation must receive more serious consideration. There may be individuals who present a risk to the community at large because they are infected and infectious and are unable or unwilling to conform their conduct in ways necessary to stop the spread of the virus. What is to be done about someone who is HIV-positive and who deliberately sets out to infect other people through sexual relations or the sharing of drug needles? What about the person who, because of limited cognitive capability or symptoms of dementia, is unable to stop dangerous conduct and continues to have unprotected sex or to frequent drug-shooting galleries? Must society sit back and allow this conduct to continue? Should some type of humane treatment facility be provided where these people could receive help but at the same time be removed from the population at large? If such a civil commitment were to be imposed, procedural safeguards would be needed. It is likely that the commitment would be for the duration of the illness; in the case of AIDS, for life. Some type of periodic review would be needed to determine the individual's continued medical status and his or her current ability and willingness to refrain from conduct that could spread the infection. Provision would have to be made for attorneys to represent these individuals at all commitment proceedings. Wherever the confinement was accomplished, appropriate treatment would have to be available, not only to address the individual's medical needs, but also to provide whatever psychological counseling or other treatment was needed so that the committed person could learn to control the behavior that could lead to spreading the disease.[50]

This type of limited segregation of those individuals who present a clear and unmistakable public health danger, where there is no other alternative to commitment, may have to be considered. It is a difficult suggestion, one that could be considered only as an absolutely last resort. The burden on individual freedom would be extreme and could be justified only if a concomitant benefit could be obtained. Moreover, the question remains whether removing these isolated individuals would have a beneficial effect in terms of stopping the epidemic.

Mandatory Public Education

One of the platitudes of the AIDS crisis is that the only weapon available to fight the disease is education. There is no vaccine, and the available treatments are only experimental. If the disease were polio, the public education program would be extensive and immediate; polio is contracted in "moral" ways.[51] AIDS is spread by sexual conduct and by sharing contaminated needles. American society is reluctant to discuss sex even in private, and the notion of a sexually explicit public campaign is very difficult to countenance. Teaching safe ways to inject drugs is anathema to the current "war" against drug use. As recently as November 1987 there has been a call by some members of the Massachusetts legislature to rescind the funds allocated to the AIDS Action Committee of Massachusetts because the committee published a brochure (not using state funds) that used explicit terms in describing "safe" and "unsafe" sexual practices.

Effective AIDS education must involve school systems. Traditionally, parents have been very concerned about sex education, preferring to control what and how their children are taught about sex. Some states are now making AIDS education a requirement of public education beginning in the elementary grades.[52] If the layers of difficulty about AIDS education are not already obvious, one additional complication needs to be mentioned. An effective means of reducing the risk of contracting HIV infection is to use a condom during sex.[53] Condoms are also a commonly used form of birth control. To advocate the use of condoms and to recommend that they be made available routinely and universally implicates the notion of urging birth control, which is contrary to the teachings of some religions.

Effective AIDS education requires some degree of effective sex education. The virus is transmitted by the "exchange of body fluids," but people need to know exactly what that means. For years, AIDS educators have been urging people to engage in "safe sex" or "safer sex." The slogans have urged "on me, not in me" and people have been advised to use condoms during intercourse. Many assumptions underlie common notions about safe sex. Some educational materials have advised that homosexuality is a cause of AIDS.

Slogans, sayings, and statements have great potential for conveying misinformation, because they generally do not employ explicit terms or refer to precise acts.

The only truly safe sex is sex in which no semen, pre-seminal fluids, or vaginal secretions are put into another person's body. That means that the only sexual activity that is safe, other than kissing, is masturbation or digital manipulation. Safer sex is sex that involves a prophylactic to prevent the infusion of potentially dangerous body fluids. AIDS education must indicate that the virus is present not just in sperm, but also in pre-seminal fluids and in vaginal secretions. That means that a condom should be put on before fellatio, and that cunnilingus is at least potentially dangerous. Homosexuality does not cause AIDS. Certain sexual acts that are frequently performed by homosexual men do present a danger of transmitting the disease. Specifically, anal intercourse is the most efficient sexual means of infusing the virus directly into the bloodstream of another.[54] Anal intercourse is a not uncommon practice among members of the heterosexual community.[55] Any indication that anal intercourse is dangerous only if performed between two men and not between a man and a woman is wrong and dangerous.

The intent here is not to provide safe sex counseling, but to demonstrate the type of explicit information that must be conveyed if it is to be of any benefit. Merely to urge the use of a condom during vaginal intercourse and not to tell people that a condom should be put on before foreplay involving fellatio is to mislead. Mention has to be made of these types of sexual practices. People have to know what is dangerous and why.

Obviously, this type of information is not generally found in elementary-school classrooms or on public-television shows. The debate about the morality of AIDS education is being waged across the country. The U.S. surgeon general has personally written a brochure explaining, in layman's terms, what is known about the disease and what is known about how to avoid spreading it.[56] The federal government will not pay for the distribution of this information to U.S. citizens because the president believes that more emphasis should be placed on sexual abstinence as the best way to prevent the spread of the disease.[57] Rep. Gerry Studds (D-Mass.), in an act of self-described desperation, has invoked his constitutional franking privilege to distribute the brochure to his constituents.[58] Others are still debating and delaying the dissemination of needed information because of not wanting to appear to be condoning sexual promiscuity.

New York City produced public service announcements aimed at providing information for the general, straight community about the potential dangers of AIDS. One commercial, showing a stylish young woman putting a package of condoms into her purse as she leaves her apartment for a night out, announces, "Don't leave home without your rubbers."[59] After the public service programs were produced, none of the three major television networks in New York City would agree to air the spots, claiming they were too risqué.[60] In the meantime, in that city more men between the ages of twenty-five and forty-four and more women between twenty-five and thirty-four are dying from AIDS each year than from cancer. Certainly, the media have the First Amendment freedom to decide what to air and what to reject. However, unless and until all parties — the government, the media, the state legislatures, and the public at large — recognize that this is a matter of life and death and agree that basic, understandable material must be disseminated widely, there will be no effective public education campaign and thousands more will die.

Housing and Employment Discrimination

Of immediate concern is whether state and federal governments will enact laws protecting those with HIV infection and AIDS from discrimination. Recently, the Supreme Court decided that communicable diseases can be considered to be handicaps within the federal Rehabilitation Act.[61] Section 504 of this act prohibits discrimination only by the federal government and by those private enterprises which receive federal funds. While it now seems fairly clear that AIDS will be considered a protected handicap under that statute, the question remains whether HIV infection will be included within the statutory ambit.[62]

Many states, including Massachusetts, have taken the position that AIDS and HIV infection are handicaps under state law.[63] Some jurisdictions have enacted statutes that specifically prohibit discrimination on the basis of AIDS.[64] Some have prohibited requiring employees or job applicants to undergo the HIV antibody test.[65]

The issue to be decided in this context is whether an employer should be able to dismiss an employee who is known to be infected with HIV or who in fact has clinical AIDS. The rights of the employer in this area generally encompass the right to hire the people of his or her choosing. Employers are understandably concerned that other employees will walk off the job if they know they are working with someone who is infected with HIV. There are fears that customers will stop patronizing shops if they know they will be waited on by a person with AIDS. Employers wonder what type of liability they will be exposed to if an employee infects someone else in the workplace. Landlords have similar issues. They are concerned that property values will drop if it is known that a person with AIDS lives in a particular apartment house, and they wonder if other units in that same building will be rentable.

Balancing the rights of landlords and employers against the rights of those stricken with AIDS is not an easy task. The various state legislatures and city councils will have to decide how the balance should be struck. The consequences are of great significance. If discrimination is permitted, it can be expected that those with HIV infection and AIDS will be denied jobs and housing. If discrimination is prohibited, it can be expected that employers and landlords will face increased costs and adverse business consequences.

Another underlying question is, Why should AIDS be treated differently than other illnesses or diseases? There is no great movement to prohibit discrimination against those with cancer or tuberculosis or hepatitis. Why should AIDS be singled out from among all diseases, even from other life-threatening, infectious diseases, for special treatment? The answer seems to be that AIDS *is* different. No other disease carries the stigma associated with AIDS. Because of the way in which AIDS first entered the United States and because of the people who were first affected, AIDS is often associated with illegal or immoral behavior. An AIDS diagnosis often carries the assumption that the patient is a homosexual man or a drug user. The hemophiliac community, while suffering greatly from HIV infection, seems to be trying to distance itself from the AIDS movement so as to avoid the stigma and discrimination commonly associated with homosexuality and drug use. The simple fact is that homosexuals and drug users have not enjoyed an elevated position in society. They have often been subjected to discrimination, and traditionally they have not had great political clout. For these reasons, there is more likelihood of discrimination against those with AIDS.

Further, the very mention of AIDS engenders fear and trepidation. The common understanding is that the disease is universally fatal. It is known to be communicable. These factors combine to make discrimination against those with the disease inevitable. Even in states that have enacted strong laws prohibiting discrimination, the instances of AIDS patients being denied housing, jobs, medical treatment, and other services are amazingly numerous.[66]

AIDS is different from other contagious diseases, and it should be treated differently.

Insurance

Debate is currently raging about the ways in which the insurance industry is attempting to protect itself from claims based on AIDS. The industry obviously is concerned lest huge numbers of new claims for life and health insurance drain its available pool of resources. Those who want protection against future infection with HIV want the benefit of insurance.

The controversy is focusing on the issue of testing. The insurance industry wants to require those applying for insurance, or at least some types of insurance (generally life and disability), to be tested for the HIV antibody. Those with positive test results would not receive insurance policies. AIDS activists are vehemently opposed to any mandatory testing as a precondition to insurance coverage. The range of approaches to this problem spans the horizon. In Washington D.C.,[67] and in California,[68] all HIV antibody testing is prohibited. New York State has announced plans to allow testing for life and disability policies but not for health insurance.[69] In Massachusetts, Insurance Commissioner Peter Hiam took the position that no testing would be permitted in the state as a precondition for receiving insurance coverage. This position was overridden by the governor, and Commissioner Hiam resigned. The new insurance commissioner, Roger M. Singer, held public hearings and promulgated regulations that would have allowed some testing for large life insurance policies, but the regulations provided that the insurance industry must protect and preserve the confidentiality of the test results and that proper counseling must be offered to those who are tested. The regulations imposed additional burdens restricting and regulating the laboratories that could conduct the testing and actually specifying which tests would be considered to be valid. The insurance industry promptly brought a legal challenge and obtained an injunction against the enforcement of the new regulations. As a result, no restrictions or requirements have been imposed on the Massachusetts insurance industry concerning the use of HIV antibody testing.

While the debate has focused on testing, the real question is, Who is going to pay the cost of the epidemic? The current controversy centers around life insurance, but the fear is that testing will next be required for health insurance as well. This conjures up images of people being unable to obtain insurance to pay their medical bills and thereby being denied medical care. If health insurance is not available, those who contract AIDS will be forced upon the public hospital system. That system is already overburdened and may not be able to withstand a large new influx of patients. The welfare system and the tax base may have to pay for the medical care of those who have been denied private insurance coverage.

The testing debate is masking the more crucial issue. If some type of insurance pool were to be created which provided coverage to everyone, regardless of HIV-antibody status, the controversy about testing would disappear. What motivates the AIDS activists is the notion that everyone must be able to receive quality medical care regardless of ability to pay. Insurance pools have been created to cover the cost of other types of ailments. The same basic approach should be pursued for AIDS. There should be a combined effort of public and private funds to guarantee that everyone will receive the necessary medical care, including medicines. In the face of the obvious dimensions of this epidemic, the only realistic solution is to spread the cost as widely as possible. To do otherwise would threaten to bankrupt any single source.

While the insurance testing debate will continue, an effort should be made to focus the discussion on the underlying issue of providing a way of guaranteeing quality medical care to all. This sounds remarkably like the perennial debate on the advisability of universal medical care, an issue that has been heatedly debated for years on the floor of Congress. AIDS has not created the issue, it has merely added to the urgency of finding a resolution.

Criminal Law Revision

An idea that can be expected to receive more attention in the near future is that of using the criminal law to fight against the spread of AIDS.

To date, only isolated efforts have been made to prosecute persons for attempting to infect others with the AIDS virus. A prosecution has been brought against a soldier who tested positive during routine military testing; it was later learned that he engaged in sexual acts with another male soldier and with a female soldier without telling either person of his HIV status and without using any form of protection.[70] Another AIDS patient was discharged from a hospital declaring that he was going to go out and infect others. He was arrested later that day, following a sexual attack on a woman; he has been charged with attempted murder.[71]

It is certainly possible to draft new statutes that would make sexual activity following a positive HIV test result criminal. These statutes could be general or could be restricted to those convicted of prostitution or other sex or drug-related crimes. The object of such statutes, to punish and deter reprehensible conduct, would be unquestionably legitimate. Of more pressing concern is whether such laws would have any appreciable impact on the spread of the disease.

The IV-drug-user community appears to be the biggest bridge between the current known high-risk groups and the mainstream of American society.[72] Many recreational drug users in middle America have sex with others who neither use drugs nor engage in high-risk sexual activity. The potential for the AIDS virus to leave the IV drug community and enter the larger pool of straight society is apparent. Intravenous drug use is already illegal in virtually every jurisdiction in the country. It must be anticipated that efforts on behalf of stricter drug enforcement will be advocated as a way of addressing the AIDS epidemic.

Of course, drugs are still commonplace even though the war on drugs has been fought for years. To increase drug enforcement efforts may do nothing more than drive the drug community further underground, making it more difficult to reach its members with appropriate educational material. Again, the proffered solution of stricter drug enforcement might look good and sound appropriate without actually being able to address the problem effectively.

Rather than urge stricter drug enforcement, some AIDS activists are recommending that free sterile needles be distributed to drug addicts so that they do not have to share dirty needles. A somewhat less controversial proposal has been to distribute small bottles of household bleach to the drug addict community which can be used successfully to sterilize needles. Even the simple notion of providing AIDS education in the IV-drug-user community causes debate, as many are urging that current or former addicts should be employed to provide the educational material. These ideas may well be beneficial, practical approaches to reaching the drug-using community. The need to reach that community is of utmost importance. The IV-drug-user category is the fastest growing segment of the HIV-infected population.[73] But all of these efforts seem to countenance drug use. To adopt any of these approaches would appear to be admitting defeat in the war against drugs. Some hard choices have to be made.

Governmental Response: Public Institutions

Federal, state, and local governments have to deal with the issue of AIDS in all of their public institutions. Policies must be put into place with respect to whether prisoners will be tested for the AIDS virus; whether schoolchildren who are HIV-positive will be taught separately; whether condoms will be distributed to youthful offenders. These issues raise many charged political and moral questions.

Prisons are particularly difficult institutions to manage. They house individuals who have committed criminal offenses and who are known to be uncooperative, manipulative, and often violent. Many prisoners have a history of drug use. Homosexual behavior is reportedly a fairly frequent occurrence behind prison bars. Prison administrators have an obligation to provide a safe environment for those who are confined against their will.[74] These considerations raise the question of whether prisoners should be tested for the HIV antibody. President Reagan has declared that all federal prisoners are to be tested.[75] The Massachusetts commissioner of correction has stated that no mandatory testing policy will be implemented in the Commonwealth.[76] Some states require testing, but only of those inmates who belong to a high-risk group, that is, homosexuals, hemophiliacs, or IV drug users.[77]

The testing question, in the context of prisons, once again hides the real issue. By itself, testing provides no answers. The real point of controversy is what is to be done as a result of the test. In some jurisdictions, prisoners who test positive will be segregated from the rest of the prison population. If such a policy of segregation is followed, there is the real possibility of creating AIDS prisons to deal with the increased number of infected prisoners. An equally troubling issue is whether HIV status is an appropriate factor to consider in determining parole eligibility.

From a practical point of view, the only reason to test prisoners is to segregate. Whether HIV infection is, by itself, a valid reason to segregate a prisoner is a serious question. If separate AIDS units were established, there would be no reason for them to be any more restrictive, nor would there be any justification for the conditions of confinement to be any more onerous. If the AIDS units were more restrictive or more onerous, the greater punishment would be due to the prisoners' medical status, not their criminal behavior. Punishing people for a medical condition would be subject to a constitutional challenge.

Those who advocate testing and segregating within prisons argue that persons who are infected with HIV present a threat to the health and safety of other inmates. They point out that prison rape is a common occurrence and that the state should not put a person into prison for a relatively minor offense when that person may be raped and infected with a fatal disease. The obvious response is that it is the rapist who should be segregated, not everyone who is HIV-positive.

Another aspect of this discussion has received little attention. While prison rape is undoubtedly prevalent, consensual and situational homosexual activity also occur within prisons. In this type of sexual encounter, it is reasonable to expect that safe sex or safer sex could be practiced. However, in prisons condoms are generally regarded as contraband, since they are often used as a means of smuggling drugs into the prison. If prison officials prohibit the introduction of condoms into the facilities, they may be viewed as obstructing the use of an effective disease preventive.

The same basic considerations pertain in governmental facilities that care for the mentally retarded. Individuals in these facilities not uncommonly have active sex lives. The state may have an obligation to provide instruction on AIDS and on ways of preventing it.

There may even be an affirmative duty to provide condoms to protect the health of the patient population. The position that the problem need not be addressed because sex doesn't occur in these facilities is simply not realistic.

Institutions for the detention of youthful offenders present particularly troubling issues. It is at least realistic to expect that some type of sexual experimentation has occurred prior to incarceration and is probably continuing within the facility. State administrators will have to decide what kinds of education programs should be implemented with regard to AIDS and sex in general. They will have to confront the issue of whether to provide condoms to minors in their care. The most likely course of conduct, and the one that is most dangerous, is simply to deny that the juveniles in these institutions engage in sexual activity.

Public schools too have to confront the issue of AIDS. Some jurisdictions have made AIDS education mandatory,[78] but the content of those educational programs has yet to be determined. Abstinence, obviously, is an effective way to prevent HIV infection, perhaps the most effective.[79] But it is unrealistic to believe that teenagers won't have sex or won't experiment with drugs. School systems could be viewed as being irresponsible if they fail to provide information on alternative means of AIDS prevention, such as the use of condoms or the use of bleach to sterilize needles after each use. In state universities and colleges, there can be no denial of sexual and drug experimentation among the student body. The notion of teaching public school students how to use condoms or how to clean their "works" is contrary to the standard concept of reading, writing, and arithmetic. It is at best a difficult problem to decide how these competing interests balance out.

Business Decisions

Businesses are finding themselves unexpectedly on the front line of the AIDS debate. Employers must decide how they will deal with employees who are HIV-positive and whether to implement an on-the-job AIDS education program. They must also decide what type of program they will provide — whether, for example, it should include information on safe sex practices and ways to sterilize needles. Clearly, these are issues that are usually not encountered in the course of normal business operations.

Employees often work closely together, sharing lunchrooms, using the same telephones, and so forth. The hypothetical example arises of an infected employee falling down, injuring himself, and bleeding, then fellow employees rushing to the rescue only to be contaminated by the infected blood. Employees are very frightened by the prospect of having to work with someone who is HIV-infected or who has AIDS. The fear even extends to working with someone who lives with an AIDS patient.

This fear is understandable. The disease is almost universally fatal[80] and the infection leads to full-blown symptoms in a high percentage of cases.[81] While a great deal is known about the disease, it is still relatively new. Many workers and employers, perceiving a known risk, find it difficult to understand why they have to subject themselves to the danger of working with or employing someone who has AIDS. In cases where employers retain an employee with AIDS, other employees are likely to walk off the job.[82] These employees could be fired for their actions, but the employer might then find it difficult or even impossible to fill their positions. If the AIDS patient were fired instead, the employer might be subject to a lawsuit alleging unlawful handicap discrimination.[83]

The solution being developed by businesses and employers is to institute an AIDS education program in the workplace before an actual problem develops, thereby reducing the anxiety level among employees. The major corporations that have developed AIDS policies have universally decided to treat AIDS as they treat other life-threatening, contagious diseases.[84] Employees are permitted to retain their jobs as long as they are able to perform the job functions and as long as they do not present a risk to others. When employees are made aware of this policy and the reasons for it, the reaction to a fellow employee actually being diagnosed is often one of sympathy rather than panic or hysteria.

As businesses prepare for AIDS education programs, they too must decide what type of education they will provide. Will the program be limited to explaining the medical and epidemiological aspect of the disease, or will safe sex be discussed? The employer may be understandably reticent, not wishing to appear to advocate sex or drug use. There may be a reluctance to have on-the-job discussion of intimate sexual practices. The employer, however, is in a particularly advantageous position to provide needed information to a large group of people.

All the concerns that employers must take into account apply with equal or greater force to labor unions or collective bargaining units. These labor organizations are dedicated to the purpose of protecting workers and furthering their best interests. The conflict between infected workers and those who fear the disease must be resolved by the unions. They will have to decide whether their primary duty is to protect the infected individual or to protect other workers who are afraid that they may be exposed to the virus. They will also have to decide whether the union itself should undertake an educational campaign, and what type of education should be provided.

The Medical Community

The medical community should not be surprised to find itself in the midst of the AIDS controversy, although perhaps the particular focus of the problem is unexpected. Certainly the debate about what drugs should be prescribed and what treatment should be recommended is normal and regularly occurs with new diseases. Even the medical testimony about whether or not AIDS is casually transmitted, while controversial, cannot be viewed as unexpected.

Part of the current debate concerns the allocation of limited resources and the types of safeguards that must be followed before a new treatment can be certified as effective. The development of AZT has highlighted this problem. First, the drug proved so successful in initial trials that the normal process by which drugs are approved had to be shortened.[85] The moral dilemma was apparent. Those treated with AZT were living, and those given a placebo were dying. There could be no moral justification for continuing to withhold a valuable form of treatment for purposes of clinical certification.

After AZT was approved, the next conundrum centered on the question of who would be able to obtain the drug, as there simply wasn't enough to go around.[86] Protocols had to be established to provide the drug to a designated group; those who were the most ill were chosen.[87] While the decision can hardly be viewed as unjust or unfair, a nagging question remains. If the drug were given to those who were healthier, that is, those whose immune systems had not broken down, would it enable them to stay healthy? Subsequent trials have indicated that when the drug is given to HIV-infected individuals who have yet to show clinical manifestations of the disease, it appears to have beneficial results and the patients are better able to withstand the drug's side effects.

Then there is the final issue generated by the first effective treatment: the matter of cost. A one-year treatment with AZT has a price tag of $10,000.[88] What happens if the drug proves to be effective and patients can't afford the treatment? Will those who can't pay be allowed to die?

While these problems have emerged because of the effectiveness of AZT, they will be repeated as new treatments develop. A mechanism must be found to make all effective treatment available as expeditiously as possible and in a manner that will not put a price tag on the right to life.

The medical community is in the midst of another AIDS controversy. Like other employers, medical-care providers may not discriminate on the basis of handicap. AIDS and HIV infection are likely to be viewed as handicaps, and, in fact, that position has already been sustained by numerous court decisions.[89] Clearly, hospitals cannot refuse to treat AIDS patients. But a question remains as to whether hospitals have to perform elective procedures on those who are HIV-positive. Repeatedly, dentists are asking whether they have to treat everyone who walks through their doors seeking care. Doctors wonder whether they can ask potential patients if they have been tested for the AIDS virus. Practitioners of all sorts are seeking legal advice as to whether they can refuse homosexual patients. The answers to these questions are governed by the civil rights statutes and other laws designed to protect the handicapped and those with AIDS.[90] The answers may be somewhat unsettling, as they generally require the medical community to accept patients and not to discriminate on the basis of their medical status or individual condition. The answers seem to require that the medical community accept the increased risk of HIV infection as part of the inherent dangers of the profession.

Another aspect of AIDS discrimination in the medical community is the firing of medical providers who are themselves HIV-positive. Hospitals, clinics, and nursing homes may well be concerned that their patients not be exposed to AIDS. To that end, isolated efforts have been made to remove HIV-positive care givers from their employment. Those efforts have generally not been successful, and the employees have won either reinstatement or monetary damages.[91]

Here again, the fear element comes into play. The doctors may fear that they are being exposed to the virus by their patients; the patients have the same fear concerning their doctors. The fear is exacerbated by the law that requires the potential exposure to be endured. This is a part of the controversy that the medical community may not be prepared to address, yet it is a problem that will only continue to grow.

Personal Lives

Five years ago, AIDS was a topic of common conversation only in certain gay bars. Now the topic is repeatedly on the cover of national news magazines. Television talk-show hosts and politicians endlessly discuss the intricacies of the disease. AIDS has entered the American consciousness. It informs many of the daily decisions that are made by everyone.

The sexual revolution has died, a victim of AIDS. Men and women — young and old, gay and straight — are not willing to risk their lives for the momentary gratification of a sensory thrill. Morality has taken a new lease on life. Increasingly, people are willing to accept the health risk associated with sexual intimacy only when there is the potential of a higher reward — commitment or marriage. People are once again dating, not simply engaging in indiscriminate sexual encounters. A person's health history is now fair game for barroom conversation, right along with his or her zodiac sign and favorite movies.

There is a growing sense of mortality. The yuppie and guppie crowds are now talking about wills, living wills, and powers of attorney. There is a new awareness that fatal diseases don't attack only the old.

While the sexual revolution may have already ended, the end of the drug culture may not be far behind. The First Lady may advocate just saying no to drugs, but the AIDS epidemic may be far more persuasive. Perhaps those who are already addicted to heroin may not be persuaded by the AIDS epidemic to stop sharing needles. It is difficult to persuade people to give up their habit because they may die from AIDS when they risk their lives every day by injecting drugs. But perhaps teenagers who are about to shoot cocaine for the first time will now pause and consider that they may be exposing themselves to a disease for which there is no known cure. AIDS may be the deterrent to drugs which has long been sought.

AIDS is also affecting organized religion. The churches and synagogues cannot ignore the fact that among the dying and ill are their clergy and their followers. No longer does simply condemning homosexual practices suffice. Religions must deal directly with sex, with sex education, with homosexuality, with drug addiction, and with traditional concepts of morality. And, for the church, these disparate elements must all be brought together into some type of cohesive body of thought.

Some organized religions have long espoused the view that the purpose of sex is procreation. Taking this view to its logical conclusion, some religious bodies have condemned those sexual activities which do not, and cannot, lead to conception. Vaginal intercourse in which a contraceptive is used has been forbidden for this reason. Anal intercourse, whether between a man and a woman or between two men, is condemned. Masturbation, too, is prohibited. These teachings lead to a troublesome paradox. The sexual activity the churches permit is one that poses a danger for the transmission of the disease.

Parents are in a very similar position. How shall they explain to their children not to engage in premarital sex and at the same time explain that if they do so, to please do it in a particular way? Parents need to find a way to morally teach their children how to sterilize the needles they use to inject drugs into their veins. They have to find a way to provide information and moral leadership at the same time.

The disease has raised its nefarious head in the home, in the church, in the schools, in the hospitals, and in doctors' and dentists' offices. It has forced confrontations with subjects that many have simply preferred to ignore. Because of the nature of the disease, concepts of morality conflict with notions of fairness. Religious doctrine is opposed to sound public health policies. And as a backdrop to the debate, the number of infected increases at a frightening rate.

Conclusion

There are no easy answers. Each issue that is presented seems to create a paradox from which there is no escape. The best hope is compassion in dealing with those who are ill and concern for the health of everyone. Education is the only weapon in the current arsenal to fight this disease. Education is the most cost-effective way of stopping the spread of the epidemic. While there seems to be universal agreement that education is the best course to pursue, the disagreement concerns what should be told. Isn't the answer to tell everything and to tell it truthfully and completely? If people know what the disease is and how it can be spread and how it can't be spread, won't they then be able to make informed and appropriate decisions concerning their own lives? It is only when people are kept uninformed, when they are denied the facts needed to make decisions for themselves, that the state has overstepped its bounds and endangered the well-being of the many.

In deciding what public health measures should be imposed, the traditional approach should be followed. The degree of intrusion into personal freedoms must be balanced against the benefit that can be expected to the public health. The medical and epidemiological realities should control, not the hysteria of the crowd. Personal rights may and will have to be sacrificed for the common good; but those rights should be compromised only when it is known that good will result in a sufficient quantity to justify the personal sacrifice.

These answers are simplistic. They espouse nothing more than basic common sense. But, perhaps for at least the moment, common sense is an appropriate guide.

Notes

1. A bill (HR 1041) was introduced in the Louisiana legislature by Rep. Alphonse Jackson (D) in 1987 which would give state health officials the power to go to court seeking the arrest of anyone with AIDS and to quarantine such persons without the right of a court hearing or bail. The bill was passed by the state House of Representatives, but the governor, Edwin W. Edwards, pledged to veto the measure if it passed the Senate. "Lousiana Governor Pledges Veto If Measure Approved," *AIDS Policy & Law* 2, no. 12 (July 1, 1987): 8–9.
2. *Korematsu v. United States*, 323 U.S. 214 (1944).
3. *Jacobson v. Massachusetts*, 197 U.S. 11 (1905).
4. See Ex Parte *Arata*, 52 Cal. App. 380, 198 P. 814 (1921) (habeas corpus proceeding challenging prostitute's detention pending compulsory testing for venereal disease); *Moore v. Draper*, 57 So.2d 648 (Fla. 1952) (habeas corpus proceeding challenging civil commitment of patient with tuberculosis).
5. See Ex Parte *Caselli*, 62 Mont. 201, 204 P. 364 (1922).
6. *Greene v. Edwards*, 263 S.E. 2d 661 (W.Va. 1980).
7. See *People* ex. rel. *Barmore v. Robertson*, 302 Ill. 422, 428, 134 N.E. 815, 817 (1922) (judicial deference afforded to decision maker).
8. Section 504, of the Handicapped Rights Act of 1973, 29 U.S.C. Sec. 701–796 (1982).
9. G.L. c. 151B, secs. 1 et seq.
10. See *Jacobson v. Massachusetts*, 197 U.S. 11, 25 (1905) (police power "must be held to embrace, at least, such reasonable regulations established directly by legislative enactment as will protect the public health and public safety").
11. Ibid.
12. *Barmore v. Robertson*, 302 Ill. 422, 134 N.E. 815 (1922) (habeas corpus petition challenging reasonableness of quarantine of carriers of typhoid basilli).
13. *Moore v. Draper*, 57 So.2d 648 (Fla. 1952 habeas corpus proceeding challenging civil commitment of patient with tuberculosis).
14. *People* ex. rel. *Baker v. Strautz*, 386 Ill. 360, 54 N.E.2d 441 (1944) (habeas corpus proceeding challenging mandatory testing of prostitute for presence of venereal disease); Ex Parte *Kilbane*, 32 Ohio St. 530, 67 N.E.2d 22 (145) (habeas corpus proceeding challenging regulation providing for mandatory testing of prostitutes and those associating with them, for venereal disease).
15. *Jacobson v. Massachusetts*, 197 U.S. 11 (1905).
16. Colorado recently enacted a law requiring doctors to report all HIV-positive blood tests to the state health department. The law allows for the quarantine of some HIV-positive people for up to

three months. "Quarantine Bill Backed by Colorado Legislature," *AIDS Policy & Law* 2, no. 8 (May 6, 1987): 4. Rep. William Dannemeyer (R–Calif.) introduced legislation to make HIV-seropositive persons reportable to public health authorities and to require mandatory HIV testing of marriage license applicants, convicted prostitutes and intravenous drug users, clients of sexually transmitted disease clinics, and some hospital patients. "Reporting, Mandatory Tests Asked in Dannemeyer Bills," *AIDS Policy & Law* 2, no. 8 (May 6, 1987): 8.

17. On April 22, 1987, Secretary of Defense Caspar W. Weinberger approved a revised AIDS policy requiring that recruits who test positive for HIV be excluded from the service. "Revised AIDS Policy Okayed; Some Sanctions Authorized," *AIDS Policy & Law* 2, no. 8 (May 6, 1987): 5.

18. *Local 1812, American Federation of Government Employees v. United States Department of State*, 662 F. Supp. 50 (D.D.C., 1987).

19. Ibid.

20. Private Adrian Morris was brought before a military court-martial charged with a crime for having engaged in sexual relations with his fiancée, a second woman, and another man without having used a condom and after he had tested HIV-positive. "HIV-Positive Private Faces Assault Charges," *AIDS Policy & Law* 2, no. 9 (May 20, 1987): 3.

21. *AIDS Update*, Lambda Legal Defense and Education Fund 18 (May 1987): 2.

22. A law was enacted in Louisiana requiring that all couples married in the state must test negative for HIV antibodies before they can obtain a marriage license. "Marriage License Tests Approved in Louisiana," *AIDS Policy & Law* 2, no. 14 (July 29, 1987): 8. A bill before the Idaho legislature (SB 1100) would require AIDS testing for marriage license applicants. A similar bill (SB 994) was presented to the Oregon legislature. *AIDS Policy & Law* 2, no. 5 (March 25, 1987): 8.

23. "Bush Opens Meeting by Endorsing Wider Testing Proposed by Reagan," *AIDS Policy & Law* 2, no. 10 (June 3, 1987): 1.

24. Allan M. Brandt, *No Magic Bullet: A Social History of Venereal Disease in the United States Since 1880*, New York, Oxford University Press, 1985, 147–149.

25. Paul D. Cleary, Ph.D., Michael J. Barry, M.D., Kenneth H. Mayer, M.D., Allan M. Brandt, Ph.D., Larry Gostin, J.D., Harvey V. Fineberg, M.D., Ph.D. "Compulsory Premarital Screening for the Human Immunodeficiency Virus," *Journal of the American Medical Association* (Oct. 2, 1987): 1757-1762.

26. Richard A. Knox, "Who should be tested," *Boston Globe*, May 17, 1987, B14.

27. Note 25.

28. *Loving v. Virginia*, 388 U.S. 1 (1967); *Zablocki v. Redhail*, 434 U.S. 374 (1977).

29. "Bush Opens Meeting by Endorsing Wider Testing Proposed by Reagan."

30. See 42 U.S.C. Sec. 269 (1944).

31. Ibid.

32. "Public Health Service Urges Ban on Immigrants with HIV Infection," *AIDS Policy & Law* 2, no. 9 (May 20, 1987): 1.

33. See Randy Shilts, *And the Band Played On*, New York, St. Martin's Press, 1987, 508–510.

34. Ibid.

35. See *Commonwealth v. Page*, 339 Mass. 313, 159 N.E.2d 82 (1959) (appeal from a commitment as a sexually dangerous person, held that an individual could not be confined in a penal setting because of his mental condition).

36. Cooper, Imrie, Penny, "Antibody Response to Human Immunodeficiency Virus After Primary Infection," *Journal of Infectious Diseases*, vol. 55 (1987): 1113–1118; Marlink, Allan, McLane, et al., "Low Sensitivity of ELISA Testing in Early HIV Infection," letter to *New England Journal of Medicine* 315 (1986): 1549.

37. See Mass. Gen. Laws ch. 90, sec. 24D.

38. Constance B. Wolfsy, M.D., "Intravenous Drug Abuse and Women's Medical Issues," Report of the Surgeon General's Workshop on Children with HIV Infection and Their Families, U.S. Department of Health and Human Services, Washington, D.C., 1987, 33.

39. Centers for Disease Control, "Public Health Service Guidelines for Counseling and Antibody Testing to Prevent HIV Infection and AIDS," *Morbidity and Mortality Weekly Report* 36, no. 31 (August 14, 1987): 512.

40. Brandt, *No Magic Bullet*, 151. See also 105 CMR 340.100 (E).

41. *People* ex rel. *Baker v. Strautz*, 386 Ill. 360, 54 N.E.2d 441 (1944); Ex Parte *Arata*, 52 Cal. App. 380, 198 P. 814 (1921).

42. *Moore v. Draper*, 57 So.2d 648 (Fla. 1952); *Greene v. Edwards*, 263 S.E.2d 661 (W.Va. 1980).

43. See *Greene v. Edwards*, 263 S.E.2d 661 (W.Va. 1980).

44. See Robert Berkow, ed., *The Merck Manual of Diagnosis and Therapy*, Rahway, N.J., Merck, Sharpe & Dohme, Research Laboratories, 1982, 127.

45. See Richard Plant, *The Pink Triangle*, New York, Henry Holt and Co., 1986.

46. Thomas C. Quinn, M.D., "The Global Epidemiology of the Acquired Immunodeficiency Syndrome," Report of the Surgeon General's Workshop on Children With HIV Infection and Their Families, 7.

47. Note 36.

48. Note 25.

49. *Boston Globe*, May 17, 1987, B14.

50. See *Commonwealth v. Page*, 339 Mass. 313, 159 N.E.2d 82 (1959).

51. *The Merck Manual of Diagnosis and Therapy*, 210.

52. On April 9, 1987, New York State announced a new public information and education program, including the development of AIDS curricula for elementary and secondary schools. "Major Education Program Launched by New York State," *AIDS Policy & Law* 2, no. 7 (April 22, 1987): 1; the Pennsylvania Board of Education unanimously approved, on May 14, 1987, a regulation requiring AIDS education in the state's 501 school districts. The regulation includes the provision that AIDS education be taught at least once each year at the elementary, junior high, and high school levels. "School Board Approves Mandatory AIDS Education," *AIDS Policy & Law* 2, no. 9 (May 20, 1987): 5.

53. Surgeon General's Report on Acquired Immune Deficiency Syndrome, 1986, 17.

54. See Warren Winkelstein, Jr., M.D., "Sexual Practices and Risk of Infection by the Human Immunodeficiency Virus," *Journal of the American Medical Association*, 257, no. 3 (January 16, 1987): 321, 323.

55. See David R. Bolling, "Prevalence, Goals and Complications of Heterosexual Intercourse in a Gynecologic Population," *Journal of Reproductive Medicine* 29 (1977): 120–124. Also see Bruce V. Voeller, "Heterosexual Anal Sex," Mariposa Occasional Papers 1B (1983): 1–8.

56. See Surgeon General's Report on Acquired Immune Deficiency Syndrome, 1986.

57. See "Dispute on Nationwide Brochure Mailing Continues Between Congress, White House," *AIDS Policy & Law* 2, no. 19 (October 7, 1987): 1.

58. "Studds mails constituents AIDS report," *Boston Globe*, May 19, 1987.

59. "New York's AIDS Ad Campaign Seen Unlikely to Succeed," *AIDS Policy & Law* 2, no. 9 (May 20, 1987): 4.

60. Ibid.

61. 29 U.S.C. Sec. 701–796 (1982).

62. See *School Board of Nassau County v. Arline*, 107 S.Ct. 1123, 1128 n. 7 (1987).

63. See *Cronin v. New England Telephone Co.*, Suffolk Superior Court, No. 80332 Memorandum of Decision and Order on Defendants' Motion to Dismiss, August 15, 1986.

64. Mayor Ray Flynn of Boston issued an executive order prohibiting discrimination in the hiring and promotion of city employees on the basis of AIDS, ARC, or HIV infection. *AIDS Update*, Lambda Legal Defense and Education Fund, no. 17 (April 1987).

65. See Mass. Gen. Laws ch. 111, sec 70F.

66. See, for example, *Chalk v. United States District Court, Central District of California*, 832 F.2d 1158 (9th Cir. 1987).

67. See "Senate Moves to Repeal DC Law Prohibiting Tests," *AIDS Policy & Law* 2, no. 19 (October 7, 1987): 3.

68. See "Aetna Concedes Mistake in Requesting HIV Waiver," *AIDS Policy & Law* 2, no. 10 (June 3, 1987): 8.

69. "New York to Ban HIV Tests for Health Insurance," *AIDS Policy & Law*, 2, no. 8 (May 6, 1987): 9.

70. "HIV-Positive Private Faces Assault Charges," *AIDS Policy & Law* 2, no. 9 (May 20, 1987): 3.

71. "HIV-Positive Man Charged with Intent to Kill," *AIDS Policy & Law* 2, no. 10 (June 3, 1987): 6.

72. Martha F. Rogers, M.D., "Transmission of Human Immunodeficiency Virus Infection in the United States," Report of the Surgeon General's Workshop on Children with HIV Infection and Their Families, U.S. Department of Health and Human Services, 1987, 17.

73. See "Needle Exchange Project Rejected by New York State," *AIDS Policy & Law* 2, no. 9 (May 20, 1987): 2.

74. See *Jones v. United States*, 534 F.2d 53, cert. denied 429 U.S. 978 (1976) (Bureau of Prisons is required to exercise ordinary diligence to keep prisoners safe and free from harm).

75. "HIV Testing in Federal Prisons," *AIDS Policy & Law* 2, no. 11 (June 17, 1987).

76. Gregory Witcher, "No AIDS Tests for inmates, state says," *Boston Globe*, May 26, 1987, 1.

77. "AIDS in Correctional Facilities: Issues and Options," National Institute of Justice, U.S. Department of Justice, Washington, D.C., April 1986, 39.

78. Note 52.

79. See Surgeon General's Report on Acquired Immune Deficiency Syndrome, 1986.

80. Ibid.

81. Public health officials consider it very likely that 100 percent of those infected with HIV will eventually develop AIDS or some other lethal manifestation of the disease. "Forum Told That HIV May Always Lead to AIDS," *AIDS Policy & Law* 2, no. 8 (May 6, 1987): 6.

82. Michael R. Brown, "AIDS Discrimination in the Workplace: The Legal Dilemma," *Case & Comment* (May–June 1987): 8.

83. Gregory M. Shumaker, "AIDS: Does It Qualify as a 'Handicap' Under the Rehabilitation Act of 1973?" *Notre Dame Law Review* (1986): 572–594.

84. "Survey Shows Few Firms Implement AIDS Policies," *AIDS Policy & Law* 2, no. 10 (June 3, 1987): 7–8. See also M. Rowe, M. Russel-Einhorn, M. Baker, "The Fear of AIDS," *Harvard Business Review* (July–August 1986).

85. Fourteen months after Phase II trials began on AZT, more than three times as many patients who took placebos had died as those taking AZT. "Mortality Rate Still Lower for Patients Taking AZT," *AIDS Policy & Law* 2, no. 7 (April 22, 1987): 2.

86. Ibid.

87. Ibid.

88. "Cost, Availability of AZT Questioned at House Hearing," *AIDS Policy & Law* 2, no. 5 (March 25, 1987): 1.

89. See *Cronin v. New England Telephone Co.; Chalk v. United States District Court, Central District of California*, F.2d (9th Cir. 1987).

90. Harvey Schwartz, Alec Gray, "Can You Say No?" *Massachusetts Medicine* 2, no. 5 (September–October 1987): 39–43.

91. Mother Frances Hospital in Tyler, Texas, offered a monetary settlement to its anesthesia director after the hospital banned him from working directly with patients. "Hospital Settles with Nurse Anesthetist Who Filed Federal Discrimination Suit," *AIDS Alert* 2, no. 5 (May 1987): 80. The Westchester County Medical Center, in New York, allegedly refused to complete the application process of an individual applying for the position of pharmacist when it was learned that he was HIV-positive. *AIDS Update*, Lambda Legal Defense and Education Fund 18 (May 1987).

"I'd like to leave you with an image that came to me quite unexpectedly last Saturday evening while strolling in the mall. It was quite hot, I'd just come from a concert, and I came upon the Vietnam Memorial. It was quiet, it was very dimly lit, there were thousands of names carved in stone — mute testaments to overwhelming sadness. I was struck by the comparisons and similarities with people with AIDS who have also died. That sense of loss, that senseless loss of life, the youth, the confusion, the pain, the suffering, the grief of the survivors."

AIDS and A-Bomb Disease: Facing A Special Death

Chris Glaser

In 1979 it was called "gay cancer," and it took the life of an acquaintance. Then "gay-related immune deficiency," or GRID, claimed neighbors, friends of friends, fellow activists. I began grief and death counseling with a segment of the population ordinarily concerned with life's ambitions and enjoyments: men in their twenties and thirties. Hospital visits and memorial services became more frequent.

By 1983, when it had come to be called AIDS, my own friends began to be affected. One was a man I dated in seminary, and I was devastated to learn of his illness only upon receiving a notice of his memorial service. Another friend, a minister, shared his struggle to survive AIDS. In our exchanges he helped me come to terms with my own anxiety about developing the disease.

I am now 36, the average age of death of a person with AIDS. As far as I know, I don't have the disease, and I have chosen not to be tested for antibodies to HIV, the virus related to AIDS. I take care of my health, am in a relationship, and follow safe-sex guidelines. Test results would not change anything for the better and the stress I'd experience if I have been exposed to the virus would be for the worse, since stress lowers immunity.

But I do not feel "safe." I am in a battle zone; I see buddies fall left and right. How can I cope with the continuing loss? Why am *I* spared? What makes me think I *will* be spared? Why would I believe I'm going to get out of this battle *alive?* Why are men with purer, more loving hearts than mine suffering with AIDS and I am not?

I share this experience, these feelings and questions with countless gay men and an increasing number of heterosexual men and women. Yet I've found it difficult to adequately express the devastating dimensions of AIDS on the gay community. Half of any therapeutic process requires putting one's experience in words, words which help me and others understand.

Preparing a sermon for the commemoration of the bombing of Hiroshima, I reread Robert Jay Lifton's analysis of the experience of Hiroshima's survivors.[1] Despite real, qualitative, and quantitative differences which forever separate the experiences, I recognize remarkable parallels between their way of coping and the gay community's coping with AIDS. I draw on the framework Lifton constructed, not only to understand the

Chris Glaser is the author of Uncommon Calling: A Gay Man's Struggle to Serve the Church, *published in 1988 by Harper & Row.*

present suffering of the gay community, but to place that suffering in context with all human suffering.

The survivors of the Hiroshima blast experienced a "permanent encounter with death," according to Lifton, which can be described in four stages. First, survivors of the atomic blast felt as if "the whole world is dying." As gay men, our encounter with death from AIDS seems endless. Not just countless friends and strangers die but our world, our newly formed and newly found community, is dying.

The second stage experienced by Hiroshima survivors was the threat of invisible contamination from radiation that "leaves behind in the bodies of those exposed to it deadly influences which may emerge at any time and strike down their victims." With the incubation period of AIDS said to be as much as ten years, we in the gay community experience a similar fear of invisible contamination which may strike at any time. Accompanying the threat of invisible contamination among Hiroshima survivors came rumors, logical and illogical. AIDS, too, has brought rumors, from its inevitability ("I've probably already been exposed") to its invincibility ("Everyone exposed to the virus dies") to its being spread through everyday contact (example: serving dinner guests with AIDS on paper plates while everyone else is served on china).

Mind and Body

The third stage comes later. Hiroshima survivors encountered it in the effects of radiation years afterward: from various forms of cancer, especially leukemia, to the birth of defective children, often mentally retarded. Lifton writes of this period, ". . . in the minds of survivors any kind of ailment, whether it be simple fatigue [or something more critical] . . . becomes associated with the atomic bomb and its related death imagery." Lifton continues, "And their problem is intensified by the continuous publicizing of chronic atomic bomb effects — or 'A-bomb disease' — by mass media and by survivor and peace organizations."

The similarity to the experience of urban gay males is stunning. If we feel fatigued, experience any ailment from a cold or flu to an infection, our thoughts immediately turn to AIDS and death. The increased publicity AIDS is receiving is necessary but it heightens our anxiety. Confronted by nagging doubts as to whether we've been exposed, we may experience psychosomatic symptoms, and the stress we experience makes us yet more vulnerable.

And what of those who love us? I intentionally lost weight a year ago, and friends in other churches still remark on it, asking *very* seriously, "Are you all right?" A father of a gay son living in New York City says it's like having a son who guards a U.S. embassy in the Middle East: Danger is always present; bad news might come at any moment.

Finally, the fourth experience of Hiroshima survivors is not really a stage, but a condition of lifelong identification with death and dying. The *hibakusha,* as they are called in Japanese, meaning "explosion-affected people," are "a tainted group," discriminated against in jobs and marriage arrangements. As a result, many hide their experience. They themselves question their right to live, because of an unconscious perception of balance which supposes one's survival has been made possible by others' deaths. The *hibakusha* experience guilt and low self-esteem. Any affirmation or enjoyment of life seems impure. They search for meaning in symbols of peace and the peace movement, yet are torn apart as a community by ideological and personal antagonisms which stem from feelings of their unworthiness of any organizational or personal success. They suspect their leaders are tainted by political motivations or personal impurity. Only those who died from the blast are pure. Even attempts to memorialize the dead, whether through art, religion, or state ceremony, prove inadequate.

Lifton's analysis here sheds light on the double stigma attached to the gay community: homosexuality as well as AIDS. Coming out of the closet as gay or lesbian is a deathlike experience, in which some expectations and dreams die, initiating a grief process for one's self and one's family and friends who must say goodbye to the individual's former image and possibilities. At the same time a new understanding and image of the person emerges, so what may first be experienced as a death is realized rather as a transformation having continuities with the past as well as the future.

Yet now the "new" person becomes part of "a tainted group" societally and risks discrimination because of homophobia. That homophobia has already imprinted guilt and low self-esteem on homosexuals, which subsequently retards the trust of both self and others needed in gay community organizing.

These dynamics intensify with AIDS. Persons with AIDS have been isolated like unhugged lepers by friends, family, and community. Many have lost jobs and housing. Many experience guilt, shame, and low self-esteem for having contracted a disease from societally disapproved sexual behavior. Small wonder many try to hide their condition in the closet from which they once emerged. Organizations and leaders who try to help are scrutinized for any impure motives or intentions or imperfect service. The broader gay community has proven incredibly loving and generous in caring for its own (as well as those who are not gay but have AIDS). Yet gay men and even lesbian women (the latter having virtually no incidence of AIDS) fall prey to society's phobia regarding AIDS, based on rumored assumptions that the entire gay community has been contaminated.

The parallels continue. Hiroshima survivors seeking medical and economic benefits sometimes felt, according to Lifton, "deeply antagonistic to both help and helper because they tend to confirm [one's] own sense of weakness and inferiority." Persons with AIDS, or "PWAs," as many refer to themselves, suffer the same dilemma. And medical and social workers have a unique opportunity to play God in the worst sense of the term in relation to AIDS, since it is shrouded in a "dirty" mystery: socially associated with sexual promiscuity and drug abuse, medically not yet fully understood and therefore not completely treatable.

Targets of Rage

Hiroshima survivors felt anger and hatred about the bomb, but had no clear focus for either anger or hate. Should they hate the United States for dropping the bomb or their own country for starting the war? Should they direct anger at the president who ordered the destruction or the bomber crew who delivered it? Similarly, the hatred and anger that surface in a person with AIDS lack obvious focus. Should he hate the person who exposed him, if known, or should he blame himself for sexually expressing himself or coming out of the closet in the first place? Was the gay community somehow responsible in its permissiveness or the broader society, which fails to support, let alone encourage, monogamous relationships for gay men?

A health care professional told me of several young men with AIDS who admitted they had no intention of refraining from sexual encounters which could endanger others' lives. "Somebody gave it to me," one declared angrily, "so I'm going to give it to somebody else!"

Throughout history, humans have struggled with the meaning of life and death. Lifton describes five modes of immortality which have helped in this struggle. But he says all five were threatened for survivors of the Hiroshima holocaust. The case of AIDS is different; the two experiences exist on separate planes. Still, Lifton's modes of immortality help us understand the unique spiritual dilemma of gay men, a dilemma whose elements will have varying configurations for other segments of the world's population that are or will be confronting this health crisis.

Modes of immortality are not just pondered when a person is dying; instead, says Lifton, they become "inner standards by which we evaluate our lives, by which we maintain feelings of connection, significance and progress." Homosexuality itself limits access to several common modes of immortality. The biological mode, living on in one's children or living on in the memory of family-like groupings (like churches), may be denied gays and lesbians. Homosexuals generally do not have children, and often are rejected by or remove themselves from family-like groups, from the biological family to the family of faith.

The theological mode of immortality is threatened by religion's condemnation, its refusal to accept homosexuality, its failure to integrate the experience into the fabric of faith. The mode of nature, the hope that nature or the species will survive us, is accessible. But the urban ghettoization of the gay community removes nature as a generally available and meaningful mode by which we evaluate our lives.

Instead, the gay community relies heavily on the two remaining modes of immortality: the mode of works and the mode of experiential transcendence. With regard to the mode of works, it is not surprising that artistic achievements, social movements, economic affluence, or spiritual insights are disproportionately associated with lesbians and gays. In regard to experiential transcendence, it is equally unremarkable that "experiential radicalism" (as Lifton names it) has swept the gay community, from sexual experimentation to human potential movements, from trend-setting fashion to spectacular entertaining.

For gay men, a diagnosis of AIDS calls into question these very modes of immortality. If one relies on the work mode, whatever achievements are to be made must be done soon, in the limited time available between medical testing and treatment on the one hand and the enforced energy conservation required to avoid fatigue and illness on the other.

And living life to its fullest, experiential transcendence, must be radically redefined. Financial resources may be restricted by medical expenses as well as loss of income resulting from giving up one's job or reducing work hours. Intake of everything from sugar to coffee to alcohol to drugs (necessary or misused) must be regulated, if not abandoned altogether, since all reduce immunity. Adequate sleep and avoidance of stress and physical exertion means a more sheltered existence. Mobility may be limited geographically by proximity to the few centers for treatment or physically by the confines of hospital room and possibly various breathing or intravenous tubes. Sexual drive may be psychologically or chemically inhibited, or find solitary or limited expression. A person with AIDS may be deprived of emotional nourishment as fearful friends hesitate inviting, visiting, touching, and hugging him. Within these narrow constrictions, not unknown to others with limiting disease or disability, blessed is the person with AIDS who can celebrate the wonders of life yet left to him.

The modes of work and experiential transcendence are not threatened simply for gay men with an AIDS or ARC diagnosis. Those who suffer "AIDS anxiety," the fear that they have been infected and will any moment manifest AIDS, are also affected. Because there have been instances in which a victim has had little or no warning of impending death from AIDS, literally dying "over the weekend" or within a month, gay men have little assurance as to longevity. As I write these words, I am aware I may not live to see this article published.

Two fears seem to dominate within AIDS anxiety: the "hassles" of debilitating illness, from loss of income to hospital stays, and an increasing fear of intimacy, since sexual intimacy communicates the virus related to AIDS. To have death associated with intimacy further inhibits gay men already socialized to avoid intimacy, first as men, and secondly as gay men who are encouraged to conceal their sexual orientation.

With the crippling of the two modes of immortality gay men have heavily depended upon, many turn to the other three. Though fathering children is out of the question for an infected man, the biological mode of immortality may find fulfillment in reestablishing or strengthening ties with family, or more dearly valuing extended non-blood-related families of friends. Some turn to nature, caring for house plants and pets, walking on the shore or at mountain retreats. And the survival of the species looms large on the agenda as the gay community prophetically forewarns the broader society of necessary precautions to avoid the spread of AIDS.

Finally, gay men also turn to the theological mode of immortality. When I helped a local AIDS service organization by providing spiritual counseling and religious referrals, few asked to speak with a minister, priest, or rabbi. Perhaps they already had such counsel, but I dare say many, if not most, felt abandoned by traditional religions because of their sexual orientation. Many have found healing in nontraditional, holistic, and positive-approach forms of spirituality. Positive imaging transforms them more than a prayer of confession, universal salvation comforts more than limited atonement, holding and hugging heal better than countless sermons, and silent meditation offers them peace wordy prayers do not. Rather than defensively rejecting such preferred alternatives, the church and temple might consider their spiritual pragmatism and hear a call to liturgical reform.

Initially dragging their feet because of a distaste for homosexuality, Christians have recently voiced concern and compassion for persons with AIDS. Some have offered special "healing services," which are to be commended as long as it's not forgotten that *every* worship service should be an opportunity for healing; that "healing" should not be confused with a desired *uniformity* of sexual orientation or lifestyle; and that healing may come in many forms, even the ultimate form of death.

Unprovidentially, some gay men and some persons with AIDS return to their abandoned religion with the same negative self-image and punitive God-image they left with as young people. I have counseled parents who've received the startling double revelation their son is gay and has AIDS. In one such case, the parents' love for their son helped them to cope not only with the information, but also to challenge Christianity's negativity on the subject. They could not believe God did not love their son as he was. But the church had done its damage: Neither I nor his parents could convince the son God loved him. He died believing and (worse) accepting AIDS as God's punishment for being homosexual.

A rumor which spread in Hiroshima claimed the bomb and A-bomb disease were a cosmic or divine retribution for past sins: the victims experiencing guilt for their own victimization. Homophobia and vestigial beliefs in God as punitive parent have contributed to similar rumors: AIDS as divine retribution generally visited upon the gay community; AIDS as punishment for individuals presumed to have lived in the "fast lane" of drugs, alcohol, and promiscuity.

Some gay men and persons with AIDS have found healing within traditional Christianity for both AIDS anxiety and AIDS itself. They have remained within the church but have challenged its views on homosexuality. Their faith makes it possible for them to see the condemn homosexuality, but judges the self-righteous who do. They do not view AIDS as God's punishment, though they may view AIDS as an opportunity for God's work to be made manifest as they reach out in compassion to care for persons with AIDS, and as they evaluate their own sexual expression to ensure it is life-giving rather than life-threatening. And they usually find support within Christian churches or organizations whose ministry focuses on gay concerns (like Metropolitan Community Churches or denominational gay/lesbian support groups) or whose ministry includes those concerns (like many congregations which more or less openly welcome lesbians and gays).

In the AIDS crisis, the urgent challenge to the broader church is not simply the need to champion compassion and care for persons with AIDS, but also the necessity of providing the resources of God's healing spirit and the family of faith for all gay and lesbian Christians. This translates into becoming a yet more inclusive and gracious church. Robert Jay Lifton's understanding of the effects of the Hiroshima bombing may inform our understanding of the effects of AIDS, from how it is experienced to how it may be transcended. My prayer is that such understanding may prompt the church to apply its Easter faith and hope to needless crucifixions of doubt and despair.

Note

1. Robert Jay Lifton, *Death in Life: Survivors of Hiroshima* (New York: Basic Books, 1982).

Medical Care of AIDS in New England: Costs and Implications

Stewart J. Landers, J.D., M.C.P.
George R. Seage III, M.P.H.

This article presents an overview of cost issues related to AIDS. Data from the Massachusetts Cost of AIDS Study are combined with epidemiological projections to estimate the cost of treating people diagnosed with AIDS in New England. Aggregate inpatient, ambulatory, and home care costs are estimated to be $96.9 million and $524.8 million through 1987 and 1991, respectively. These estimates represent a relatively small percentage of total health care costs for all illnesses over the same time period.

The authors find that the cost of treating AIDS does not affect all health care providers uniformly and therefore argue that appropriate measures must be developed to assist those impacted disproportionately. Reduction of inpatient hospital days through the creation of subacute care centers, subsidy programs for medical care providers serving large numbers of uninsured or underinsured AIDS patients and education to prevent new cases are recommended to continue the availability of medical care for people with AIDS.

The rapidly growing number of AIDS cases in the United States has generated an increased interest in the cost of treating patients with HIV infection. Projections of future cases — the number is expected to exceed 270,000 for the nation as a whole by 1991 — are a warning to legislators, insurers, employers, health care and policy planners, hospital administrators, private practitioners, and health care activists to prepare for the economic impact of AIDS.[1] One of the most frequent questions asked of public health officials regarding treatment programs for people with AIDS is, How much will it cost?

The health care needs of people with AIDS are usually considered from the perspective either of cost or of utilization. With regard to cost, the key questions are, How much will it cost? Who will pay the cost? To what extent can society afford to pay the cost? From the perspective of utilization, the important issues are related to the availability of resources: What types of resources do AIDS patients need? Are these resources available currently? Will they be available to meet future demand?

Stewart J. Landers is project director of the Massachusetts Cost of AIDS Study. George R. Seage III is the senior AIDS epidemiologist for the Boston Department of Health and Hospitals and is principal investigator of the Massachusetts Cost of AIDS Study.

Questions about cost and utilization of services merge in the areas of planning and budgeting. While there is little doubt that the resource utilization and the accompanying cost of treating people with AIDS are large and will get significantly larger, it is also likely that, given adequate planning, cost-effective resources can be identified to meet this need.

In this article, the authors stress that information about cost is critical to planning for the provision of AIDS care. The text is divided into three main sections. The first section reviews information currently available on the cost of services in New England, specifically in Massachusetts. Inpatient, ambulatory, and home care costs are described. The indirect costs of care are discussed. These indirect costs include some hidden costs that may represent the largest costs of the epidemic. Changes in the cost of treating people with AIDS are discussed. The section concludes with estimates of the cost of treating AIDS in New England up to 1988 and cumulatively through 1991.

The second section describes the payer mix of AIDS patients and the anticipated impact of the projected AIDS crisis on each type of payer. People with AIDS must do battle with private and public insurance programs to receive coverage for their care. Public and private insurers, as well as hospitals providing free care, struggle to act responsibly in the face of this epidemic without overextending themselves financially.

The third section discusses the implications of health care costs in planning for the provision of health care for people with AIDS. The section addresses issues of insurability, cost containment, and prevention, and targets specific areas where planning is necessary to provide humane, comprehensive, and quality care to persons with AIDS.

The Cost of Treating Patients with AIDS

The initial report on the cost of treating patients with AIDS estimated a cost of $147,000 per patient.[2] Subsequent studies in San Francisco and Massachusetts found that medical care costs were significantly lower.[3, 4] A review of cost studies by the federal Office for Information Technology reported lower costs in studies from Maryland, New York, New Mexico, Alabama, Minnesota, Florida, and California.[5] Research from a hospital in Virginia[6] and the first two national studies with a wide sample of data[7, 8] provide further confirmation that direct medical care costs are lower than the initial estimate, probably in the range of $20,000 to $60,000.

Cost in Massachusetts

In Massachusetts, a study to determine the costs of treating AIDS was begun in February 1985. The study was sponsored by the state Department of Public Health and was conducted by the public health AIDS program of the Boston Department of Health and Hospitals. In that study, the authors of this article and their colleagues evaluated forty-five AIDS patients seen at the New England Deaconess Hospital between March 1984 and February 1985.[9]

Inpatient and outpatient medical and billing records were reviewed to obtain cost, utilization, and demographic data. Data from the Massachusetts Rate Setting Commission were used to convert inpatient charges to costs. Charges for ambulatory care were converted to costs through the use of Blue Cross customary reimbursement rates.

On the basis of these data, the researchers calculated an average hospitalization cost of $14,189 and an average length of stay of 21 days per hospitalization. To answer a variety of questions, the authors also calculated cost per patient per annum (twelve-month period) as $46,505, and costs per case, from diagnosis to death, as $50,380.[10]

Analyses of the data also yielded the number of hospitalizations per patient as 1.6; hospitalizations per patient per annum, 3.3; hospital days per patient, 33; and hospital days per patient per annum, 62.

Components of Inpatient and Ambulatory Care

In the aforementioned cost study, the researchers analyzed the components of inpatient and ambulatory care to determine where the medical expenses of treating AIDS patients are concentrated. The results of this analysis (table 1) show that inpatient costs, constituting 89 percent of total costs incurred by AIDS patients, are dramatically higher than ambulatory costs.

Total ancillary services, including laboratory services, were responsible for 47.9 percent of all inpatient care costs for the patients with AIDS studied. This percentage for ancillary services is not unusual for patient care costs generally. However, the high laboratory component of ancillary services is greater for AIDS patients than for non-AIDS patients. Room and board (routine and intensive care) and laboratory services comprised the two largest categories of cost, representing 45 and 22 percent, respectively, of total inpatient care costs.

Cost for laboratory services and cost of professional services accounted for 56 and 16.9 percent, respectively, of all ambulatory care costs. The large percentage of cost in laboratory services is related to the close monitoring of patients' immune status for diagnostic and palliative purposes.

Home Care and Support Services

Very few studies have analyzed both the cost and the cost-effectiveness of services that allow people with AIDS to spend more time at home and, presumably, less time in acute care settings. However, a study of thirty-seven pediatric AIDS cases in New York City identified 1,909 hospital days that the researchers labeled "social admissions" — that is, patient days in acute inpatient care facilities resulting from lack of appropriate available placement.[11] These so-called social admissions represented 31.2 percent of hospital days for this cohort of pediatric AIDS cases. Thus, if adequate services were available outside the hospital, the number of hospital days could be drastically reduced for this cohort.

A San Francisco study of both paid and volunteer home care services showed that home care was significantly less expensive than hospital-based care.[12] Among the resources evaluated was a home-based hospice program. This program provided a range of home care services to persons with AIDS which enabled them to spend most of the duration of their illness, including the terminal stage, at home. For the 165 persons with AIDS who received care under this program, the study found that they required an average of 47 hospice days per person, at an average cost of $4,401 per patient. The average cost per day of hospice care was $94, compared to an inpatient cost per day at San Francisco General Hospital of $773.[13] Additional data from San Francisco estimate the cost of acute inpatient care at $800/day; subacute care at $500/day; skilled nursing facility at $300/day; residential hospice at $100/day; and nonmedical group residence at $50/day.[14]

To evaluate home care needs and utilization, clients of the AIDS Action Committee of Massachusetts were surveyed.[15] A questionnaire was mailed in the spring of 1986 to 115 clients of the AIDS Action Committee and was returned by 43 individuals. The purpose of

Total Cost per Patient for AIDS Medical Care*

Total Cost by Components

Service Area	Cost (U.S. $)	(%)
Inpatient cost	22,097	(89.2)
Outpatient cost	1,907	(7.7)
Outpatient cost (related to research protocol)	760	(3.1)
Total	24,764	(100)

Inpatient Cost by Components

Service Area	Cost (U.S. $)	(%)
Room cost	9,176	(41.5)
Laboratory	4,786	(21.7)
Pharmacy	2,958	(13.4)
Supplies	1,126	(5.1)
X-ray	1,099	(5.0)
Professional cost	1,016	(4.6)
Intensive-care room cost	845	(3.8)
Therapy	622	(2.8)
Operating room cost	454	(2.1)
Miscellaneous	15	(0.1)
Total	22,097	(100)

Outpatient Cost by Components

Service Area	Cost (U.S. $)	(%)
Laboratory	1,493	(56.0)
Professional charges	452	(16.9)
Surgery	254	(9.5)
Pharmacy	229	(8.6)
Therapy	136	(5.1)
X-ray	64	(2.4)
Miscellaneous	29	(1.1)
Emergency room visits	11	(0.4)
Total	2,668	(100)

*George R. Seage III, Stewart Landers, et al., unpublished data from study of cost of treating 45 AIDS patients at New England Deaconess Hospital 1984–85.

the questionnaire was to determine the average weekly utilization of home care services. The results indicate that 65 percent of respondents used or needed some home care services. The researchers determined a mean utilization cost of $107 per week, applying Blue Cross reimbursement rates to estimate the cost of these home care services. Assuming that persons with AIDS receive home care except when they are hospitalized, the cost of home care services for a person with AIDS from diagnosis to death may be estimated to be $4,985.[16]

This figure may be based on an underestimation of home care utilization. Those individuals needing the greatest amount of care were the least likely to respond to a questionnaire. However, the estimate is almost identical to the estimated cost of home-based hospice care in San Francisco and may be used as a rough approximation of home care costs. A thorough, population-based study of the utilization of home care health services by AIDS patients needs to be performed.

Indirect Costs

Scitovsky and Rice have divided the indirect costs of AIDS into two types: morbidity costs (productivity lost on account of illness) and mortality costs (future earnings lost for those who die prematurely).[17] They estimated the total direct and indirect cost of AIDS in the United States in 1985 alone to be $4.8 billion. Of this cost, the researchers calculated $3.9 billion, or 81 percent, as indirect costs. Thus, while indirect costs are less obvious in terms of impact upon the health care system, the overall economic impact of such indirect costs is immense.

Mortality costs account for 94 percent of indirect costs. These costs are very high, owing to the young age of AIDS patients and the associated large numbers of years of life lost. Not included in this accounting is the fact that many persons with AIDS may not pay premiums to health insurance, taxes, Social Security, and so on, during what are usually a person's most productive years.

Other indirect costs related to the cost of AIDS include added infection control precautions, nursing care, and supplies, as well as complex case management services.[18] The difficulty of caring for AIDS patients consists in increasing personnel costs, owing to the need for additional support services for personnel. This article will not include the indirect costs of AIDS in its projections of direct medical care costs in New England.

Changes in the Cost of Treating AIDS

The cost of providing medical care to a person with AIDS is not static. There is evidence that the cost may be declining. New and costly therapies for persons with AIDS, as well as experience in the treatment of AIDS, will affect the cost of care.

Evidence of reduction in cost. In July 1985, the study of the cost of treating persons with AIDS in Massachusetts expanded to include five hospitals and to evaluate patient utilization over the two-year period March 1984 through February 1986.[19] Two hundred and forty patients were enrolled over the two-year period. This cohort represented 55 percent of all AIDS patients alive in Massachusetts during the study period. The cohort was representative of all AIDS patients reported to the Massachusetts AIDS Surveillance Program with regard to risk group status, gender, geographical distribution, and race.

Preliminary data on cost over the two-year period showed a decline in total inpatient and outpatient cost from year one to year two at each of the five hospitals studied. The researchers attributed the observed decrease both to shorter lengths of stay (mean reduced from 19.2 days/hospitalization to 15.7 days/hospitalization) and to a decrease in the mean number of hospitalizations (mean reduced from 2.2 hospitalizations/patient to 1.9 hospitalizations/patient). Future analysis of these data will attempt to evaluate additional factors related to the decline in cost, such as the availability of support services and home care programs.

The effect on cost of AZT. As antiviral and other therapies are developed, the direct medical care cost of treating AIDS is likely to change. One therapeutic agent that may have a significant impact on cost of care is the drug Azidothymidine (AZT). It is uncertain whether use of this drug, which has been shown to decrease the frequency of life-threatening pneumonia in AIDS patients, will increase or decrease utilization of health care services.[20] AZT may reduce the length of stay for AIDS-related hospitalizations and the overall number of hospital days for AIDS patients, by decreasing the severity of opportunistic infections. AZT may also keep AIDS patients healthier longer and allow them to continue working longer.

On the other hand, by allowing patients to survive more bouts of *Pneumocystis carinii* pneumonia (PCP), AZT may result in more lifetime hospitalizations and an increased number of total hospital days. In addition, physicians may become more aggressive in their treatment, knowing there is a drug that may significantly extend the patient's life once any immediate crisis is forestalled.

One thing is certain: AZT is an expensive drug. A one-year supply of AZT is currently estimated to cost between $8,000 and $10,000.[21] Once on AZT, an AIDS patient needs to continue taking the drug as long as he or she is alive, unless serious side effects occur.

Experience with AIDS patients. The extent of an institution's experience with AIDS patients may alter the cost of services to persons with AIDS for a number of reasons, including familiarity with the disease; adoption of an oncological modality of treatment; and recognition of the particular out-of-hospital services that AIDS patients may require.

The lack of familiarity with the care required by persons with AIDS may lead to unnecessary cost expenditures. A report on the provision of medical care at U.S. public and private teaching hospitals found that 15 percent of responding hospitals had not yet treated an AIDS patient.[22] Familiarity with the care and support that persons with AIDS require will reduce the number of hospital days, the use of intensive care, and the application of unnecessary diagnostic techniques.

As AIDS is a new and thus far terminal illness, AIDS care may utilize a range of different treatment modalities. For example, an alternative to the inpatient hospital model is the oncological or hospice model. This model, developed for terminally ill cancer patients, attempts to maximize comfort for the afflicted individual and minimize aggressive or intrusive diagnostic and therapeutic measures. AIDS patients receiving hospice care are much less likely to be placed under intensive care — an unpleasant (albeit potentially life-prolonging) and costly form of care.

The availability of support services and home care can make a difference in the length of hospitalizations and the overall cost. In some cases, discharge planners need to familiarize themselves with the services and support groups already available to persons with AIDS. However, the absence of such services in many local communities may prevent the implementation of an effective and realistic home care plan.

Estimating Cost in New England

For purposes of estimating direct medical care costs per case, the authors have combined the mean inpatient and ambulatory cost per case, $50,380, and the mean estimated home care cost, $4,985. Our estimated total direct medical care costs per case are $55,365.

The number of AIDS cases diagnosed to date in New England is based on case reports to the Centers for Disease Control (CDC) by the six New England states as of November 23, 1987 (see table 2). Nationally, more than 270,000 cases are expected by the end of 1991. Massachusetts has consistently reported 2 percent of the national cases, and this percentage is used to estimate the case load in Massachusetts cumulatively through 1991. Projections for the other five New England states are based on the total number of cases each state has reported cumulatively to November 23, 1987, and the percentage of New England cases each such total represents. Using these calculations, the total direct medical care cost is $524.8 million for persons with AIDS diagnosed in New England during the ten-year period 1981 to 1991.

Who Will Pay? A Look at the Payers

With an estimate of $524.8 million needed to pay for the direct medical cost of treating persons with AIDS in New England through 1991 (see table 2), the most important questions are, Who is and who will be paying for this, and who will pay in the future? The simple, if somewhat naive, answer, of course, is that we all pay for the cost of treating AIDS, either through health insurance premiums, federal and state tax dollars for Medicare and Medicaid, or local tax revenue that provides services to the uninsured or reimbursements to hospitals for free care and bad debt. The reason this point of view is naive is that the exact payer mix matters greatly to each potential payer. Insurers wish to reduce their exposure to high costs; holders of private insurance policies do not want their premiums to rise; and government health care budgets need to remain responsive to a wide variety of political interests. In essence, AIDS costs highlight the classic confrontation between the private versus the public sector.

Analysis of the payer mix is key to measuring the impact of policies that will shift the cost of caring for AIDS patients among payers. The Massachusetts cost study found that 47 percent of people with AIDS had Blue Cross, 18 percent had commercial insurance, 18 percent had Medicaid, and 18 percent had no insurance.[23] These data differ from the data presented by Andrulis and Beers et al. in their nationwide study. They reported that for hospitalizations in the Northeast region, only 12 percent were reimbursed by private insurance. Instead, 65 percent of patients had Medicaid, 17 percent had no insurance, and 11 percent had Medicare, received veterans' benefits, were prisoners, or were classified as "other."[24]

Table 2

AIDS Cases and Costs* in New England States

State	AIDS Cases Diagnosed to 11/23/87[a]		AIDS Cases Diagnosed to 1991[b]	Cost of AIDS Diagnosed to11/23/87 (in $millions)[c]	Cost of AIDS Diagnosed to 1991 (in $millions)[c]
Massachusetts	997	(57.0%)	5,400	55.2	299.0
Connecticut	521	(29.8%)	2,822	28.8	156.2
Rhode Island	105	(6.0%)	569	5.8	31.5
Maine	57	(3.3%)	309	3.2	17.1
New Hampshire	49	(2.8%)	265	2.7	14.7
Vermont	21	(1.2%)	114	1.2	6.3
Totals	1,750	(100.0%)	9,497	96.9	524.8

*Costs include hospital inpatient, hospital outpatient, and home care costs.

NOTE: Projections are likely to vary by as much as 50 percent; any variation between these projections and those found in other articles is due to different assumptions about the number of infected persons, the spread of infection, and the rate at which those infected will progress to AIDS.

[a] *AIDS Weekly Surveillance Report — United States,* United States AIDS Program, Center for Infectious Diseases, Centers for Disease Control, November 23, 1987, 2.

[b] W. M. Morgan and J. W. Curran, "Acquired Immunodeficiency Syndrome: Current and Future Trends," *Public Health Reports* 101, no. 5 (September–October 1986): 461.

[c] Costs data are based on George R. Seage III, Stewart Landers, Anita Barry, et al., "Medical Care Costs of AIDS in Massachusetts," *Journal of the American Medical Association* 256, no. 22 (December 12, 1986): 3107.

sachusetts study was comprised predominantly of white, gay men, most of whom were working at jobs that provided health insurance at the time they became ill. Andrulis and Beers et al. studied costs at public hospitals and teaching hospitals, and their Northeast region includes New York and New Jersey as well as New England. The number of persons with AIDS in New England who rely on the public health system may range from 36 percent to almost 90 percent.

Private Insurers

Concern about AIDS costs is not uniform among private insurers. Some private payers are devising strategies to reduce their exposure to AIDS-related costs. A quick look at the rise of widespread health insurance, as well as its recent decline, sheds light on the concerns of the industry.

The growth of health insurance in the United States from the time of World War II to the present is well documented by Rashi Fein, an expert in medical economics at the Harvard School of Public Health:

> [By 1977,] over 80 percent of total health insurance premiums went for the purchase of group coverage and over 95 percent of all group insurance was provided in the employment context. Furthermore, almost 90 percent of all U.S. employees worked in firms that provided health insurance plans and over 90 percent of employees in those firms were eligible for the insurance.[25]

However, Fein also notes:

> In 1977 over 99 percent of workers in firms with over 1,000 employees had an employment-related health insurance plan, compared with only 55 percent of workers in firms with 25 or fewer employees. . . . In general, workers in smaller and nonunionized firms were less likely to have employment-related group coverage.[26]

Group health insurance is usually provided without any physical exam or laboratory testing. After a fixed waiting period, the employee is covered regardless of any preexisting conditions he or she may have. As a member of a group insurance plan, an individual cannot be denied coverage as a result of HIV testing or other prescreening method employed by insurers for persons seeking individual coverage.

Under the Consolidated Omnibus Budget Reconstruction Act of 1985 (COBRA), persons covered by group health insurance policies in companies of twenty or more employees have the right to continue insurance for a period of eighteen months following termination of employment.[27] Individuals must pay the full cost of premiums. COBRA also requires that individuals are informed of this right, which enables AIDS patients to prolong the time period during which their financial resources are protected from the cost of high medical expenses.

In the 1980s, a significant decline in the availability of group health insurance has occurred. To protect against rising costs, employers frequently exclude family members and part-time employees from group health policies or require higher co-payments, leaving fewer individuals covered by insurance.

Furthermore, a growing number of companies, especially larger firms, no longer offer commercial policies and are self-insuring. Eighty-five percent of firms with more than forty thousand employees and 70 percent of firms with between twenty and thirty thousand employees are now self-insured.[28] Self-insured groups are covered under the federal Employee Retirement Income Security Act (ERISA) and are exempt from state regulation. There has been no federal initiative to protect insurance coverage for persons with AIDS; therefore, employers that are self-insured have greater discretion regarding decisions to test for the AIDS antibody or to not cover AIDS at all. In addition, because these employers are not subject to state attempts to pool higher health insurance risks, they undermine the limited experimentation with shared risk pools.

Health Maintenance Organizations (HMOs), a relatively new entrant into the health care market, have shaped health care policy significantly. HMOs are concerned that HIV-antibody-positive persons with a choice of insurers will select HMOs to reduce the high co-payments required by many traditional health insurance policies.

Public-Sector Insurance

The reduced availability of private health insurance underscores the importance of Medicaid as an insurer of last resort for AIDS patients in New England. Medicaid eligibility is dependent upon income and assets. If a person has assets in his or her name, those resources must be depleted in order for that individual to qualify. States have a wide variety of criteria for Medicaid eligibility. For example, Andrulis and Beers et al. found that only 15 percent of AIDS cases in the South are paid for by Medicaid.[29] This figure is attributed to the restrictive Medicaid eligibility requirements common among southern states.

Individuals under age sixty-five become eligible for Medicare after they have received Social Security Disability Insurance (SSDI) for twenty-four consecutive months, followed by a processing period of three to five months. However, the median conditional probability of survival from date of diagnosis with AIDS is 347 days.[30] Thus, most persons with AIDS never qualify for Medicare. In 1985, Massachusetts determined that an AIDS diagnosis is a presumptive disability, which qualifies persons with AIDS for SSDI. However, with the recently expanded case definition, certain AIDS diagnoses, including wasting syndrome and dementia, no longer automatically qualify an individual for SSDI.

Currently, Medicare pays for the care of approximately 1 to 2 percent of AIDS patients in Massachusetts, but it could pay for more. There exists a waiver of the two-year Medicare waiting period for individuals with certain types of renal disease. If a similar waiver were available for AIDS patients, the cost of treating them would shift dramatically from Medicaid to Medicare, and consequently from the state to the federal government. Further analysis is necessary to demonstrate the magnitude of this cost shift if the waiting period were eliminated or if it were reduced to six, twelve, or eighteen months.

Implicit in a state-controlled program is the power to determine what will or will not be covered. Such decisions are likely to reflect political as well as medical realities. The decision of a Medicaid program to pay for AZT, for example, is likely to depend as much on political will as on economics. Medicaid in Massachusetts, as in most states with large and visible advocacy groups representing persons with AIDS, has decided that it will pay for AZT.

Free Care

Despite the availability of Medicaid and the advent of client advocates to help people enroll in publicly funded programs, many individuals continue to fall through the cracks and seek medical care without any insurance coverage. In Massachusetts, a reimbursement system (Chapter 572) was established to cover hospital losses resulting from free care. The system, which expired October 1, 1987, allowed hospitals to set charges in excess of expenses in order to cover free care. Some other New England states do not reimburse hospitals for free care.

A large number of persons with AIDS do not have health insurance and therefore tax the system to reimburse free care. Thus, the AIDS epidemic has a disproportionate impact on those hospitals seeing the greatest numbers of AIDS patients. Boston hospitals reported 79 percent of Massachusetts cases, although only 47 percent of Massachusetts cases actually reside in Boston. The concentration of cases at these hospitals invalidates the equations previously used to compensate these institutions.

The AIDS epidemic will increase the need for services among uninsured, underinsured, and Medicaid patients. For hospitals that continue to provide care for indigent patients, this epidemic will mean a rise in free care. Government must ensure the willingness and financial ability of hospitals to care for indigent patients.

Issues Affecting Cost and Treatment

The direct medical care costs of treating persons with AIDS present a challenge to the fiscal planning efforts of health care planners in New England. In relation to overall national health expenditures, the actual cost of treating persons with AIDS is small. Scitovsky and Rice estimate that in 1991, AIDS will represent 1.4 percent of estimated national medical care costs.[31] This relatively small percentage could be absorbed if it were distributed evenly across all insurers and providers of care. However, in order to tame the rise in health care costs, access to health care has become unevenly distributed in society. The health care industry is developing new methodologies for cost containment. In the process, certain population groups — such as family members — have effectively been denied access to medical care; some employers provide very limited options that deny employees full coverage. These disenfranchised groups are already taxing the public health care system. With the addition of AIDS treatment, certain providers may be totally crippled.

A new movement to protect access to health insurance is developing nationwide in response to the cost containment practices in the health care industry. Advocates of compassionate health care must couple arguments for wider access to care with plans for cost containment. Without cost containment, plans to increase access to health insurance do not appear to be politically viable. In Massachusetts, Governor Dukakis has led a movement for universal health insurance but as of this writing has not succeeded in passing legislation for this purpose.[32]

Until some form of universal health insurance is enacted, the marketplace for health care will become increasingly restrictive. For persons with AIDS or who are infected with HIV, the available options may become fewer as the need for insurance becomes greater. In the next section, we look at the developments in health insurance which affect persons with AIDS or at risk for AIDS. The section concludes with suggestions for reducing the adverse economic impact of AIDS on the health care system.

Developments in Health Insurance

Various developments in health insurance may alter the source of payments as well as the cost of care. HIV antibody screening will shift responsibility for the cost of caring for AIDS from private insurance to the public sector. Insurance coverage of subacute care facilities will shift medical care services to less cost-intensive alternatives. Shared risk pools are one mechanism for maintaining private insurer involvement in the care of persons with AIDS.

HIV antibody testing. Insurers have sought the right to screen applicants for health insurance for evidence of HIV infection. Screening for HIV antibody status has not been initiated for group health insurance, since no eligibility screening practices are currently in place for group plans. If insurance losses due to AIDS become unmanageable, insurers may increase efforts to screen for HIV infection under group plans. In Massachusetts, hearings on proposed regulation of the use of the HIV antibody test reflected widespread consensus among all constituencies, except insurers, against the use of the test for health insurance eligibility.[33] This view is consistent with a widespread opinion in Massachusetts that health insurance is a necessity and should be considered a basic individual right.

The Massachusetts Division of Insurance had, until September 1, 1987, prohibited insurers from using the HIV antibody test at all. The division then promulgated and adopted regulations allowing limited use of the test for individual life and disability insurance plans. The regulations also provided for limited confidentiality of test results and for required counseling of persons who tested positive. Upon challenge by the insurance industry, a preliminary court decision held that the regulation is an invalid exercise of power by the insurance commissioner.[34] At the present time, it is uncertain whether courts will recognize an administrative or regulatory ban on antibody testing without special enabling legislation.

Fairness and excessive losses are the main arguments offered by insurers to justify screening out HIV-infected individuals for health insurance. Insurers argue that if they are forced to assume the high cost of insuring HIV-infected persons, individual premiums will increase. Any rise in premiums, they contend, will force individuals who are struggling to maintain individual policies to give up those policies. Therefore, if the insurability of individuals with HIV infection or AIDS is protected, other individuals may be deprived of health insurance. Furthermore, since insurance companies currently refuse insurance to "bad risks" — such as former cancer patients, women with certain types of benign cysts,[35] and others — insurers argue it would be unfair to insure HIV-infected persons who are comparably bad risks. However, state governments, for public policy reasons, have successfully constrained insurers from using other tests, including those which indicate the presence of sickle cell, Tay-Sachs, and hemoglobin C traits.[36]

Insurers are so adamant about the preceding arguments that to avoid state regulations against HIV testing, they are attempting to use other methods to screen applicants without using HIV testing per se. Some insurers have already utilized screening criteria as diverse as marital status, residence or zip code, medical history, beneficiary, and living arrangements to screen out persons who are potentially at risk for AIDS.[37]

The use of HIV screening threatens to create a class of individuals likely to be subject to discrimination in various aspects of life. Persons with AIDS or who are perceived to be at risk for AIDS have suffered discrimination in employment, housing, accommodations, and parental rights.[38] Use of HIV screening by insurers increases the risk of discrimination, particularly since safeguards to protect the confidentiality of information collected by insurance companies are inadequate. The failure of the federal government to protect individuals from discrimination on the basis of their HIV antibody status creates an atmosphere that discourages use of the antibody test.

Coverage of home care, hospice, and other forms of subacute care. Strategies need to address the coverage of cost-effective methods of caring for AIDS patients, including home care, hospice, group residences, skilled nursing facilities, and subacute care units.

As noted in the first section of this article, the daily costs of care for these services are significantly lower than acute inpatient cost.

Medicaid programs in each state may apply for a waiver that would allow the program to develop more effective reimbursement plans for a particular disease. New Jersey has received such a waiver for AIDS and has established a system for reimbursing those out-of-hospital services which are required to care for patients with AIDS in the most humane and cost-effective manner.

Beginning in FY'87, Massachusetts allocated funds to eight home health care agencies, in order to assist the agencies in developing services for persons with AIDS. The grants have been used for staff training, education, and outreach programs. The grant recipients have argued that insufficient reimbursement is still a major impediment to effective delivery of services to persons with AIDS, and have looked to insurers, primarily Medicaid, to reevaluate the services for which home health care agencies may seek reimbursement.

Case management is another approach that is receiving increased attention as a cost-effective way of coping with specific medical problems. Under this approach, a case manager helps develop a strategic plan for the patient. For example, in the case of AIDS patients, a case management approach may involve educating the family and friends in order to help them overcome fears of the disease and help them enable the patient to remain at home as long as possible. Blue Cross of Massachusetts has adopted a case management system for elderly patients but has not implemented the program for persons with AIDS. A study of the effectiveness of case management for AIDS patients is under way at the AIDS Medical Resource Center in Illinois.[39]

Shared risk pools. The problem of "uninsurables" is not a new one, and, as indicated earlier, other classes of individuals have had difficulty obtaining health insurance. In order to maintain private insurer involvement in coverage of high-risk individuals, thirteen states have passed legislation establishing risk pool programs.[40] Under these programs, private insurers contribute to a pool that provides health insurance to individuals at high risk for various diseases. The premiums are generally higher than normal, and government subsidies keep them within an affordable range. The programs have not been very successful. In 1986, the seven operating risk pools enrolled only twenty-one thousand people, and all but one of the pools lost money.[41] The addition of AIDS patients as beneficiaries of the pool would exacerbate this situation further.

Access to insurance is hampered for persons with AIDS not only because of unavailability, but also because of cost of premiums, since an AIDS diagnosis is often accompanied by loss of employment and of the ability to pay for insurance. Therefore, shared risk pools *alone* are unlikely to solve the problem of providing health insurance for persons with AIDS, and may need to be combined with a subsidy or coupon-type program to allow persons with AIDS to purchase such insurance.

Suggestions for Managing the Cost of Caring for People with AIDS

Reduce acute inpatient care days. Acute inpatient care constitutes the largest single component of the direct medical care costs of AIDS patients. It is necessary to reduce acute inpatient care as much as possible without compromising the quality of care each patient receives. Reduction of inpatient care may be accomplished by establishing an organized, well-trained, and reimbursable continuum of care.

Physicians must be trained to recognize the opportunistic infections associated with AIDS in a timely way. They must be familiar with the latest treatments, particularly those which allow patients to be treated at home or at subacute care facilities.

Subacute levels of care — including skilled nursing facilities, home health care, hospice programs, and group residences — must be developed through the utilization of new or existing resources. Reimbursements must be flexible enough to make such facilities economically feasible.

Target specific medical care providers for assistance. Those institutions or insurers which provide the greatest amounts of unreimbursed care must be identified, and subsidies must be provided to enable the continued delivery of these services. Owing to matters of geography, philosophy, or reputation or to referral networks, certain institutions are likely to care for disproportionately high numbers of AIDS patients who are uninsured or underinsured. Adequate systems must be developed to determine who is being disproportionately impacted as well as the extent of shortfalls related to AIDS care. Accurate assessments of the extent of unreimbursed care will assure the most cost-effective distributions of subsidies or program funds.

Strengthen AIDS education. Education about AIDS must be strengthened to prevent new cases. While our projections through 1991 indicate a situation that appears to be economically manageable, worst case scenarios through 1995 and beyond may present a far less manageable situation. Reducing the number of new infections and thereby reducing the number of new AIDS cases is an important and extremely cost-effective strategy.

Conclusion

The cost of treating people with AIDS, estimated to be more than $500 million for cases diagnosed in New England over the ten-year period 1981 to 1991, is an increasing burden for society and especially for the health care industry. However, this cost is only a small percentage of overall health care costs and, with proper planning, can be managed.

The largest component of AIDS health care costs is acute inpatient care, and the largest part of inpatient care costs consists of room and board. Ambulatory care and home care are significantly less expensive alternatives.

Paying for AIDS is made more difficult by the patchwork nature of the current health care reimbursement system and distribution of services. Many persons with AIDS are uninsured or underinsured, or may lose their insurance coverage during the course of their illness. Various strategies may be implemented to maintain or perhaps expand insurance coverage for people with AIDS. However, insurers, including Medicare and Medicaid, will oppose any plan that increases their share of AIDS coverage.

Particular insurers or health care providers may find themselves overburdened as they become the primary care centers for AIDS patients. Public and teaching hospitals in New England are likely to be burdened the most by the AIDS epidemic.

To guard against the deterioration of health care services for people with AIDS, the authors recommend reduction of acute inpatient care through the development of alternative levels of care, including subacute care, skilled nursing facilities, hospice programs, group residences, and home health care; the development of targeted subsidies or programs to relieve severe pressures on particular insurers or health care providers; and the strengthening of education to slow the growth of the AIDS epidemic.

The Massachusetts Cost of AIDS Study is a project of the Community Infectious Disease Epidemiology Program (CIDEP) at the Boston Department of Health and Hospitals and the Boston University School of Public Health in Boston, Massachusetts. The project was supported by a grant from the AIDS Research Council of the Massachusetts Department of Public Health and the Boston Department of Health and Hospitals. The authors wish to acknowledge Paula V. Kaminow for her editorial assistance with the manuscript.

Notes

1. W. M. Morgan and J. W. Curran, "Acquired Immunodeficiency Syndrome: Current and Future Trends," *Public Health Reports* 101, no. 5 (September–October 1986): 461.
2. Ann M. Hardy, Kathryn Rauch, Dean Echenberg, et al., "The Economic Impact of the First 10,000 Cases of AIDS in the United States," *Journal of the American Medical Association* 255, no. 2 (January 10, 1986): 210.
3. Anne A. Scitovsky, Mary Cline, and Philip R. Lee, "Medical Care Costs of Patients with AIDS in San Francisco," *Journal of the American Medical Association* 256, no. 22 (December 12, 1986): 3103.
4. George R. Seage III, Stewart Landers, Anita Barry, et al., "Medical Care Costs of AIDS in Massachusetts," *Journal of the American Medical Association* 256, no. 22 (December 12, 1986): 3107.
5. Jane E. Sisk, "The Cost of AIDS: A Review of the Estimates," *Health Affairs* (Summer 1987): 5–21.
6. Lisa G. Kaplowitz et al., "Hospital Costs of Patients with AIDS in Richmond, Virginia," Poster Presentation TP.208 at the Third International Conference on AIDS (June 1987), Washington, D.C.
7. Edmund J. Graves and Mary Moien, "Hospitalizations for AIDS, United States, 1984–85," *American Journal of Public Health* 77, no. 6 (June 1987): 729–730.
8. Dennis P. Andrulis, Virginia S. Beers, et al., "The Provision and Financing of Medical Care for AIDS Patients in U.S. Public and Private Teaching Hospitals," *Journal of the American Medical Association* 258, no. 10 (September 11, 1987): 1343–1346.
9. Seage et al., op. cit., at 3107.
10. Seage et al., op. cit. The authors used the following formulae to derive various estimates of cost:

    Cost per patient = inpatient and outpatient cost = $24,764

    $$\text{Cost per patient per annum} = \frac{\sum_{1}^{N}\left(\dfrac{\text{Cost per patient} \times 12}{\text{\# months in study}}\right)}{N} = \$46{,}505$$

    To calculate the total inpatient and outpatient costs of treating an AIDS patient (cost per case), we multiply the per annum cost by the average life expectancy from diagnosis to death, estimated to be thirteen months. See Ann M. Hardy et al., op. cit., at 210.

    Cost per case = cost per patient per annum times survival time (13/12 of a year) = $50,380
11. James D. Hegarty et al., "Medical Care Costs of Children with HIV Infection in Harlem," Presentation Th.11.3 at the Third International Conference on AIDS (June 1987), Washington, D.C.
12. Peter Arno, "The Nonprofit Sector's Response to the AIDS Epidemic: Community-based Services in San Francisco," *American Journal of Public Health* 76, no. 11 (November 1986): 1325–1330.
13. Scitovsky et al., op. cit., at 3104.
14. Robert T. Chen, "Integration of Chronic Care Services," Presentation V.D. at AIDS National Conference (November 1987), San Francisco.

15. Stewart Landers, George R. Seage III, unpublished data based on survey of people with AIDS conducted May 1986 in conjunction with the AIDS Action Committee of Massachusetts.

16. To estimate the total cost of home care services, the authors assume that persons with AIDS incur the average cost of home care each week they are not hospitalized. Since average hospital days per patient per annum = 62, the number of weeks not in the hospital per annum = 43 (52 weeks – 9 weeks). Thus, the cost of home care per patient per annum = 43 x $107 = $4,601. Using the average survival time of 13 months (see note 10), the average cost of home care per case = $4,985.

17. Anne A. Scitovsky and Dorothy P. Rice, "Estimates of the Direct and Indirect Costs of AIDS in the United States, 1985, 1986, and 1991," *Public Health Reports* 102, no. 1 (January–February 1987): 5–16.

18. Jesse Green, M. Singer, and N. Wintfeld, "The AIDS Epidemic: A Projection of Its Impact on Hospitals, 1986–1991," Poster Presentation MP.205 at the Third International Conference on AIDS (June 1987), Washington, D.C.

19. George R. Seage III, Stewart J. Landers, Anita Barry, et al., "Costs of Medical Care for AIDS in Massachusetts: Trends Over a Two-Year Period," Poster Presentation WP.210 at the Third International Conference on AIDS (June l987), Washington, D.C.

20. Margaret A. Fischl et al., "The Efficacy of Azidothymidine in the Treatment of Patients with AIDS and AIDS-Related Complex," *New England Journal of Medicine* 317, no. 4 (July 23, 1987): 187–188.

21. Emily H. Thomas and Daniel M. Fox, "The Cost of AZT," *AIDS and Public Policy Journal* 2, no. 2 (Spring–Summer 1987): 17. Burroughs-Wellcome has announced a 20 percent price reduction in the cost of AZT as a result of its increased capacity for manufacturing the drug.

22. Andrulis et al., op. cit., at 1343.

23. Seage, Landers, et al., op. cit., note 4 at 3107.

24. Andrulis et al., op. cit., at 1346.

25. Rashi Fein, *Medical Care, Medical Costs: The Search for a Health Insurance Policy* (Cambridge, Mass.: Harvard University Press, 1986), 153.

26. Ibid.

27. Consolidated Omnibus Budget Reconciliation Act of 1985, Public Law 99-272.

28. Peter S. Arno, "The Economic Impact of AIDS," *Journal of the American Medical Association* 258, no. 10 (September 11, 1987): 1377.

29. Andrulis et al., op. cit., at 1346.

30. Richard Rothenberg et al., "Survival with the Acquired Immunodeficiency Syndrome," *New England Journal of Medicine* 317, no. 21 (November 19, 1987): 1299.

31. Scitovsky and Rice, op. cit., at 5.

32. Bruce Mohl and Richard A. Knox, "House leader delays action on health bill," *Boston Globe,* December 29, 1987, 1.

33. Massachusetts Division of Insurance Public Hearing on Proposed Regulations Governing HIV-Related Testing and the Use of AIDS-Related Information for Life and Health Insurance (211 CMR 36.00), August 4-5, 1987.

34. *Life Insurance Association of Massachusetts v. Singer,* Mass. Superior Ct., Suffolk Cty., CA No. 87–5321.

35. Nora Zamichow, "Coverage denial called unjustified," *Boston Globe,* August 18, 1986, 40.

36. Benjamin Schatz, "The AIDS Insurance Crisis: Underwriting or Overreaching?" *Harvard Law Review* 100, no. 7 (May 1987): 1798.

37. Ibid., at 1787.

38. Ibid., at 1784.

39. Gordon Nary, director, AIDS Medical Resource Center, Illinois, written correspondence, June 15, 1987.

40. Schatz, op. cit., at 1796.

41. Arno, op. cit., note 28, at 1377.

AIDS and New England Hospitals

Jesse Green, Ph.D.
Neil Wintfeld, Ph.D.
Madeleine Singer, M.P.H.
Kevin Schulman, B.S.

The Centers for Disease Control projects that nine thousand persons with AIDS will be alive in New England in 1991, representing a sevenfold increase from 1986. Our analysis indicates that more than 2 percent of medical/surgical beds in New England will be used for AIDS care by 1991, representing 766 fully occupied hospital beds. The direct cost of providing hospital care to New England's AIDS patients is projected to be $195.2 million in 1991, reflecting 3 percent of all hospital inpatient costs in the region.

AIDS treatment is very unevenly distributed among hospitals in New England. Just twenty hospitals (8 percent of short-term general hospitals in the region) provided over 60 percent of the care required by all AIDS patients in New England in 1986. If this trend continues, nearly 5 percent of all the beds available in these twenty institutions will be required for AIDS care by 1991.

Alternatives to inpatient care are an important means of limiting the demands the AIDS epidemic places on inpatient care facilities. A number of outpatient AIDS clinics have been established in New England hospitals, including clinics at Yale-New Haven Hospital and Rhode Island Hospital. However, skilled nursing facilities in New England, as in other parts of the country, are not prepared to care for AIDS patients. Similarly, the development of in-home services for AIDS patients is just beginning in New England.

Hospital planning for New England should begin addressing the need to expand alternative care services. Hospitals may begin by developing an integrated system of inpatient care with outpatient clinics and by designing units or multidisciplinary teams to care for AIDS patients. But even the best case management and discharge planning efforts cannot succeed if there is no place outside the hospital for AIDS patients to go. Each state needs to look closely at its capacity to provide long-term care, hospice care, and home care in order to fill gaps where they exist.

The authors are affiliated with the NYU Medical Center, where Dr. Jesse Green is director for research, Dr. Neil Wintfeld is senior research analyst, and Madeleine Singer is research analyst. Kevin Schulman was a research associate at the medical center; he is now a medical student there.

AIDS cases have been reported in every state in the nation, and although the preponderance of cases to date have occurred in New York City and San Francisco, national projections indicate that by 1991, more than 80 percent of AIDS cases will occur outside these two areas of concentration. While current estimates indicate that AIDS cases utilized nearly one million days of inpatient care nationwide in 1986, projections for 1991 show AIDS patients requiring more than 5 million days of inpatient care.[1] This is nearly 60 percent more inpatient care than motor vehicle accident victims or lung cancer patients required in 1980. The six New England states are projected to have 9,020 live AIDS cases in 1991, representing more than 5 percent of the nation's AIDS cases.

In order to assess the impact of the AIDS epidemic on hospitals in New England, projections of inpatient bed days, inpatient beds, and inpatient costs were constructed for each of the six New England states. Estimates of three basic parameters are necessary to produce these projections: number of AIDS cases alive during the time period (prevalence); number of days of inpatient care required per patient; and the average daily cost of care for AIDS patients.

Methods

The number of bed days of care is defined as the product of prevalence and days of care per case, and an inpatient bed is defined as an acute care bed occupied for a full year (bed days/365). Inpatient costs are defined as the product of estimated days of care and the average daily cost of care.

W. Meade Morgan of the Centers for Disease Control (CDC) developed a model for projecting the prevalence of AIDS on the basis of cases reported between January 1983 and April 1986. The model projects 174,000 prevalent AIDS cases nationally in 1991.[2] At our request, Morgan assisted us in breaking down the prevalence projections by state.[3] Table 1 displays these projections for the New England states.

The first study of AIDS treatment costs with a national scope was conducted by Andrulis et al.[4] The study included a sample of 169 public and private teaching hospitals, representing over one-third of the AIDS-related hospital admissions in the United States in 1985. The Andrulis survey included 11 New England hospitals, reflecting 233 AIDS admissions and more than seven thousand days of inpatient care for 134 AIDS patients. Andrulis found that AIDS patients in New England used an average of thirty-one hospital days in 1985. In our projections for New England, we have used this thirty-one-day estimate for hospital days per patient alive in a year.

The cost of care per day for AIDS hospitalizations has been estimated in a number of studies. Scitovsky found $887 per day (charges) at San Francisco General Hospital;[5] Seage found $666 per day (costs) at New England Deaconess Hospital.[6] Andrulis estimated $635 per day (costs) from his survey. We have relied on Andrulis's estimate but have increased it by 10 percent for the increased levels of nursing care associated with AIDS patients. The daily cost of care used in our analysis was $698. The adjustment for nursing care was added because several studies have found intense levels of nursing care required by AIDS patients. A study of nursing care for AIDS patients at the New York City Health and Hospitals Corporation found, for example, that AIDS cases required 40 percent more direct nursing care than other medical-surgical patients.[7] Other studies have found that AIDS patients require as little as 28 percent and as much as 100 percent more nursing-care hours than the average patient.[8] The cost adjustment applied above assumes that

Table 1

Projections of AIDS Prevalence in New England, 1986–1991

State	Prevalence in 1986 (est.)	Percent of New England Cases, 1986	Percent of U.S. Cases, 1986	Prevalence in 1991 (est.)
Maine	50	4.21%	0.16%	425
New Hampshire	31	2.61	0.10	276
Vermont	12	1.01	0.04	106
Massachusetts	656	55.27	2.11	4,346
Rhode Island	81	6.82	0.26	722
Connecticut	357	30.08	1.15	3,145
New England	1,187	100.00%	3.82%	9,020

NOTE: Prevalence estimates rounded to nearest case. On the advice of W. Meade Morgan of the Centers for Disease Control, the original prevalence estimates were increased by 20 percent to account for underreporting and underascertainment.

Source: Projections based on CDC data on AIDS cases reported between January 1983 and April 1986.

AIDS patients use 40 percent more nursing care than other patients and that nursing represents 25 percent of total inpatient costs.[9]

Hospital Bed Need and Costs for AIDS in New England: 1986–1991

We project that there will be 9,020 persons in New England with AIDS alive in 1991, more than a sevenfold increase from 1986 (see table 1). More than 80 percent of the cases in New England will be concentrated in Massachusetts and Connecticut, but New Hampshire, Vermont, Maine, and Rhode Island, with far fewer cases, will still have sufficient numbers to present local hospitals with a major challenge. For example, prevalent cases in New Hampshire are estimated to increase from 31 in 1986 to 276 in 1991; in Rhode Island, prevalent cases are estimated to increase from 81 in 1986 to more than 700 in 1991. Thus, Rhode Island in 1991 may well have as many AIDS cases as Massachusetts had in 1986.

The increases in case load will have substantial impacts on hospital utilization. We project that in 1991 AIDS patients will require more than 279,000 bed days of inpatient care in New England (see table 2). This represents 765 fully occupied hospital beds. This is as many hospital beds as were occupied by AIDS patients in New York City in 1986.[10] While a quarter of 1 percent of medical/surgical beds in New England were used for AIDS treatment in 1986, projections show this growing more than sevenfold to nearly 2 percent of medical/surgical beds in 1991 (see table 2).

The cost of providing care to New England's AIDS patients is projected to be $195.2 million in 1991, reflecting 3 percent of all hospital inpatient costs in the region (see table 3). This is substantially more than utilization levels in 1986, when an estimated $25.7 million was spent on inpatient AIDS care, reflecting .39 percent of total inpatient costs.

The impact of AIDS is projected to vary across the six New England states. In Connecticut, we expect that by 1991, 3.2 percent of all medical/surgical beds will be dedicated to AIDS treatment (table 2). This is a higher proportion of AIDS beds to total medical/surgi-

Table 2

Hospital Use by Persons with AIDS in New England, 1986 and 1991

State	Hospital Bed Days for AIDS 1986	Hospital Bed Days for AIDS 1991	Hospital Beds Occupied 1986	Hospital Beds Occupied 1991	Percent of Medical/ Surgical Beds Needed for AIDS, 1991*
Maine	1,550	13,175	4	36	1.0%
New Hampshire	961	8,556	3	23	0.9
Vermont	372	3,286	1	9	0.6
Massachusetts	20,336	134,726	56	369	1.8
Rhode Island	2,511	22,382	7	61	1.9
Connecticut	11,067	97,495	30	267	3.2
New England	36,797	279,620	101	765	1.9%
United States	928,584	5,057,136	2,545	13,854	1.9%

*Percentages calculated on the basis of the number of medical/surgical beds reported in *Hospital Statistics 1986*, American Hospital Association, Chicago, Ill.

cal beds than was found in either New York City or San Francisco in 1986.[11] AIDS patients in Rhode Island and Massachusetts are projected to use just under 2 percent of all medical/surgical beds in each state in 1991. In Massachusetts, AIDS cases are projected to account for more than 2.5 percent of all inpatient hospital expenses in 1991, and in Rhode Island, for nearly 3.5 percent of these expenses in 1991. With only 106 cases projected, Vermont will experience slightly more than one-half of 1 percent of its medical/ surgical beds being used for AIDS in 1991.

A Few Hospitals Treat Most of the AIDS Cases

In discussions with hospital associations and health officials, it has become clear that AIDS treatment is very unevenly distributed among hospitals. The Massachusetts Hospital Association, for example, did pioneering work on the concentration of AIDS cases in their AIDS task force report.[12] The research showed that 57 percent of all AIDS discharges in Massachusetts were from just three hospitals. At one of these hospitals, extrapolation of present trends indicated that as many as 30 percent of its beds could be filled by AIDS patients by 1991.

We obtained information concerning the concentration of AIDS cases for each of the six New England states and assessed this problem for the region as a whole. Nine hospitals (3 in Massachusetts and 6 in Connecticut) currently are treating nearly half the region's AIDS cases, and 20 hospitals out of the 246 short-term general hospitals in New England are currently treating more than 60 percent of the region's AIDS patients (see table 4). In some states, the level of concentration is even more intense. For example, in Rhode Island, 3 hospitals are treating 90 percent of that state's cases; and in Maine, 2 short-term general hospitals out of a total 42 in the state (4.8 percent of the state's short-term general care hospitals) reportedly are treating 90 percent of that state's AIDS cases.

If this trend continues, these institutions will be particularly hard hit by the proliferation of AIDS cases. By 1991, if the current distribution remains unchanged, the 20 "high concentration" hospitals in New England are projected to provide more than 175,000 bed

Table 3

Hospital Inpatient Treatment Costs for AIDS as a Percentage of Total Hospital Inpatient Costs, 1986 and 1991

State	Total Inpatient Costs in General Hospitals*	Hospital Inpatient Costs for AIDS 1986	Hospital Inpatient Costs for AIDS 1991	AIDS Cost as a Percent of Total Inpatient Cost, 1986	AIDS Cost as a Percent of Total Inpatient Cost, 1991
Maine	$ 467,325,108	$ 1,081,900	$ 9,196,150	0.23%	1.97%
New Hampshire	364,169,829	670,778	5,972,088	0.18	1.64
Vermont	191,800,350	259,656	2,293,628	0.14	1.20
Massachusetts	3,520,031,352	14,194,528	94,038,748	0.40	2.67
Rhode Island	457,831,391	1,752,678	15,622,636	0.38	3.41
Connecticut	1,512,310,982	7,724,766	68,051,510	0.51	4.50
New England	$ 6,513,469,013	$ 25,684,306	$ 195,174,760	0.39%	3.00%
United States	$118,681,479,000	$648,152,000	$3,529,881,000	0.55%	2.97%

**Hospital Statistics 1986,* American Hospital Association, Chicago, Ill.

Table 4

Concentration of AIDS Cases in New England Hospitals, 1986

State	Total Short-term General Hospitals in State*	Number of Hospitals in Which AIDS Is Concentrated	Percent of State's AIDS Cases Treated in These Hospitals 1986	Total Number of Beds in High-Concentration Hospitals*	Percent of Total Beds Needed for AIDS in High-Concentration Hospitals, 1986	Percent of Total Beds Needed for AIDS in High-Concentration Hospitals, 1991
Maine	42	2	90%	716	0.50%	4.53%
New Hampshire	29	5	90	1,438	0.19	1.44
Vermont	17	1	68	491	0.14	1.25
Massachusetts	105	3	57	2,020	1.58	10.41
Rhode Island	15	3	90	1,272	0.50	4.32
Connecticut	38	6	60	3,786	0.48	4.23
New England	246	20	63%	9,723	0.65%	4.96%

**American Hospital Association Guide to the Health Care Field,* 1986, American Hospital Association, Chicago, Ill.

days of care to AIDS patients, requiring nearly 5 percent of all the beds available in these hospitals (see table 4). At the state level, the 3 high-concentration hospitals in Massachusetts would need to devote more than 10 percent of their combined beds to AIDS care. Since the current average occupancy rate for all patients at these 3 hospitals is nearly 85 percent, the care requirements for AIDS patients would bring these hospitals very near to 100 percent of capacity. In Rhode Island, where the projected 1991 AIDS prevalence is less than one-fifth the level in Massachusetts, the high-concentration hospitals are projected to devote 4.32 percent of beds to AIDS care. These hospitals currently have an average occupancy rate for all patients of greater than 80 percent, so AIDS care will have a significant effect on their operations. A similar situation exists in Connecticut, where 60 percent of AIDS cases are projected to utilize more than 4 percent of total beds in 6 of the state's 38 short-term general hospitals, and in Maine, where 90 percent of AIDS cases are projected to use more than 4.5 percent of beds in just 2 of the state's 42 short-term general hospitals. The high-concentration hospitals both in Maine and Connecticut currently have average occupancy rates, for all patients, of nearly 80 percent.

Even in states like Vermont and New Hampshire, where AIDS prevalence is low, the high-concentration hospitals will have four to six beds devoted to AIDS in 1991, more if the impact of AIDS-related complex (ARC) is added. The need for four to six full-time beds for AIDS has a significant impact on a hospital. The possibility of a dedicated AIDS unit will need to be addressed urgently in the high-concentration hospitals, even in very low prevalence states.

Additional Epidemic-Based Costs for New England Hospitals

Several factors that were not included in the estimates just described are likely to affect the level of inpatient care for AIDS patients — most notably, the use of the hospital by patients with ARC; the migration of AIDS patients to New England from other states; and the requirement for hospitals to implement universal precautions for all patients.

The preceding analysis focused exclusively on inpatient resource utilization by AIDS patients. While AIDS is the last and most serious stage of HIV infection, earlier manifestations of infection, such as ARC, sometimes involve hospitalization. Estimates of the proportion of all HIV-related hospital bed days that are for ARC rather than AIDS have ranged from 23 to 46 percent.[13] These studies suggest that estimates of hospital utilization which focus exclusively on AIDS, as strictly defined, may substantially understate the hospital-care requirements of HIV-infected individuals.

Reports from several state health departments and AIDS coordinators in New England indicated that AIDS patients may frequently obtain treatment outside the state in which the case was originally diagnosed. For example, the state health department in New Hampshire reported that at least 20 percent of AIDS patients in the state received some of their care in Boston. There are many anecdotal reports that patients go to Boston in order to obtain therapy under a research protocol. In-migration to New Hampshire and Vermont was also reported for patients in the final stage of the disease who "came home to die." The surveillance system for reporting AIDS cases to the CDC records only the location where a patient was first diagnosed. Therefore, any increases in AIDS prevalence in New England due to migration will not be reflected in CDC data.

Recently, the CDC recommended that "blood and body-fluid precautions should be consistently used for *all patients,*" regardless of their HIV status.[14] This entails widespread use of gloves, gowns, masks, goggles, and puncture-resistant containers. The Massachusetts Hospital Association has estimated the direct material costs for these precautions at $3.35 million for Massachusetts, with much larger costs anticipated as a result of decreased productivity in operating rooms and increased requirements for hazardous waste disposal procedures. Regional estimates of the increased costs associated with these problems are not currently available but may constitute a significant incremental cost to hospitals due, indirectly, to the HIV epidemic.

Alternatives to the Hospital

Alternatives to inpatient care for AIDS patients are often cited as the best way to reduce unnecessary inpatient care and treatment costs. Early in the epidemic, San Francisco General Hospital developed a model of care which involved close coordination between an inpatient unit and a broad array of outpatient community-based services, including counseling, hospice, home care, and housing services.[15] New York State has developed a multidisciplinary AIDS program, the Designated AIDS Care Center Program, which creates incentives for hospitals to coordinate services in and out of the hospital through a case management model. The Robert Wood Johnson Foundation and the Health Resources Service Administration (HRSA) have made extensive grants to twenty-four areas to facilitate coordination and expansion of community-based services. An AIDS service demonstration grant has been awarded by HRSA to the Fenway Community Health Center in Boston. The federal Health Care Financing Administration (HCFA) is encouraging states to apply for Medicaid waivers to include home and community-based services to AIDS patients on a disease-specific basis.

A number of AIDS clinics have been established in New England hospitals which provide outpatient and physician services. Rhode Island Hospital in Providence and Yale-New Haven Hospital in Connecticut have established ambulatory care clinics to treat people with AIDS. Yale-New Haven Hospital has three AIDS clinics that provide primary care and consultative visits. A total of 144 HIV-positive patients are currently registered at the Rhode Island Hospital outpatient clinic. The clinic received 666 outpatient visits between January 1986 and June 1987. In Massachusetts, it is estimated that about 7 to 10 percent of the AIDS patients in the state are currently utilizing ambulatory care services.[16] In addition, there are undoubtedly a large number of persons with ARC who are using ambulatory care services in Massachusetts.

The development of in-home services for AIDS patients who require basic care in activities of daily living is just beginning in New England. The local hospice organizations and the Visiting Nurse Association (VNA) are now providing important in-home services for AIDS patients. Home-care services are being provided to AIDS patients by the Maine Hospice Council, and data from the Department of Public Health in Massachusetts suggest that about 20 percent of the AIDS patients are receiving in-home care, usually provided by hospice and the VNA.[17] Home care for AIDS patients is also being provided by the VNA in Connecticut. The only freestanding hospice in Connecticut, the Connecticut Hospice in Branford, has two beds assigned to AIDS patients.

Active community organizations in New England are playing an important role in servicing the needs of AIDS patients. For example, Rhode Island Project AIDS, the AIDS Action Committee in Boston, and the Maine AIDS Project are providing services such as counseling, advocacy, personal care assistance, case management, and housing assistance. The AIDS Action Committee in Boston has been in existence since 1983. It is staffed with 600 volunteers working with 45 paid staff members, and a budget of $1.75 million. Approximately 65 percent of the AIDS cases in Massachusetts have utilized the services of the AIDS Action Committee.[18] The Maine AIDS Project provides a buddy program and a hotline service to approximately half of the cases diagnosed with AIDS in Maine. It is staffed with about 150 active volunteers and 2 full-time staff members. As was discovered in San Francisco, Los Angeles, and New York, these volunteer agencies and their support are vital to assuring quality care for AIDS patients.

patients in New England. For example, in Maine an outpatient clinic is in the process of being established at the Maine Medical Center in Portland. The medical center is also affiliated with a project to establish a live-in center in Portland which would accommodate seven to nine AIDS patients who need care in a sheltered environment. The state has also appropriated $300,000 for patient-care coordination. In Massachusetts, money has been allocated to fund eight community agencies to provide home care to people with AIDS and to support the costs of a residential program for children with AIDS, and funding is proposed to support two new hospice facilities.[19] An interagency monitoring system for the treatment of AIDS patients is being proposed in Connecticut. One of the objectives of the project is to explore alternative delivery sites; another is to encourage public and community agencies to respond to these approaches for treating AIDS patients.[20]

The New England states are facing obstacles in the provision of alternative care for AIDS patients. A report from a major teaching hospital in Connecticut stated, for example, that significant numbers of AIDS patients requiring basic nursing services had extended inpatient stays, owing to the lack of an alternative facility. One AIDS patient with dementia at this hospital occupied an acute care medical bed for two years because of the absence of alternative care. Vermont, a state with a relatively small number of AIDS cases, is also facing the lack of alternative treatment sites for AIDS patients.

Skilled nursing facilities (SNFs) may not be prepared to handle AIDS patients. Issues about placement include the lack of available beds and insufficient infection control precautions. Massachusetts has had difficulty placing AIDS patients in nursing home beds because of a shortage of these beds in the state and the general problem of placing a thirty- to forty-year-old AIDS patient in an SNF, where the average age is over eighty.[21] In Connecticut, the ad hoc Committee on AIDS Economic Impact reported that "it is extremely difficult, if not impossible, to admit AIDS patients to a skilled nursing facility."[22] State planning agencies in Connecticut and Massachusetts are considering the alternative of setting aside skilled nursing or subacute care beds for AIDS patients in an acute care setting, not in a long-term care facility.[23]

Discussion

As AIDS patients compose larger and larger proportions of the hospital inpatient population, their impact on hospital operations is becoming more pronounced. AIDS patients require more nursing care than the average medical/surgical patient, and they require careful infection control procedures.[24] The presence of significant numbers of AIDS patients also engenders the need for staff training and increases the level of required housekeeping service. Moreover, as occupancy rates approach full capacity, the entire range of hospital services and departments feel the impact.

AIDS presents a host of issues to hospitals which become more critical as the volume of patients increases. Staff concerns must be dealt with sensitively. But even with precautions being taken, needle sticks and other accidental exposures will occur. Hospitals need to develop approaches for counseling and follow-up for staff who have such exposures. Physician concerns about exposure sometimes reach levels where they may affect access to care. As AIDS cases increase, these problems are bound to arise in many hospitals. In addition, there will be heightened concerns about confidentiality, quality of care, discharge planning, hiring, and financial effects. AIDS has an impact on nearly every department of the hospital. Even the presence of a few cases requires much rethinking of established procedures on the part of hospital departments and staff. Perhaps the most important thing hospital administrators and state officials can do is to anticipate the impact of this growing problem and begin now to develop the plans, policies, and procedures necessary for coping. Among the first set of issues that must be addressed are the means to distribute more evenly among hospitals the burden of treating AIDS patients and to plan for the facilities needed to provide alternatives to hospital care.

As the number of AIDS cases begins to increase in areas of currently low prevalence, efforts to train and educate local hospitals to care for AIDS patients need to be encouraged. Massachusetts predicts that by 1991 most counties in the state will have more than fifty AIDS cases.[25] Programs need to be funded to develop educational tools and conduct training sessions so that expertise can be shared among physicians, nurses, and administrators.

AIDS is beginning to affect the operation of all hospitals. Implementation of the recent CDC precaution recommendations, described earlier, involves educating employees about HIV transmission and prevention; providing equipment and supplies to prevent transmission; monitoring adherence to recommendations; and developing institutional policy and guidelines for universal precautions.

Hospital Planning for the Epidemic

Hospital planning for New England should urgently begin to address the need of AIDS patients for alternatives to acute care services. Hospitals may begin by developing an integrated system of inpatient care with outpatient clinics. Some hospitals may designate units or multidisciplinary treatment teams to handle a large number of AIDS patients. States may seek funding to develop out-of-hospital services, such as a grant from the Medicaid Home and Community-Based Services Waiver Program of the federal Health Care Financing Administration. States that need to address the issue of fragmentation of care may be encouraged to utilize a case management approach to the care of AIDS patients which coordinates AIDS inpatient care with outpatient treatment, home care, and housing assistance. The case management program may result in the reduction of inpatient service utilization and may help assure appropriate outpatient care. However, even the best case management and discharge planning efforts cannot succeed if there is no place outside a hospital for AIDS patients to go. Each state needs to look closely at its capacity to provide long-term, hospice, and home care and to fill gaps where they exist.

State planning for the epidemic should be addressing the differences in resource utilization which are based on the risk group mix in the state, which affects hospitalization patterns and the spread of the epidemic. A state such as Connecticut, where intravenous drug users (IVDUs) represent 29 percent of the cases and have become the primary source of new AIDS cases, may need a different model of inpatient and outpatient care than Maine, which has primarily a male homosexual AIDS population. A state with a large IVDU AIDS population must deal with the possibility of longer lengths of stay, a need for housing assistance to place the patient after discharge from the hospital, and a reliance on public-sector funding for services.

It is encouraging that all states in New England have established an AIDS task force, either through the local hospital association or through the state government. A thorough report prepared by the Massachusetts Hospital Association AIDS Task Force has assessed the impact of AIDS on the hospital industry in Massachusetts in order to identify gaps in services and prepare for the increasing number of cases in the future. There is a great need for planning and program development by the New England states to assure that services will be delivered to AIDS patients as the epidemic widens and as its impact on the health care delivery systems of these six states becomes more profound.

Notes

1. J. Green et al., "Projecting the Impact of AIDS on Hospitals," *Health Affairs* 6, no. 3 (Fall 1987): 19–31.
2. W. M. Morgan and J. W. Curran, "Acquired Immunodeficiency Syndrome Current and Future Trends," *Public Health Reports* (September–October 1986): 460.
3. W. M. Morgan, AIDS Program, Center for Infectious Diseases, Centers for Disease Control, personal communication, October 1987.
4. D. P. Andrulis et al., "The Provision and Financing of Medical Care for AIDS Patients in U.S. Public and Private Teaching Hospitals," *Journal of the American Medical Association* 258, no. 10 (11 September 1987): 1343–1346.
5. A. A. Scitovsky, M. Cline, and P. R. Lee, "Medical Care Costs of Patients with AIDS in San Francisco," *Journal of the American Medical Association* 256, no. 22 (12 December 1986): 3101–3106.
6. G. R. Seage et al., "Medical Care Costs of AIDS in Massachusetts," *Journal of the American Medical Association* 256, no. 22 (12 December 1986): 3107–3110.
7. J. I. Boufford, "AIDS and the Public Hospital System in New York City," paper presented at the Project HOPE Conference on the Socioeconomic Impact of AIDS on Health Care Systems, Washington, D.C., 25–31 March 1987.
8. Greater New York Hospital Association, "Study of Routine Costs of Treating Hospitalized AIDS Patients," executive summary, April 1986, 3. M. F. Belmont, "St. Luke's–Roosevelt Hospital Center Study: Resource Utilization by AIDS Patients in the Acute Care Hospital," final report summary, submitted to the Health Services Improvement Fund, Inc., December 1985, 25. L. D. Trace, "The Total Cost of Nursing Care for Patients with AIDS," *Patients and Purse Strings II* (New York: NLN Press, forthcoming).
9. Our descriptions of inpatient resource utilization may appear to differ from the analyses by Landers and Seage which also are presented in this volume. Despite their apparent differences, the analyses are fundamentally consistent. Landers and Seage use an incidence-based approach and estimate annualized costs cumulatively through 1991. Our estimates reflect prevalence-based estimates, and estimate hospital utilization during a calendar year. For example, Landers and Seage describe overall days of hospitalization per year to be 62 days. Our estimate of 31 days per case alive in a year appears quite different but is actually consistent, because Landers and Seage have annualized their estimate to adjust for the number of months subjects were in the study. Landers and Seage report an average of 1.6 hospitalizations at 21 days each, which yields 33.6 days of hospital care. This is the number that should be compared with our 31-day estimate. Our estimate was based on hospitals throughout New England, while Landers and Seage base their estimate of days of care on one hospital; this accounts for the small discrepancy between these two estimates. Similarly, Landers and Seage report inpatient costs per patient of $22,097, which compares closely with our estimate of $21,638 per patient. Finally, the estimates of the regional impact of AIDS presented by Landers and Seage reflect *cumulative* costs based on cumulative incidence through 1991, while our descriptions of the regional impact of AIDS are based on prevalence estimates for 1986 and 1991 and reflect costs and utilization for each of those two calendar years.
10. J. Green et al., "Projecting the Impact of AIDS on Hospitals," 22.
11. Ibid.

12. Massachusetts Hospital Association, "Report of the AIDS Task Force of the Massachusetts Hospital Association," September 1987.

13. New York University Medical Center, unpublished data. B. Green, Greater New York Hospital Association, written communication, July 1987.

14. Centers for Disease Control, "Recommendations for Prevention of HIV Transmission in Health Care Settings," *Morbidity and Mortality Weekly Report* 36, no. 2S (21 August 1987): 5s.

15. P. S. Arno, "The Nonprofit Sector's Response to the AIDS Epidemic: Community-Based Services in San Francisco," *American Journal of Public Health* 76, no. 11 (November 1986): 1325–1330.

16. Massachusetts Hospital Association, "Report of the AIDS Task Force Subcommittee on Delivery Systems," September 1987, 3.

17. Ibid.

18. Massachusetts Senate Post Audit and Oversite Bureau, "Acquired Immune Deficiency Syndrome (AIDS) in Massachusetts: Prevention, Patient Care and Cost," April 1987, 3–4.

19. Massachusetts Hospital Association, "Report of the AIDS Task Force Subcommittee on Delivery Systems," 16.

20. Connecticut Hospital Association, "The AIDS Project Progress Report," 1987, 1.

21. Massachusetts Hospital Association, "Report of the AIDS Task Force Subcommittee on Delivery Systems," 15. B. C. Vladeck, *Unloving Care: The Nursing Home Tragedy* (New York: Basic Books, 1980), 13.

22. Connecticut Hospital Association, "The AIDS Project Progress Report," 4–5.

23. Ibid. Massachusetts Hospital Association, "Report of the AIDS Task Force Subcommittee on Delivery Systems," 15.

24. J. Green et al., "Projecting the Impact of AIDS on Hospitals," 25–27.

25. Massachusetts Hospital Association, "Report of the AIDS Task Force of the Massachusetts Hospital Association," 5.

[illegible]

[illegible]

[illegible] 1988: 1326–1328.

16. [illegible] Task Force [illegible]

17. [illegible]

18. [illegible] April 1987), 3–4.

19. [illegible] the AIDS Task Force [illegible]

20. [illegible] Progress Report," 1987, 1.

21. [illegible] AIDS Task Force [illegible]

22. [illegible] "The AIDS [illegible] Progress Report," 4–5.

23. [illegible] AIDS Task Force [illegible]

24. [illegible] the Impact of AIDS [illegible]

25. [illegible] the AIDS Task Force [illegible]

A Crisis in Insurance

Benjamin Lipson

As the life and health insurance industry evaluates its long-term financial goals, the cloud of Black Monday — October 19, 1987, the day the stock market collapsed — blurs its cherished investment income projections. With investment portfolios under siege, mutual life insurance companies and stock companies alike are wary of making policy-pricing miscalculations that could prove to be disastrous. As if that weren't enough, one single disease — acquired immunodeficiency syndrome — looms as the most serious threat to life and health insurers for the remainder of this century. The spread of the new disease has caused insurers to adjust their underwriting requirements by insisting on tests for the AIDS antibody as a precondition for obtaining insurance. Increasingly, life insurance companies are prepared to curtail the availability of insurance in states that place restrictions on testing for insurance purposes. There are also important privacy issues that must be adequately addressed if systematic abuse of the individual's right to privacy is to be avoided.

The liability insurance industry has been in crisis since the early 1980s, when soaring prime rates and double-digit investment returns led insurance companies, with their huge pools of capital, into the equity, investment, and other riskier markets. What's more, they decided that by dropping the prices on insurance products, they could attract even more premium dollars to invest.

That cash-flow underwriting of the early 1980s, fueled by double-digit interest rates and aggressive marketing, gave way to a limited availability of liability insurance and significant rate increases.

Doctors started to leave the practice of medicine. Municipal pools and parks and youth hockey rinks were closed. Children's products were taken off the market. The availability of goods and services providing comfort, recreation, and the necessities of life was threatened, and to this day many tavern owners are closing their premises because they cannot

Benjamin Lipson is a Boston-based life broker and insurability consultant. He writes a weekly column, "Insurance," for the Boston Globe *and is the author of* How to Collect More on Your Insurance Claims—Legally.

obtain adequate, affordable liability insurance.

While this was going on five years ago, an inflationary spiral was evolving which dramatically increased the cost of litigation and health care — major factors involved in the payment of liability losses. This coincided with a heightened public awareness of consumer rights in liability situations. Many lawsuits were generated and many claims were filed as the public decided to get its full share of compensation for the pain and suffering of an accident or for a product failure.

Then interest rates began to drop. Property and liability insurers found themselves in a crisis. They had to increase premiums and eliminate writing certain classes of business, such as medical malpractice, product liability, and pollution liability.

Making things worse were increasingly liberal court interpretations that delivered liability judgments never before contemplated. Imagine a New Year's reveler leaving a house party, crashing his automobile into a tree, and ultimately suing the homeowner, his host. Lawyers have been successful in suits in which it was shown that the homeowner was careless in overseeing the dispensing of alcohol.[1]

Improved 1987 operating figures for the property and casualty insurance companies reflected the results of their stringent underwriting practices. Happily, the situation is still improving, with rate relief available for consumers. The trend seems to be reverting to more reasonable rates in the property insurance field and for certain liability coverages, other than medical malpractice, products, and pollution coverage.[2]

Will a Frightened Industry Want to Respond to Legitimate Consumer Concerns?

The AIDS crisis is confounding the impact of this otherwise positive trend. As a result of this unprecedented disease, American consumers are finding it riskier to purchase adequate, affordable life and health insurance without giving away one of their most precious possessions, their privacy. Insurance companies, long the exemplars of corporate achievement, now have to contend with the impact of AIDS on the total mortality among their clients, a risk not contemplated when most of their insurance was sold and underwritten. Employers, worried about the infection spreading among their work force, have begun looking for loopholes in their fringe benefit packages, long a vested right for the U.S. worker. And, given the skyrocketing growth of AIDS cases, life and health insurance companies have begun to wonder how long they will be able to offer even the self-insured forms of coverage.

The biggest problem in the AIDS crisis — for the insurance industry — is viability in the face of a swelling claims experience. The biggest problem for consumers, however, is protecting themselves from the insurance industry as it decides how it is going to cope with the crisis. The early returns are not good for consumers. Instead of facing up to the problem, the insurance industry is treating the issue with benign neglect. Consumers' rights to privacy have been abused by secret testing for AIDS. Worse, people with other conditions — coronary artery disease, high blood pressure, cancer, diabetes, alcoholism, and mental illness, histories that ordinarily would not have prevented them from buying insurance, even if at a higher premium — are the victims of AIDS-related discriminatory practices spreading throughout the industry.

In the case of preferred risks, persons who have nothing significant in their medical histories are being asked to document in great length and detail minor sore throats and colds. Heretofore, these conditions were not considered by underwriters. But given the AIDS mentality, underwriters now fear the worst and are constantly vigilant about any condition, no matter how slight or how remote, in the event that it could be a by-product of the AIDS antibody.

Persons with controllable hypertension, successful recoveries from bypass surgery, and histories of elevated cholesterol and other abnormal blood chemistries are being looked at closer than ever, and are being accorded few accommodations by underwriters, who would prefer to err on the side of caution in the rating of substandard risks to compensate for any adverse mortality that could develop from AIDS-related claims for insureds already on the books.

In evaluating all of this turmoil, one must take cognizance of the pressures being applied to the insurance industry today. Gone is the era when the actuarial tables ruled, when policy sales leaped from year to year, and when the masses faithfully remitted their premiums, all to the glory and profit of the underwriters. Actuarial tables, commonly representing valid statistical data of the past combined with current actuarial assumptions about life expectancy, could be relied upon to predict future mortality — until now. They have been predictors of the future, but they have no accurate actuarial measurement of the adverse mortality of AIDS-related claims which could develop from not only risks on the books, but individuals who are tested and who could acquire the disease in the future.

Today, some companies are wondering how long they can last. Consider TransAmerica Occidental Life, whose senior vice president David Gooding has stated publicly that from 1982 to 1986 the AIDS risk in life insurance cost the industry twenty times what it would assume for a person who was healthy according to insurance industry standards.

Early in 1986, Gooding told the National Association of Insurance Commissioners that insurance companies must adopt new, carefully thought out policies and practices if they were to remain solvent and meet the claims of tens of millions of policyholders.[3]

Given the threat of AIDS-related claims, coupled with insurers' use of junk bonds, state regulators have begun to take notice. In January 1987 the New York State Insurance Department acted to better monitor the solvency of insurers in order to guarantee that funds would be available to provide the benefits promised to consumers. Authorizing Regulation 126, the department now requires life insurers to match assets with liabilities when evaluating annuities, annuity benefits, and guaranteed-interest contracts.[4]

New York, which was the first state to implement such stringent measures, felt they were necessary in order to prevent the occurrence in the insurance industry of something similar to a run on a bank. Regulation 126 assumes increased significance as long as insurers continue to use junk bonds as the investments backing the projected yields of certain insurance products.[5]

The required methodology is complex and highly technical and necessitates the use of various scenarios and projections by the actuaries to determine the insurance company cash flow when there are various fluctuations in interest rates and different demands for surrenders. The practice is intended to establish the appropriate safeguards to prevent a future drain on company surplus.

Meanwhile, the insurance business goes on. Companies continue to issue life and health policies with the full legal, moral, and fiduciary obligation to their stockholders to make a profit and underwrite prudently. Companies can, by right, accept and reject risks and set premiums according to sound underwriting practices. But this process does not include the right to condone a system that misleads, deceives, or abuses the privacy rights of any insurance applicant. This is the AIDS era, however, and there have been deceptions and abuses.

While the broad effect of AIDS on the insurance industry concerns both life and health coverage, the way in which this disease will impinge upon both companies and individuals who are struggling to provide health care to the afflicted is especially poignant. There is no better way to understand the personal impact of AIDS than by reading a letter like the following one, from an anonymous Boston reader of my column, "Insurance":

> My lover has AIDS. I think I could be a carrier of the AIDS antibody, but I have no intention of taking any blood tests. A positive test result would serve no useful purpose.
>
> My lover and I have insurance questions, as he is reaching the point where he can no longer work full-time. He plans to leave the state to return to his place of birth to die. I wish to relocate there with him. This will involve a change of jobs on my part. We're worried about the future of our health-care insurance and have questions about our coverage. We already know he will face thousands of dollars of expenses and I could be in the same boat, someday. It is difficult to get a direct answer from any credible source. We get a different story from everyone we speak to. We fear breaches of privacy if we make formal requests for the information we need. He is covered under an HMO (health maintenance organization) plan, I'm covered by Blue Cross–Blue Shield. Can you help us?[6]

This letter underscores the truly devastating human cost of AIDS. Imagine how the panic will grow as AIDS spreads more widely, into the heterosexual population, and millions of people suddenly begin to wonder who will pay for their medical costs, their living expenses, and the expenses and costs of their families. AIDS will become synonymous with another ugly word — bankruptcy. In fact, in many cases, it already has. Consider the following statistics:[7]

- The average medical costs associated with AIDS are $97,000 *per patient*. Recent studies found that average lifetime costs range from $45,000 in special managed-care situations to up to $140,000.

- As of January 18, 1988, the cumulative number of AIDS cases reported in the United States was 51,361. Of that number, 28,683 are known to have resulted in death, 56 percent of the total.

- By the end of 1991, 270,000 cumulative cases of AIDS will have been reported in the United States, 179,000 of them fatalities (58 percent). In a 1986 survey, the American Council of Life Insurance (ACLI) attempted to measure the extent of AIDS-related claims. Companies writing 46 percent of the life and health insurance coverage in the United States responded. Adjusting the figures to cover 100 percent of the people in the market, it is estimated that AIDS-related death claims in 1986 were about $292 million.

- The average AIDS death claim on individual policies was $30,500, compared with the average claim of $7,300 on all policies. (The lower figure represents policies that have been on the books for thirty years or more and whose value is unadjusted for inflation.)

The average group life claim has been $27,000 for AIDS-related cases; the average group health claim has been $13,800. The ACLI has said that the cost of health care associated with AIDS claims varies from $45,000 on the West Coast to $140,000 on the East Coast; the average claim is about $97,000, according to 1986 estimates.[8]

Insurance consultant Barbara Lautzenheiser is a former vice president of the Phoenix Mutual Life Insurance Company and a past president of the National Association of Actuaries. In a speech to life insurance underwriters in New Orleans in the spring of 1987, she detailed a chilling cost scenario:

> Assume that 100 men who are infected with the AIDS virus are issued insurance because of the insurance company's inability to test for the infection. Assume each is age 34 and purchases $100,000 of term insurance, the cheapest form of coverage that builds no cash values. The average premium for the next seven years for that form of coverage is $199 per year. Assume none of these persons dies for the whole of seven years, then 20 percent die (the lowest percent expressed by the Centers for Disease Control). The total death benefit payable is 20 x $100,000 equals $2 million.
>
> How can the insurance company afford to pay out $2 million when all it has collected is $139,300?[9]

And if this is not chilling enough, consider the facts quoted by Lautzenheiser from a January story in the *Navy Times* citing military research that suggests AIDS may kill 99.9 percent of those who are exposed to the AIDS virus.[10]

Comments by Dr. James Mason, director of the federal Centers for Disease Control (CDC) in Atlanta, Georgia, seem to confirm the degree of severity reported by the *Navy Times*. "If we observe these infected individuals long enough," said Dr. Mason, "a figure approximately 100 percent of those infected will develop symptoms of this disease, which is eventually fatal."[11]

That deadly prospect has the gay male community, especially in California, in a panic, Lautzenheiser told the audience of underwriters in New Orleans. "Their greatest concern is testing itself, because of fear of losing their jobs if the employer finds out they tested positive; fear of the test results being recorded by name, so that there is a list that can be subpoenaed and those on the list quarantined." Further, she said, "the issue now is money, through health insurance to pay their health-care costs and through health insurance to pay their 'partner's' health-care costs. Money will become even more important as the size of the gay community becomes smaller and their less costly self-support system vanishes."

Lautzenheiser had a warning for her insurance audience: The gay community is large and influential, and it votes. Many gay men donate substantial amounts of money to politicians who support their cause. Moreover, the gay male bloc is only one special-interest group. "What will the diabetic or cancer foundations do when they find out they have to pay substandard rates or can't get insurance when those infected with the AIDS virus can get insurance at standard rates?" she asked. "What about those with multiple sclerosis, muscular dystrophy, epilepsy, or any of the other diseases, particularly those which get high television visibility? Can't you see a Labor Day Telethon on how Jerry's Kids were discriminated against by the insurance industry?"[12]

These comments make an implicit statement about the cost of insuring a person with AIDS: Once a person has AIDS, it doesn't abate. He or she is always faced with the almost certain probability of dying. Therefore, a person with AIDS is uninsurable. In the case of heart attacks, for instance, there are all types and severities. People who have coronary attacks have the potential to recover; after five to eight years of recovery, they can usually buy insurance at standard rates. Depending on how young they are when the disease begins, diabetics have a more difficult time buying insurance. Juvenile diabetics are virtually uninsurable because of their high mortality rate. Persons between the ages of twenty and forty-five will pay heavy extra premiums; those between the ages of forty-five and sixty will pay moderate extra rates; persons over sixty will pay near-standard rates. Once a person is "rated" for diabetes, however, the surcharge is never removed.

Other temporary conditions that can cost extra premiums are hypertension, elevated cholesterol, and elevated triglycerides. In cases such as these, a change in lifestyle, a loss of weight, and strict adherence to a medical regimen can often result in an improved condition. That's usually enough of a reason for the insurer to consider reducing or eliminating any extra premium being charged.

AIDS cases, however, don't get less expensive, at least not yet. Consequently, the only recourse for many families and friends of persons with AIDS is to find ways to offer support. In Boston, the gay male community has, to its credit, provided help with specific activities. The AIDS Action Committee held fund-raisers and distributed more than $150,000 in FY'87 for direct financial assistance. Additionally, the committee provided many basic services not available from professionals, such as transportation, a meals-on-wheels program, practical home care and counseling services, and support from volunteer nonprofessionals.

In San Francisco, the gay male community has conducted similar volunteer programs. A California study showed that the cost of care for AIDS patients in San Francisco in their final eighteen months of life averaged $52,000 to $74,000, well below the national figure of $147,000 and the state's $65,000 to $110,000.[13]

The solution for most long-term AIDS sufferers is turning to government assistance. Most find themselves on welfare soon after beginning to suffer the most debilitating effects of the disease. Nationally, about 40 percent of AIDS patients turn to Medicaid, and their dependence becomes absolute on support such as food stamps, local welfare programs, Social Security Disability, and Supplemental Security income.

Nor is insurance the total answer to AIDS-related expenses, the sufferers and their families have found. One agency in New York City, Gay Men's Health Crisis, estimates that fewer than 30 percent of its clients with private health insurance will receive payments for prescription drugs. This statistic becomes more relevant to the AIDS patient as new and costlier drugs are developed each year. Treatments with AZT, a new drug that some say holds the best hope yet for treating AIDS, can cost up to $10,000 annually.[14]

The Testing Dilemma

Nowhere in the AIDS dilemma is the push-pull between business and humanitarian interests more evident than in the debate about testing. Insurance underwriters, bound by their responsibilities to directors and investors, will continue to press for unlimited testing. Rights activists, concerned that testing is a potential threat to civil liberty, will continue to call, at the very least, for limitations to general testing. Consultant Barbara Lautzenheiser has urged life insurance underwriters to work to block any legislation to ban AIDS testing. According to Lautzenheiser, any interference with AIDS testing poses a major threat to the risk classification system upon which the insurance industry bases its ability to approve or deny an application for insurance. With antitesting laws in place in California, Wisconsin, and Washington, D.C., she says, some companies have simply stopped issuing life insurance. "Washington, D.C.'s legislation is so severe — not even allowing a non-AIDS-specific test, called the T-cell test — [that a] Harvard University study reports that of the sample they took, 80 percent of the life insurance companies have ceased writing [policies] in the district. . . . California still allows the T-cell test, but one company announced on April 1 that it has withdrawn from that state, too."[15]

It remains to be seen whether company pullouts are for real or whether they are just a threat aimed at securing leverage with state legislatures and insurance commissioners who may be considering similar actions. It is expected that several state legislatures and insurance regulators will be called upon to act on some form of testing for their states during 1988. Testing, unfortunately for our civil liberties, is the insurance industry's most accurate method of identifying who among their potential policyholders is an AIDS threat. Every New England state except Connecticut has proposed legislation that, while controlling or limiting test procedures, would in fact allow testing to take place. In Massachusetts, an attempt by Insurance Commissioner Peter Hiam to be protective about AIDS testing eventually cost him his job.[16]

The practice of using blood testing as a general underwriting requirement on cases involving $1 million or more came about ten years ago, when life insurance companies discontinued the practice of requiring two examinations on two different days by two different medical examiners. Applicants complained about the inconvenience of the procedure and said that the second examination was simply a duplicate of the first. Worse, some companies discovered that they were being charged for a second examination that in fact had not been done. Underwriters decided that blood tests could give them more information and more protection than a second examination.

It became common, if a life insurance applicant had a history of an abnormal blood chemistry — indicative of diabetes, elevated cholesterol, gout, or an abnormal liver function — for a blood test to be taken at the time of the insurance examination. In that way, the company could determine whether there was any change in the applicant's condition. The underwriting of health insurance differs significantly from underwriting of life insurance. Most health insurance is issued on a group basis. For smaller groups, this usually covers all employees, without any medical examinations or blood tests, but with a "preexisting exclusion rider." This rider means that certain conditions that existed at the inception of a person's employment, or eligibility for group health coverage, will be covered only when a predetermined waiting period expires. The "contestable period" can be from three months to three years. (The use of the preexisting exclusion by health insurance underwriters, particularly at claim time, has always been a source of irritation for consumers who do not understand its beneficial significance. There have been cases in which consumers, at the time of application, have had cancer, AIDS, or cardiovascular ailments and have been unaware of these conditions, which would have escaped detection and treatment had there been no test.) For most larger groups, or in some health maintenance organizations, there is guaranteed-issue insurance, without any exclusions for claims and benefits due to preexisting conditions.

A relatively small amount of health insurance is sold on an individual basis. The pricing of individual health insurance does not lend itself to the use of physical examinations and blood testing as underwriting requirements. Rather, these cases are underwritten on the basis of medical information provided by the applicant. The applicant is asked to detail past and present illnesses and to provide the names and addresses of hospitals and doctors consulted.

From this information, health insurance underwriters can determine whether the applicant is eligible for coverage, is required to pay a penalty surcharge, or must be assigned a longer waiting period for a preexisting condition.

In December 1987, because of the exclusion-clause problems with insurance companies, Attorney General James Shannon of Massachusetts proposed a change in the preexisting conditions clause of that state's accident and health (A & H) insurance policies — a change that would make it harder for A & H insurers to deny coverage on this basis.[17] Shannon claimed that this change was based upon model language developed by the National Association of Insurance Commissioners.

In mid-1986, fearing the adverse effect of AIDS mortality, life insurers began to reduce the financial threshold at which blood tests would be required, even if there was no history of any abnormality to justify such testing. The testing threshold by December 1987 became $100,000 for most life insurers writing business in Massachusetts. On a number of cases in the fall of 1986, some companies were already using this lower threshold on smaller policies to get the client's blood and test it, without his or her informed consent, for the AIDS antibody.[18]

I brought this to the attention of Commissioner Hiam, who said he would enforce his strict regulation banning blood testing and that he would look into this new development. He had made it clear in the past that testing for the AIDS antibody would not be tolerated in Massachusetts. Most insurers complied with the regulation, but others continued the practice, as a way of testing the insurance commissioner's authority to tell them how to conduct business. If they conceded to Hiam on an arbitrary ruling, they reasoned, then they could eventually lose control of their underwriting prerogatives.[19]

In March 1987, Ronald N. Shehade, manager of American Para Professional Systems of Wellesley, a company that draws blood samples for testing, told me: "Laboratory technicians in the field no longer have control over the blood samples. The lab does not acknowledge receipt of the sample, they do not furnish us or you [the insurance applicant] with the results, nor can we or you obtain these results."

Writing about this situation a year ago, I advised consumers to confirm with their insurance agents which tests have been requested from the laboratory, while keeping in mind that the tests vary by company.[20] (Today, however, some laboratories will provide a confirmation describing the tests that might be done.)

At worst, by attempting to influence blood-testing requirements and procedures, some insurers are ignoring the root causes of the disease. Some of them are hiding their heads in the shifting sands of circumstance, pain, and desperation. AIDS is here to stay. If a fail-safe blood test, one that completely eliminated false-positive results, were ever to become available, insurance companies would be in a better position to justify their legitimate concerns about blood screening for the AIDS antibody being a component part of the life underwriting process.

Nevertheless, when testing is a requirement for life insurance, insurers should be more candid with their applicants, telling them just what they expect from persons who buy insurance and why they have established those underwriting guidelines which are in use. They should make it clear to all applicants exactly what will be done with their blood sample after it is drawn, even though in Massachusetts, such disclosure is not mandatory. They should explain the reasons for and the types of tests to be performed by the laboratory on the samples drawn. Most important, they should explain to the insurance applicant how they will guarantee the protection of his or her privacy as reports of the test filter down through the underwriting process.

These things are necessary not only for the financial protection of the public, whose loved ones may — almost certainly will — feel the sting of the AIDS crisis, but also for the protection of the companies that must insure them as well. This is a situation in which the survival of the insurance industry is at stake. The most certain element in all of this is that the future can't be left to insurance industry management, which at times speaks out of both sides of its mouth — crying poverty when looking for legislative help, then becoming aggressive and throwing out the rate books when competing for a sale.[21]

From December 1986 to June 1987, representatives of the insurance commissioner's office carried on negotiations with the insurance industry to develop a fair and equitable blood-testing policy in Massachusetts. In a proposed compromise, insurers would be allowed to underwrite their business and eliminate and screen any applicant who might have AIDS, while preserving the rights of individuals who knowingly agreed to submit to the test.

Negotiations broke down, and because of the politics involved, Hiam resigned on the eve of the issuance of Governor Michael S. Dukakis's blood-testing plan. That plan was opposed by the industry, because it required blood testing in applications for more than $100,000 of life insurance and imposed an onerous administrative burden on companies to enforce the very rigid requirement of privacy and confidentiality spelled out in the proposed regulation. Persons applying for less than $100,000 do not face a mandatory blood test requirement.

Consumer groups opposed the plan, primarily because of the privacy risks involved in submitting to blood testing. In my newspaper column, I suggested to the governor an alternative that would make available insurance that would exclude any death benefit if death were due to AIDS and for which no blood testing would be required.[22]

Insurers licensed to do business in Massachusetts (with one exception) opposed the concept. They felt that once a policy was in effect for more than two years, they could not contest the circumstances surrounding the death and its preceding events. The companies charged that doctors declared other causes of death, such as pneumonia and various forms of cancer, to mask real cause of death — AIDS — in an attempt to protect the family's privacy.

Proponents of an AIDS exclusion option say it would save insurance companies millions of dollars spent on testing procedures, laboratory fees, lengthy investigative consumer reports, and costly underwriting practices. These funds would then be available to reduce the cost of insurance for all consumers. No insurance industry–related job would be lost, and the insurance companies would continue to invest millions of dollars in the economy through their financing, building, and investments. Opponents of eliminating coverage for AIDS say that once a policy has gone beyond the "contestable period," the insurer has no right to investigate the circumstances surrounding a death. This is a problem because, in many cases, death certificates for AIDS in fact do not tell the true story.

Further, opponents argue, consumers who have no reason to believe they are infected with AIDS would no longer be inhibited from applying for life insurance because of the potential adverse consequences of a test. After insurance had been issued, there would be nothing to prevent an individual from taking an AIDS antibody test on a confidential basis. Even better, individuals with the AIDS antibody, who ordinarily would not be able to buy life insurance, would be able to insure themselves for accidental death or for death caused by other illnesses, such as stroke, heart attack, or cancer.

Apart from the obvious medical and psychosocial impact of the disease, what better deterrent could a person have to avoid behavior that could result in AIDS than the knowledge that life insurance would become void upon death? What better educational technique could the federal government implement than loss of life insurance for policyholders who develop AIDS?

Savings Bank Life Insurance adopted my recommendation, and it was approved by the new insurance commissioner, Roger M. Singer, when he promulgated another set of AIDS-testing regulations, after two days of hearings (which brought considerable opposition). As of December 1987, Savings Bank Life Insurance had written more than $1.7 billion of life insurance coverage on Massachusetts residents which excludes coverage for AIDS.

In early October 1987, the Massachusetts Superior Court granted the life and health insurance industry a preliminary injunction against Singer's AIDS regulations. Under the order, the commissioner was prevented from implementing and enforcing his testing rules.[23]

"Failure to issue the injunctive relief prayed for will subject the plaintiffs to a substantial risk of irreparable harm," the court said. "This loss will be immediate and consist of not only unquantifiable economic losses, but loss of good will, deprivation of property rights, and a restraint of the plaintiffs' ability to compete."

The ruling continued: "There is also a serious question raised that the regulation is in violation of the Equal Protection provision of the U.S. Constitution, as well as an unconstitutional delegation of legislative powers under the Massachusetts Constitution."

Perhaps as a warning about the uncertainties of the legal process, the court also remarked: "It appears clear that there is a substantial possibility that the plaintiffs will be successful after a full hearing on the merits."[24]

Now that the battle lines are drawn, insurance applicants are at the mercy of the insurers, who say they are only exercising their legitimate rights and are testing for the AIDS antibody whenever possible.

This controversy can be expected to be played out in the courts for some time. No matter what decision is reached in the Massachusetts Superior Court, it is virtually certain that the case will ultimately land in the U.S. Supreme Court.

The insurance industry is bringing its heavy guns to battle in the Massachusetts courts. It believes that Massachusetts is a bellwether state in the insurance industry — as Massachusetts goes, so goes the nation.

Appreciating the potential liability exposure involved in blood testing, various insurers, including John Hancock, Northwestern, and Massachusetts Mutual Life Insurance Company, have prepared self-serving brochures that are handed to applicants to assuage any concern about the reliability of the testing and the confidentiality of the results. A look at "Why Am I Being Tested?" — a portion of a Mass Mutual brochure issued late in 1987 — illustrates the point:

> *Question:* Am I being tested because Mass Mutual thinks I have AIDS?
>
> *Answer:* No. In fact, the Company believes it very unlikely. It is anticipated that the overwhelming percentage (well over 99 percent) of the AIDS antibody tests performed will be negative. [This would seem to underline the concern that there will be false-positive test results.]

Under "What If My Blood Test Comes Back Positive?" we find:

Question: Will positive results from the AIDS antibody test also be sent automatically to the MIB [the Medical Information Bureau, a supersecret and highly computerized industry information clearinghouse whose headquarters are in Westwood]?

Answer: Yes, but the HIV antibody test results do not have a specific code; they fall under a catchall code used for any blood abnormality that does not have a code of its own. This code indicates that an abnormality has been found, but does not specify which type.

This answer by Mass Mutual, which represents the industry's current practice, puts people who have blood abnormalities that are not terminal or life-threatening in the same category as a carrier of the AIDS antibody, a pure and simple form of reverse discrimination.

To Peter Hiam, the insurance industry's early call for widespread testing demonstrated its panic. Cognizant of the enormous social and economic implications of a positive AIDS test, not to mention the high potential for a false-positive or false-negative test result, Hiam banned testing in Massachusetts. Barbara Lautzenheiser was well aware of Hiam's actions: "Apparently the Massachusetts Insurance Commissioner doesn't read the newspapers," she chided in her New Orleans speech last spring. "As of April 20, there were 34,513 cases [of AIDS]. That's 2,531 since March 9. That's 60 new cases per day," said the concerned insurance consultant. What was worse, she said, the Centers for Disease Control expected up to 18,000 new cases of AIDS in 1986. Actually, there were only 13,197 new cases that year.

"The number of cases is still doubling," said Lautzenheiser, "but only over 24 months instead of every year. Just think of what I've said — *only* every 2 years doubling instead of every year. That's still horrendous. . . . I don't think the insurers are reacting in haste. I think they are reacting in waste — wasted time for action."[25]

Further proof that the insurance industry is well within its rights to call for testing, Lautzenheiser said, was that the gay male community — the group with the highest risk factor — has called for the greater availability of insurance for AIDS victims, even if the insurance is offered on a more expensive assigned risk pool concept, if testing positive is not considered a preexisting condition. However, "[homosexual men] do not want testing to be a surrogate for classification by sexual orientation," Lautzenheiser said.

Now contrast Lautzenheiser's views with those of Massachusetts state representative David B. Cohen, writing in the *Boston Globe* in August 1987. Citing figures developed by his office in the summer of 1987 from statistics available from the Massachusetts Division of Insurance, Cohen said the following:

> There is little evidence to support giving AIDS tests to applicants for life insurance. For all of the dire predictions that a flood of AIDS-related death claims would sweep insurers into insolvency, the fiscal impact of the disease on the industry has been minuscule. In Massachusetts, out of more than $1.5 billion in death claims, only $551,000 has been related to AIDS. This amounts to about 15 cents per policy per year. While insurers are quick to point out that the incidence of AIDS may triple by 1991, even a tenfold increase in claims payouts in that time would still amount to only $1.50 per policy per year. At the same time, it costs $50 per policy to test for the AIDS virus.[26]

An illustration of the "great debate" going on about the AIDS testing issue came in June 1987 in an edition of the *Sunday Boston Herald*.[27] The editors contrasted, on a single tabloid page, the viewpoints of pro- and anti-testing advocates. Calling for use of "all appropriate tools at our disposal" to help the nation meet the AIDS crisis was William Bennett, the U.S. secretary of education. Warning that public health can be guarded only "by protecting confidentiality and prohibiting discrimination" was U.S. Rep. Henry Waxman, the Democrat from California.

The salient points of argument from the article:

> *Bennett:* Even if routine testing drove a few individuals underground, this would have to be balanced against the crucial need for information that more widespread testing would produce for individuals and for society, information that would save lives.
>
> *Waxman:* We cannot expect people to respond to medical advice if in doing so they jeopardize their jobs, housing, insurance, privacy, children, families and their futures. Misuse of testing and test results could damage the nation's ability to study and understand the AIDS epidemic. What we know about the disease we know because gay men and AIDS patients have volunteered to cooperate with research. If misguided testing drives these people underground, it will only prolong the epidemic.
>
> *Bennett:* Precautions can be taken to guard against violating confidentiality, particularly in identifying sexual partners. This is already being done in many states in cases involving venereal disease.
>
> *Waxman:* Testing policy is uncertain. While the Public Health Service has issued statements opposing discrimination against people who test positive, the Justice Department says discrimination is legal and not the government's problem, even when based on irrational fears. The mixed policy means only individuals who either have nothing to lose or already have the disease will seek testing. Persons who might have been exposed to AIDS and those who might be infectious will avoid testing.
>
> *Bennett:* AIDS tests are not unreliable. In the rare case where a false positive result occurs, this can be resolved by using a follow-up test.
>
> *Waxman:* The test does not indicate who is sick. It pinpoints most, but not all, persons who have been exposed and who are probably infectious. Because the disease is transmitted only by sex and blood, the medical usefulness of tests is limited to blood banks, the individual tested and his or her sexual partners.

In a summation, Waxman stated his fears about a "nightmarish" situation: "Black-market blood tests, forged ID cards, bribed officials, safe houses and fugitives," all the result of the tyranny of mandatory testing. "A testing policy that does not guarantee that test results will be used fairly and respectfully will be recognized as the house-to-house search that it is. Programs that test, fire and quarantine people will make our America into Anne Frank's Europe," the congressman wrote.

With all the controversy that the issue has created, with differing opinions expressed by consumers, government, and the insurance industry, the health insurance industry, meanwhile, continues to worry about statistics that estimate claims costs in AIDS cases can run up to $100,000 a year per case. While health insurers realize they are already covering active workers who are carriers of the AIDS antibody, they say a greater threat is posed by giving insurance to new applicants who could be known or unknown carriers of AIDS.

Blue Cross–Blue Shield, whose health insurance covers 55 percent of the Massachusetts market, says that, for now, it has no plans to require testing for AIDS. It will continue to pay for the treatment and hospitalization of AIDS and any FDA-approved medications, including AZT. That coverage is subject to the terms and conditions of the individual subscriber's coverage.

According to Dr. James Young, vice president and medical director of Blue Cross–Blue Shield in Massachusetts, handling this problem in any other manner, including blood testing, would be contrary to the mission and role of Blue Cross in the marketplace. Blue Cross, he notes, was established to spread the actuarial risks throughout its entire membership.[28]

Consumers should not expect such generous treatment from the commercial health insurers. These companies have fiduciary obligations to operate profitably, and they can be expected to attack the AIDS problem on two fronts. Existing business, they say, will experience significant rate increases, more restrictive waiting periods, and tougher pre-existing exclusion riders for new employees. They will also attempt to make policy deductibles a percentage of an employee's income. Finally, commercial insurers will attempt to require AIDS blood tests for new employees in certain health insurance programs.

The informational authorization you provide when applying for insurance will also take on new meaning in the AIDS era. Few insurance applicants realize that when they sign an insurance application they also sign a privacy release that relates not only to information on the form itself, but also to facts that may be uncovered during the investigation of their medical history.

The typical authorization seems simple enough: "I hereby authorize any licensed physician, medical practitioner, hospital, clinic or other medically related facility, insurance company, any medical information bureau or other organization, institution, or person having any records or knowledge of me or my health to give the insurance company any such information. A photocopy of this signed authorization shall be valid as the original." In plain English, this statement means: "I authorize anybody with any knowledge about me to give this knowledge to the insurance company." Nowhere does it limit information strictly to the applicant's insurability or ability to pay premiums. The validity of the authorization is not time-limited on most authorization forms.

Consumers who decide to go forward with their insurance should ask ahead of time to see the blood authorization forms and should ask clarifying questions. They are entitled to determine ahead of time what test is deemed necessary by the insurer and whether it includes an AIDS antibody test. If the AIDS antibody test is going to be taken, the company should say so. It should not hide behind the phrase "such testing as may be deemed necessary."[29]

The important thing here is that, while insurance companies have a right to remain financially viable, consumers have a right to know what is going to happen to their privacy and what is going to happen to their blood. After that information has been ascertained, consumers can decide whether to buy insurance from a particular company or whether to find another company that does not require a blood test.

The Privacy Issue

There is no question that once a person admits on an insurance application that he or she has taken an AIDS test, insurance underwriters will always consider that person's health suspect. The underwriter will want to know the reason for the test. Was the applicant concerned that sexual promiscuity caused exposure to the AIDS virus? Was the decision to take the test due to a blood transfusion? Did another underwriter require the test because of the consumer's lifestyle? Whatever the answers, the key to the privacy issue, from an insurance point of view, is understanding that underwriters are trained to err on the side of caution.

In an attempt to help settle the emotional outcry about AIDS, the National Insurance Commissioners Association has created an Advisory Committee on the disease. A member of the committee has offered the following guidelines for testing:

- Prior informed consent must be secured from the applicant regarding the antibody test.
- Insurance companies must apply the test on a nondiscriminatory basis, not on the basis of sexual orientation.
- Health insurance should be available for all persons who test positive.
- All insurance companies should set a specific minimum amount of insurance above which testing would be mandatory.
- Insurance companies should be allowed to test only if the laws of the particular state do not require reporting positive test results to the state health department.

The committee is also concerned that sexual orientation should not be used by insurance companies to make underwriting decisions. Some suggested guidelines for medical and lifestyle questions to be used by insurers are as follows:

- The marital status or living arrangements of insurance applicants should not be used to establish the applicant's sexual orientation.
- The question of gender should not be used to help determine the sexual orientation of the applicant or for further investigation of the applicant.
- Insurance companies should not establish "redlined" districts in which coverage would be denied, as is sometimes done in underwriting fire insurance.
- No applicant for life or health insurance should be rejected because he or she has sought advice or counsel about AIDS from health care professionals.

These are all good suggestions and would go a long way toward settling the AIDS panic that is appearing in more and more segments of American society, both private and commercial. There is no doubt that people who seek insurance have a right to be concerned. If an insurance company in Massachusetts requests a blood test, chances are excellent that the applicant's blood sample will be tested for AIDS. In Kansas, the Home Office Reference Laboratory, whose facilities are used by 85 percent of the nation's insurers, confirmed this in 1986. Several dozen of the more than three hundred companies operating in

Massachusetts, the laboratory said, were requesting AIDS-related tests without the applicants' knowledge.[30]

If there is nothing in an insurance applicant's background to justify such a blood test, and if the insurance seeker wants to avoid the stigma associated with AIDS testing, several options are available. A blood test taken by the applicant's own physician, during an annual checkup, say, is usually acceptable. The applicant should check with different insurers for their testing policies. And there's nothing wrong with the applicant's personal physician using his or her office laboratory to perform the test. Finally, applicants can insist that the insurance company provide them with a letter certifying that the company will not test their blood for the AIDS antibody.

The harsh reality of the privacy issue in the AIDS era, however, is that the implicit confidentiality between doctor and patient may no longer exist. This issue was discussed as early as 1985 in a Washington publication, the *Privacy Journal,* which saw four distinct categories of threats to confidentiality:

> First, one's status as a patient with the disease; second, results of blood test possibly showing that an individual carries the AIDS virus and may spread the disease, even though he himself does not have it and may never have it; third, one's identity as a donor of blood, a confidential status now threatened because infected blood transfusions are thought to be one way in which the disease spreads; and finally, one's sexual preference.[31]

The journal makes the point that "everybody seems to want to know who the AIDS patients are," and reminds us that in earlier times, lepers were required to wear warning bells.[32] (That was really an invasion of privacy!)

Perhaps the biggest threat to privacy comes with the increasingly prevalent insurance or job application question, "Do you engage in homosexual activities?" The appearance of AIDS on the medical and insurance horizon gave justification to a horde of officials who would like to have just this sort of information for their files. The tragedy, the *Privacy Journal* notes, is that "this comes at a time when one's sexual preference had just been generally accepted as one's own business, even though there are few, if any, statutes or court decisions recognizing such a right of confidentiality."[33]

Lack of confidentiality in medical records is another issue that has blossomed along with the AIDS epidemic. Despite the alleged protection of medical records, particularly those records which are involved in underwriting life and health insurance, there is no guarantee that such derogatory information can be kept secure. The most prominent keeper of such information for the insurance industry, the Medical Information Bureau, has frequently asserted that its information has not been used in any way that is harmful to insurance applicants.

Founded in 1902, the MIB has stored in its Boston computer information on more than 12 million Americans. If you discount the data-processing system the Social Security Administration uses for programs like Medicare, the MIB probably qualifies as the largest information network in the medical field. Insurance companies that belong to the MIB — those which write most of the life insurance in the United States — can receive your file in less than thirty minutes, at a cost of less than $1 per inquiry. Part of the authorization on a policy application is permission for the insurance company to go to the MIB for your file — and for the company to give the MIB a report on you.

The MIB says that this information exchange is necessary to provide insurance companies with safeguards against those who may hide medical facts about themselves in order to gain lower premiums than they would ordinarily be assigned. The MIB does not record specific underwriting decisions, but it does record the content of specific insurance company reports. It maintains that strict rules guarantee confidentiality within its organization and among its member companies, and that it makes every effort to keep its files accurate.

Despite these guarantees, the MIB cannot be depended upon to protect personal privacy, according to some privacy advocates who have criticized the agency. The insurance companies say that the bureau maintains numerous secret codes through which it can enter a derogatory note about an insurance applicant. Yet the MIB refuses to make known to consumers either the conditions that call for such an entry or the codes themselves. According to Neil Day, MIB president, it is in the public's best interest not to have the code list and related data made public. This policy, he says, is consistent with the MIB's primary concern: the high level of confidentiality the agency says it has maintained for many years.

Unlike the federal government, the insurance industry does not classify underwriting data and consumer files with any degree of sophisticated security protection or safeguard from access by any unauthorized personnel. There are no shredders who destroy sensitive medical and mental health information and all types of blood test results. Blanket, unlimited authorizations can be photocopied at any time.

The Federal Privacy Act of 1974 created the Privacy Protection Study Commission. For two years, the panel conducted a review of individual privacy rights which included an examination of the medical-record-keeping practices of the insurance industry. Reporting to President Jimmy Carter in 1977, the commission said its findings and recommendations could serve to safeguard a person's right to be fairly treated, and to be spared unwarranted intrusion.

A major recommendation of the commission's report was that no insurance company should ask, require, or induce an individual to sign any statement authorizing any individual or any institution to disclose information about him or her unless that statement was specific as to its expiration date, which should be reasonable — not to exceed one year, and, in the case of life insurance and noncancelable or guaranteed-renewable health insurance, two years after the date of the policy.

That recommendation has been implemented in a handful of states, including Virginia, California, and Connecticut, as part of state privacy laws. Thus far, Massachusetts has refused to enact similar privacy legislation. This may change, however, when the 1988 state legislature considers a bill filed by the state Insurance Department called the Insurance Information and Privacy Protection Act. This law would pertain to all forms of insurance — life, health, disability, property, and casualty.

The law would protect all data obtained by an underwriter as an applicant sought insurance. Limitations pertaining to informed consent and time periods have been recommended for applicants' medical authorization forms. And the manner in which personal information can be collected by third parties has been defined, with protection afforded the consumer.

Some insurers have voluntarily amended required authorization forms to conform to provisions mandated in states with privacy laws. Most insurers doing business in Massachusetts, however, still require consumers to sign authorization forms that have no expiration date.

And so, the abuse of consumers' privacy goes on in Massachusetts, as insurers continue to use unauthorized practices to detect potential AIDS cases. How can applicants be expected to trust insurers when their record of deceit is known? What the consumer comes away with is the knowledge that the investigatory authorizations they sign are misleading and deceptive and carry erroneous implications that the signer has given the insurer consent.

Now that the Massachusetts courts have sided with the insurance industry and have prevented the implementation of Insurance Commissioner Singer's more cautionary AIDS blood-testing policy, the deadly antibody is fair game for all insurers selling life insurance. Even consumers applying for modest amounts of life insurance are going to be threatened. There will be the usual blood profile — previously the only requirement in million-dollar cases or where there was suspicion of an abnormal blood chemistry. But now there will be an AIDS test and, in some cases, a drug screening.

The insurers' position, as noted earlier, is that liver cancer, diabetes, and kidney diseases have been discovered during a blood screen, conditions that would not have been spotted were it not for the threat of AIDS. If the consumer is going to be given a free test that could reveal life-threatening problems, they argue, isn't the AIDS test worth the risk?

The answer is, not really. Consumers can have blood tests taken by their personal physician and avoid the potential loss of privacy, the effect of an unauthorized disclosure of false positives, and the impact on their insurability and employment.

Until legislation is enacted to clarify these authorization forms, all consumers are in jeopardy. For example, the form provided by the Prudential Insurance–owned GIB Laboratories of Newark, New Jersey, says the following:

> The blood drawn from you today will be sent to GIB Laboratories, where it will be subjected to such testing as deemed necessary or desirable by the requesting insurance company. This may include testing for human T-cell lymphotropic virus-type III antibodies, associated with acquired immunodeficiency syndrome (unless precluded by law). The results of the testing will be reported to the requesting insurance company for use by it and/or its affiliates in considering you for insurance. These results may also be reported to any reinsurer, to other companies to whom you apply for insurance or submit claims, and to the Medical Information Bureau for the use and purposes set forth in the notice on your application for insurance.

The form provided by the insurance industry's largest blood-testing facility — the Home Office Reference Laboratory — tells you that HORL will perform some or all tests (if permitted by law) on the basis of standing instructions from the insurance company. The tests include blood profile, T-cell count and ratio, hemoglobic ALC, apoliproprotein, full drug screen, CBC, and HIV (HTLV-III) antibody screen.

Again, there is an attempt to deceive the applicant. If the standing instructions from the insurance company call for a full drug screening and an AIDS antibody screening, the consumer should be told. He should not be misled into thinking that because he has led a clean life, the insurer will not test his blood for drugs or the AIDS antibody.

Searching for Solutions

With AIDS-related discord growing daily among the public, the insurance industry, and the industry's regulators, government agencies have attempted to develop solutions to the problems that the disease presents to all segments of society. None of these efforts have been completely successful; some have been rejected or modified to the point where matters have returned to pre-action status in several states. There is no easy solution. Whatever attempts are made to track the disease and provide for its costs are bound to meet with civil and human rights objections, regulatory and health service omissions and violations of policy, and violations of policies already established by existing statutes. The courts, indeed, have not heard the last of the AIDS issue.

If insurance companies are to be believed, the only legitimate concern underlying their demands to test life insurance applicants for AIDS is an effort to avoid insuring individuals with a limited life expectancy. No one, even unfortunates who have the dread disease, can quarrel with that reasoning. The public realizes that no insurer wants to write fire insurance on a burning building.

But until the federal government or state governments can establish pools to provide life insurance for uninsurable applicants — carriers of AIDS and persons who have terminal cancer and other terminal conditions — these persons will have to seek coverage through guaranteed-issue forms of group insurance, or make other arrangements to protect their estates.

However important it may be, the issue raised by the insurers in the AIDS-testing controversy — the need to underwrite for a profit and to protect policyholders and shareholders from adverse financial consequences — is not their entire concern. This is a public relations ploy used to conceal the real issue.

An examination of the Dukakis administration's proposed testing regulations, whose implementation is ultimately dependent upon the decision of the courts, shows that insurers not only want to keep out AIDS-infected applicants, but also persons whose lifestyle includes promiscuous sexual behavior or drug use that could ultimately result in becoming infected with the virus. The thirty-three-page proposal, in fact, represents the potential for the greatest bad for the greatest number of persons. The section entitled "Prohibited Practices" contains the crux of the regulations:

- No insurer shall make any underwriting decision on the basis of nationality, sexual orientation or proxies for sexual orientation such as lifestyle, living arrangements, marital status, beneficiary designation, employment, and residence. This means an applicant may not be denied insurance coverage, charged an additional premium or be requested or required to submit to AIDS-related tests on the basis of any of these factors. To the extent that employment, residence, or marital status [is] used in a manner that is clearly unrelated to sexual orientation, it may be used for underwriting purposes to the extent such use is permitted under any other applicable law or regulation.

- No insurer shall seek to elicit, either directly or through an investigation conducted by another on its behalf, any information designed to determine an applicant's sexual orientation. It is also the insurer's duty to inform its staff and any other support organization about any such information included in any report or otherwise communicated.

- Insurers shall not use the fact that an individual has sought or received counseling related to AIDS or AIDS-related complex to deny coverage or otherwise evaluate insurability. Insurers are prohibited from seeking information specifically related to AIDS or ARC counseling either on an application or in the course of their investigations.

Included in the proposed regulation is an elaborate provision designed to safeguard the confidentiality of all information pertaining to AIDS-related blood testing. Severe penalties are recommended for violation of these provisions. That's all fine, but what about protection of the confidentiality of results of other types of blood tests and other records pertaining to consumers' physical and mental health which represent a component part of their life insurance file? These are those sensitive psychiatric histories, confinements in alcoholic rehabilitation clinics, coronary and cancer histories, and blood tests involving abnormal blood chemistries.

Insurers in Massachusetts, meanwhile, continue to duck and dodge the AIDS bullet. Some insurers plan to avoid becoming embroiled in controversy and costly lawsuits by increasing the size of their minimum policy to $125,000 or $150,000, well above the minimum testing requirement threshold. To avoid attacks by the civil libertarians, they will be forced to determine the lifestyle risk solely on the basis of the blood test results. In another move we'll see more of, group life insurance underwriters who are denied the opportunity to test applicants for AIDS can be expected to substantially reduce the amounts of guaranteed-issue life insurance coverage provided under their contracts. And the cost of term insurance — a temporary, inexpensive coverage — for applicants under age forty can be expected to dramatically increase in order to compensate insurance companies for the added costs of blood tests and confidentiality compliance in the proposed Massachusetts regulations.

Finally, consumers who relied on their group insurance for the major portion of their life insurance protection will have to turn to the individual market, one that will effectively be discriminating against the young buyer of smaller policies. Policies in amounts of $100,000 or less will be scarce, and the cost of term policies that will be available can be expected to increase by as much as 50 percent.

In the absence of any short-term medical breakthrough that could provide a cure for AIDS, we can only hope that the Massachusetts courts will resolve the testing issue before them so that the rights of Massachusetts insurance consumers will be protected. This means that whenever insurers intend to test for the AIDS antibody, consumers should be so advised. Only responsible, experienced blood laboratories should be used, and every effort should be employed to preserve the confidentiality of the test results.

In a decision that is indicative of the income that AIDS screening could develop, Transamerica Occidental Life earlier this year said that it is going to finance and will be part owner of a new testing laboratory for insurance companies.

James Dederer, Transamerica senior vice president, said that his company's initial startup capital contribution will be approximately $9 million. He said that the new laboratory, one of three in the United States that will serve insurance companies exclusively, will focus on future markets as the demand for services increases. Transamerica is teaming up with Jim Osborn, who pioneered the use of blood profiles in underwriting and was the founder of the Home Office Reference Laboratory, which he sold in 1983 to Business Men's Assurance Company.

Osborn said that in 1987, approximately 1 million tests were performed for insurance purposes, generating about $1 million in revenues. "If most insurance companies shift to testing at the $100,000 level, a trend which is already well under way," he noted, "the potential market will be over 5 million tests annually."

The Life Insurance Marketing Research Association reports that only about 2 percent of the 17.1 million life insurance policies written in 1985 provided coverage of $300,000 or more, while 25 percent were for $100,000 or more. Some have estimated that AIDS screening alone could produce $500 million a year in the testing business within a few years.[34]

Despite assurances from David Carpenter, chairman and chief executive officer of Transamerica Occidental, that confidentiality is a critical factor, particularly with the AIDS crisis, and that precautions will be taken to ensure such privacy, the very fact that at least two insurers could have access to blood-testing results — as could happen when Transamerica tests for other insurers — raises additional legitimate consumer concerns about privacy.

Industry spokesperson Barbara Lautzenheiser was asked whether entry to a blood-testing file by another insurer would be considered a conflict of interest and a detriment to consumer interest — since the risk of privacy abuse would increase because both the insurance company being applied to *and* a competing insurer would have access to the test results. She responded that because of consumers' legitimate concerns, Transamerica would be extra-sensitive to the need for adequate privacy controls and confidentiality.

As we approach the presidential nominating conventions of the Democratic and Republican Parties, one has to wonder how many of the candidates may have already foregone the opportunity to purchase additional life insurance, the need for which has been created by campaign debts incurred and the risks inherent in the job they seek. No doubt, they have been reluctant to take the required insurance company blood test to determine the presence of the AIDS antibody, because of the fear that a false-positive result could immediately destroy their candidacy.

Notes

1. Benjamin Lipson, "A sharp eye on the bar helps reduce holiday liability blues," *Boston Globe,* 26 November 1987.
2. Joseph Albert, president, J. S. Albert International, Needham, Massachusetts, quoted in the *Boston Globe,* 14 December 1987.
3. Lipson, "AIDS: Industry Survival Is At Stake," speech, Laventhol & Horwath 1987 Insurance Crisis Conference, New York City, April 1987; reprinted, *National Underwriter,* 23 March 1987, 21–25.
4. Robert J. Callahan, chief, New York State Actuarial Bureau, at enactment of Regulation 126.
5. Ibid.
6. Lipson, "AIDS coverage like getting fire policy on burning building," *Boston Globe,* 12 March 1987.
7. U.S. Public Health Service, *Public Health Service Plan for the Prevention and Control of AIDS and the AIDS Virus,* Report of the Coolfront Planning Conference, 4–6 June 1986, 5.
8. Interview, Robert Waldron, director, American Council of Life Insurance, New York office, January 1988.
9. "Insurers Told to Fight AIDS Tests Bans," *National Underwriter,* 25 May 1987, 23.
10. "AIDS Virus Spreads to Philippine Prostitutes," *Navy Times,* 5 January 1987.
11. "AIDS, a Medical Update," a speech by Dr. James Mason, director, Centers for Disease Control, presented at the 1987 Annual Meeting of the American Council of Life Insurance, Washington, D.C., 1987.
12. Ibid., 29.
13. Phyllis Schiller Myers, *Journal of American Society of CLU & ChFC,* May 1987, 78.

14. Roger Ricklefs, "AIDS Victims Find That a Death Sentence Leads First to Poverty," *Wall Street Journal,* 5 August 1987, 1.

15. *National Underwriter,* 25 May 1987, 22.

16. *Boston Globe,* 9 July 1987, 1.

17. *Standard* (Quincy, Mass.), 18 December 1987, 5.

18. Michael Kranish, "AIDS testing assailed by insurance chief," *Boston Globe,* 29 November 1986, 1.

19. Douglas M. Bailey, "State vows to fight insurer AIDS tests," *Boston Globe,* 25 December 1986, 1.

20. Lipson, "Agents face ethical dilemma in the AIDS era," *Boston Globe,* 12 March 1987.

21. Lipson, Laventhol & Horwath speech.

22. Lipson, "An open letter to Dukakis: There is a way out of AIDS-testing dilemma," *Boston Globe,* 9 July 1987.

23. Judge Robert Steadman, *Boston Globe,* 3 October 1987, 1.

24. Ibid.

25. *National Underwriter,* 25 May 1987, 23.

26. "AIDS insurance hysteria," *Boston Globe,* 29 August 1987, 15.

27. "AIDS: To test or not to test?" *Boston Herald,* 28 June 1987, 34.

28. Lipson, "AIDS claims expected to have effect on health coverage, too," *Boston Globe,* 2 April 1987.

29. "Testing for AIDS could become part of insurers' tests," *Boston Globe,* 19 November 1987.

30. Kranish, "AIDS testing assailed by insurance chief."

31. "In the AIDS epidemic, confidentiality takes a beating," *Privacy Journal,* Washington, D.C., September 1985.

32. Ibid.

33. Ibid., 4.

34. *National Underwriter,* 11 January 1988.

Postscript

On June 10, 1988, the Massachusetts Superior Court upheld the state's regulations that limit insurance companies' testing of applicants for exposure to the AIDS virus. The regulations ban testing of applicants for health insurance and for any group health, life, and disability insurance. However, the state allows insurance companies, under tightly controlled conditions, to require the blood tests of applicants for individual life insurance and noncancelable disability insurance for policies in excess of $100,000. Insurers are required to write life insurance policies of up to $100,000 without testing applicants for the AIDS virus. The insurance industry is appealing the decision. Meanwhile the state's regulations remain in effect.

"And I don't know what my life expectancy is going to be, but I certainly know the quality is improved. I know that not accepting the shame or the guilt or the stigma that people would throw on me has certainly extended my life expectancy. I know that being very up-front with my friends, and my family and coworkers, reduced a tremendous amount of stress, and I would encourage people to be very open with friends and if they can't handle it then that's their problem and they're going to have to cope with it."

We Were There

Irene Burns

Irene Burns and Robin Macdonald are friends. Neither knew Mitchell Holsman or Gretta Wren. And neither did Mitchell or Gretta know each other. All four live and work in New York City — Irene as a telecommunications consultant; Robin as a paralegal; Gretta as an office administrator; and Mitchell as a fashion designer — and all four were friends of John Krieter. It was the love inspired by that friendship that brought them together to care for him. He died of AIDS on January 24, 1988.

John Krieter was as close to me as my brothers (though my parents never had the opportunity to meet him). John was one of those wonderful souls you take immediately into your heart. John died of AIDS three weeks ago. I loved him very much.

I learned a great deal caring for John. I want to tell you some of what I learned because you'll need it. Every day the profile of the person with AIDS (PWA) looks more and more like someone you know. Some of your colleagues, friends, and family may be a part of the vast reservoir of HIV-infected persons. Just as you and I may be. We can't pretend this happens only in Africa, or Hollywood. John nearly died in my apartment. My neighbors are dying in theirs and so are yours.

John started to lose his sparkle about six months ago, shortly after the death of a good friend of his. I tried to talk to John about his health several times and each time he changed the subject. AIDS was not going to be discussed as a possibility by John. We'd both known people who had died of this disease. We'd seen only deterioration, dementia, and tortured souls. This was just not an option for John. I'd heard him say many times, "If I got AIDS I'd kill myself before I'd have you watch me be eaten alive — wondering what it was you used to love about me."

On December 12, John attempted suicide. He hadn't been to a doctor but he knew he had AIDS. We all knew. But no one else did. Even the woman who regularly gave John massages and who saw him shortly before his suicide attempt did not detect the ravaging changes taking place in his body.

Irene Burns is a telecommunications consultant in New York City and serves as a member of the board for the Writers' Theatre.

Before I go further, let me introduce the rest of the cast of characters: Mitchell, Gretta, and Robin. We call ourselves the FN's (Florence Nightingales).

I knew Robin, though I had only met Gretta and Mitchell. Robin and I are like sisters. I knew just what to expect from Robin. When my older sister had an accident that resulted in brain surgery, I learned from Robin's care for her what it means to be a care giver. Robin's mother worries about the deer every time there is a storm in Maine, and Robin is a chip off that beautiful old block. I expected her to be sad, solicitous (of John and the FN's), and soul-searching — reaching deep down into her soul and ours to pull up knowledge and nerve endings we didn't know were there. Yes, I knew just what to expect from Robin, and I am so happy for John (and for me) that we got just what I'd expected.

Mitchell and Gretta were enigmas. I guess I expected Mitchell to wilt. I knew of her history with agoraphobia. It was John's strength and determination that had pulled her through her roommate's death and her separation from her husband — all in the last six months. He couldn't pull her through this one, and I didn't see how she could possibly make it. I couldn't have withstood what she had and then added this to it.

I guess I expected Gretta's participation to be sporadic, at best. After all, her grandmother, aunt, and uncle had all died within the last three months. How much could a person take? No, I wasn't counting on any support from Mitchell and Gretta.

Fortunately, I was right about Robin and couldn't have been more wrong about Mitchell and Gretta. I wasn't the only one with low expectations, though. We four FN's have talked many times about our preconceived notions of one another. Sometimes it's great to be wrong.

We proved the whole *is* greater than the sum of its parts.

Ordinarily, the folks on twenty-four-hour duty are members of the patient's family. Well, we became an instant family. There is nothing like forced intimacy to strip one of safety shields and expose strengths and weaknesses with flashing neon signs. We read one another's signals as if we'd been doing it all our lives. One person's weakness would be instantly offset and overshadowed by another's strength. The balancing act was like nothing I'd ever experienced before . . . let alone with strangers.

Among many things that made this group unique, we were all self-employed. Our consultancies included law, telecommunications, fashion, and office administration. Though none of us is financially independent, we were each in the very fortunate position of being able to tell our clients that we were unavailable, circumstances dictated a higher priority. When I said that we were on twenty-four-hour duty, I meant just that. None of us got more than a few days' work done in six weeks. Every one of us borrowed money to live on while we worked for John.

We had new jobs now. Gretta was in charge of research. Mitchell kept John focused on the game plan and ran interference with all the friends and family. Robin kept us tuned in to the power centers within us waiting to be tapped. My job was to keep in touch with the medical and social services staff.

We were all in charge of comic relief.

Comedy was always important to John. Discussing tragic topics like AIDS was not. Only after the suicide attempt could we talk AIDS. Finally! But not with finality. The day after he tried to kill himself, John moved into my apartment. He was there for two days. I can't describe adequately what it was like to have him there. In the daytime, we talked about AZT, about extending life a little longer, about going to Trinidad and getting a tan. We talked about doing a few more things on borrowed time. We had hope.

But there are some things I just can't describe. Like the nights — the coughing, the fevers, the chills, the nightmares. I can't do it. I lack the control over language to make it clear, and I don't have enough control over my emotions to look back on that horror clearly.

We knew we had to hurry up, but we did think there was still time. Within forty-eight hours after John's suicide attempt, the doctor said he thought the pneumonia, clearly evidenced on John's x-ray, was PCP. The drugs for treating PCP would be rough on John's system if that wasn't what he had, so the doctor wanted a confirmed diagnosis before starting him on so severe a protocol. A mixed blessing, uncertainty is.

My studio apartment is also my office. I had business meetings scheduled there, and John felt too uncomfortable to stay. He left my apartment and moved in with Mitchell and Robin. He wasn't leaving there, he said, till he and Mitchell were on their way to Trinidad.

Despite his rapid deterioration, John insisted on not going to the hospital. Two days after moving in with Mitchell and Robin — and with two of us struggling to hold him down on the bed to control his convulsing — he looked at us and asked, "I'm not shaking badly, am I?" John had gotten slowly sicker over four days, but in only an hour and a half he had gone from quite sick to very nearly dead. We called an ambulance.

When you live in New York, you are never surprised at being treated like a nonperson. When I called 911, I expected to wait a long while, then have the folks in blue arrive with gloved paramedics and display overt aggression toward this obvious AIDS patient and us lepers who were with him. I was very wrong. Again.

The police and ambulance arrived within ten minutes. And these people were wonderful! They couldn't take John to the private hospital his doctor was affiliated with because it was not one of the nearby hospitals. That was a policy I'd forgotten about. I asked them to carry John downstairs and put him in our car so that we could drive him to the hospital. God bless these guys, they didn't treat me like the lunatic I was for even suggesting that. Very calmly, they explained that he wouldn't make it without immediate oxygen. We called the doctor to arrange for a private ambulance, and the paramedics asked to speak with him so they could report on John's vital signs before he was moved. The police and paramedics stayed with us till the other ambulance arrived. The police repeatedly apologized, saying they all wished they could do more for these guys (PWAs). The cops took each of us aside just to make sure we were coping. They were just amazing.

Their support and concern came from their AIDS experience. They knew what John's fate was likely to be; they had seen this many times before. Rather than distance themselves, they were right there with us on the most human and humane level. They'd sure earned the title "New York's finest." That they were.

I can't imagine what horrors would have been in store for us had that first contact outside our close-knit group been with people whose only exposure to AIDS was the TV commercials even I find frightening, and I'm well schooled in this disease. What happens in small towns where they think AIDS is transmitted like a cold? When someone you love is dying in your arms, the very last thing you need is a medical professional who is afraid to pick him up.

We were so very lucky.

The rollercoaster ride began in the Emergency Room. Mitchell came out and told us that John had been asked for permission to intubate him, should that become necessary, and he had refused. I went in and asked John if he understood what the doctor had said. I said, "They want your permission to bring the oxygen closer to where it is needed. If you don't get enough oxygen through the mask, because your lungs are clogged by the pneumonia, they want to put a tube of oxygen directly in your lungs until the medication can clear them enough to get oxygen normally. Did you understand that that is what they were asking you?" He said, "Get the doctor." When the doctor came in, John said, "I didn't understand." I looked at the doctor, who said nothing, then at John. I said, "Doctor, John is telling you that he did not understand the request for permission to intubate him. He is giving you permission to do that whenever you deem it necessary. Is that right, John, is that what you mean?" He just said, "Yeah, I didn't understand." Of course he didn't — he wasn't getting enough oxygen to his brain.

I've replayed that conversation in my mind I don't know how many times. It seems direct and straightforward enough on the surface. But where is the acknowledgement that this "tube of oxygen" is external life support — that it is extraordinary means? Where is the acknowledgement of the conversations we'd had months before about not living by machine? The text seems direct and nonjudgmental, but text doesn't have a tone of voice. I did. I obviously thought a tube of oxygen was a good idea. Did I owe John mention of external life support? This was the man who had said he'd rather take his own life than rot away in a hospital.

That was the beginning of what became a recurring question. When do you turn the machines on? And how, after that, do you decide to turn them off?

The first five days John was in the hospital, he was on a breathing machine. When he was taken off it, we were so excited we could barely contain ourselves. As we were walking out of the hospital, Mitchell took one look at the empty, shiny marble hallway, dropped her bags and did an Olympic-caliber cartwheel, complete with the royal wave finish. All she wanted to know was whether her legs were straight. Now, one of the things a person learns about me within minutes of meeting me is that I have a very loud belly laugh. Seeing Mitchell's spontaneous cartwheels tickled my funnybone so much I was afraid they were going to admit me to the psychiatric ward.

When we got out of the building and went to cross the street, Mitch gave a devilish grin, dropped her bags again, and did six continuous cartwheels across York Avenue. Oh, how I wish I could communicate to you the absolute joy that gushed out of me at the sight of her perfect performance. Remember, this public display, public spectacle, came from an agoraphobic. One who just couldn't reign in her happiness. From then on, all good news was judged by whether it warranted one cartwheel or more — and if more, how many.

There was a lot that was funny. The FN's kept the jokes coming, and even when the breathing machines forced John to write what he wanted to say on the back of computer printouts, his wit kept sparking us on.

Forty-eight hours after John was admitted to the hospital the first time, we all had to deal with being told he had a 15 to 40 percent chance of living through this bout with PCP (still the unconfirmed diagnosis). Forty-eight hours after that, he was off the breathing machine and out of intensive care, and we were told the *Pneumocystis* was 90 percent gone.

Rollercoaster? You bet.

AZT. Hope. We made new flight reservations for Trinidad. We brought John bathing suits that were gifts from my sister and another of his friends and had a map of Trinidad framed and perched it on his table.

Gretta, the head of the FN research department, had done her homework. We'd started reading wonderful stories of PWAs "Surviving and Thriving with AIDS." (That is a great publication put out by the PWA Coalition and available through the New York City Gay Men's Health Crisis, and it ought to be required reading for everyone! Okay, "everyone" is too much. Just people over the age of sixteen.)

It took the four of us working full-time to "manage" John's illness. We had to pay his bills, get him on Medicaid, give away his fish, make and receive hundreds of phone calls, keep people from visiting when he didn't want anyone to see a machine breathing for him, get people to visit when our jokes couldn't get a laugh out of him, clean his house of dirt and pre-suicide depression, and do so many other things.

We never minded cleaning his spit or bedpans or missed bedpans, because we loved him. I can't imagine how that gets done by a stranger. It's a loving act that requires real family. What happens to the PWAs who don't have someone who loves them right there when these things need attending? John had a hard time accepting our help. He needed it and he took it. But it wasn't easy for him to accept his dependency. Even when he couldn't eat by himself, he wouldn't let a nurse feed him. We could do it as long as it was no big deal. His willingness to fight was tied to his image of himself. He needed constant support from people who knew what his self-image was and who fed it the right food at the right time.

After twenty-one days in the hospital, John was told he could go home. Waiting in the lounge for John's discharge papers, we all laughed about Mitchell's now-legendary cartwheels and how they had begun. We told John about strangers walking up to Mitch and saying, "Thank you. I really enjoyed that!" and he wanted a command performance. She did a cartwheel for him right there in the lounge and he shook his head and said, "Slower, Mitchell, your skirt didn't have time to fall and show your panties." She actually did a cartwheel in slow motion (showing off the black, lace-trimmed dance pants I'd given her especially for the occasion).

Twelve hours, four sets of blood work, and two x-rays later, John was discharged.

Life and death. Such extremes.

Last summer, a very dear friend of mine came alarmingly close to dying of cancer. John hated how that affected me. He kept saying, "Deal with it!! If the bitch dies, she dies. That's it now. Go on." Neither of us could say, "If he dies, he dies," when it came to John's turn. It wasn't that easy. We *had* to "deal with it!"

Before John died, I thought I would exercise the same choices he did. That included a preference for suicide if I learned I had AIDS. Most people I know say they would never want to be kept alive by machine. I've changed my mind about AIDS, suicide, and life-support machines. Our survival instinct can't be summoned in the abstract. My feelings about "living wills" (legal instructions to next of kin regarding life-support systems) are very different now. I don't want to be Karen Ann Quinlan, but I don't want to miss a chance at more quality time either.

John had been out of the hospital just six days before we took him back to the Emergency Room. He died twelve days later. We didn't know that the first stay in the hospital was just our warm-up exercise for this one. Now it really got tough.

He understood the question about the tube of oxygen all too well this time, and he wanted no part of it. DNR (Do not resuscitate) instructions were reaffirmed daily — when the medical team could find John lucid for a few moments.

I can't begin to really describe what this time was like. This was hell.

The virus had gone to his brain. Some of his hallucinations seemed fun and inviting. Then there were the others. We tried not to think about what he must have been seeing when he twisted his face muscles so as to be unrecognizable and shook his head — and everything else — and whispered, "No! No!" The first day he probably had two hours, all told, of being consciously with us. That number decreased daily. The coughing now brought up blood the size and consistency of golf balls.

Once, after filling a spit cup of blood balls, he said, "Save that. I want to give it to Troop and Patty." Then he looked at me with abject horror on his face and whispered, "I know." He'd heard himself ask for a gift of blood for his friends, and he was horrified that this had happened to him. I just smiled and rubbed his feet and told him a story.

My worst nightmares are the ones that include him saying, "I know," with that tortured look on his face. That was the hardest moment for me. I was glad that I had majored in theater and was able to look as though nothing had happened when, in fact, I was as horrified by his unwelcomed knowledge as he was.

I left town three days before John died. A few days before that, John had given me a hard time for not being better prepared for this business trip. I had to go. I knew I was saying goodbye to him before I left.

What could be harder than what we had just been through? Leaving. Being with people who didn't understand at all and didn't want to hear about it. Abandoning Robin, Mitchell, and Gretta. Needing them.

As Robin says, "The hits just kept on coming."

Now what?

Some of us fear, late some nights — before the nightmares start — that we may have contracted AIDS from cleaning spit cups, or from other, less elegant caretaker duties. Gloves aren't always available, or convenient. We weren't careless, certainly, but we weren't always following the strictest of standards either. Irrespective of that fear, none of us, given the chance, would have done anything differently. No, that's not true. We can each think of instances where we would have done more.

Preparing for this article, we all discovered something terribly important. We're still a family. When John died, the force that had brought us together, the goal we had had in common, went too. None of us knew if the FN's needed to be a group anymore. As we talked of writing about our experiences, we found ourselves back in the automatic pilot mode — picking each other up, filling in the holes — finding that delicate balance. John's legacy holds something very different for each one of us. And something very much the same. He left us each other.

We've learned wonderful things . . . about each other and about ourselves. We've learned horrible things . . . about AIDS, certainly, but also about "the system."

AZT costs $800 a month. It takes several months to get a Medicaid application approved. Many PWAs don't have months! John died just five and a half weeks after visiting a doctor who couldn't make a definite diagnosis of AIDS. Five and a half weeks!

When John's doctor prescribed AZT, John's Medicaid had not yet come through. He didn't have $800 to pay for the drug. Neither did we.

But we did have Maryann, the system's greatest gift. Maryann called us four hours after we left the Emergency Room. She introduced herself as a social worker on staff at the hospital, then said, "Now, tell me what can I do for you." I told her that the first question John had asked from behind his oxygen mask was, "Who is going to pay for all of this?"

She said, "I know, I've already seen him."

When John was released from the hospital after his first stay, Maryann stressed that her job wasn't over just because he was no longer a patient there. She insisted that we call her if she could help in any way. When the doctor handed me the AZT prescription, I called Maryann. She had already submitted the appropriate forms for Medicaid. She had researched city and state programs that would cover medical expenses until Medicaid kicked in. Her preparations for the AZT prescription began two weeks before the doctor wrote it. She told me one day that in the preceding two days she had made forty phone calls about funding just for John (and he was not the first PWA she had supported). Forty phone calls!

I bet you think that's an exaggeration. She told me about the calls. These weren't repeated messages to the same folks. She had initiated and completed forty *different* phone conversations on John's behalf. Just in the preceding two days.

She uncovered a program that allowed the manufacturer of AZT to provide the drug at no cost until government funding was available. But they needed a letter from her and one from the doctor. John needed AZT. Now! How were we going to get through the two weeks till the paperwork was processed?

She said, "I'll ask the hospital to pay for it. I'm going upstairs right now with the request in one hand and my resignation in the other. They'll have to accept one of them. Call me back in ten minutes."

She didn't have to resign. The hospital gave us the AZT.

This woman is obviously quite extraordinary. How many social workers would — or even could — place forty phone calls in two days and put their job in jeopardy to get medication for a stranger?

Every PWA needs a Maryann. We got one. What in hell do other people do? Why is it that this woman *had* to work that hard to find ways to help one man when thousands are in the same situation?

I'm as deeply angry for needing Maryann as I am grateful for having her.

Maryann succeeded in allaying John's fears about being thrown out of the hospital because he couldn't pay the bill, but nobody came to talk to him about any other fears he might have. It's probably safe to assume that someone who has attempted suicide and then winds up on a toboggan ride to hell needs professional counseling. But, that isn't part of the program.

We were lucky. Again. John had a client who is a psychologist. We called and asked her to please visit him in the hospital. She was more than glad to do it. He could talk to a friend. He would never have requested of the hospital staff that they send in a psychiatrist. What do PWAs do without friends who are mental health professionals?

Friends pulled through on so many fronts.

Another friend helped us get around a policy that probably makes a lot of sense — unless it backfires, as it did on us. The Gay Men's Health Crisis does an exemplary job in providing information about and support for PWAs. Twenty pages of praise would still be inadequate recognition (so just send them your money so they can keep it up). But even this wonderful organization suffers from imperfections.

In order to arrange for John to be visited by someone who had firsthand experience with AIDS, the request had to come from him — the PWA — not from friends. John was scared. The only people he'd known with AIDS were dead or dying. All had suffered horribly, and he was afraid to see someone else with the disease. He desperately needed to replace those perceptions if he was going to be able to continue the fight. Those were the notions which went along with suicide. They had to be replaced by the image of someone surviving and thriving with AIDS, and there are a lot more of those people around than any of us had realized.

We couldn't arrange a visit, and he wouldn't arrange one.

Thankfully, a friend told us about someone visiting from LA who had gone to the Gay Men's Health Crisis and said, "I have AIDS and I'm happier and healthier than I've ever been in my life. I'd like to spread some sunshine. How can I visit some PWAs in the hospital? They know the 'before' picture, I'd like to show them what happens after the makeover." He was told that wouldn't be possible until after he had taken some training to qualify as a counselor. When our mutual friend heard that one, he sent this imported ray of sunshine our way. We needed his mind and his heart, not a certificate.

John was visited by that PWA and his psychologist friend on the same day. (Mitchell's arms got pretty tired from the cartwheels this occasion warranted.) These two visits made a tremendous difference to John . . . to all of us.

What happens to PWAs who don't have these strokes of luck? Why do we call it "luck" when some attention is paid to the nonmedical effects of AIDS?

The FN's did extensive research. Considering how much is not known about AIDS, we were quite surprised to find that a vast amount of information is available. We read studies on numerous drugs and treatment programs. We read about many PWAs surviving and thriving. We read those things and were then shocked to discover that the physicians treating John had not. They were anxious to do so once we brought the data to their attention.

When John was in the Emergency Room the second time, we had to insist upon seeing the attending physician. We couldn't get the nurse, head nurse, or resident to acknowledge the interaction that possibly might result from administering aspirin to reduce John's fever. I talked to them about the possible effects on his blood work or the diminished efficacy of the AZT, or both, were he to be given aspirin or acetaminophen. When the attending arrived, he was, understandably, annoyed at being summoned. When we explained why, he looked at me and said sarcastically, "Where did you hear that?" I said simply, "I read it here, in the insert that came with the AZT. You'll find it under the heading 'Contraindications.'" He read it. His demeanor changed immediately. He thanked us and changed the order to Tylenol, knowing now what to watch out for.

I'm sorry to say that this is just one of our examples.

We learned a great deal that goes beyond our personal experience. We learned about patient advocacy. In this case, it took four full-time FN's to support the medical, financial, psychological, and mundane needs of one PWA.

Regrettably, we fear that this knowledge will be more than character building. We know we will need to call upon it again.

The dignity of this article belongs to Padraig O'Malley; the precision of its expression belongs to Toni Jean Rosenberg; and the indignity of AIDS death belongs to us all.

The Role of Education in AIDS Prevention

George A. Lamb, M.D.
Linette G. Liebling, M.S.P.H.

The severity of the current AIDS epidemic, combined with the lack of successful biological interventions, necessitates an active educational program as the primary intervention strategy. Health education theories abound, but relatively little definitive application of these theories has been made to the issues involved with HIV transmission: sexual behavior and the sharing of intravenous drug apparatus. Significant behavior changes have occurred in some people, but the consistency of the behavior change may be difficult to sustain. Thus, the authors suggest that health education should be delivered repeatedly in culturally acceptable language and format, by community leaders, and through many different approaches (churches, schools, media, and so on). Finally, because of the limited definitive evidence regarding these approaches with respect to AIDS, considerable resources should be provided to evaluate these strategies and to revise programs on the basis of the evaluations.

The acquired immunodeficiency syndrome (AIDS) has exploded in New England just as it has throughout the nation and the world. This generation of citizens is witnessing an epidemic of frightening proportions, with more than fifty thousand U.S. cases reported between June 4, 1981, and January 4, 1988, and a mortality rate of over 50 percent in AIDS patients. In addition to the morbidity and mortality, there has been unprecedented hysteria and fear of contagion, leading to isolation of persons with AIDS and their friends and families. Finally, since most of those afflicted are either minorities, homosexual men, or illicit intravenous drug users (IVDUs), or a combination of these, a social isolation has often resulted as well. This is somewhat reminiscent of what occurred in response to recognition of the epidemic of sexually transmitted diseases (STDs) at about the turn of the century.[1]

Despite the sudden emergence of the illness and its dreadful consequences, knowledge

Dr. George A. Lamb is deputy commissioner of the City of Boston Department of Health and Hospitals and is professor of pediatrics and public health at the Boston University School of Medicine. Linette G. Liebling is AIDS Program specialist at the JSI Research and Training Institute in Boston and is the former AIDS coordinator for the City of Boston Department of Health and Hospitals.

about the problem has accumulated very rapidly. The basic epidemiology was conveyed by 1985 with descriptions of high-risk groups;[2] the human immunodeficiency virus (HIV) was identified by 1984;[3] a moderately specific and sensitive antibody test was developed in the same year;[4] the genetic structure of the virus(es) was identified by 1985;[5] and in 1987, prototype vaccines were developed and Phase I testing was begun.[6]

However, it is not likely that a vaccine will be available for several years. First, the virus changes its structure frequently, thus complicating the task of vaccine production and testing. Second, protective antibodies have not been conclusively established. Third, the efficacy of a vaccine may be difficult to establish, since the incubation period of the disease appears to be lengthy. Similarly, safety may be hard to prove, since the genetic material may have long-term oncogenic (cancer-producing) properties. Finally, difficult practical and ethical problems will undoubtedly arise in testing candidate vaccines.

A second potential preventive strategy could be the use of drugs either to block infections (for example, amantadine for influenza A) or to stop the progression of the infection from the asymptomatic stage to illness. Despite intensive efforts, the prospect for such drugs is not considered good. To this point, drugs are available which seem to slow the progression of the illness, but drugs for prevention do not seem to be within view.

Because of the difficulty in developing preventive biological approaches with vaccines and drugs, considerable emphasis has been placed on the other obvious focus for the prevention of HIV infection; that is, education about the agent and methods for lessening or eliminating the possibility of transmission.

Early in the epidemic, homosexual community groups responded to information about the virus by adopting and recommending sexual practices that would reduce its transmission. Specifically, organizations in San Francisco, Los Angeles, New York, and Boston provided information on "safer sex" practices.[7, 8, 9] More recently, and perhaps facing greater resistance, those involved with intravenous (IV) drug users and the subject of AIDS have been providing information on the safer use of needles by drug users; that is, practices that may restrict the spread of HIV in this high-risk group.

What are the prospects for success in the effort to reduce the spread of infection through health education? This question and the public policy issues that are related to it are the focus of this article.

Health Education Theory

In general, health education has achieved considerable visibility during the last two or three decades. At least in part, its growing popularity is due to the recognition that many serious and prevalent illnesses (for example, lung cancer, heart disease, injuries) are either caused by or related to negative lifestyle behaviors (cigarette smoking, overeating or inadequate nutrition, lack of exercise, and drug use, primarily).

The initial efforts of the health professions to educate individuals at risk usually involved a combination of information about the risk behaviors and prescriptions for behavior changes. Not surprisingly, individuals did not often respond positively to these initiatives.[10, 11, 12] In fact, compliance with behavior-change prescriptions was less than with drug prescriptions. Many individuals involved with the risk behaviors do not even enter the health care system until the behaviors are very well established or the disease is already present.

As physicians and nurses were becoming increasingly aware of their ineffectiveness as health educators, social scientists were developing cogent theories to guide us in the development of potentially more effective health education strategies. Many of these theories could serve as the basis for our education strategies in the battle to prevent AIDS.

The Health Belief Model is one such theory. It is based on six variables that are assumed to predict behavior: (1) perceived susceptibility to a health threat; (2) perceived severity of the consequences of the threat; (3) the individual's evaluation of the efficacy of possible behavior change; (4) the perceived costs of possible actions; (5) the presence or absence of cues to action, such as symptoms or mass media communications; and (6) demographic, structural, and social-psychological factors that act as "enabling" factors.[13] In general, research supports the validity of this approach, but the approach assumes a rational basis for behavior. Unfortunately, sexual activity and drug use, the two areas of behavior that pose the greatest risk of transmitting HIV, are often spontaneous acts that may not be under rational control.[14] Moreover, fear, as it relates to becoming infected with or passing on the virus, may also affect otherwise rational behavior. For example, the fear of illness in HIV-positive individuals may lead to depression and increased sexual contacts rather than to "safer sex." Also, some reports indicate that seropositive and even ill individuals may continue to engage in unsafe, multiple contacts as a method of retribution aimed at those who infected them.

A second theory is the Fear Drive Model.[15] This has been less well studied but suggests that fear creates feelings of dysphoria which most people would choose to relieve by reducing the fear. Thus, the fear component has been conceptualized as the crucial motivating factor. As with the Health Belief Model, though, the changes that are induced tend to be small, and the usefulness of this approach in AIDS prevention is unclear. In dealing with AIDS, however, we must recognize that a great deal of fear is often present and that it must be considered in the development of health education strategies; otherwise, the educational messages will not be heard.

Howard Leventhal has noted that if a threat is overpowering, it may lead to a breakdown in a person's self-esteem, thereby reducing the person's ability to cope. He adds, "The level of fear stimulated by the information at the time of exposure seems to be irrelevant," he says, "but exposure to information about threat can lead to action if accompanied by behavioral planning."[16] The mere provision of information is not enough, Leventhal concludes; steps must be offered to empower people to change behavior.

The Dual Process Model, developed by Leventhal and his colleagues, suggests that people react both cognitively and emotionally to health messages that arouse fear. Individuals first attempt to evaluate the particular threat, then select and rehearse specific steps to avoid the threat. Empirical data are not available to judge the potential impact of this model on the spontaneous behaviors of drug use and sex.

A fourth approach, Social Learning Theory, would seem to serve as a potentially important framework for health education about AIDS.[17, 18] Albert Bandura stresses the importance of the reciprocal relationship between behavior and the environment; in everyday life, behaviors alter environmental conditions and are in turn altered by the very conditions they create. However, the environmental information has to be presented in a way that is understandable to the individual and that fits within that person's life experiences. This means that health education information has to be delivered in a culturally acceptable and understandable format and by a person with whom the individual can identify. Social Learning Theory has served as the basis for the successful health education approaches of cardiovascular disease prevention, but its applicability to AIDS prevention is untested.

The advent of the acquired immunodeficiency syndrome and the current limits of biological approaches lead us to reexamine health education theory and its applicability to the problem of AIDS. Although there have been anecdotal claims of success, few studies exist which definitively demonstrate the effectiveness of educational interventions in reducing or eliminating the spread of HIV. This lack of evidence stems partly from the overall milieu of fear in which educational programs exist — a fear that may be altering behaviors both positively and negatively. Overall, there would seem to be risk-reduction attempts both in sexual behavior and in the sharing of apparatus among intravenous drug users.[19]

The first group to have been affected is comprised of homosexual and bisexual men. This group still represents the largest number of cases. This group was also the earliest to develop health education messages and suggestions for effective behavior-change strategies. The threat of AIDS and the information disseminated about the spread of the virus have resulted in significant behavior changes in nearly all aspects of sexual behavior among many members of this community.

In a study conducted in New York City in 1985, homosexual males reported a 48 percent decline in kissing; a 60 percent decline in passive and active oral-genital sex; a 98 percent decline in swallowing a partner's semen; and a 75 percent decline in passive and active anal intercourse.[20] Fifty-one percent of those interviewed reported that they no longer engaged in receptive rectal ejaculation. Studies in San Francisco report similar declines.[21] Support for these self-reported behavior changes comes from epidemiological reports of declining rates of gonorrhea of the rectum and throat.[22]

Unfortunately, it is unclear whether these behavior changes are due to the more-structured health education programs or to the marked increase in fear generated by the media and by word-of-mouth information.

In research at a Denver clinic for sexually transmitted diseases, behavior change reported by homosexual males was statistically greater than that reported by heterosexual males. It would appear that successful change of behavior is in part due to the change in cultural definition of what is "appropriate" or acceptable behavior among gay men in the age of AIDS.[23] In the epicenter cities of AIDS, the homosexual communities have been successful in redefining intimacy, and this message has been consistent in all prevention programs. For example: Alterations of acceptable behavior in bathhouses and gay bars has occurred because of pressure from the gay community as well as legal action in some cases. Reports from Ansell Marketing, Inc., one of the largest condom manufacturers in the United States, indicates that sales have increased 10 percent yearly in each of the past two years.[24] This may be a reflection of behavior change among gay men, although specific data to support this hypothesis are not available. Illicit intravenous drug users comprise the second largest group to have been affected by AIDS. Fear may not be effective as a motivational strategy for behavior change with members of the IVDU group, whose fatalistic acceptance of the risk of death is seemingly an accepted part of their lifestyle. Yet reports indicate that IVDUs are learning about AIDS and adjusting their habits to reduce transmission of the virus.

In a 1984 study conducted with fifty-nine IVDUs in New York City, 93 percent of the respondents knew that intravenous drug users were at risk for AIDS.[25] In a similar study conducted by Peter A. Selwyn, in 1985, 97 percent of IVDUs interviewed acknowledged needle sharing as a risk factor (N = 261).[26] Both studies reported behavioral changes. In the first group, 59 percent reported behavioral change: 31 percent reported cleaning needles; 29 percent, a reduction in the sharing of works; and 51 percent, that their friends had also changed behavior. In Selwyn's group, 60 percent reported some behavior change regarding needle use; logistic regression analysis indicated that persistent needle sharing was associated with lower scores on an AIDS knowledge questionnaire. Forty-eight percent had decreased their number of sex partners or were using condoms. The population groups represented in these studies had been exposed to AIDS information and counseling in their methadone maintenance programs, either through outreach efforts or through the corrections systems. It must be noted, however, that these self-reports of behavior change do not adequately reflect or evaluate a final education/intervention program.

Health Education Policy

At this point in the AIDS epidemic, health education is the only viable alternative to preventing the spread of infection, given the unlikely prospect of effective vaccines or drugs, or both, in the near future. Unfortunately, the scientific basis for effective health education approaches is not as sound as we would like; its status probably reflects, at least in part, the heavy emphasis on research in the biological rather than the social sciences over the last many decades. Nevertheless, the evidence shows that the two highest risk groups in the United States, homosexual/bisexual men and intravenous drug users, can receive educational messages about AIDS and learn from them. Further, at least among homosexual men there has been a significant decrease in high-risk behaviors. A great deal remains to be done, however, and significant change among IVDUs has yet to be established.

Of primary importance to the authors is the development of an overall federal policy, with appropriate funding, to promote a systematic educational strategy that is both credible and feasible. In this regard, one strategy must not be selected at the expense of another. Evidence from other discussions (about heart disease, for example) suggests that multiple approaches work synergistically. At the same time, all approaches that are used need to be continuously evaluated and modified as new knowledge about AIDS is gained in the area of social science. Although an analogous process is used in acquiring biological information about AIDS, the approach is less well accepted with respect to the social science aspects of AIDS, and there may be fewer available and experienced scientists to do the research.

The need to provide appropriately explicit information that does not interfere with either individual or group cultural beliefs may present the most formidable difficulty in the implementation of an educational approach. Examples include concerns that education in the use of condoms fosters the continued practice of engaging in sex with multiple partners (either homosexual or heterosexual) and that teaching drug users to clean syringes and needles with bleach condones the practice of drug use. However, all health education theories and models recognize the importance of clear and unambiguous messages. In particular, Social Learning Theory would suggest that the messages need to be relevant to the environment in which a person lives. Further, the Dual Process Model suggests that behavior change is more likely when behaviors are understandable and can be rehearsed. This supports the idea that the mere provision and distribution of information are not adequate for changing behavior. If the information is provided within an environment (that is, social structure, culture) that is enhancing, behavior change may more likely follow. An effective education program needs to address the affective as well as cognitive areas of learning. Additionally, these behaviors need to be augmented with other strategies for change. The experience of British troops in World War II serves as an example. When troops were given a message advising sexual abstinence, 20 percent of five thousand troops on leave in Paris became infected with syphilis. A second approach was more successful: some troops were issued condoms in addition to information, and subsequently only 3 percent of three hundred thousand troops visiting Paris became infected.[27] What we learn is that while educational strategies are of value, prevention programs that consist only of pleas for abstinence may not be as successful as programs that include counseling strategies to emphasize "safer" types of sexual contact. These strategies should be supported by access to the means of protection (for example, distribution of condoms or sterile needles and syringes, or both). For these and other reasons, the authors believe that specific federal policies should be developed and implemented at once.

Of equal importance to a national policy and message is the need to implement supplementary approaches at the state and local levels. This may be more difficult to do uniformly in a free and democratic society, where different states and localities have varying incentives and financial resources. However, our evaluation of the health education theories and research supports the notion that behavior change is more likely when individuals receive the same or similar messages from multiple sources. Thus, each locality should develop programs for educational messages about AIDS, to be delivered via the mass media, the schools, the churches, community agencies, health providers, and whatever other avenues and approaches are available to communities. The examples of the heart disease prevention programs would appear to be good and successful models. These programs have been based largely on Social Learning Theory, described earlier, and include health education material delivered in a culturally acceptable format, delivered through several channels (for example, church, school, media, doctors) and involving community leaders. However, we must recognize that these local programs should be commenced at once in order to have maximal opportunity for success. We must also understand that these programs will need to be modified with experience, and that they will be expensive. Federal guidance and support will be essential, but regional and state direction may be necessary if the federal direction continues to be unsatisfactory.

Conclusions

Relatively little definitive information is available regarding the effectiveness of health education in decreasing or eliminating HIV transmission. Nevertheless, since this is the only current available strategy, we must continue these preventive approaches, which are based on available theory and previous experience with other health problems. Also, these programs need to be formally evaluated in order to redirect prevention strategies in the future. Federal, state, and local policies and resources will need to be allocated with this in mind.

Notes

1. Allan M. Brandt, *No Magic Bullet: A Social History of Venereal Disease in the United States Since 1880* (New York: Oxford University Press, 1985).
2. James W. Curran, W. Meade Morgan, et al., "The Epidemiology of AIDS: Current Status and Future Prospects," *Science,* 229 (1985): 1352–1357.

3. M. Popovic, M. G. Sarngadharan, et al., "Detection, Isolation, and Continuous Production of Cytopathic Retroviruses (HTLV-III) from Patients with AIDS and Pre-AIDS," *Science,* 224 (1984): 497–500.

4. M. G. Sarngadharan, M. Popovic, et al., "Antibodies Reactive with a Human T-lymphotropic Retrovirus (HTLV-III) in the Serum of Patients with AIDS," *Science,* 224 (1984): 506–508.

5. Robert C. Gallo and Flossie Wong-Stall, "A Human T-lymphotropic Retrovirus (HTLV-III) as the Cause of the Acquired Immunodeficiency Syndrome," *Annals of Internal Medicine,* 103 (1985): 679–689.

6. Deborah Barnes, "Broad Issues Debated at AIDS Vaccine Workshop," *Science,* 236 (1987): 255–257.

7. June E. Osborn, "AIDS, Social Sciences, and Health Education: A Personal Perspective," *Health Education Quarterly,* 13, no. 4 (Winter 1986): 287–299.

8. John L. Martin, "The Impact of AIDS on Gay Male Sexual Behavior Patterns in New York City," *American Journal of Public Health,* 77, no. 5 (May 1987): 578–581.

9. Donald E. Riesenberg, "AIDS-prompted Behavior Change Reported," *Journal of the American Medical Association,* 255, no. 2 (1986): 71–72.

10. Richard F. Gillum and Arthur J. Barsky, "Diagnosis and Management of Patient Noncompliance," *Journal of the American Medical Association,* 228, no. 12 (1974): 1563–1567.

11. Anthony L. Komaroff, "The Practitioner and Compliant Patient," *American Journal of Public Health,* 66, no. 9 (1976): 833–835.

12. David D. Schmidt, "Patient Compliance: The Effect of the Doctor as a Therapeutic Agent," *Journal of Family Practice,* 4, no. 5 (1977): 853–856.

13. Paul D. Cleary, Theresa F. Rogers, et al., "Health Education About AIDS Among Seropositive Blood Donors," *Health Education Quarterly,* 13, no. 4 (Winter 1986): 317–330.

14. Carol-Ann Emmons, Jill G. Joseph, et al., "Psychosocial Predictors of Reported Behavior Change in Homosexual Men at Risk for AIDS," *Health Education Quarterly,* 13, no. 4 (Winter 1986): 331–346.

15. Howard Leventhal et al., "The Impact of Communications on the Self-Regulation of Health Beliefs, Decisions, and Behaviors," *Health Education Quarterly,* 10 (1983): 3–28.

16. Howard Leventhal, Daniel Meyer, and David Nernz, "The Common Sense Representation of Illness Danger," in *Medical Psychology,* vol. 6, ed. S. Rachman (Elmsford, N.Y.: Pergamon Press, 1980): 11.

17. N. H. Becker, *The Health Belief Model and Personal Health Behavior* (Thorofare, N.J.: Slack, 1974).

18. Albert Bandura, *Social Learning Theory* (Englewood Cliffs, N.J.: Prentice-Hall, 1977).

19. Don C. Des Jarlais and Samuel R. Friedman, "HIV Infection Among Intravenous Drug Users: Epidemiology and Risk Reduction," *AIDS,* 1 (1987): 67–76.

20. John L. Martin, "The Impact of AIDS on Gay Male Sexual Behavior Patterns in New York City," *American Journal of Public Health,* 77, no. 5 (1987): 578–581.

21. Leon H. McKusick, W. Horstman, and Thomas J. Coates, "AIDS and Sexual Behavior Reported by Gay Men in San Francisco," *American Journal of Public Health,* 75 (1985): 493–496.

22. "Update: Acquired Immunodeficiency Syndrome (AIDS) — United States," *Morbidity and Mortality Weekly Report,* 33 (1984): 661–664.

23. Thomas A. Petermann and James Curran, "Sexual Transmission of Human Immunodeficiency Virus," *Journal of the American Medical Association,* 256, no. 16 (1986): 2222–2226.

24. Ansell Marketing, Inc., personal communication between Linette G. Liebling and Lou Brenner, senior vice president, Personal Products Division, February 27, 1987.

25. Samuel R. Friedman, Don C. Des Jarlais, and Jo L. Sotheran, "AIDS Education for Intravenous Drug Users," *Health Education Quarterly,* 13, no. 4 (1986): 383–393.

26. Peter A. Selwyn, Cheryl Feiner, et al., "Knowledge About AIDS and High-Risk Behavior Among Intravenous Drug Users in New York City," presented at a meeting of the American Public Health Association (APHA), Washington, D.C., November 18, 1985.

27. Petermann and Curran, "Sexual Transmission of Human Immunodeficiency Virus."

Behavioral Change in Homosexual Men at Risk for AIDS: Intervention and Policy Implications

Susanne B. Montgomery, Ph.D.
Jill G. Joseph, Ph.D.

With more than fifty thousand cases of acquired immunodeficiency syndrome (AIDS) diagnosed since its initial recognition in 1981 and no cure or vaccine in sight, experts agree that prevention is of the utmost importance. Yet very little research has investigated how existing social-psychological and health behavioral knowledge can be applied to the special circumstances of programmatic responses to AIDS. One of the central aims of our own research group has been to describe the psychosocial determinants of successful behavioral risk reduction among homosexual men, the largest affected group. This work is reviewed and its implications for the development of intervention programs and public health policy are discussed.

The first report of life-threatening, untreatable, and unexplained immune suppression in otherwise healthy young male homosexuals appeared in 1981.[1, 2, 3, 4] Most AIDS cases have been concentrated in urban centers such as New York City, Miami, Los Angeles, and San Francisco. Since the first recognition of AIDS in 1981, the study of this disorder has progressed rapidly, largely through investigation of cases arising in specific high-risk groups, such as homosexual men, intravenous drug users, and hemophiliacs. Most of these cases have also resided in the urban epicenters of the epidemic.[5] As of January 18, 1988, more than 51,361 people in the United States had developed the syndrome as defined by the Centers for Disease Control (CDC). More than half the persons who have developed AIDS have already died, and the three-year mortality rate is 90 percent. Even more disturbing are estimates from the CDC and the World Health Organization (WHO) that as many as 1.5 million people in the United States and between 5 million and 19 million worldwide are already infected with human immunodeficiency virus (HIV).[6] Most experts agree that the AIDS cases reported so far represent only the beginning of a much larger epidemic.[7]

That AIDS has occurred mostly in young adults, who ordinarily comprise the healthiest

Dr. Susanne B. Montgomery is assistant professor of epidemiology in the Department of Health and Safety Studies at the University of Illinois at Urbana-Champaign. Dr. Jill G. Joseph is assistant professor of epidemiology in the School of Public Health at the University of Michigan and is the principal investigator of the Coping and Change Study.

segment of the population, has serious implications. Recent studies have identified AIDS as the fastest growing cause of premature death as measured by potential years of life lost.[8] For example, in New York City, the leading cause of death among men between twenty and thirty-nine years of age is AIDS. It is also disturbing that, in the United States, blacks and Hispanics represent nearly 39 percent of all cases.[9] Not only is the number of AIDS cases among minorities disproportionate, but blacks and Hispanics also survive for a shorter time after having been diagnosed with the syndrome.[10, 11]

The first public health efforts to prevent the spread of the then still unknown HIV were initiated in 1983, when blood-collection agencies requested that persons known to be at risk for AIDS (for example, homosexual men) voluntarily stop donating blood.[12] In addition, community-based organizations of homosexual men soon made the AIDS problem one of their main concerns. They urged their constituency to comply with the blood banks' request, and soon began developing "safe sex" guidelines based on the available epidemiological evidence that AIDS was a sexually transmitted disease associated with certain identifiable risk behaviors.[13]

Epidemiologically, the highest risks are associated with intravenous drug use and certain sexual practices: among gay men in particular, unprotected (without a condom) receptive anal intercourse,[14, 15] especially in combination with multiple, casual partners. Perinatal transmission (occurring at about the time of birth) is also well documented. Serologic surveys of asymptomatic members of risk groups have revealed a high prevalence of infection with HIV, ranging from 40 to 70 percent of homosexual men in San Francisco and from 50 to 60 percent of intravenous drug users in New York City and northern New Jersey.[16, 17] Transmission by casual social contact, such as handshaking or face-to-face conversation, is not known to occur. Even in settings of close personal care of AIDS patients at home, transmission has not occurred when proper precautions were taken. [18]There is also no documented evidence that insect vectors (for example, lice and mosquitoes) or vaccines (such as hepatitis B vaccine) are implicated in HIV transmission.

Certain key features make control of AIDS difficult: First, the infection is spread predominantly through sexual contact, and second, there is a period of infectivity, lasting months or years, in which a person is often unaware that he or she is carrying the virus. [19]Since a large proportion of seropositive asymptomatic persons have been shown to be viremic (having the AIDS virus in the blood), all seropositive individuals, whether symptomatic or not, must be presumed to be capable of spreading this infection until it is proven otherwise.[20] Further, it appears that once an individual has been infected with HIV, the virus remains in the body indefinitely.[21]

In a thorough review, Osborn concludes that "the most attractive opportunity for coping with the AIDS epidemic is prevention. If transmission is not interrupted by medical, behavioral, or other modifications, there seems no doubt that those in high-risk groups will uniformly become infected."[22] Therefore, the main task of public health today is to prevent infection of people not yet infected with HIV. The population has to be educated about the syndrome, its transmission, and the consequences of engaging in behaviors that will put themselves or others at risk for infection. Ways have to be found to *motivate* people to change their behavior. One cannot assume that knowledge and education alone will provide the necessary motivation. It is therefore increasingly important to develop frameworks that can serve as the theoretical and empirical bases for programs through which messages about prevention and behavior change can be delivered and evaluated more successfully. Behavioral patterns among those at risk for AIDS must be carefully described. The behavioral risk reduction that has already occurred then has to be analyzed in order to detect relevant factors that may explain such change. In this context, it will be necessary to describe the relationship of personal beliefs and attitudes to behavior. The challenge is to find modes through which society can best encourage risk reduction without further exacerbating the social stigma associated with high-risk behavior.[23]

Literature from the behavioral sciences should help inform this critical preventive effort. If necessary, new research should address the special issues that arise in this situation — issues that pose a set of circumstances and psychosocial concerns with which most health-related research has not yet dealt. Not only is a person at risk threatened with a potentially fatal condition, but AIDS carries its own unique set of stigmatizing consequences. Moreover, AIDS is linked to sexual and drug use behaviors that are often poorly understood and inadequately discussed in the public domain.

Altering any personal health-related behavior is often extremely difficult. Nevertheless, much insight has been provided by behavioral-science approaches, particularly in the field of health behavior and related sociological and psychological disciplines. In many cases, simply being aware that benefits will ultimately result from behavior modification does not suffice to change established behavioral patterns that often provide certain intrinsic rewards for the individual. Those seeking to change their behavior may theoretically agree that change is necessary yet find this knowledge insufficient for permanent adoption of the suggested lifestyle. However, considerable progress has been made, both theoretically and practically, in identifying successful motivation and behavior-management approaches to modifying lifestyle.[24] In some instances, this may entail helping people to develop new perspectives about their lives and demonstrating how the behavior/lifestyle change is consistent with continued pleasure or enjoyment. The key is to develop alternatives that are both feasible and ultimately sufficiently rewarding so that they themselves serve as a motivation for the maintenance of change.[25]

As discussed earlier, epidemiological studies link behavioral patterns to the development of AIDS. For example, one of the earliest studies of Kaposi's sarcoma and AIDS in homosexual men concluded that the variable most strongly associated with the illness was "fast lane" sexual practices, in particular anonymous sexual encounters with many different partners. Other risk factors included exposure to feces during sex and a history of other infectious diseases such as hepatitis B. On the basis of such early research and of ongoing investigation that validated them, behavior-change recommendations were issued by the CDC.[26] Thus, "safer sex" guidelines have been developed which urge homosexuals and heterosexuals potentially at risk for transmission of HIV to avoid the exchange of "bodily fluids," particularly semen, during sexual activity.[27] Common sexual practices that would put a person at risk have been described, and individuals are encouraged to avoid or modify them, for instance through the consistent and careful use of condoms along with a spermicide containing Nonoxynol-9.[28]

Numerous epidemiological/behavioral research studies are being conducted among homosexual men, and all of these report that considerable behavioral change has occurred in this particular high-risk group.[29] Most of the work investigating behavioral change in response to AIDS among homosexually active males is being conducted in a few cities; all of this work focuses on describing sexual behaviors linked to risk-reduction recommendations, such as frequency of receptive/insertive anal intercourse; use of condoms or spermicide, or both, during anal intercourse; and number of sexual partners. Regardless of whether a high-, medium-, or low-risk population was studied, major declines in the prevalence of receptive anal intercourse were documented.[30, 31, 32] Although the use of condoms is increasing, this practice is not yet either universal or consistent. A trend toward reduced numbers of sexual partners is generally observed.[33, 34, 35] Risk reduction appears to be occurring more frequently through the modification, rather than the elimination, of particular sexual activity. Longitudinal data generally indicate more individual recidivism and instability than are suggested by aggregate changes.

In the relatively short time since AIDS was recognized as a major health threat (and, more important, since behaviors have been clearly identified as risk factors), little published research has become available describing the predictors and determinants of the behavioral change. The few studies that document behavior change do not generally investigate what *leads* to such change.[36, 37, 38] This article will review work conducted by our group during the past few years to describe both the magnitude and determinants of behavioral risk reduction in a cohort of homosexual men. These findings, and the theoretical constructs underlying them, will be discussed specifically in terms of their relevance to program and policy development.

Health Behavior Theory

During the past two decades, considerable theoretical and empirical work has been done in order to understand the psychosocial predictors of health-promoting behaviors.[39] Although more than a dozen separate models of health behavior are described in the literature, a review conducted by Cummings, Becker, and Maile points out that they all share a common set of conceptual elements.[40] These are accessibility of care; evaluation of care; perception of symptoms and threat of the disease; social-network characteristics; knowledge about the disease; and demographic characteristics.

It seems unlikely that the very complex issues of AIDS-related behavioral change would be thoroughly addressed by any one model. Nonetheless, our group decided to identify a core model of potential predictors. The Health Belief Model (HBM) was chosen, as it incorporates all the dimensions discussed above while leaving theoretical room for appropriate expansion.[41] Other models that were considered applicable and were reviewed for that purpose include Fishbein and Ajzen's theory of reasoned action; fear arousal models; subjective utility; and the Triandis Intention Model.[42]

The Health Belief Model and Its Applicability to the AIDS Crisis

According to the Health Belief Model (HBM), preventive health behaviors are a function of an individual's perceptions of four factors: (1) personal vulnerability to acquiring a disease; (2) the severity of the disease; (3) a feasible path of action that can be taken to prevent disease; and (4) the benefits versus costs of the potential action. For the model to apply, there must be a general concern about health, and cues must be provided in order to focus the individual's attention on a specific set of preventive behaviors (examples of such cues are information supplied through the mass media or advice given by a health care professional).[43] This model was developed in the early 1950s by a group of social psychologists in an attempt to explain the "widespread failure" of people to accept the concept of disease prevention, for example, screening for the early detection of asymptomatic disease (such as Tay-Sachs disease and breast self-examination) and vaccination behavior.[44] The model was derived from a well-established body of psychological and behavioral theory (particularly value-expectancy approaches and theory about "decision making under conditions of uncertainty").[45] As with most value-expectancy approaches, the Health Belief Model suggests two common determinants of impulse to action: (1) "valence," which is the value placed by an individual on a particular outcome or goal, and (2) "subjective probability," the individual's perception or estimate that a particular action will produce the desired outcome.[46] In summary, the HBM hypothesizes that people will not become motivated to undertake preventive action unless they are psychologically ready. Readiness is defined by the extent to which individuals have minimal knowledge; think of themselves as potentially vulnerable; see the disease as sufficiently threatening; are convinced of the efficacy of the preventive activity; and have minimal barriers to undertaking change.[47] The HBM also acknowledges the importance of sociodemographic variables. However, it is hypothesized that these variables influence the decision to undertake a preventive action only indirectly by influencing the individual's perceptions.

In a review of the relevant health education theory, Lamb and Liebling[48] point out that sexual activity is a spontaneous act and may not always be under rational control, which may limit the applicability of the HBM in this context. Also, in a recent review, Berkman notes that whether conditions for successful behavior change are fulfilled and whether a person then engages in risk-reducing behaviors rather than maladaptive modes of coping depend, among other things, on a person's social support networks, socialization experiences, beliefs regarding self, and the reinforcements of the environment.[49] Given Berkman's remarks and the earlier mentioned limitations of the model, it was felt necessary to expand the model to include such relevant psychosocial dimensions as social support, AIDS-related stresses, personality and coping characteristics, and mental health.

This expanded model was used to investigate data from approximately a thousand homosexual men at risk for AIDS who participated in both an HIV natural history study — the Chicago-based Multicenter AIDS Cohort Study (MACS)[50] — and the Coping and Change Study (CCS), the behavioral/psychosocial investigation that formed the basis of this article. The challenge was to determine whether the HBM and an expanded set of predictors explained behavioral change in a population subgroup of homosexual males that based part of its identification on the very right to pursue a lifestyle that now puts them at risk.

Approximately 95 percent of MACS participants agreed to take part in the concurrent supplemental psychosocial study. All findings reported in this article are limited to a subset of individuals who participated in four assessments between 1984 and 1986. The members of this cohort are largely white (93 percent); in their mid-thirties; well educated (average education attainment 16.4 years); and have a mean income of $24,922.[51] Ninety-three percent of the men reported being in a "primary relationship" with another man, and well over 95 percent described themselves as exclusively homosexual. Although it cannot be presumed that participants in this study are representative of all homosexual men in Chicago, they do resemble closely white male homosexuals diagnosed with AIDS as well as cohorts being studied elsewhere.[52, 53]

Methods and Results of Behavioral Data

A self-administered questionnaire in the Coping and Change Study asked participants to report frequency and type of sexual activity as practiced with a variety of partners, ranging from one's primary sexual partner to anonymous sexual partners. The questionnaire inquired about behaviors during the preceding month, a time span that is sufficiently short to permit accurate recall but long enough to reduce the intra-individual variability of sexual behavior.[54]

Across the two years of study, there was a consistent reduction in "risky" behaviors, such as receptive anal sex or contact with multiple sexual partners, and an overall increase in preventive behaviors, such as condom use during anal sex. In order to meaningfully summarize a variety of sexual behaviors that could lead to HIV exposure, a summary Risk Index (RI) was constructed.[55] Duplicate ELISA and Western blot assay data were available for all participants.[56] This information was used to validate the self-reported risk information and indicated that the men generally provided accurate data. It was also apparent that, generally speaking, there are two broad risk groups: (1) those who are celibate or who are avoiding receptive anal sex, and (2) those who continue to engage in receptive anal intercourse.

It is clear that during the two-year observational period, extensive aggregate risk reduction occurred. Risk reduction strategies that are preferred over celibacy include eliminating receptive anal sex, becoming monogamous, and using condoms. Individual change exhibits considerable variability, with approximately 60 percent of the men demonstrating a consistently low-risk or improving pattern over the course of the two-year investigation. However, it is worrisome that approximately 25 percent of all homosexual men in this cohort do not consistently practice safer sex, although they at least occasionally do so.[57] In addition, a small group consistently engages in high-risk behaviors with multiple sexual partners. It should be acknowledged that this overall description fails to take into account certain other changes. For example, men who have dramatically reduced their number of sexual partners but still engage in unprotected anal sex are classified as "consistently" at high risk. Nonetheless, the increasing seroprevalence of HIV infection in the male homosexual population suggests that the somewhat stringent definitions of the summary Risk Index are appropriate. Simply reducing the number of one's partners in the environment of rising seroprevalence may not lower risk of infection at all. Similar concerns have been raised by Martin.[58] He points out that although many of the respondents he observed changed some aspect of their behavior, it is disturbing that many do not change their behavior *completely.* He argues that if the epidemic is to be successfully contained, this group of nonchangers and recidivists has to be the target of special intervention efforts.

We realized, therefore, that it was of particular importance to describe the psychosocial predictors of successful change and its maintenance. As did other research groups, we found sociodemographic characteristics to be important initial screening devices to target special "higher" risk groups.[59, 60] Younger respondents are less likely either to initiate positive changes or to maintain them once initiated. Another finding points to the protective or helpful nature of being in a "primary" relationship. Although age and primary relationship are often related, the fact that both of these variables were significant in a multivariate model indicates that they are independently related to risk reduction. Education level is similarly important, with a higher level being predictive of positive behavioral changes. Finally, the special importance of the findings that nonwhite respondents are significantly less likely to successfully change or to maintain changes, or both, has to be stressed. This finding is especially noteworthy, because there were few nonwhite respondents (thus limiting statistical power) and because these respondents, as part of a major research effort, had above-average, consistent, and similar access to risk-reduction information, as did the white respondents.

It is apparent that preventive programs among homosexual men should target their intervention efforts at higher-risk men. Programs should be developed to accommodate less-educated individuals, and special efforts should be made to reach younger and nonwhite homosexual men. These latter individuals have been the hardest to reach for any intervention effort. Nonetheless, the crisis of AIDS may increase the likelihood of success. For example, a recent review suggests that intravenous drug users, a demonstrably disadvantaged group, are altering their drug-using and needle-sharing behaviors in response to the threat of AIDS.[61] After identifying the subgroups most in need of intervention, the next task is to specify the program content most likely to facilitate behavioral risk reduction. In order to do so, the determinants for risk reduction in the cohort with whom we are working will be examined for their applicability to the development of intervention programs.

The Special Issue of Perceived Risk and Mandatory Testing

Many existing or proposed public health programs assume that it is useful to make individuals aware that they are "at risk." A further assumption is that the perception of being at risk in turn leads to appropriate behavioral changes. This is the main argument advanced in the cause of mandatory testing. The research evidence on the issue is, at best, sketchy. In a forthcoming study of HIV antibody testing and subsequent behavior change, Mayer et al. found that the observed behavioral changes were the same whether respondents were knowingly seropositive or seronegative or had chosen not to obtain their serologic results.[62] Although few of the men in our study had requested information regarding their antibody status, the perceived risk of AIDS was assessed from everyone. Longitudinal analyses demonstrated that an increased perception of risk either had *no* effect on behavior or was negatively associated with risk reduction. This issue was specifically investigated in another report from our research group.[63] On the whole, there was no evidence that in the investigated group of men such a perception of risk was related to subsequent positive changes in behavior or to the development of other health beliefs that might facilitate such behavioral risk reduction. On the contrary, evidence showed that those who perceived themselves to be at increased risk subsequently had increased barriers to behavioral risk reduction and experienced a range of psychological and social distress. In a group already burdened by the complex behavioral, social, and psychological demands of the AIDS epidemic, this has potentially serious consequences. For example, psychological and social distress may ultimately reduce adherence to behavioral risk reduction guidelines or may disrupt maintenance of already established, positive behaviors. Other research efforts investigating the consequences of voluntarily being told one's HIV antibody status observed that persons choosing to be told tended to be initially the most functional and psychologically healthy individuals. However, once they were informed that they were seropositive, there was a deterioration in overall mental health.[64] These effects were observed *despite* the fact that all those seeking disclosure of their antibody status were counseled about the meaning of the result. In conjunction with our findings that depression is a predictor of behavioral recidivism, this should lead to caution regarding mandatory implementation of HIV antibody testing.

Other Important Psychosocial Variables Explaining Behavioral Change

Personal predispositions and reactions were also assessed for their relationship to behavioral risk reduction. An increased sense of personal mastery also predicted successful behavioral risk reduction. As might be expected, those who have a "doom orientation" were less likely to change their behavior positively. Coping styles also differentiated the two groups. Instead of coping with the threat of AIDS through active problem solving, persons who were less successful tended to cope by denial. This response may help relieve psychological distress but has demonstrably adverse effects on behavior. However, it is possible that coping styles can be taught and therefore altered. A program designed to improve skills that may be helpful in "unlearning" behaviors could address these issues. Such a program would, of course, need to confront the potential pessimism regarding behavioral change among those who are already seropositive. Unfortunately, no epidemiological evidence is yet available which clearly indicates the value of behavioral change in altering HIV natural history for these individuals. However, the potential benefits derived from reducing further exposure to HIV and other immunosuppressive agents could be emphasized. This might enable homosexual men to realistically assess their risk status in a more constructive and optimistic way.

Another powerful predictor of positive behavioral change was whether or not social norms were perceived to be consistent with behavioral recommendations. Unfortunately, our research indicates that the group at highest risk is also a group that is less a part of the homosexual male community. Such individuals tend to "detach" themselves from the problem by being less involved in the community, knowing less about AIDS, having fewer friends with AIDS, and denying themselves an emotional reaction to the crisis. These findings highlight the special value of intervention programs that *arise from* the targeted subculture or community. Community-based groups may be better able to reach their own marginal members, increase personal identification with the larger "at risk" group, and simultaneously provide culturally appropriate information. Furthermore, such groups often have comprehensive AIDS-relevant services that are focused both on behavioral risk reduction and on psychological needs. This would seem desirable, as data emerging from our group suggest that these two domains are, in fact, interrelated. Not only is an emotion-focused coping style predictive of subsequent risk reduction, but those with less psychological distress are also less likely to positively change their behavior. Taken together, these findings may indicate that accepting and dealing with psychological issues are part of facilitating behavioral risk reduction.

It is not enough to get people to change. AIDS may never go away. Behavioral change, if it is to have any impact on the containment of this disease, has to be consistent. People will have to change their behavior in such a way that they will be able to maintain these behavioral changes for the rest of their lives. Unlike behavioral changes undertaken to address chronic diseases, incomplete change or brief recidivism can be deadly in the case of HIV transmission. Therefore, recommendations to be more "careful" in choosing sexual partners or to have unprotected anal sex only with a monogamous partner, for example, are extremely dangerous, because they promote a sense of false security. It must be stressed that the control of HIV transmission requires adequate behavioral changes that are applied consistently. Recidivism can be as hazardous as never changing. The frequently observed phenomena of transitory backsliding and incremental change are unfortunately unacceptable in the case of AIDS. Therefore, as mentioned above, the development of programs designed to maintain and support existing behavioral changes is absolutely essential.

It is apparent that further efforts to identify the individual and social determinants of behavioral risk reduction should be undertaken. More important, the results of such research should be applied in the development of intervention programs and should then be carefully evaluated. With no cure or vaccine currently available, our only preventive tool is behavioral risk reduction. We must design the best prevention programs possible, which means carefully utilizing the existing and available theories and data. A program that is based on the insight gained from research rather than on unrelated or only slightly similar experiences can more adequately address the real issues involved in trying to change a behavior as complex, central, and reinforcing as human sexuality.

Notes

1. M. S. Gottlieb et al. P. carinii pneumonia and mucosal candidiasis in previously healthy homosexual men: Evidence of a new cellular immuno-deficiency. *New England Journal of Medicine* 305: 1425–1431, 1981.
2. A. E. Friedman-Kier et al. Kaposi's sarcoma and P. carinii pneumonia among homosexual men: NYC and California. *Morbidity and Mortality Weekly Report* 30: 205–208, 1981.
3. M. S. Gottlieb, H. M. Schanker, P. Fan, A. Saxon, J. D. Weisman, I. Posalki. Pneumocystic pneumonia: Los Angeles. *Morbidity and Mortality Weekly Report* 30: 250–252, 1981.
4. D. T. Durack. Opportunistic infections and Kaposi's sarcoma in homosexual men. *New England Journal of Medicine* 305: 1465–1467, 1981.
5. J. E. Groopman, P. A. Volberding. The AIDS epidemic: Continental drift. *Nature* 307: 211–212, 1984.
6. World Health Organization (WHO). Number of AIDS Cases by Country and Continent (handout). Third International Conference on AIDS, Washington, D.C., 1987.
7. R. Brookmeyer, M. H. Gail. Minimum size of the AIDS epidemic in the United States. *Lancet* 1320–1322, December 6, 1986.
8. A. J. H. Stevens, E. S. Searle, G. P. A. Winyard. AIDS and life years lost: One district's challenge. *British Medical Journal* 294: 572–573, 1987.
9. Public Health Service Plan for the Prevention and Control of AIDS and the AIDS Virus. Report of the Coolfront Planning Conference, June 1986.
10. Centers for Disease Control. Additional recommendations to reduce sexual and drug abuse related transmission of human T-lymphotropic virus type III/lymphadenopathy-associated virus. *Journal of the American Medical Association* 255 (14): 1843–1849, 1986.
11. G. Weston. AIDS in the black community. *Black/Out* 1, 2: 13–15, 1986.
12. J. Pindyck, A. Waldman, E. Zing, et al. Measures to decrease the risk of AIDS transmission by blood transfusion: Evidence of blood donor cooperation. *Transfusion* 25: 3–9, 1985.
13. Bay Area Physicians for Human Rights Scientific Committee: AIDS Risk Reduction (pamphlet). San Francisco Bay Area Physicians for Human Rights, 1983.
14. J. J. Goedert, M. G. Sarngadharan, R. J. Biggar, D. M. Winn, M. H. Greene, D. L. Mann, R. C. Gallo, et al. Determinants of retrovirus (HTLV-III) antibody and immunodeficiency conditions in homosexual men. *Lancet* 2: 711–716, 1984.
15. J. E. Groopman, K. H. Mayer, M. G. Sarngadharan, D. Ayotte, D. Allen, R. C. Gallo. Seroepidemiology of human T-lymphotropic virus type III among homosexual men with the acquired immunodeficiency syndrome or generalized lymphadenopathy and among asymptomatic controls in Boston. *Annals of Internal Medicine* 102: 334–337, 1985.
16. S. H. Weiss, H. M. Ginzberg, J. J. Goedert, et al. Risk Factors for HTLV-III Infection Among Parenteral Drug Users (abstract). Twenty-second Annual Meeting of the American Society of Clinical Oncology, Los Angeles, May 1986.
17. H. W. Jaffe, W. W. Darrow, D. F. Echenberg, et al. AIDS in a cohort of homosexual men: A 6-year follow-up study. *Annals of Internal Medicine* 103: 210–214, 1985.

18. G. H. Friedland, B. R. Saltzman, M. F. Rogers, et al. Lack of transmission of HTLV-III/LAV infection to household contacts of patients with AIDS or AIDS-related complex with oral candidiasis. *New England Journal of Medicine* 314: 344–349, 1986.

19. E. D. Acheson. AIDS: A challenge for the public health. *Lancet* 662–666, March 22, 1986.

20. Centers for Disease Control. Update: Acquired immunodeficiency syndrome on the San Francisco cohort study, 1978–1985. *Morbidity and Mortality Weekly Report* 34: 573–575, 1985.

21. R. C. Gallo, S. Z. Salahuddin, M. Popovic, et al. Frequent detection and isolation of cytopathic retrovirus (HTLV-III) from patients with AIDS and at risk for AIDS. *Science* 224: 500–503, 1984.

22. J. E. Osborn. The AIDS epidemic: Multidisciplinary trouble. *New England Journal of Medicine* 314 (12): 779–782, 1986.

23. K. H. Mayer. The Epidemiologic Investigation of AIDS. Hastings Center Report, August 1985, pp. 12–15.

24. H. B. Kaplan, R. J. Johnson, C. A. Bailey, W. Simon. The sociological study of AIDS: A critical review of the literature and suggested research agenda. *Journal of Health and Social Behavior* 28 (2): 140–157, 1987.

25. Institute of Medicine. *Health and Behavior: Frontiers of Research in the Biobehavioral Sciences.* D. A. Hamburg, G. R. Elliott, D. L. Parron (Eds.). National Academy Press, Washington, D.C., 1982.

26. Centers for Disease Control. Prevention of acquired immune deficiency syndrome: Report of interagency recommendations. *Morbidity and Mortality Weekly Report* 32: 101–104, 1983.

27. C. E. Koop. Surgeon general's report on acquired immune deficiency syndrome. *Public Health Reports* 102 (1): 1–3, 1987.

28. Centers for Disease Control. Additional recommendations to reduce sexual and drug abuse related transmission of human T-lymphotropic virus type III/lymphadenopathy-associated virus. *Journal of the American Medical Association* 255 (14): 1843–1849, 1986.

29. J. L. Martin. The impact of AIDS on gay male sexual behavior patterns in New York City. *American Journal of Public Health* 77: 578–581, 1987.

30. L. McKusick, J. A. Wiley, et al. Reported changes in sexual behavior of men at risk for AIDS, San Francisco, 1982–1984 AIDS behavioral research project. *Public Health Reports* 100 (6): 622–629, 1985.

31. J. L. Martin. AIDS risk reduction recommendations and sexual behavior patterns among gay men: A multifactorial approach to assessing change. *Health Education Quarterly* 13: 347–358, 1986.

32. W. Winkelstein, M. Samuel, N. S. Padian, J. A. Wiley. Selected sexual practices of San Francisco heterosexual men and risk of infection by the human immunodeficiency virus. *Journal of the American Medical Association* 257: 1470–1471, 1987.

33. McKusick et al., 1985.

34. Martin, 1987.

35. Winkelstein et al.

36. Martin, 1986.

37. McKusick et al., 1985.

38. J. G. Joseph, S. B. Montgomery, C. A. Emmons, R. C. Kessler, D. G. Ostrow, C. B. Wortman, K. O'Brien, M. Eller, S. Eshleman. Magnitude and determinants of behavioral risk reduction: Longitudinal analysis of a cohort at risk for AIDS. *Psychology and Health* 1: 73–96, 1987.

39. M. H. Becker, L. A. Maiman. Models of Health-Related Behavior. *Handbook of Health, Health Care, and the Health Professions.* D. Mechanic (Ed.). Free Press, New York, 1983.

40. K. M. Cummings, M. H. Becker, M. C. Maile. Bringing the models together: An empirical approach to combining variables used to explain health actions. *Journal of Behavioral Medicine* 3 (2): 125–145, 1983.

41. George A. Lamb and Linette G. Liebling review the HBM as to its applicability to health education practice in AIDS prevention in "The Role of Education in AIDS Prevention," published in this issue of the *New England Journal of Public Policy.*

42. See a review by John P. Kirscht, Preventive health behavior: A review of research and issues. *Health Psychology* 2 (3): 277–301, 1983.

43. M. H. Becker. The Health Belief Model of personal health behavior. *Health Education Monographs* 2: 324–508, 1974.

44. I. M. Rosenstock. Historical origins of the Health Belief Model. *Health Education Monographs* 2: 328–335, 1974.

45. Becker, Maiman.

46. L. A. Maiman, M. H. Becker. The Health Belief Model: Origins and correlates in psychological theory. *Health Education Monographs* 2: 326–353, 1974.

47. I. M. Rosenstock. Why people use health services. *Milbank Memorial Fund Quarterly* 44: 94–124, 1966.

48. Lamb, Liebling.

49. L. F. Berkman. The Relationship of Social Networks and Social Support to Morbidity and Mortality. *Social Support and Health.* S. Cohen and S. L. Lyme (Eds.). Academic Press, New York, 1985, 241–262.

50. Participants in the here discussed Coping and Change Study (CCS) were recruited from a cohort of approximately one thousand homosexual men who were enrolled in the Multicenter AIDS Cohort Study (MACS) in Chicago. This collaborative biomedical study, funded by the National Institute of Allergy and Infectious Diseases (NIAID) and the National Cancer Institute (NCI), was designed to investigate the natural history of AIDS by collecting biannual medical and laboratory data from study participants. All participants in the Chicago MACS were invited to enroll in the psychosocial investigation discussed here. For more information about the MACS, please refer to D. Kaslow, D. G. Ostrow, and the Multicenter AIDS Cohort Study (MACS): Rationale, organization, and selected characteristics of the participants. Paper presented at the Society for Epidemiologic Research Meetings, Pittsburgh, June 1986.

51. C. Emmons, J. G. Joseph, R. C. Kessler, C. Wortman, S. B. Montgomery, D. Ostrow. Psychosocial predictors of reported behavior change in homosexual men at risk for AIDS. *Health Education Quarterly* 13 (4): 331–345, 1986.

52. R. Anderson, J. Levy. Prevalence of antibodies of AIDS-associated retrovirus in single men in San Francisco. *Lancet* 1 (8422): 217, 1985.

53. D. Ostrow, C. Emmons, N. Altman, J. G. Joseph, J. Phair, J. Chmiel. Sexual behavior change and persistence in homosexual men. Paper presented at the International Conference on AIDS, Atlanta, Ga., June 1985.

54. J. G. Joseph, S. B. Montgomery, R. C. Kessler, D. G. Ostrow, C. A. Emmons, J. P. Phair. Two-year-long longitudinal study of behavioral risk reduction in a cohort of homosexual men. Paper presented at the Third International AIDS Conference, Washington, D.C., June 1987.

55. On the basis of CDC guidelines, respondents' answers to various questions regarding sexual activities were quantified in a summary Risk Index in the following way:

Level 1: No Risk: Celibate: yes.

Level 2: Low Risk: Either if respondent was monogamous and had receptive anal sex with a condom, *or:* if respondent was nonmonogamous but had no receptive anal sex.

Level 3: Modified High Risk: Either if respondent was monogamous but had receptive anal sex without a condom, *or:* if respondent was not monogamous but had receptive anal sex with a condom.

Level 4: High Risk: If a respondent was not monogamous and did not use a condom during anal intercourse.

56. J. Parry. An immunoglobulin G capture assay for antihuman T-lymphotrophic virus type III/LAV and its use as a confirmatory test. *Journal of Medical Virology* 19 (4): 387–398, 1986.

57. CDC, 1983.

58. Martin, 1986.

59. McKusick et al., 1985.

60. Winkelstein et al.

61. M. H. Becker, J. G. Joseph. AIDS and behavioral change to reduce risk: A review. In press, *American Journal of Public Health.*

62. K. Mayer, J. McCusker, J. Zapka, A. M. Stoddart, J. S. Avrunin, S. P. Saltman. HIV antibody test disclosure and subsequent behavior. Forthcoming, *American Journal of Public Health.*

63. J. G. Joseph, S. B. Montgomery, C. A. Emmons, J. P. Kirscht, R. C. Kessler, D. G. Ostrow, C. B. Wortman, K. O'Brien, M. Eller, S. Eshleman. Perceived risk of AIDS: Assessing the behavioral and psychological consequences in a cohort of gay men. *Journal of Applied Social Psychology* 17 (3): 231–250, 1987.

64. L. McKusick, T. J. Coates, J. A. Wiley, S. F. Morin, R. Stall. Prevention of HIV infection among gay men and bisexual men: Two longitudinal studies. Paper presented at the Third International Conference on AIDS, Washington, D.C., 1987.

Introducing AIDS Education in Connecticut Schools

William Sabella, M.P.H.

Most of the nation's schoolchildren are not infected with the AIDS virus (HIV). Since AIDS is a preventable disease, no one need become infected. In order to protect themselves, everyone, including children, must understand exactly how HIV is and is not contracted. The message of prevention, however, is controversial, since it must include advice on safer sex and drug use.

In 1984, Connecticut was forced to face the issue of a child with HIV infection entering school. The state responded by creating guidelines for prevention of disease transmission in schools and by subsequently developing an AIDS curriculum. Obstacles to AIDS education in school include inability to decide upon curricular content as well as political concerns on the part of school administrators. In Connecticut, committee representatives of state and local agencies of health and education and of academia are working together to overcome these obstacles.

As of December 7, 1987, 580 cases of AIDS had been reported in Connecticut. This figure represents approximately 1.2 percent of the total cases nationally. Children under thirteen years of age make up 3.2 percent of the total cases in Connecticut, compared to 1 percent nationally. The state ranks fifth in the nation in identified cases of AIDS in women. Thirty-five percent of the state's adult cases are in heterosexual intravenous drug users, compared to 17 percent nationally.

Infectious-disease experts at the National Institutes of Health and the Centers for Disease Control estimate that nationally, in comparison to those persons who have AIDS, there are 5 to 10 times as many people with AIDS-related complex (ARC), and 50 to 100 times as many who, if their blood were tested, would prove to be human immunodeficiency virus (HIV) antibody-positive and probably infected with the disease. We do not know whether the proportions among children are the same as among adults. We do know that many infected children will be well enough to attend school, and many of them present school policy problems. Most children with HIV infection have experienced

William Sabella is AIDS education coordinator/counselor at Yale-New Haven Hospital in Connecticut and is a lecturer at the Yale School of Public Health. He was formerly coordinator of AIDS education for the Connecticut State Department of Health Services.

transmission from their mother in utero. The principal school policy issue concerning these children is their admission to school. I shall not, in this article, be addressing that issue. I have focused my attention, instead, on how to prevent future infection in the vast majority of our students, who are currently uninfected and often not yet at risk.

Need for Education of Youth

Everyone needs to understand that AIDS is a preventable disease. No one, youth or adult, need become infected with HIV. In order to get the prevention message across, adults must face up to certain facts:

1. Some of our youth are sexually active with their own or the opposite gender or will be in the near future, and many will experiment with illicit drugs.

2. Any prevention message must be explicit and sensitive enough to provide youth with the necessary skills to protect themselves and their partners, including safer sex practices, proper condom use, and safe drug practices. Abstinence must be stressed.

In Connecticut, the age range with the most new AIDS cases reported in 1987 was the group between twenty and twenty-nine. Because of the long incubation period (the time between viral infection and the demonstration of symptoms), it can be assumed that many of these people may have become infected while still teenagers. The following facts, recently compiled by the Connecticut State Department of Education, are indicators of teenage sexual activity in Connecticut:[1]

- In 1987, there were more than 2,300 cases of sexually transmitted diseases in fifteen- to nineteen-year-olds and more than 200 cases in ten- to fourteen-year-olds.

- In 1985, 45 percent of new patients (4,601) at the state's Planned Parenthood clinics were seventeen years of age or younger.

- Thirty-three percent of all clients at Planned Parenthood clinics in Connecticut (15,615 persons) were nineteen years old or younger.

- Connecticut hospitals and clinics performed 5,448 abortions on young women in the nineteen-year-old age group.

Teenagers who are engaging in unprotected sexual activity now or who do so as they reach adulthood will be the AIDS cases of the 1990s. The goal of public health and education is to prevent those infections *now.*

Each child in this country has the right to a public education. Children need to understand the circumstances that make it safe to be in a classroom with a schoolmate who has AIDS or ARC or who is infected with HIV. School administrators, parents, teachers, and community are responsible for educating themselves about precise behaviors that may transmit HIV; only in this way can all children attend school in an environment that is conducive to learning and that avoids irrational fears and bigotry.

An important question is, Where can youth who do not attend school be reached? Many adolescents at greater risk for AIDS in Connecticut are not necessarily enrolled in school. In the past, dropouts, runaways, and unemployed youth have been difficult to reach. Innovative methods need to be devised. For example, AIDS-information programs could be developed with the cooperation of video game parlors, movie theaters, and youth groups.

With respect to children who do attend school, there are obstacles to providing education about AIDS. The decision to teach about AIDS in schools has probably already been made in districts that have comprehensive health curricula or in those with existing "family life" programs. A common question arises among educators: At what age should students be exposed to AIDS education? The problem of deciding can delay the implementation of effective programs.

Misinformation on the part of the general public, including parents, teachers, and school administrators, has exacerbated the problem. Because of sensationalism on the part of the press, AIDS is considered largely a disease of homosexual men and intravenous drug users. The epidemiological term "risk groups" has been used too freely to describe the types of people who get AIDS. Consequently, those in the community at large, including youth, have denied that AIDS is a disease they could get. Lack of concern has created an attitude that AIDS is someone else's problem.

Any discussion of AIDS prevention requires open discussion of sexual activity, including sexual orientation, drug practices, and prostitution. Few teachers are comfortable discussing such issues. How can we expect comprehensive programs to develop without the aid of teachers who are willing to discuss the facts and the complicated social problems that are associated with AIDS?

The concept of traditional family values is intimately entwined with the refusal of some school districts to provide education about AIDS. Some districts consider discussion of AIDS immoral and irreligious. There is a great fear of offending church groups and parents, many of whom believe that any discussion of sex or drugs will promote such behavior. To complicate matters, some communities are blessed with very vocal individuals of extreme conservative/moralist viewpoints.

Not a small problem is the fear of political consequences for careers of school administrators. An administrator's position is often dictated by the will of the community. Some administrators have much to lose by not advocating the will of parents. In certain instances, a superintendent may have taken a public position against teaching about AIDS. It may be difficult to reverse that decision without losing face.

Working Together to Provide AIDS Education

It is the duty of both state education and health officials to work together to develop AIDS education programs that will be acceptable to the community and that will halt HIV transmission. In 1984, a Connecticut child with ARC was denied admission to a New Haven public school. The superintendent of schools was not convinced of the safety of having such a child in a classroom. The response of the state Departments of Education and Health Services was the development of a task force that produced guidelines published jointly by the two departments in April 1985. The guidelines state that each child in Connecticut has a "Constitutional right to a free, suitable program of educational experiences." After task force members learned about AIDS, and after much compromise, a unanimous decision reached by active task force members stated that "as a general rule, a child with AIDS/ARC should be allowed to attend school in a regular classroom setting." The guidelines have served as a model for school boards throughout the country.[2]

The Stratford/Bridgeport Survey

In 1986, a survey was undertaken to determine the knowledge, attitudes, and beliefs of Connecticut's high school students concerning AIDS. The effort was organized by a Yale epidemiologist in conjunction with the state Department of Health Services and two local school and health districts.[3] The group determined that many students were misinformed about basic AIDS facts. Most students said they wanted to learn more about AIDS; half said they wanted to learn in school. Many said they wanted to learn from a nurse, doctor or teacher, lectures, talks, radio, television, and, not surprisingly, videos. Most did not want to read about AIDS. An education intervention program was developed and implemented. Local physicians and teachers were trained by this author. These teams were provided with educational materials and a video to inform students of their misconceptions and answer their questions.[4] Another survey of young people, done by Ralph J. DiClemente, Jim Zorn, and Lydia Temoshok, has revealed a marked variability in knowledge about AIDS.[5]

On September 30, 1986, with the aid of information garnered from the Stratford/Bridgeport School Survey, an outline for an AIDS curriculum was presented at a Yale University seminar.[6]

By late 1986, the overwhelming demand for AIDS education materials for students resulted in the creation of another joint task force. This second effort, which included representatives from health agencies and from school and community organizations, resulted in the development of a curriculum for secondary schools, which was modeled after the guidelines presented at the September Yale conference.

In addition to distributing the curriculum to all school districts in Connecticut, the state Departments of Education and Health Services have worked together to train representative teachers for each region in the state in the use of materials. The resource packet contains background information, learning objectives, pre- and post-test video resources (which include a discussion guide), and transparency masters. (Learning objectives can be found in appendix A at the end of this article, on page 342.) Even though the curriculum is not mandated, by June 1987 it was estimated that 90 percent of Connecticut's high school students had received some form of AIDS education.[7] The task force has begun to address the development of programs for younger children. A K-8 curriculum is expected by the spring of 1988.

Public pressure and the individual commitment of state officials to implement an AIDS education program quickly was responsible for Connecticut's timely institution of education programs for older children. In order to educate all children effectively, though, AIDS curricula materials must be incorporated into a comprehensive health education program that is acceptable to the community.

In September 1987, the Connecticut State Department of Education was awarded one of the nation's first AIDS education cooperative agreements with the federal Centers for Disease Control. The department plans to formulate AIDS education programs for kindergarten through the twelfth grade and increase the number of schools that will incorporate them into comprehensive health education/prevention programs. Detailed evaluation plans are now being implemented.[8]

Questions of Content and Substance

What should AIDS education include, and at what age? Surgeon General C. Everett Koop has suggested that AIDS education be taught beginning in kindergarten and extending through the twelfth grade.[9] The message of prevention for secondary-school children must include specific advice on how to keep HIV from entering the body. Most dangerous behaviors include anal and vaginal intercourse and sharing blood-contaminated needles. The virus survives in blood, vaginal secretions, and semen. The prevention messages must stress abstinence from sex and drugs as the first line of defense; both kinds of abstinence are viable alternatives for many adolescents, even though lifelong sexual abstinence is rarely acceptable. Without the message of abstinence, few school boards will tolerate an AIDS curriculum.

In order to prevent cases of AIDS among teenagers of the 1990s, sexually active and drug-using children and those who are considering these activities must immediately acquire positive life skills and the knowledge necessary for responsible decision making and behavior. The community must understand the need for and must support AIDS education/prevention programs. Secondary-school children must understand that sex without condoms and sharing injection equipment are dangerous to them and their partners.

Skills for implementing safety concepts would best be developed in a context of a comprehensive health education curriculum that underscores the relationships between personal behavior and health. Information about AIDS and other sexually transmitted diseases should be included. Assertiveness training, decision making, the ability to say no, and responsibility for one's behavior should be stressed.

Children who are in the sixth or seventh grade are in what the author considers the "gray area" of AIDS education. Some eleven- or twelve-year-old children are completely oblivious of sex or drugs, or both. Others are somewhat sophisticated. During one of my first school lectures on AIDS, one seventh-grader asked, "What about oral sex?" while other students remained glassy-eyed and disinterested. Teachers of this age range should be particularly sensitive to the degree of sophistication that is present.

The least well developed AIDS education has been for elementary grades. Why teach AIDS at such an early age? The most obvious answer is that children do not grow up in a vacuum. They listen to adult conversation, watch television, and talk to older children. Unless they understand the basics of AIDS, ignorance will beget unnecessary fear and anxiety. Young children should understand that to be in a classroom with an HIV-infected classmate is not dangerous. They should also be aware of infectious diseases in general. Educators should explain to them how they can use good hygiene to prevent many diseases.

Early interventions should include the development of self-esteem and self-worth, and the cultivation of individual abilities. Why do we, as a society, shape homophobia and perpetuate pressures that lead to drug abuse? By not addressing these issues in a progressive fashion, we risk causing unhealthy behavior patterns in adolescents which may continue into adulthood.

Any AIDS message aimed at kindergartners through twelfth-graders must appeal to youth. Videos, role-playing, and peer education are examples of successful techniques. Of course, the message should be ethnically and culturally sensitive.

Who Will Deliver the Message?

The message about AIDS, delivered to children, must be handled by individuals who are credible and who are comfortable with the material. In Connecticut, even though hundreds of teachers have been trained, few feel comfortable teaching about AIDS, especially answering questions about it. Teachers who are not comfortable answering AIDS questions should never feel compelled to do so. They probably would answer inappropriately. Both the state Department of Health Services and Department of Education still get requests for "experts" to teach the children. There is no easy solution to this problem. A technique that might be helpful: identify those teachers who are comfortable teaching about AIDS and publicize their presence among faculty and students. These teachers, who are already willing to talk to students about AIDS, could be provided with telephone numbers of local AIDS service organizations; names of speakers' bureaus; locations of anonymous counseling/testing sites; and names of knowledgeable and sensitive physicians and clergy who are willing to provide AIDS services. Given such information, these teachers could be an effective resource during the initial training of other teachers.

Teachers in Connecticut who are most comfortable with AIDS issues are those who have already taught family life programs. This group includes health educators, school nurses, and physical education teachers. Ultimately, the responsibility for AIDS education of youth must be borne by teachers. The burden cannot be borne by "experts" outside the school system. Parents will not bear the burden, or may be too ignorant of the facts themselves to do so. Sometimes, parents are too religiously or culturally restricted. Seminars for parents and teachers about the need to talk to children about AIDS and how to do so may present the opportunity to discuss sexuality, hygiene, and other sexually transmitted diseases besides AIDS.

Reaction of the Connecticut Community

Ironically, the greatest obstacle to AIDS education has been parents. In order for AIDS education to be allowed in the schools, parents and community first need to understand AIDS. This means that they need to have their questions answered by a credible professional, usually at a community forum. Parents need to hear that we are trying to save the lives of children. Even among health care providers and public health professionals, only a few are effective in presenting this information at public forums. It behooves organizers of such events to select speakers carefully. In Connecticut, the most effective presenters have included public health professionals such as nurses and health educators who are comfortable answering AIDS questions. Panel discussion is often useful. Including a person with AIDS or a family member of someone with AIDS can be particularly effective, since it humanizes the issues. Because of discrimination, few people with AIDS have been brave enough to come forward. However, in Connecticut, two individuals made videotaped presentations before they died. Both of these videos have been invaluable in helping Connecticut's residents accept the AIDS reality.

What Has Yet to Be Done?

There is no time to wait. The challenge seems formidable, but what needs to be done can be broken down into manageable tasks. Connecticut is fortunate. The state Department of Education has already begun to implement all of the following projects through a cooperative agreement with the Centers for Disease Control.[10]

- AIDS education programs need to be translated into Spanish and disseminated throughout Connecticut's Hispanic community.

- Regional workshops should be implemented for youth in prisons and detention centers.

- A survey of the extent of youth-oriented AIDS education in Connecticut should be implemented.

- All education interventions should be evaluated, using pre- and post-test survey instruments.

- After education interventions, a survey measuring attitude and knowledge change among teachers, students, and parents should be implemented.

Connecticut communities whose consciousness has already been raised through AIDS education efforts understand the importance of AIDS prevention advice for teenagers *now.* Other states should learn from Connecticut's experience. The availability of an AIDS curriculum sanctioned by two state agencies allowed secondary-school officials and parent/teacher organizations to discuss the issues. The author believes that dissemination of an elementary school curriculum will have the same effect.

If we as a nation do not succeed immediately in informing and motivating our youth, they will pay the penalty with their health and their lives.

General Answers for AIDS Learning Objectives

Goal 1 **Each student will be able to describe the spectrum and natural history of AIDS.**

Objectives: **The student will be able to**

- define the acronym AIDS.

  AIDS is an acronym for acquired immunodeficiency syndrome. AIDS is a disease that breaks down a part of the body's immune system, leaving a person vulnerable to a variety of unusual, life-threatening illnesses.

- identify the cause of AIDS.

  AIDS is caused by a blood-borne virus called HIV. These all refer to the same virus, which is also called the AIDS virus.

- define AIDS virus infection and the asymptomatic carrier state.

  This is when a person has a positive antibody test. This means that the person has been exposed to the virus. These people have no signs or symptoms of any illness; however, they are presumed to be infectious. The number of these people who will go on to develop ARC or AIDS is unclear at this time.

- define the spectrum of disease caused by the AIDS virus.

  Following the asymptomatic carrier state, the next stage is ARC (AIDS-related complex). At this stage, a person is positive for the AIDS virus and in addition may have some symptoms, including slight fever; night sweats; swollen glands (neck, armpits, groin); unexplained weight loss; diarrhea; fatigue; and loss of appetite. Opportunistic infection (for example, *Pneumocystis carinii* pneumonia) is not present.

  The next stage is AIDS, whose signs and symptoms include unexplained, persistent fatigue; unexplained fever, shaking chills, and/or drenching night sweats lasting longer than several weeks; unexplained weight loss of more than ten pounds; swollen glands (enlarged lymph nodes, usually in the neck, armpits, or groin) that are otherwise unexplainable and that last more than two months; pink or purple flat or raised blotches or bumps occurring on or under the skin, inside the mouth, nose, eyelids, or rectum; persistent white spots or unusual blemishes in the mouth; persistent diarrhea; persistent dry cough that has lasted too long to be caused by a common respiratory infection, especially if accompanied by shortness of breath.

  In addition to these, a person is positive on the antibody test and develops opportunistic infections or diseases.

Goal 2 **Each student will understand how the AIDS virus affects the human immune system.**

Objectives: **The student will be able to**

- explain the role of the T-helper cell in the immune system and how it is affected by the AIDS virus. An explanation follows.

  Lymphocytes are white blood cells that play crucial roles in the immune system. Lymphocytes are divided into two groups: B-lymphocytes (B-cells) and T-lymphocytes (T-cells).

  T-cells are further divided into T-helper cells and T-suppressor cells.

When antigen invades the body, the T-helper cells send a message to the B-cells to start antibody production. In people infected with the AIDS virus, the virus specifically invades and destroys the T-helper cells. As a result, antibody production and other defense mechanisms are impaired. Because of the decrease in the number of T-helper cells, the person becomes more susceptible to a wide range of infections.

- define *antigen* and *antibody* and discuss their relationship.

  Antigen is something that invades the body and is seen by the body as being "foreign" or "nonself."

  Antibody is what our body makes in response to antigen (foreign invader or nonself). Specific antibody is made in response to the specific antigen, with the intent of ridding the body of this foreign invader.

  In the case of AIDS, the antibodies that are made in response to this infection do not kill the virus. Therefore, the presence of antibody is a sign of infection, not immunity.

- explain the significance of a positive or a negative antibody test.

  The AIDS antibody test is an inexpensive screening test developed to protect the blood supply. By showing the presence or absence of antibody to the virus, the test tells whether a blood specimen has been infected with the AIDS virus. The test is also used to screen donor semen for artificial insemination, and it is recommended for other organ donations to protect recipients of organ transplants. Some individuals have taken the antibody test to determine whether or not they have been infected by the AIDS virus.

  A positive antibody test means that a person has had exposure to the AIDS virus and that antibody has been produced in response. It does not mean that a person has AIDS or that he or she will necessarily go on to develop AIDS. A person with a positive test must assume that he or she is capable of passing the virus on to others.

  A negative antibody test may mean that the person has not been infected with the virus *or* that the person has been infected but has not yet produced antibodies.

Goal 3 **Each student will be able to describe the transmission of the AIDS virus.**

Objectives: **The student will be able to**

- list and explain the ways in which AIDS is transmitted.

  AIDS is not easily transmitted from person to person. It is transmitted by the blood, semen, or vaginal secretions of an infected person. AIDS is spread by sexual contact and needle sharing. Blood, semen, or vaginal secretions of one person must enter the bloodstream of another person. Intravenous (IV) drug users who have the virus may also transmit it sexually. The virus may be transmitted from infected mother to infant, before or during birth.

- list misconceptions about AIDS virus transmission.

  The infection is not spread through casual, nonsexual contact with persons infected with the virus, ARC, or AIDS. AIDS cannot be contracted by the act of donating blood.

- identify "risky behaviors" that increase the chances of getting AIDS. These behaviors include
  - vaginal and anal sex without condoms.
  - oral sex.
  - sharing needles during IV drug use.

AIDS virus infection.

Objectives: **The student will be able to**

- describe the decisions that individuals must make in order to prevent AIDS transmission. These include the following:
    - Seek AIDS information and share this information with family and friends.
    - Abstain from risky behaviors (see explanation under objectives for Goal 3).
    - Always use a condom during sexual intercourse.
    - Do not use IV drugs; if one does use such drugs, he or she should enter a treatment program.
    - Do not share needles.
    - Do not have sex with multiple partners. Know your sex partner and whether he or she is at risk for AIDS.
    - Do not share razors or toothbrushes.
- explain how an individual may play an active role in bringing the AIDS epidemic under control.
- stay informed about AIDS.
- identify resources for information regarding AIDS.
- describe current methods of control of AIDS virus infection, including drugs or other treatment modes.
- know that there is no vaccine and that experimental drugs such as AZT may control infection but are not cures.
- educate family and friends and follow the suggestions listed above.

Special thanks are extended to Elizabeth Veit of the Connecticut State Department of Health Services for writing these student learning objectives.

Notes

1. Elaine Brainerd, Connecticut State Department of Education, telephone conversation with author, September 1987.
2. Joint Task Force, "Prevention of Disease Transmission in Schools: AIDS," Connecticut State Departments of Health and Education (Hartford, 1984).
3. S. Helgerson, L. Peterson, W. Sabella, et al., "Junior and Senior High School Students' Knowledge About AIDS: They Want to Learn More and Want to Learn It in School." Manuscript, October 1987.
4. The title of the video is *Sex, Drugs and AIDS* (O.D.N. Productions, New York City).
5. Ralph J. DiClemente, Jim Zorn, Lydia Temoshok, "Adolescents and AIDS: A Survey of Knowledge, Attitudes, and Beliefs about AIDS in San Francisco," *American Journal of Public Health* 76 (12): 1443–1445 (December 1986).
6. William Sabella and Jane Burgess, "AIDS and the School-Aged Child, A Seminar," Yale University (New Haven, 1986).

7. Elaine Brainerd, Veronica Skerker, Connecticut State Department of Education, telephone conversations with author, October 1987.
8. Elaine Brainerd, Connecticut State Department of Education, telephone conversation with author, November 1987.
9. C. Everett Koop, M.D., "Surgeon General's Report on Acquired Immune Deficiency Syndrome," U.S. Public Health Service (Washington, D.C., 1986).
10. Elaine Brainerd, Connecticut State Department of Education, telephone conversation with author, November 1987.

"The only thing I'd really like to stress is in my coming to know a lot of people who have been beating the odds, or as someone said, not having AIDS properly. There do seem to be a few common threads, and humor is obviously one of them. We all have to lighten up a little bit, because we all can't be grim and sad all of the time, we can't cry all of the time. The other fact is, and I think the three words Body, Mind, and Spirit really say it, finding ways to have your support system encompass all those areas. And taking time to make the search. My experience is that there are an awful lot of people out there to support you and what you do have to do is ask."

Human Immunodeficiency Virus in Intravenous Drug Users: Epidemiology, Issues, and Controversies

Donald E. Craven, M.D.

Intravenous drug users are the second most common risk group for acquired immunodeficiency syndrome (AIDS) in the United States, and they account for approximately 25 percent of the cases. Drug users may spread human immunodeficiency virus (HIV) by sharing contaminated drug injection paraphernalia and through sexual contact; women who use drugs can transmit the virus to their children. The rapid spread of HIV in this risk group and the fact that intravenous drug users are a source for heterosexual and perinatal transmission underscore the need for immediate intervention. In addition, many drug addicts are poor, have limited career possibilities, and lack health insurance, which leaves the cost of hospitalization and treatment to the public sector.

In the absence of a vaccine or an effective chemotherapy, efforts to prevent the spread of HIV must be focused on education, behavior modification, and drug treatment. Drug-treatment programs with a strong emphasis on HIV education should be available to all drug users. Community outreach programs will be difficult and expensive to initiate, because drug addicts have no formal organization or community AIDS prevention groups. To prevent the spread of HIV, federal, state, and local resources will have to be employed in conjunction with a community infrastructure dedicated to stopping drugs, providing effective drug treatment, and educating active drug users on methods of AIDS prevention. Intervention strategies for controlling the spread of HIV among active intravenous drug users should include teaching them safer sex practices and encouraging them to seek drug treatment and stop needle sharing. In addition, such strategies should be accompanied by information about needle disinfection and access to sterile needles.

> There is no area in which there is so much mystery, so much misunderstanding, and so many differences of opinion as in the area of narcotics.
>
> — President John F. Kennedy
> Address to White House Conference on Narcotics and Drug Abuse, September 1962

Dr. Donald E. Craven is associate professor of medicine and microbiology at the Boston University School of Medicine; associate professor of epidemiology and biostatistics at the Boston University School of Public Health; and director of AIDS Public Health Activities, City of Boston, Boston City Hospital.

labeled drug abuse the number one health problem in the United States. The report asserted that "more than 20,000,000 Americans use marijuana regularly, approximately 8,000,000 to 20,000,000 are cocaine users, about 500,000 are heroin addicts, 1,000,000 are regular users of hallucinogens and 6,000,000 people abuse prescription drugs."[1] The AIDS epidemic has exponentially increased the concern over drug use. Intravenous drug use is now the second most common risk factor for AIDS transmission in the United States,[2] and the use of oral and intravenous drugs has been implicated in the transmission of human immunodeficiency virus in gay men.[3]

Intravenous drug users (IVDUs) are universally regarded as outcasts, and public disdain toward them is widespread. Anti-narcotics crusader Richmond Hobson summarized public sentiment toward this group nearly fifty years ago: "Most of the daylight robberies, daring holdups, cruel murders and similar crimes of violence are now known to be committed chiefly by drug addicts, who constitute the primary cause of our alarming crime rate. Drug addiction is more communicable and less curable than leprosy. Drug addicts are the principal carriers of vice diseases and with their lowered resistance are incubators and carriers of the streptococcus, pneumonia, the germ of flu, of tuberculosis and other diseases. . . . Upon this issue hangs the perpetuation of civilization, the destiny of the world and the future of the human race."[4] In the past, society has tended to ignore the problem of drug use, but the close association between AIDS and intravenous drug use has escalated the problem to a level that cannot be dismissed.

In less than a decade, AIDS has become the number one public health concern in the United States. It has had a greater impact on our health care system than virtually any other infectious disease in our history. The issues of AIDS touch the most sensitive nerves of our legal, moral, and social fiber. Discussion of such subjects as patient confidentiality, the use of the HIV antibody blood test for screening, and ways to respond to the epidemic invariably ignite controversy. Within a short period, AIDS has transformed our traditional public health approaches to epidemic control.[5] Because there is no vaccine or effective chemoprophylaxis against HIV infection at the present time, epidemic control measures must consist mainly in education and behavior modification programs. Behavior modification will be a formidable task for all risk groups, but it will be especially difficult for intravenous drug users.

Although the problems of drug addiction and those of AIDS are separate, they are still closely related, and intervention strategies must consider the two sets of problems together. This article will examine the epidemiology of HIV infection in intravenous drug users, and will discuss selective issues and controversies surrounding the formulation of health policy to contain the spread of HIV. Problems related to intravenous drug users in Massachusetts, the New England state with the highest number of reported AIDS cases, will receive special emphasis. It is painfully obvious that the solution to the spread of HIV infection in intravenous drug users will not be quick or simple. We are facing a colossal problem with catastrophic implications that require immediate, multifaceted, and cost-effective intervention strategies.

Intravenous Drug Users

Between HIV-infected homosexual males and the intravenous drug user there are several notable differences that are critical to understand (table 1). The term *drug user* refers to any person who uses psychoactive substances outside the framework of the medical sys-

Table 1

Summary of Notable General Differences Between Intravenous Drug Users (IVDUs) and Homosexual Males (HSMs) with Infection Due to Human Immunodeficiency Virus (HIV)

Characteristic	IVDUs	HSMs
Sex	Male/female	Male
Usual sexual preference	Female	Male
Race	Minorities > white	White > minorities
Employed	No	Yes
Socioeconomic class	Middle/lower	Middle/upper
Average educational level	High school	College
Health insurance	None/Medicaid	Private
Access to health care	Limited	Good
Criminal record	Possible	No
Social structure	Fragmented	Intact
Support groups	Rare	Available
Psychosocial problems	Common	Variable
Advocacy groups	Sparse/ineffective	Numerous/effective
Access to AIDS information	Limited	Good

Sources: See article notes 9, 11, 12, and 13.

tem.[6] The National Institute of Drug Abuse (NIDA) estimates that there are between 350,000 and 400,000 active intravenous drug users in the United States. Perhaps as many as 10 million Americans have used cocaine, and estimates from NIDA suggest that most cocaine users have injected it intravenously at least once.[7]

Information on patterns of drug use has been limited to studies of patients entering drug treatment programs.[8] Of the 11,623 clients who self-administered intravenous drugs and who participated in the 1983 Treatment Outcome Prospective Study (TOPS) at the Research Triangle Institute in North Carolina, 73 percent were male, 45 percent were white, and 76 percent were between the ages of twenty-two and thirty-five.[9] Most of the participants were in methadone maintenance or detoxification programs or in therapeutic communities. As expected, nearly all of the heroin users, compared to approximately half of the cocaine users, administered drugs intravenously. About half of the heroin users and 20 percent of the cocaine addicts used drugs daily. These data suggest that large numbers of intravenous drug users could be at risk for HIV.

Traditional stereotypes of heroin addicts and cocaine users are disappearing or changing.[10, 11, 12, 13, 14, 15] Two reasons for this are changes in the drug culture and the recent trend toward polydrug use. Intravenous drug users comprise a wide spectrum of persons and personalities. Characteristics of the addict may vary with the type of drug used, geographic area, social class, and the local drug culture. The addicted person may be a teenager, an athlete, an artist, a businessperson, or a prostitute — in short, nearly anyone. Drugs may be injected daily, on weekends, or at parties. The addict may inject alone, with another person, or with a group.

Some addicts are employed and work regularly; others have a drug habit that consumes their entire life. For some drug users, maintaining a habit that costs $100 to $400 per day is a full-time job, one that requires "copping" (stealing and reselling) about two to four times this amount to pay for the habit.[16] In some cases, the economics and social interactions associated with the use of heroin may provide a welcome escape from routine life. Addicts who survive on the street must be active, skillful, and clever.

Most people do not appreciate that drug addiction is a serious psychological and physiological disease. The drive to sustain a habit or to avoid opiate withdrawal is powerful, and does not preclude stealing from loved ones or becoming involved in violent crime. William Burroughs, a well-known author and drug addict, referred to addiction as a disease caused by the "junk virus": "Junk is the ideal product . . . the ultimate merchandise. No sales talk necessary. The client will crawl through a sewer and beg to buy. . . . He does not improve and simplify his merchandise. He degrades and simplifies the client. He pays his staff in junk. . . . A dope fiend is a man in total need of dope. Beyond a certain frequency need knows absolutely no limit or control. . . . You would lie, cheat, inform on your friends, steal, do *anything* to satisfy total need."[17]

Cocaine is a more social drug than heroin and therefore is more likely to be associated with needle sharing. Because the effect of cocaine is short-lived, users often require frequent injections of small doses. Groups of cocaine users may share needles and syringes until the supply of drug is exhausted. About 40 percent of cocaine users snort the drug, 30 percent freebase, and about 20 shoot the drug intravenously (figures may vary between cities).[18] Heroin addicts may also "shoot" cocaine intravenously[19] or use the two drugs together ("speedballing"). In a recent study conducted in New York City, approximately 70 percent of the addicts attending a methadone maintenance clinic reported that they had also used cocaine.[20]

Cocaine holds a special appeal for the white middle-class male, who is usually employed and is well educated. The use of cocaine is often associated with bursts of energy and high levels of productivity, followed by periods of little activity.[21, 22] Many cocaine addicts use alcohol, sedatives, or heroin to relieve the mood change that follows the cocaine euphoria. The desire to repeat the cocaine "high" and avoid the "post-high depression" may lead to an obsession to get the drug regardless of the risk involved.[23] In a survey of 500 cocaine users who called a hotline, 455 said they had stolen money from their employers, family, or friends to support their habit: more than half had used up at least

Table 2

Possible Methods of Transmission of Human Immunodeficiency Virus (HIV) in Persons Who Have Intravenous Drug Use as a Risk Factor

Blood Transmission	
	Contaminated needles, syringes, or cookers
	Needle sharing
	Use of shooting galleries
Sexual Transmission	
	Homosexual male intravenous drug user
	Female sexual partner of an intravenous drug user
	Intravenous drug user prostitute
Perinatal Transmission	
	Transplacental exposure
	Exposure to HIV-infected genital secretions or blood
	Breast milk contaminated with HIV

Sources: See article notes 23 and 29.

half of their savings; half were in debt; and 42 percent had lost their financial assets.[24] A large number had also lost a loved one, a job, or a friend. Twenty-eight percent had participated in illegal activities to obtain their drug. Clearly, drug addiction is a serious disease with many implications.

Epidemiology

Risk Factors for Intravenous Transmission

A drug user can transmit HIV intravenously or sexually; women who use drugs can transmit the virus perinatally to the fetus or newborn (table 2). Blood transmission of HIV may occur by using or sharing contaminated drug injection paraphernalia ("works"), such as needles, syringes, or "cookers" (figure 1).[25] A cooker is most often a bottle cap that is used by the addict to heat tap water in which to dissolve the heroin prior to injection. Transmission of HIV probably requires repeated exposures to small amounts of HIV on

Figure 1

Intravenous Drug Paraphernalia and Bleach Bottle for Disinfection

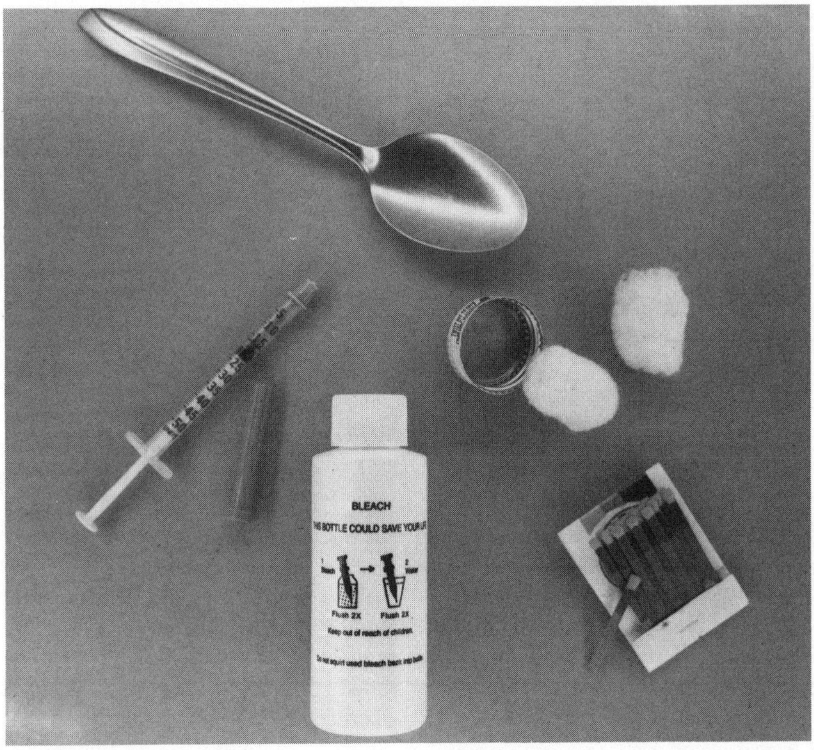

Depicted are a syringe; a needle; and a "cooker" (spoon or bottle cap), in which tap water is heated to dissolve the heroin; and cotton, which is placed in the cooker to remove particulate matter before the drug is drawn in to the syringe. Also shown is a sample bottle of bleach, which is used by some addicts to disinfect drug paraphernalia.

Risk Factors Associated with Acquisition and Transmission of Human Immunodeficiency Virus (HIV) Among Intravenous Drug Users (IVDUs) and Their Sexual Contacts

Risk Factors Associated with IV Drug Use
Number of drug injections
Number of days of needle sharing
Number of needle-sharing partners
Number of HIV-antibody-positive needle-sharing partners
Use of shooting galleries
Sharing of cookers
Not being in drug treatment

Other Risk Factors
IVDU as sexual partner
Prostitution
No barrier precautions (use of condoms)
Geographic location (reservoir of HIV)
Minority (black or Hispanic) IVDU

Sources: See article notes 23, 27, 28, 29, and 33.

drug injection paraphernalia.[26] Seropositivity to HIV has been correlated with several risk factors (table 3), including amount of needle sharing, number of needle-sharing partners, and number of days of needle use.[27, 28, 29, 30, 31] HIV transmission has also been correlated with the use of "shooting galleries."[32, 33] A shooting gallery is a place where an addict goes to shoot drugs or to have drugs administered.[34, 35, 36] There is usually a small fee to enter; drug injection paraphernalia may be rented or purchased; and addicts with scarred and damaged veins can have drugs injected by a "street doctor" (usually an addict or an ex-addict). Unfortunately, the works that are sold, rented, or used by the street doctor may be contaminated with HIV. Efforts to control the spread of HIV by the intravenous route should focus on discouraging both intravenous drug use and sharing of drug paraphernalia; if these efforts are not successful, intravenous drug users should be taught proper methods of disinfection or should be given access to sterile syringes.

Risk Factors for Sexual Transmission

It is difficult to separate intravenous spread of HIV from sexual transmission. HIV is present in semen[37, 38] and in female genital secretions.[39, 40] Ample evidence shows that HIV can be transmitted from males to females, and data suggest that female-to-male transmission occurs as well.[41, 42, 43] Transmission of HIV may not be as efficient as transmission of other sexually transmitted diseases,[44] and seropositivity appears to be associated with exposure to multiple sexual partners,[45, 46] with specific host factors,[47] or with intrinsic differences in strains of HIV.[48] The use of condoms to prevent HIV infection has not yet been studied in sufficient detail, but it is likely that condom use will reduce the frequency of HIV transmission.[49, 50] Strategies for containing the sexually transmitted spread of HIV in drug users would include abstaining from sexual relations, limiting the number of sexual partners, or using condoms and other types of safer sex practices. In contrast to other risk groups, intravenous drug users need to alter behavior with respect to both intravenous and sexual transmission of HIV.

AIDS in Intravenous Drug Users

As of January 1, 1988, approximately fifty thousand cases of AIDS had been reported to the Centers for Disease Control (CDC). Of these patients, about half have succumbed to their illness.[51] Intravenous drug use was the sole risk factor in 17 percent of the total number of cases; both intravenous drug use and male homosexuality/bisexuality were risk factors in another 8 percent of the cases. Thus, intravenous drug use, either alone or in combination with other risk factors, accounts for more than 25 percent of the AIDS cases in the United States. On the basis of the revised (September 1987) CDC definition of AIDS,[52] the number of cases has increased by about 15 percent. It is possible that more intravenous drug users will be among these newly defined cases.

As noted above, the number of AIDS cases among intravenous drug users varies by geographic region. Overall, the incidence of AIDS in intravenous drug users is higher on the East Coast than on the West Coast. New York City and the areas of New Jersey that surround New York City have reported the highest rates of AIDS in intravenous drug users in the United States.[53] In fact, intravenous drug users now account for more than 40 percent of the reported AIDS cases from New York City.

In Massachusetts, as of January 1, 1988, more than twelve hundred cases of AIDS had been reported.[54] Intravenous drug use was the sole risk factor in 12 percent of the cases, and 5 percent of the cases were reported among homosexual/bisexual males who also had a history of intravenous drug use. Most Massachusetts cases have been reported in the greater Boston area, but foci of cases have also been reported in Springfield, Holyoke, Worcester, and New Bedford. Of great concern is the increase in AIDS cases among intravenous drug users which has been reported in Massachusetts over the past three years (figure 2). In 1987 in that state, intravenous drug users accounted for 20 percent of the AIDS cases, compared to 13 percent in 1986. The number of AIDS cases in female intravenous drug users in Massachusetts is increasing dramatically, and minorities constitute a disproportionate number of IVDU AIDS cases in the state (table 4).

It is important to emphasize that reported cases of AIDS account for only a fraction of the population who are infected with HIV. In addition, there is an extensive incubation

Figure 2

Massachusetts Resident AIDS Cases in Intravenous Drug Users by Sex

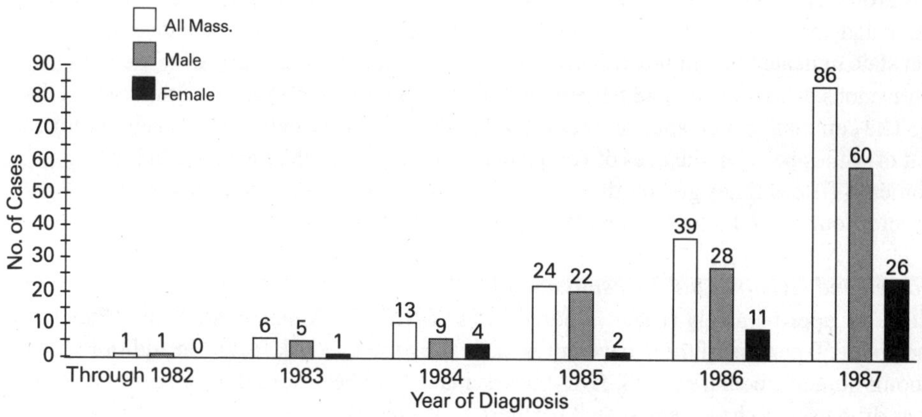

Source: Data provided by Beverly Heinze-Lacey, AIDS Surveillance Unit, Massachusetts Department of Public Health and Boston Department of Health and Hospitals.

Table 4

Summary of AIDS Cases in 157 Intravenous Drug Users According to Race and Sex Which Were Reported in Massachusetts as of December 15, 1987

	White (%)	Black (%)	Hispanic (%)	Total (%)
Male	26 (57)	54 (77)	40 (98)	120 (77)
Female	20 (43)	16 (23)	1 (2)	37 (23)
Total cases	46 (29)	70 (45)	41 (26)	157 (100)

Source: Data provided by Beverly Heinze-Lacey, AIDS Surveillance Unit, Massachusetts Department of Public Health and the Boston Department of Health and Hospitals.

period before the onset of clinical disease. It is estimated that for every case of AIDS that is reported, there are approximately fifty more cases of HIV infection.[55]

Seroprevalence data may provide more accurate information about the number of persons infected with the virus. Numerous rates of HIV antibody seropositivity have been reported.[56] Of course, the seroprevalence rate will vary with the specific type of population sampled. For example, the prevalence of HIV antibody will probably be higher among active drug users in the inner city than in drug users who are in drug treatment. Seroprevalence data from New York City suggest that HIV is present in 40 percent or more of the estimated two hundred thousand intravenous drug users there.[57, 58] In Boston, there are an estimated sixteen thousand intravenous drug users. Among eighty-nine persons in the methadone treatment program at Boston City Hospital in 1986, the seroprevalence rate was approximately 15 percent, compared to a rate of about 28 percent for hospitalized addicts without AIDS.[59] Therefore, the author estimates that about 25 percent of the sixteen thousand drug users in Boston may be infected with HIV in 1988.

Intravenous Drug Use, AIDS, and Minorities

A disproportionate percentage of minorities in the United States have intravenous drug use as the reported risk for AIDS.[60] Although minorities comprise only 20 percent of the total population in the United States, about 40 percent of the AIDS cases have occurred in this group. In Massachusetts, minorities constitute approximately 10 percent of the population and approximately 25 percent of the AIDS cases.[61] Cumulative data through 1987 in that state indicated that minorities accounted for 78 percent of the 120 AIDS cases in male intravenous drug users and 48 percent of the cases in female intravenous drug users (table 4). The cumulative incidence of AIDS among blacks in Massachusetts is nearly six times that of whites between the ages of fifteen and forty-nine, and the incidence in black women is fifteen times greater than in white women.[62] These data point to the need to target resources and intervention efforts toward minority groups.

Women and Heterosexual Transmission of HIV

There are approximately fifteen hundred cases of AIDS in women in the United States,[63] and about 50 percent of these have intravenous drug use as a risk factor. In addition, among women who have AIDS, five times as many have been sexual partners of intravenous drug users as have been sexual partners of gay men.[64]

Intravenous drug users represent the largest number of heterosexuals infected with HIV in the United States.[65] These persons are an obvious bridge for heterosexual transmission of HIV. More than 90 percent of intravenous drug users are heterosexual, and more than 80 percent are sexually active.[66] Unfortunately, accurate data on heterosexual spread of HIV in drug users are difficult to assess because of the confounding by drug use.

Perinatal and Pediatric AIDS

Female drug users and female sexual partners of male drug users are an important source for perinatal transmission of HIV.[67] Nearly 30 percent of intravenous drug users are women, and of these, nearly all are in their prime childbearing years.[68] HIV may be transmitted in utero or in the period just after delivery, through contact with infected blood or genital secretions. Breast milk has also been suggested as a mode of transmission. Infection rates of children born of HIV-positive mothers may vary from zero to 65 percent.[69, 70, 71] As of January 1, 1988, more than 77 percent of the 737 cases of pediatric AIDS in the United States had occurred in minority children, most of whom had mothers who were intravenous drug users or who were the sexual contact of an intravenous drug user.[72] In Massachusetts, 56 percent of the 18 cases of pediatric AIDS have occurred in minorities, and most of these children have had a parent who was an intravenous drug user.[73]

AIDS in Prostitutes

Male and female prostitutes who use intravenous drugs are also a major group at risk for acquiring and transmitting HIV in the United States.[74] Approximately 30 to 50 percent of female intravenous drug users are also involved in prostitution.[75, 76] Although female prostitutes in Africa appear to have a high prevalence of HIV without drug use as a risk factor, data from the United States suggest that in this country, the use of intravenous drugs was strongly correlated with HIV seropositivity.[77] Seroprevalence rates for HIV varied from 1 to 57 percent for prostitutes, depending on the geographic region, the incidence of AIDS in women, the use of intravenous drugs, and the use of condoms. Rates of seropositivity were 25 percent for black and Hispanic prostitutes who used IV drugs, compared to 7.7 percent for black and Hispanic prostitutes who did not use drugs; rates were 10.2 and 2.4 percent, respectively, for white prostitutes.[78]

AIDS in Prisoners

As of 1986, 766 cases of AIDS had been reported from correctional facilities nationwide.[79] Approximately 75 percent of the cases were reported from the "mid-Atlantic region," and most have intravenous drug use as a risk factor.[80] The limited available data suggest that the rate of transmission among all inmates is 1 percent.[81]

Health Policy Issues for Controlling the Spread of HIV

> There have been as many plagues as wars in history; yet always plagues and wars take people equally by surprise . . .
>
> When war breaks out, people say: "It's stupid; it can't last long." But though a war may well be "too stupid," that doesn't prevent its lasting. Stupidity has a knack of getting its way . . .
>
> A pestilence isn't a thing made to man's measure; therefore we tell ourselves that pestilence is a mere bogy of the mind, a bad dream that will pass away. But it doesn't always pass away . . . it is men who pass away.
>
> —Albert Camus
> *The Plague*

Unfortunately, the response of public health officials to the AIDS epidemic has been characterized by a great deal of confusion. The issue of containing the spread of HIV infection in intravenous drug users has been no exception, and few steps have been taken to address it. Obviously, the problems are complex and often controversial. Part of the controversy stems from ambivalent feelings on the part of politicians and public health officials toward drug users, addiction, and AIDS. These feelings may translate into a lack of strong moral, social, or economic commitment to education, treatment, and rehabilitation programs for intravenous drug users.

Health policy for the control of HIV in intravenous drug users needs to be targeted in three general areas. First, specific efforts are needed to educate the public about the explosive nature of HIV infection among intravenous drug users. It must be made clear that this group is a natural bridge for spreading the virus heterosexually and perinatally to children. Special efforts are needed to discourage persons from trying drugs. Second, addicts who are using drugs should be informed and urged to enter drug treatment programs. For the remaining group of active users who do not want to enter drug treatment, there should be risk-reduction programs to stop needle sharing, teach proper disinfection of works, provide access to sterile needles, and emphasize that HIV can be transmitted sexually as well as by dirty needles. A summary of possible intervention strategies for intravenous drug users is given in table 5.

Education and Risk Reduction

Education and risk-reduction programs are critical for controlling the spread of HIV in

Figure 3

Interactions Between AIDS Intervention Programs Based on Drug Treatment, Risk Reduction, Education, and Counseling

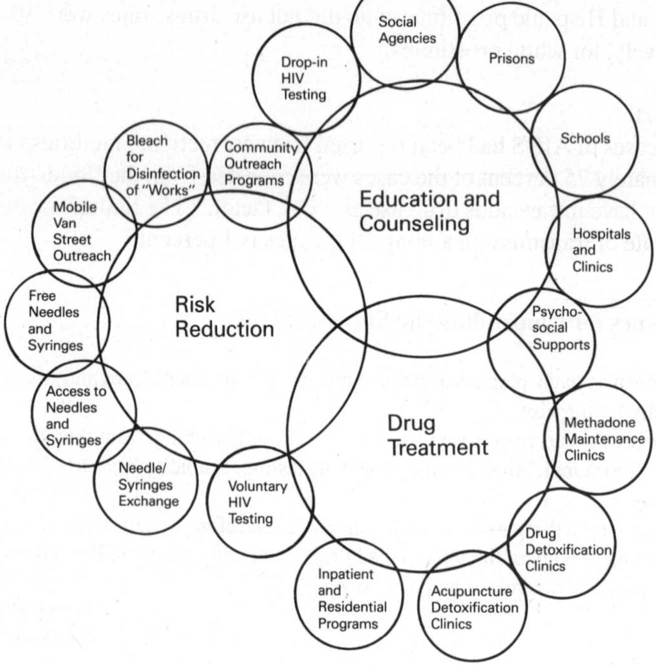

Table 5

Possible Strategies for Controlling the Spread of Human Immunodeficiency Virus (HIV) Among Intravenous Drug Users (IVDUs)

Education

Education of the general public
Prevention programs targeted at schools, dropouts, and high-risk areas
Culturally appropriate education and prevention programs
Education of IVDUs about prevention and risk reduction
Emphasis on double risk of IV drug use and sexual transmission
Efforts to alter drug culture
Multifaceted programs with credibility and community outreach

Drug Treatment

Better access to drug treatment
New and more diverse treatment
More customized treatment programs
Better rehabilitation after treatment
Preferential admission of HIV-antibody-positive IVDUs
Better access to HIV testing and counseling
Special programs for pregnant addicts

Prevention of Parenteral Transmission of HIV

Needle-syringe disinfection with bleach
Access to sterile needles
- Needle exchange
- Sale of sterile needles without prescription

Change in state laws regarding possession of needles
Closing of all shooting galleries
Elimination of drug use in prisons
Available anonymous and confidential HIV antibody testing with support, counseling, and education

Prevention of Sexual Transmission of HIV

Access to and/or distribution of condoms
Access to birth control
Available counseling and HIV antibody testing
Evaluation, counseling, and education of sexual partners

Legal Intervention

Strict enforcement of drug-trafficking laws
Higher penalties for possession of IV drugs
Mandatory education for drug users, prostitutes, prisoners
Mandatory education and listing of "johns"

Sources: See article notes 9, 11, 23, 27, 28, 29, 82, 86, 89, 90, 91, 92, 93, 94, 101, and 104.

the intravenous drug user. At the present time, it is essential that these programs be properly designed, implemented, and evaluated. Current AIDS education and risk-reduction programs need to be expanded and integrated into existing drug treatment and community outreach programs (figure 3). Many of these programs, however, are wrapped in a bureaucracy that may prevent effective use of resources. Designing specific intervention programs for intravenous drug users is difficult; costly, because the programs need to be customized; and often controversial.

While AIDS action groups in the United States have successfully educated gay men, drug addicts are often less compliant and less interested in being educated. They also have no advocacy group to disseminate information. Drug treatment centers appear to be the logical site for initiating contact with drug addicts and providing them with education about AIDS. All intravenous drug users entering treatment should be informed of HIV transmission and transmission prevention. They can receive this information from drug counselors or from recovered addicts who have been trained as counselors. In general, intravenous drug users respond better to the personal approach than to being given a pamphlet on AIDS. Videos on risk reduction may be an even more effective educational tool. Introductory courses on AIDS are offered to counselors and intravenous drug users on a regular basis by the National Institute of Drug Abuse, AIDS action committees, and some public health departments.

In many cities, there is a sense of urgency about instituting education and risk-reduction programs while seroprevalence rates are relatively low. Thus, the risk of waiting must be weighed against the need for scientific proof of a program's efficacy. Scientific or well-designed studies are difficult to perform on intravenous drug users, but recent data indicate that it is possible to educate drug users about AIDS and to modify their behavior.[82, 83, 84]

Knowledge of AIDS and its routes of transmission were evident in a 1985 study of intravenous drug users in jail (N=115) and in methadone maintenance (N=146) and found that 97 percent of both groups knew that sharing needles could transmit AIDS virus.[85] Sixty percent of the intravenous drug users in methadone treatment had used risk-reduction methods, of which decreased needle sharing was the most common; 42 percent stated that they had stopped sharing needles, and 24 percent reported decreased needle sharing. Behavior change was less evident among incarcerated intravenous drug users; 23 percent stated that they had stopped needle sharing, and 38 percent reported decreased needle sharing. Data from Friedman et al. in New York City found that 59 percent of the intravenous drug users interviewed had adopted new behaviors, such as using clean needles, disinfecting needles, and reducing needle sharing.[86] Further data from New York and New Jersey indicate that drug users appear to be switching from injecting cocaine and heroin to smoking it.[87] In San Francisco, AIDS is a topic of "grave concern" for intravenous drug users. Biernacki and Feldman have reported that intravenous drug users want to learn how to protect themselves and, more specifically, how to sterilize drug paraphernalia.[88]

Efforts to reach IVDUs not in treatment are necessarily labor-intensive. To be effective, such efforts require establishing intervention programs in such places as hospitals, clinics, jails, prisons, and court-mandated rehabilitation centers, and at welfare and unemployment offices. Participation in an education program on AIDS risk reduction should be mandated for persons charged with soliciting or prostitution and as a condition for release from jail or prison. The message at each site must be clear, concise, and nonjudgmental. It can be delivered personally, by video, or — probably less effectively — through well-designed pamphlets. Messages about AIDS prevention should be displayed on community billboards and on signs in stores, subways, and buses. The messages should discourage drug use, provide access to help, and, where it is culturally appropriate, be posted in foreign languages.

Many drug users are aware that sharing needles and using contaminated works present risks. However, the possibility of acquiring or transmitting HIV sexually is not widely appreciated among this group, and therefore sexual preventive strategies are not commonly used. Specific efforts will be required to teach intravenous drug users that unprotected sexual intercourse, exposure to multiple sexual partners, and ignoring safer sex guidelines are important factors for HIV transmission. This may be the most difficult task to accomplish.

Community outreach programs that educate and encourage active drug users to seek drug treatment need to be established.[89] Health officials in New Jersey have successfully linked risk reduction for AIDS with drug treatment by distributing coupons that addicts can use for drug detoxification.[90] These coupons eliminate co-payment by the intravenous drug user for drug treatment. Recovered drug addicts can be trained as health educators and can be used to disseminate information about AIDS in the drug-using community. The message should be simple and nonjudgmental: Stop drugs and seek treatment; don't share needles, syringes, or cookers; use bleach to disinfect all drug paraphernalia.

Mobil vans appear to offer an effective method of community outreach. They are less costly than traditional programs but need to be further evaluated. In Amsterdam, methadone and information about AIDS are distributed by van,[91] and in New Jersey, mobil vans are staffed by physicians and social workers who provide medical information and referrals.[92] Because intravenous drug users often congregate in certain areas in the city, mobil vans may provide the optimal vehicle for control of HIV among this population.

Recently, the National Institute of Drug Abuse provided several community outreach demonstration projects with funds to conduct comprehensive prevention programs for intravenous drug users.[93] These programs will stress the importance of avoiding drugs, seeking drug treatment, disinfecting drug paraphernalia, and practicing safer sex. Although it is not clear what impact these programs will have on the course of the AIDS epidemic in this population, the approach seems promising, in that education and prevention are the only tools currently available. Failure to initiate these prevention programs, particularly when seroprevalence rates are low, could prove to be a costly mistake.[94]

The schools are of critical importance as a locus for disseminating information about AIDS. Special efforts should be made to reach school dropouts. In the Boston Public Schools, more than 40 percent of the students who start high school do not finish. This is probably the group who are most at risk for running away, starting to use drugs, or engaging in prostitution as a means of support; thus, individuals in this group are probably at the highest risk for contracting AIDS.

Grants from the Centers for Disease Control to establish AIDS educational programs in schools have been awarded to twelve cities, including Boston. Multifaceted intervention — including traditional methods of teaching, peer teaching, the use of videos, and so on — is needed in order to provide basic information about AIDS and HIV infection. Appropriate and timely intervention may provide an effective deterrent against dropping out and thus against acquiring HIV infection.

Drug Treatment Programs

Access to drug treatment is a cornerstone for controlling the spread of HIV. Drug treatment programs are the most logical site to begin education and risk-reduction programs for intravenous drug users. Many drug treatment programs, however, have not instituted effective AIDS education, nor are they equipped to care for HIV-infected patients and their psychosocial needs. In Massachusetts, opportunities for drug treatment are insufficient, and there are long waiting periods for different treatment facilities, especially for women, who traditionally have had a more difficult time finding placements in rehabilitation programs.

Fortunately, intravenous drug users appear to fear AIDS enough to change or modify their behavior and reduce risk by entering drug treatment. According to Des Jarlais et al., more than 50 percent of the drug users seeking drug treatment cited fear of AIDS as one reason for entering treatment.[95]

In New York City, about 100 drug treatment programs care for thirty thousand persons, which accounts for about 15 percent of the total number of addicts there.[96] In Boston, there are an estimated sixteen thousand intravenous drug users and about 900 treatment slots. There is a severe shortage of drug treatment facilities in nearly all U.S. cities, owing in large part to insufficient funds, lack of treatment sites, and poor use of existing facilities.

Nationally, methadone maintenance programs have been the mainstay of outpatient treatment programs for the past twenty years.[97] Methadone does not produce sedation or euphoria but reduces the craving for narcotics. In essence, methadone stabilizes the life of many addicts, and removes them from the daily hustle of the search for drugs. The counseling and support that accompany methadone treatment are a critical part of most programs. Methadone is dispensed daily in most clinics, and is administered under the observation of clinic staff. Many clinics monitor urine samples of patients to determine whether the intravenous drug user is still injecting drugs, because some addicts continue to use drugs while they are on methadone.

In Amsterdam, methadone is distributed cost-free by mobile van. Addicts are carefully observed to make certain that they ingest the drug.[98] This type of program appears cost-effective; facilitates access to drug treatment; maintains contact with the addict; and obviates the problems of establishing detoxification or methadone maintenance clinics in the neighborhood. Mobil vans may not provide the necessary social support, but can refer patients to Narcotics Anonymous or other groups. It is questionable whether this type of program would be accepted in the United States.

There is a great deal of controversy in the United States about whether the aim of treatment should be methadone maintenance or complete nonuse of drugs, particularly in view of the high relapse rates and continued drug use among persons on methadone maintenance.[99] Despite the high relapse rates, Dole and Nyswander report that the lives of many patients who are on methadone maintenance are more stable and more productive, since the patients are free of the constant craving for heroin and thus have stopped engaging in the criminal activities associated with its use.[100] The heroin addict may not be medically cured, but if he is integrated into society and is less likely to contract or spread AIDS virus, the treatment should be considered successful.[101, 102]

Testing for HIV Antibody

Because of the dearth of drug treatment slots, many public health and drug rehabilitation programs have decided to selectively admit addicts who are HIV-antibody-positive. This provides an incentive for voluntary HIV testing, but, ironically, access to testing is limited.

The importance of HIV testing as an impetus for the intravenous drug user to modify or change behavior is unclear at this time. Many public health officials argue that all intravenous drug users should consider themselves HIV-positive, refrain from sharing needles, and practice safer sex. Others argue that an individual's knowledge of his or her HIV antibody status may reinforce the use of condoms, limit the number of sexual partners, and eliminate the sharing of drug paraphernalia. Studies in gay men and limited studies in intravenous drug users suggest that there is a wide spectrum of behavioral responses to HIV testing.[103, 104, 105, 106] Recent data from Kings County Hospital in Brooklyn reveal a wide range of psychological reactions to HIV testing in intravenous drug users, and indicate that psychological reactions are apparent more frequently and are more severe in female intravenous drug users than in gay men.[107] Many of these female intravenous drug users had a documented increase in drug use following HIV testing. The use of voluntary HIV testing for drug users in treatment remains moot and requires further evaluation.

In general, intravenous drug users have not used the state-run alternative HIV test sites, which offer free and anonymous blood testing for HIV, perhaps because of the need to make appointments for testing several weeks in advance.[108] In order to improve access to HIV antibody testing for drug users, the Massachusetts Department of Drug Rehabilitation and the Boston Department of Health and Hospitals have opened an anonymous drop-in HIV counseling and testing program called Project Trust at Boston City Hospital for intravenous drug users, their sexual contacts, needle-sharing partners, and families. Project Trust also provides education, support groups, and referral for drug treatment.

With respect to programs for HIV antibody testing, it is important to realize that the screening test for HIV has limitations and that false-positive and false-negative results may be obtained.[109] The number of false-positive screening tests in intravenous drug users is likely to be lower than in healthy blood donors, but the number of false-negative tests would probably be greater.

HIV antibody testing in pregnant intravenous drug users raises particular issues. In Boston, New York City, and New Jersey, pregnant addicts are given priority for treatment slots, and some drug treatment programs are specially equipped to deal with the pregnant addict. However, testing for HIV may have an adverse effect on the addicted mother. Cancellieri et al. suggest that approximately 44 percent of their pregnant addicts who had HIV testing had serious psychiatric sequelae and increased their use of "crack" during their pregnancy.[110] Four of the sixty HIV-tested patients who were followed in the study required psychiatric hospitalizations for acute psychoses or suicidal or homicidal behavior following their binges with cocaine. In addition, pregnant intravenous drug users often avoided testing until after their abortion. In our experience at Boston City Hospital and in the experience of others, many HIV-seropositive pregnant intravenous drug users in whom an elective abortion is possible choose to continue their pregnancy, in spite of the risk of fetal infection.[111, 112]

Voluntary HIV testing, with appropriate counseling, should be made available to all prisoners and their sexual contacts. However, few programs for voluntary testing have been established in prisons, and data concerning the acceptance and efficacy of those programs which do exist are sparse.

In many U.S. cities, prostitutes have access to voluntary HIV blood testing in clinics for sexually transmitted diseases. In some U.S. states, such as Nevada, and in Amsterdam, licensed prostitutes must routinely be screened for HIV antibody.[113] In data that have been gathered on the subject of prostitution in the United States, HIV seropositivity has correlated with intravenous drug use and absence of condom use.[114] Because prostitutes are a sexually active population, it would be reasonable for health departments to set up education and voluntary testing programs for them and to work with prostitutes' unions, where they exist, in this process. In New Jersey, women arrested for prostitution undergo mandatory HIV testing. Some public health officials believe that educational programs and voluntary testing should be offered to "johns," or individuals caught soliciting.

Disinfection of Drug Paraphernalia

The primary emphasis of all educational materials for intravenous drug users is to stop using drugs and seek drug treatment. Secondarily, there should be a clear message not to share needles, to stay away from shooting galleries, and, if necessary, to disinfect needles and syringes with bleach. Given the limited access to needles and syringes in most U.S. states, many public health officials have supported efforts to distribute educational material on proper disinfection of drug paraphernalia. Limited laboratory data indicate that HIV is killed by heat; by many household disinfectants such as bleach and rubbing alcohol; by spirits such as vodka or wine; and by dish-washing detergent.[115, 116] Boiling syringes is inconvenient and removes the silicon lubricant from the plunger. Therefore, use of Clorox has been recommended as an effective, safe, and convenient method of disinfection. Bottles of household bleach, with instructions for proper use, are now being distributed in Massachusetts, New Jersey, New York, California, and Maryland, along with hotline numbers that can be called for information about disinfection procedures.

Access to Sterile Needles and Syringes

Data from Des Jarlais et al. indicate that there is a demand for sterile needles in New York,[117] but laws limiting access to needles and syringes prohibit the sale of needles without a prescription. Heated debates are in progress over the importance of access to sterile drug paraphernalia in limiting the spread of AIDS. Proponents of distributing free needles and syringes or instituting needle exchange programs argue that high rates of HIV are present in many states that limit access to free needles, and that preventing one case of AIDS would more than pay for these programs. Opponents of the policy argue that distributing free needles would encourage intravenous drug use and would not be useful to most addicts, because needle sharing is part of the drug culture and the means for disinfection are widely available.

In Canada and some European countries, needles and syringes can be purchased without a prescription. In many places where this policy prevails, seroprevalence rates are low, but whether the rates are the result of the policy or of cultural differences and a smaller reservoir of virus is unclear. Greater access to needles and syringes in U.S. states would require decriminalization of drug paraphernalia possession.

There are thirteen different needle and syringe exchanges in Amsterdam.[118] The latest data indicate that 350,000 needles and syringes were exchanged there in 1986, and that needle sharing was reduced with no attendant increase in the patient load on drug-free treatment programs. Positive experiences with needle exchange programs have also been reported from Sydney, Australia, and from Liverpool, England.[119, 120] Investigators in these studies emphasize that the programs provide a means of continuing education through constant contact with active drug users who do not want to be in treatment but who also do not want to acquire or transmit HIV. Needle exchanges are a logical site for providing free condoms, spermicides, and leaflets on safer sex and drug use.[121] Advocates acknowledge that these programs would reach only a portion of the drug user population and emphasize that the approach should be incorporated into a more comprehensive strategy for risk reduction.

Quarantine

Quarantine has been a traditional means of preventing the spread of plague and smallpox. However, in comparison to AIDS, each of these diseases had a limited incubation period, and the duration of each was usually short. HIV infection is usually asymptomatic, and it is not transmitted casually. Quarantining persons with HIV would require mass screening, with all of its attendant complications, including follow-up screening for false negatives and an enormous amount of money to provide care for the 1 million to 2 million people in the United States who are probably HIV-infected and who will remain infected for life. For these reasons, and because AIDS is a preventable disease, quarantine is an unacceptable strategy.

Cost of Treating Drug Users Who Have Aids

The cost of treating an AIDS case in the United States varies among geographic regions and among hospitals. Estimates of the medical care costs per AIDS patient vary between $47,000 and $147,000.[122, 123] These estimates do not include indirect costs for precautions; the cost of Azidothymidine (> $10,000 per year); laboratory costs for transfusions; laboratory expenses to monitor treatment with Azidothymidine; the costs of treating the addiction; or the support services needed to care for this population. Moreover, the estimates do not include those hospitalization costs which precede the diagnosis of AIDS. Recent data suggest that patients with ARC and, possibly, intravenous drug users who are HIV-positive are also more likely to have recurrent bacterial infections that require hospitalization.[124]

The CDC's projected increase in AIDS cases for 1991,[125] coupled with the potential rapid spread of HIV transmission among intravenous drug users,[126] translates into huge costs for AIDS treatment, let alone for treating drug addiction. Data suggest that 30 percent or more of seropositive intravenous drug users will eventually develop AIDS,[127] and that more than 70 percent of intravenous drug users who develop ARC will require medical attention. These estimates indicate that the medical costs for treating this population could be staggering. Furthermore, in contrast to many gay males, most heroin addicts do not have health insurance or support systems (table 1). This results in longer hospitalization and more costly post-hospital care,[128] and it underscores the importance of effective health policy programs for the intravenous drug user.

Conclusion

In the absence of a vaccine or an effective chemotherapy to cure or prevent HIV infection, efforts to prevent AIDS must focus on education and on behavior modification. The intravenous drug user is at risk both through drug use and through sexual contact with infected partners. Moreover, the addict has to deal not only with the threat of AIDS, but also with his or her own addiction. Intravenous drug users now comprise the second highest risk group for AIDS in the United States. Women, children, and minorities are widely affected as well. Therefore, intervention programs, which need to include risk-reduction strategies and drug treatment, must explain the risk factors in each of these groups. The challenge is formidable, and programs will need to be creative, multifaceted, and culturally appropriate. Social prejudice, political barriers, and economic constraints will only prolong the epidemic and magnify the risk for others.

This article was supported in part by a grant from the Massachusetts Department of Health.

Notes

1. B. Freemantle. *The Fix: The World Drug Trade.* Tom Doherty and Associates, New York, N.Y., 1987, p. 2.
2. Center for Infectious Diseases, Centers for Disease Control, AIDS Program. *AIDS Weekly Surveillance Report — United States,* December 28, 1987.
3. D. G. Ostrow, M. Van Raden, L. Kingsley, et al. Drug use and sexual behavior change in a cohort of homosexual men. Presented at the Third International Conference on AIDS, Washington, D.C., June 1–5, 1987:157.
4. Note 1, p. 15.
5. D. M. Fox. AIDS and the American health polity: The history and prospects of a crisis of authority. *Milbank Quarterly.* 1986; 64:7–33.
6. H. M. Ginsburg. Intravenous drug users and the acquired immunodeficiency syndrome. *Public Health Reports.* 1984; 99:206–211.
7. K. Leishman. Heterosexuals and AIDS: The second stage of the epidemic. *Atlantic.* February 1987: 39–58.
8. Note 6.
9. S. G. Craddock. Drug use before and during drug treatment: 1979–81. TOPS admission cohorts. Research Triangle Institute, Research Triangle Park, N.C., November 1983.
10. Ibid.
11. E. Preble, J. J. Casey, Jr. Taking care of business: The heroin user's life on the street. *International Journal of Addictions.* 1969; 4:1–24.
12. Mark S. Gold, M.D. *800-Cocaine.* Chapter 2, "Profile of the cocaine user." Bantam Books, New York, N.Y., 1984, pp. 7–13.
13. S. Cohen. *The Substance Abuse Problems,* vol. 1. Haworth Press, New York, N.Y., 1981.
14. William S. Burroughs. *Naked Lunch.* Grove Press, New York, N.Y., 1959.
15. E. Drucker. AIDS and addiction in New York City. *American Journal of Drug and Alcohol Abuse.* 1986: 12:165–181.
16. Note 11.
17. Note 14, p. xxxix.
18. Note 12.
19. Note 13.
20. Note 15.
21. Note 12.
22. Note 13.
23. Ibid.
24. Note 12.
25. G. H. Friedland, R. S. Klein. Transmission of human immunodeficiency virus. *New England Journal of Medicine.* 1987; 317:1125–1135.
26. Ibid.
27. Ibid.

28. R. E. Chaisson, A. R. Moss, R. Onishi, et al. Human immunodeficiency virus infection in heterosexual intravenous drug users in San Francisco. *American Journal of Public Health.* 1987; 77:169–172.

29. S. H. Weiss, H. M. Ginzburg, J. J. Goedert. Risk factors for HTLV-III infection among parenteral drug users. *Proceedings of the Society of Clinical Oncology.* 1986; 5:3.

30. E. E. Schoenbaum, P. A. Selwyn, C. A. Feiner, et al. Prevalence and risk factors associated with HTLV-III/LAV antibodies among intravenous drug abusers in a methadone program in New York City. Presented at the Second International Conference on AIDS, Paris, June 23–25, 1986.

31. D. C. Des Jarlais, S. R. Friedman. HIV infection among intravenous drug users: Epidemiology and risk reduction. *AIDS.* 1987;1:67–76.

32. Note 25.

33. Note 31.

34. Note 25.

35. H. M. Ginsburg. Intravenous drug abusers and HIV infections: A consequence of their actions. *Law, Medicine and Health Care.* 1986;14:268–272.

36. M. W. Vogt, D. J. Witt, D. E. Craven, et al. Isolation of HTLV-III/LAV from cervical secretions of women at risk for AIDS. *Lancet.* 1986;1:525–527.

37. D. D. Ho, R. T. Schooley, T. R. Rota, et al. HTLV-III in the semen and blood of a healthy homosexual man. *Science.* 1984; 226:451–453.

38. G. J. Stewart, J. P. P. Tyler, A. L. Cunningham, et al. Transmission of human T-cell lymphotropic virus type III (HTLV-III) by artificial insemination by donor. *Lancet.* 1985; 2:581–584.

39. Note 36.

40. C. B. Wofsy, J. B. Cohen, L. B. Hauer, et al. Isolation of AIDS-associated retrovirus from genital secretions of women with antibodies to the virus. *Lancet.* 1986;1:527–529.

41. T. C. Quinn, J. M. Mann, J. W. Curran, P. Piot. AIDS in Africa: An epidemiologic paradigm. *Science.* 1986; 234:955–963.

42. C. Franzen, M. Jertborn, G. Biberfield. Four generations of heterosexual transmission of LAV/HTLV-III in a Swedish town. Presented at the Second International Conference on AIDS, Paris, June 23–25, 1986.

43. L. H. Calabrese, L. V. Gopalakrishna. Transmission of HTLV-III infection from man to woman to man. *New England Journal of Medicine.* 1986; 314:987.

44. Note 25.

45. J. K. Kreiss, D. Koech, F. A. Plummer, et al. AIDS virus infection in Nairobi prostitutes: Spread of the epidemic to East Africa. *New England Journal of Medicine.* 1986; 314:414–418.

46. N. Clumeck, P. Van de Perre, M. Carael, et al. Heterosexual promiscuity among African patients with AIDS. *New England Journal of Medicine.* 1985; 313:182.

47. L. J. Eales, K. E. Nye, J. M. Parkin, et al. Association of different allelic forms of group-specific component with susceptibility to, and clinical manifestation of, human immunodeficiency virus infection. *Lancet.* 1987;1:999–1002.

48. K. Dahl, K. Martin, G. Miller. Differences among human immunodeficiency virus strains and their capacities to induce cytolysis or persistent infection of a lymphoblastoid cell line immortalized by Epstein-Barr virus. *Journal of Virology.* 1987; 61:1602–1608.

49. M. A. Fischl, G. M. Dickinson, G. M. Scott, et al. Evaluation of heterosexual partners, children, and household contacts of adults with AIDS. *Journal of the American Medical Association.* 1987; 257:640–644.

50. J. Mann, T. C. Quinn, P. Piot, et al. Condom use and HIV infection among prostitutes in Zaire. *New England Journal of Medicine.* 1987; 316:345.

51. Note 2.

52. Revision of the CDC surveillance case definition for acquired immunodeficiency syndrome. *Morbidity and Mortality Weekly Report.* 1987; 36:1S.

53. J. P. Koplan, A. M. Hardy, J. R. Allen. Epidemiology of the acquired immunodeficiency syndrome in intravenous drug users. *Advances in Alcohol and Substance Abuse.* 1986; 5:13–23.

54. Massachusetts Department of Public Health/Boston Department of Health and Hospitals. *AIDS Newsletter.* August–September 1987; 3(8).

55. U.S. Public Health Service, Centers for Disease Control. Coolfront Report. *Public Health Reports.* July–August 1986;101(4).

56. Centers for Disease Control. Review of HIV infection in the United States. *Morbidity and Mortality Weekly Report.* December 18, 1987; 36(Supp. 6).

57. T. J. Spira, D. C. Des Jarlais, M. M. Marmor, et al. Prevalence of antibody to lymphadenopathy-associated virus among drug detoxification patients in New York. *New England Journal of Medicine.* 1984; 311:467–468.

58. S. Maayan, R. Backenroth, E. Rieber, et al. Antibody to lymphadenopathy-associated virus/ human T lymphotropic virus, type III in various groups of illicit drug abusers in New York City. *Journal of Infectious Diseases.* 1985;152:843.

59. D. E. Craven, D. J. Witt, M. S. Hutchison, et al. Prevalence of antibody to human immunodeficiency virus in intravenous drug users in Boston (unpublished date, 1987).

60. Centers for Disease Control. Acquired immunodeficiency syndrome (AIDS) among blacks and Hispanics. *Morbidity and Mortality Weekly Report.* 1986; 35:655–656.

61. Note 54.

62. Ibid.

63. Note 2.

64. Note 60.

65. Note 25.

66. Ibid.

67. Note 60.

68. Note 15.

69. G. B. Scott, M. A. Fischl, N. Klimas, et al. Mothers of infants with the acquired immunodeficiency syndrome: Evidence for symptomatic and asymptomatic carriers. *Journal of the American Medical Association.* 1985; 253:363–366.

70. Centers for Disease Control. Recommendations for assisting in the prevention of perinatal transmission of human T-lymphotropic virus type III/lymphadenopathy-associated virus and acquired immunodeficiency syndrome. *Morbidity and Mortality Weekly Report.* 1985; 34:725–732.

71. F. Chiodo, M. Ricchie, P. Costiglola, et al. Vertical transmission of LAV/HTLV-III. Presented at the Second International Conference on AIDS, Paris, June 23–25, 1986.

72. Note 60.

73. Note 54.

74. Centers for Disease Control. Antibody to HIV in female prostitutes — United States. *Morbidity and Mortality Weekly Report.* 1987; 36:157–161.

75. Note 6.

76. Note 15.

77. Note 74.

78. Note 43.

79. Centers for Disease Control. Acquired immunodeficiency syndrome in correctional facilities: A report of the National Institute of Justice and the American Correctional Association. *Morbidity and Mortality Weekly Report.* 1986; 35:195–199.

80. Bureau of Communicable Disease Control, New York State Department of Health. *AIDS Surveillance Monthly Update.* September 1985.

81. Maryland Division of Correction. AIDS Press Conference, December 19, 1985.

82. D. C. Des Jarlais, S. Tross, S. R. Friedman. Behavioral changes in responses to AIDS. In *AIDS — Acquired Immunodeficiency Syndrome and Other Manifestations of HIV Infection: Epidemiology, Etiology, Immunology, Clinical Manifestations, Pathology, Control, Treatment and Prevention.* G. P. Wormser, R. Stall, E. J. Bottone (eds.). Noyes Publications, Parkridge, N.J., 1987, pp. 1053–1070.

83. New York study: Cost for caring for IVDA with AIDS is higher than for homosexuals. *AIDS Alert.* 1986;1(11):200.

84. P. A. Selwyn, C. P. Cox, C. Feiner, et al. Knowledge about AIDS and high-risk behavior among intravenous drug users in New York City. Presented at the Annual Meeting of the American Public Health Association, Washington, D.C., November 18, 1985.

85. Ibid.

86. S. R. Friedman, D.. C. Des Jarlais, J. L. Sothern. AIDS health education for intravenous drug users. *Health Education Quarterly.* 1986;13:383–393.

87. Note 82.

88. P. Biernacki, H. Feldman. Ethnographic observations of IV drug use practices that put users at risk for AIDS. Presented at the Fifteenth International Institute on the Prevention and Treatment of Drug Dependence, Amsterdam, the Netherlands, April 6–11, 1986.

89. W. E. McAuliffe. Intravenous drug use and the spread of AIDS. *Governance: Harvard Journal of Public Policy.* September 1987; 55–60.

90. J. J. Jackson, L. Rotkiewicz. A coupon program: AIDS education and drug treatment. Presented at the Third International Conference on AIDS, Washington, D.C., June 1–5, 1987:156.

91. E. C. Buning. Prevention policy on AIDS among drug addicts in Amsterdam. Presented at the Third International Conference on AIDS, Washington, D.C., June 1–5, 1987:40.

92. J. H. Rutledge, R. Conviser. The need for innovation to halt AIDS among intravenous drug abusers (IVDA) and their sex partners. Presented at the Third International Conference on AIDS, Washington, D.C., June 1–5, 1987:139.

93. Note 89.

94. Ibid.

95. Note 82.

96. Note 15.

97. S. E. Nichols. Methadone maintenance and AIDS (unpublished data, 1987).

98. Note 91.

99. R. G. Newman. Methadone treatment: Defining and evaluating success. *New England Journal of Medicine.* 1987; 317:447–450.

100. M. Pollack, M. A. Schiltz, B. LeJeune. Safer sex and acceptance of testing: Results of a nationwide annual survey among French gay men. Presented at the Third International Conference on AIDS, Washington, D.C., June 1–5, 1987.

101. Note 99.

102. V. P. Dole, M. E. Nyswander. Heroin addiction: A metabolic disease. *Archives of Internal Medicine.* 1967;120:19–24.

103. B. Willoughby, M. T. Schechter, W. J. Boyko, et al. Sexual practices and condom use in a cohort of homosexual men: Evidence of differential modification between seropositive and seronegative men. Presented at the Third International Conference on AIDS, Washington, D.C., June 1–5, 1987: 5.

104. Note 102.

105. A. Pesce, N. Negre, J. P. Cassuto. Knowledge of HIV contamination modalities and its consequence on seropositive patients' behavior. Presented at the Third International Conference on AIDS, Washington, D.C., June 1–5, 1987: 60.

106. C. B. Wofsy. Human immunodeficiency virus in women. *Journal of The American Medical Association.* 1987; 257:2074–2076.

107. F. R. Cancellieri, J. Fine, S. Holman, et al. Psychologic reactions to HIV-spectrum disease: A comparison of responses (unpublished manuscript, 1987).

108. J. Harris, R. Carr, T. Ford, T. Broadbent. Trends and utilization of Massachusetts Alternative Test Site Program. Presented at the Twenty-seventh Interscience Conference on Antimicrobial Agents and Chemotherapy, New York City, October 4–7, 1987, Abstract no. 696.

109. K. B. Meyer, S. G. Pauker. Screening for HIV: Can we afford the false positive rate? *New England Journal of Medicine.* 1987; 317:238–241.

110. Note 107.

111. Note 28.

112. Note 106.

113. Note 45.

114. Ibid.

115. S. Jain, N. Flynn, E. Keddie, et al. Disinfection of IV drug paraphernalia using commonly available materials: Hope for controlling spread of HIV among intravenous drug users? Presented at the Third International Conference on AIDS, Washington, D.C., June 1–5, 1987:42.

116. L. S. Martin, J. S. McDougal, S. L. Loskowski. Disinfection and inactivation of human T lymphotropic virus type III/lymphadenopathy-associated virus. *Journal of Infectious Diseases.* 1985;152:400–403.

117. D. C. Des Jarlais, S. R. Friedman, W. Hopkins. Risk reduction for the acquired immunodeficiency syndrome among intravenous drug users. *Annals of Internal Medicine.* 1985;103:755–759.

118. A. D. Wodak, K. Dolan, A. Imrie, et al. HIV antibodies in needles and syringes used by intravenous drug users. Presented at the Third International Conference on AIDS, Washington, D.C., June 1–5, 1987: 41.

119. Ibid.

120. R. Newcombe. The Liverpool syringe exchange scheme for drug injectors: A preliminary report. *Mersey Drugs Journal.* 1987; 6:8–10.

121. Ibid.

122. G. R. Seage, S. Lander, M. A. Barry, et al. Medical care costs of AIDS in Massachusetts. *Journal of the American Medical Association.* 1986; 256:3107–3109.

123. A. M. Hardy, K. Rauch, D. Echenberg, et al. The economic impact of the first 10,000 cases of acquired immunodeficiency syndrome in the United States. *Journal of the American Medical Association.* 1986; 255:209–216.

124. D. J. Witt, D. E. Craven, W. R. McCabe. Bacterial infection in patients with AIDS and ARC. *American Journal of Medicine.* 1987; 82:900–906.

125. Note 55, pp. 341–348.

126. Note 57.

127. Note 82.

128. Note 83.

Minorities and HIV Infection

Veneita Porter

This article discusses a preliminary comparison of responses to AIDS in ethnic communities and their basis in previously established support systems. The importance of public policy and its connection to racism and cultural insensitivities are discussed as they relate to communities of color at risk. Particular attention is paid to problems of communication and to the ethics involving confidentiality.

The AIDS crisis has emphasized the definite distinction between race and class in the United States. In order to see clearly the crisis as it is viewed in poor minority communities, primarily the Black and Latino/Hispanic communities, as well as its effects on them, it is necessary to look at how AIDS was originally connected with the gay male population when the epidemic first hit the United States in the early 1980s. The segments of the minority populations spoken of in this article are largely poor and working-class socioeconomic groups. Problems of poverty, coupled with poor medical maintenance and IV drug use, have existed in these communities for long periods of time; the occurrence of AIDS has simply compounded preexisting conditions among these populations.

Initially, discussions surrounding AIDS focused on the gay male population, mainly in large cities. AIDS was originally named GRID, gay related immune deficiency, because of the large number of those infected with the disease who were gay. Men in San Francisco were exhibiting clinical symptoms such as extreme weight loss, cancerous lesions normally found only in elderly men of Mediterranean descent, and unexplained pneumonias. Their deaths were swift and largely unexplainable. The disease baffled doctors, who were unable to diagnose it and who feared its potential spread.

AIDS also presented the media with a whole new range of possibilities. Here was a disease whose causes seemed closely related to the unexplored world of gay male sexuality. Here were indications of a world that middle America had known very little about. This world began to surface in the press, which initially defined the gay male community as made up of bars, restrooms, and public bath facilities, all of which became public domain for the media. Gay men who once had been thought of as leaders in the sexual

Veneita Porter is executive director of Rhode Island Project AIDS and is a board member of the National AIDS Network.

revolution were now seen as lepers, as people became familiar with the theories surrounding the epidemic.

Yet for all this media attention, many stories were left untold. The typical profile of a person with AIDS was a white male usually residing in San Francisco or New York. Among the general public, many understood the concept of "high risk" and felt safe. Ethnic minority communities that had already dealt with the burden of a higher incidence of hypertension, infant mortality, and cancer than the white population breathed a sigh of ill-timed relief. Investigating the likely place of origin for AIDS, scientists identified the virus as first coming from Africa, mostly the central and eastern regions, and Haiti.

Indeed, the Centers for Disease Control (CDC) in Atlanta, Georgia, initially focused on Haitian immigrants as potentially identifiable carriers of the virus and placed them on its list of high-risk populations. When Haitians were first thought to be a risk group in the United States, the backlash against them was felt severely in the major cities. Haitian stores were put out of business, Haitian children were refused admittance to school, and Haitian domestics lost their jobs.[1] In an area clouded with apprehension and varying degrees of knowledge, the public response in the majority communities was based on fear, lack of information, and sometimes racism. Here was a disease that was closely linked with gay male sexuality and its environments and with African and Haitian immigrants, communities from which most of mainstream America felt separate. In the seven years following the first identification of AIDS in the United States, little was done to focus on the fact that AIDS is everyone's disease. It has only been during the past two years that this message has begun to be carried to the minority populations.

Minority health issues and health maintenance have become increasingly important in light of the AIDS crisis. The statistics are startling: while constituting 12 and 6 percent of the U.S. population, respectively, Blacks and Latinos/Hispanics account for 25 and 14 percent, respectively, of all diagnosed AIDS cases. As such, people of color represent 39 percent of the reported cases of AIDS but make up only 18 percent of the general population.[2]

In any population where poverty is a cofactor, poor health maintenance, high infant mortality, drug use, and a high incidence of sexually transmitted disease all play a large role in making poor communities, especially poor ethnic communities, a breeding ground for many types of disease. Surprisingly, it was not until recently, with the leadership of U.S. Surgeon General C. Everett Koop, that public health authorities clearly stated that people of color needed much more information about AIDS than they were receiving.

The combination of misinformation and apathy in the culture of most poor communities has contributed to the disproportionate number of people with AIDS in these communities. According to Dr. Beny E. Primm, who runs the Urban Resources Program in Manhattan and Brooklyn, "People just feel 'I'm not an IV-drug user or a bisexual, it's not gonna get me.' But that's not the case. There are so many closet bisexuals and drug users, and former drug users who now are leading heterosexual lives, and infectious to others. It is totally alarming."[3]

Drug use, high infant mortality rates, high unemployment, low literacy rates, and other difficulties have stressed poor communities to the breaking point. Given inadequate social and medical services, and in some cases inadequate school systems, in addition to these problems, the fatigue that is experienced can only be compounded by the AIDS crisis.

On the other hand, the response of the vast majority of the gay male and lesbian population to this health crisis has been admirable. The swift and efficient mobilization of financial and emotional resources with which homosexuals have met the ever rising numbers of people affected by AIDS both within and outside their own community has given an important reminder to public policymakers about how a disease should be handled from its onset. Washington's lack of response is a clear reminder of what can happen when any problem is ignored for too long. Yet it is well to examine the resources that the gay community has had at its disposal.

Organized and highly functional groups of gay men and lesbians often reside in highly concentrated areas of industrial and urban growth. These groups range from political to religious to social and sometimes ethnic. How visible and active these groups are may well depend on how liberal or flexible their surrounding environments are. Yet even in the most conservative of cities, there exist functioning gay networks from which individuals can derive support. Examples are the agencies in New York, San Francisco, and Boston which formed with the onset of the AIDS crisis. In these cities, the pressure to create a working system of individuals and institutions willing to combat the spread of AIDS was somewhat eased by the already existing networks within the gay communities.

These organizations should be kept in mind when one examines ethnic minorities and the AIDS crisis. In most poor communities, urban or rural, minority community centers have been losing ground since the early seventies. It has only been with the resurgence of interest in minority health during the past five years that any of the centers have remained open. When the AIDS health crisis was recognized in gay communities, there were already existing support systems; in minority communities, such systems were weak or nonexistent. Now the minority community is being asked to create information agencies and support systems to meet the needs of people ill with a disease denied by that very same community. Furthermore, the community-based organizations started at the onset of this health crisis began with a certain clientele in mind. Built primarily by and for white men to serve a defined client population, these organizations were ill prepared to serve an evolving client population — one that includes people of culturally, linguistically, and ethnically different backgrounds.

How is it possible to break through cultural bias and effectively inform minority communities about behavior and risk factors?

When AIDS was first talked about in the gay community, it was a given that one needed to discuss with candor and openness one's sexual experiences, one's sexual agenda, and one's sexual preference. Gay men who had been leaders in the sexual revolution talked honestly and openly about their sexual identities and what needed to change in terms of behavior in the AIDS crisis. But in minority communities, this discussion has been a long time in coming. Among Black women, who are thirteen times as likely to get AIDS as their white counterparts,[4] the idea of sexual candor, or of sexual agendas, has been kept in the closet. There is a certain reluctance among individuals in ethnic communities to be openly gay or lesbian or for women to express sexuality in general. In Latino/Hispanic communities, the idea of women discussing sexuality may be perceived as unfeminine and perhaps immoral.

In speaking to people of color, the issues of homosexuality and bisexuality are usually best avoided. It is less threatening and more effective to concentrate on the issues of family, women, infants, and children when talking to communities where these populations are most at risk. "Minority agencies have sometimes been hesitant to fund and implement AIDS-related programs for fear [such programs are] being perceived as homosexual activities," says Norm Nickens, a representative of the San Francisco Human Rights Commission.[5]

In communities that have a strong religious tradition, the discussion of sexual behavior by either sex is not welcomed. Minority bisexuals and homosexuals, it seems, must make a choice between their sexual and cultural identities.

Thus, there are two hidden problems in the ethnic communities: one, the unwillingness or inability to deal with open sexuality, and two, the church's or leading cultural institution's refusal to accept or even confirm homosexuality or bisexuality as part of its community make-up. So a cultural bias influencing health policy issues exists, and there is some difficulty in bridging the chasm between the gay community, which may engage in frank discussion of sexual practices and behaviors, and an ethnic community where such practices are not even acknowledged. Yolanda Serrano of ADAPT, a group of volunteers — many of them former addicts — who visit shooting galleries with prevention literature, says, "To overcome the barriers posed by cultural tradition, political suspicion, and personal anxiety is an immense, forbidding task. What we need is massive, constant education for this message to get across. It has to be constant, otherwise it's not going to work."[6]

This gulf must be crossed to allow the second step of discussion — what those behaviors and risk factors are.

AIDS presented an entirely different face when Black women who were partners of IV drug users or who were IV drug users themselves were also identified as persons with AIDS in the minority communities. Those communities were then confronted with new difficulties besides the reluctance to discuss the problem and the lack of information. Serrano states that she has seen the "pandemonium" in Black families when AIDS strikes: their isolation from neighbors and friends and the rigidly defined roles that make it difficult for women to negotiate safe sex. The disease itself may exhibit symptoms differently in people of color. There has been some initial medical evidence that people of color in larger cities have a much shorter period from time of diagnosis to death than their white counterparts.[7] Existing problems, such as insufficient funding for medical research in minority communities, have already started to take a toll upon the ever growing numbers of people with AIDS. If there are insufficient funds to begin with in a community, a health crisis compounding this lack makes the stress more widely felt.

So what happens when a service agency built on one sort of model is asked to expand its services to deal with another sort of model?

The first step is to examine government response to the AIDS crisis. It is only during the last two to two and a half years that the Centers for Disease Control has put the issues of minorities and AIDS on its funding agenda. Racism, both institutionally and on a community basis, has been a problem within the health care community for some time. When coupled with the AIDS issue, racism can be an extremely powerful tool. Community agendas for medicine, research, and public health policy differ greatly from community to community and from general public policy concerns.

The gay male community has had a strong voice in making its AIDS agenda heard, ensuring that health officials and their government counterparts understand that human rights and gay civil liberties should go hand in hand in the AIDS crisis. Such political mobilization has not been matched in minority or ethnic communities. Minority communities must quickly and effectively learn to combine health coalitions and political coalitions in order to survive in this health crisis.

Government, community, and health officials must also address the problems of illiteracy and cultural influences in linguistic minorities if they are to deal effectively with the issue of health maintenance in poor communities.

"All Latinos are not the same," says Alex Compagnet, president of Salud, a new health organization in the District of Columbia which is focusing on AIDS prevention. "We come from different countries and we have different customs and traditions and levels of education, and too many programs have failed to realize that. We need education that is culturally relevant, by Latinos for Latinos."[8]

Producing informative educational materials that are culturally sensitive and linguistically accurate is a time-consuming process for service agencies. Their success in this endeavor will be a measure of how effective they can be in the long term in dealing with a health crisis in poor or ethnically different minority communities. A Spanish translation of an English-language brochure discussing symptoms of AIDS is ineffective if it shows pictures of gay white men to an audience of Latino/Hispanic mothers. Messages must be presented to audiences in a culturally sensitive manner. Animation, drawings, and audio- and videotapes need to be used to reach ethnic minorities. Commercials, bus posters, resource manuals, and radio and television public service announcements are a few of the simple but effective ways that have been tried in some communities to reach these populations. Street outreach workers are a necessary aid in dealing with communities where social clubs or civic organizations do not play a major role.

It is important to be culturally aware of the community and to address the culture within its context. Often in poor communities, children are the only lifeline people have to the world. When legacies of money, educational endowment, and property are not available, children may provide the only positive community alternative. Thus, women of childbearing age who become ill with AIDS and die will leave certain irreversible legacies in terms of community loss. As more and more people of color are affected by drugs, and as their sexual partners are being affected by drugs and AIDS, the future of the minority group is in peril.

"Sometimes in our culture," says Salud president Compagnet, "we speak of sex as something we have to hide, but SIDA [the Spanish acronym for AIDS] is a crisis that's affecting our community, and we have to take care of ourselves. Otherwise, many of our families will be affected and will disappear."[9]

There is no denying that people of color are just beginning to wake up to the issue of AIDS in their communities. But how quickly will this awakening spread? Is there a way in which government officials and policymakers can speak directly and clearly to this population? If so, what long-lasting effect will this have on public policy?

Certain Black and other minority groups, such as the church and fraternal organizations, have yet to recognize AIDS as part of their civil rights agendas. Discrimination and AIDS go hand in hand largely because of the stigma attached to the behaviors associated with transmission of the virus. The Black and Latino/Hispanic middle classes, which may possess the technical and financial resources to launch educational campaigns, have resisted acknowledging that the spread of HIV infection has something to do with sexual behavior. To overcome the barriers posed by cultural tradition and political suspicion, it is important to understand that civil rights in the AIDS battle are intimately linked to the survival and nurturance of the minority community as we now know it. The fact that all communities will have to deal with AIDS in the next several years is becoming commonplace knowledge.

Considering the problems of massive education in communities that have yet to be reached, such as low literacy populations, prison populations, people who may not have English as their first language, and young people who may be making sexual decisions in the next few years, the job of AIDS education is enormous. Despite the possible encroachment on their civil rights and the threat of AIDS and ethnic and racial discrimination, the call to become more involved has yet to be sufficiently heard by communities of color. The fact that reproductive rights, prisoners' rights, and poor people's rights in general are integrally linked with AIDS and the rights of people with AIDS has not been recognized by the vast majority of the ethnic community. The bottom line regarding ethnic communities' civil rights — access to education, access to fair housing, and access to equal paying jobs — is affected by public policy and private-sector policies on AIDS and discrimination. If mothers and fathers can be turned away from public housing because of their HIV status, whether they are Black, white, or yellow is no longer a consideration. When the government in Washington says that AIDS-related discrimination is acceptable in some circumstances, whether the person being discriminated against is Black or white is moot. When HIV and antibody testing are routinely done without patients' consent in hospitals, the color of the patient is not important. When people can be denied access to housing, jobs, and medical help because of their HIV status, civil rights take on an entirely new and different meaning. People in the human health industry have known for a long time that the contents of medical records — possibly containing HIV test results — of prisoners, welfare recipients, and people on any kind of disability or insurance assistance can become common knowledge. Inappropriate access to medical records was a problem before AIDS, and this problem has increased now that HIV status is part of the picture.

Military recruits, welfare recipients, and prison inmates are examples of persons whose records are often given inappropriate access. If three times as many people of color as whites show up HIV-positive in military recruiting records, they are subject several times over to loss of employment potential in a population that is already heavily unemployed.[10]

With respect to the poor and the disabled, medical confidentiality is a myth. The individuals concerned must have access to the knowledge of their rights of confidentiality. If not, those rights will not be granted. An article published last year in the *American Journal of Public Health* warned that "the screening of selective populations involves the systematic collection of sensitive health care information. HIV infection is associated with sexual practice and drug use, universally regarded as confidential, and HIV-infected people are predominantly members of risk groups subject to persistent prejudice and discrimination."[11]

Related to the question of confidentiality of medical records is the possibility of mandatory HIV testing in the prison population. Prisoners are known to have very few rights, less medical assistance and less access to medical benefits than those not incarcerated, and very little voice in the community at large. How the issue of mandatory testing of the largely ethnic and closed prison population is decided is sure to affect the rights of the general community to which prisoners will eventually return.

Both public health officials and minority community members must realize that simply because prisoners are behind walls does not mean that medical information and AIDS information should not reach them. Prisoners are woefully uneducated about safer sex techniques and about the role of drug-injection equipment in the spread of the AIDS virus. Prison officials' refusal or reluctance to discuss issues of homosexuality and drug use inside prison walls must be resolved. Limitations on the education of prisoners in the ways of safer sex and risk reduction put the families and communities who are on the outside waiting for them to return home at much greater peril than public officials realize. The very fact that the communities behind walls are mostly ethnic makes one wonder about the level of concern among public and prison officials with respect to the increasing needs of minority and ethnic populations.

In examining the possibilities for policy change, it is necessary to consider current national policies that will disproportionately affect people of color. All of the problems of poor minority communities make clear that in order to combat this disease and its further spread in the ethnic community, a joint effort will be required on the part of government policymakers and the members of minority communities.

What will encourage government officials and minority community members to join together to present a unified educational message and voice in the battle against AIDS?

Health policy agendas, public policy agendas, and community agendas will naturally differ. The benefit of every individual is important, but how those benefits are to be obtained will have to be resolved through lengthy discussions. Ethnic communities have every reason to be nervous, suspicious, and circumspect regarding the government's official intervention in their daily and intimate lives, and to view it as cause for both concern and education. The other issue that compounds the problem is that health centers currently operating under shrinking financial budgets are ill equipped to service the growing needs of HIV-infected clients. Minority communities, which have over and over again seen government and federal monies come into their communities only to be pulled out six or twelve years later, will naturally be suspicious when new monies are introduced to combat AIDS. Contracts involving long-standing obligations to these communities, as well as increased and supplemental fundings as AIDS case loads grow, must be part of public policy planning for ethnic minorities.

An important part of joining forces against the AIDS epidemic is experienced managerial assistance. Minority educational programs that have existed on sustenance funding should be encouraged to have financial and program planning, program administrators, and ongoing evaluation and assessment of the manner in which their agency and community needs are being met. Evaluation of management, along with productive, ongoing criticism, is a necessary component of any program-funding development. Simply because agencies are located in ethnic minority cultures does not mean that these managerial assistance packages should be neglected.

The question of women and AIDS demands the attention and concern of the minority population. Separate agencies and separate programs are needed for HIV-positive women, their children, and their families. AIDS in the ethnic community is a disease of families and cultures. People do not exist in a vacuum, and policymakers who have been working only with gay white men have recognized the limitations of this approach. In the past, the reproductive rights of women of color have, through mandatory sterilization programs, been violated. Such discriminatory practices are not a solution to the spread of AIDS in the minority family. The promotion of pre- and postnatal care for minority mothers and their babies must continue to be developed hand in hand with AIDS education and prevention.

Churches, community centers, and other existing social supports in an ethnic community must all be included in planning on public policy levels. No one should be left out in the battle against this disease. It is not just in medical but in all emotional and social environments that communities are hard hit by AIDS. Some positive steps are being taken in such states as Florida and Rhode Island, where the National Institutes of Health have made large minority grants available to local organizations. Ongoing epidemiological studies will be necessary in all minority communities.

Is AIDS a different disease in poor minority populations? Why is it that people of color with AIDS die so much sooner than their white counterparts? Is the rate of ongoing sexually transmitted diseases an issue? Is poverty a cofactor for AIDS? Is poor health maintenance from birth to death an ongoing factor? Why is it that women with AIDS die so much sooner than their male counterparts? Is there something that history or the history of medicine has not accurately looked into when considering sexually transmitted diseases and the minority community?

One public official stated that he had no idea how many people of color were currently involved in the testing of drugs to combat AIDS. Such ignorance must be stopped. Some national agendas and some baseline numbers need to be set in the involvement of minorities in AIDS protocols. Drug addiction and drug complications have long been used as an excuse to keep minorities out of medical protocols, perpetuating the stereotype that many people with AIDS have gotten the disease through involvement with drugs. CDC statistics clearly show that this is not true. The history of IV drug use and its interactions with AIDS and AIDS complications is an important epidemiological study, but other facts must also be examined. It has taken a long time to realize that AIDS is a medically complicated disease, and it has taken just as long to realize that it is also a socially and ethnically complicated disease. Added to this are complications of political agendas as they affect public policy.

Involving minority communities and giving them self-empowerment is the only way to effectively fight AIDS. Public health will continue to be an evolving population issue as communities begin to discover solutions to their immediately apparent problems, and to identify seemingly hidden ones. For example, Arturo Olivas, director of Cara a Cara (Face to Face), a Los Angeles–based AIDS prevention organization, found that in the Latino/Hispanic community, "programs that focus on women to try and get men to use condoms won't work. We're trying to make it the macho thing to do. The theme of a new poster campaign aimed at Latin men features a male face that is half human and half skeleton. The message: 'AIDS Attacks Even the Most Macho.'"

Similarly, it is an ex-IV drug user who, understanding the intricacies of that community, can best talk about what it's like to be part of that culture. And people with AIDS, through their willingness to share their experience of the disease, may be the best advocates of prevention. It is hoped, however, that it will be the survivors in a healthy minority community who will provide examples of the effectiveness of safer sex, safer needle use, abstinence, and condom use programs.

In ethnic communities, sound public policies and politics must be used to heal the wounds that have been suffered in relations between some of the community-based organizations, AIDS agencies, and government policymakers. Eight years into the epidemic, answers are still coming too slowly. In order to know the facts and act on them effectively, minority populations must hear the message and learn to empower themselves so that they can face an existing problem and become part of an evolving solution.

Special thanks to Robin Bradford and Tom Menard.

Notes

1. Leonard A. Eisner, *Fair Employment Report* (December 1983): 206.
2. Centers for Disease Control, "AIDS Among Blacks and Hispanics in the U.S.," *Morbidity and Mortality Weekly Report* 35, no. 42 (October 24, 1986): 655–666.

3. Dr. Beny E. Primm, in Richard Goldstein, "AIDS and Race, A Hidden Epidemic," *Village Voice*, March 10, 1987, p. 25.

4. Mary Guinen, "Epidemiology of AIDS in Women in the U.S. (1981–1986)," *Journal of the American Medical Association* 257, no. 15 (1987): 2039–2049.

5. *Exchange* 4 (May 1987): 2.

6. Yolanda Serrano, in Goldstein, "AIDS and Race," p. 27.

7. Dr. Wayne Greaves, "People of Color: The Discriminatory Impact," *The Report from the New York City Commission on Human Rights* (September 1986): 3.

8. Alex Compagnet, in Sandra G. Boodman, "Everyone Talks about AIDS — but Hispanics," *Washington Post Weekly Report,* January 4–10, 1988, p. 31.

9. Ibid.

10. Randall Stone Burner, "Risk Factors in Military Recruits in HIV-Positive Antibody," *New England Journal of Medicine* 315, no. 21 (1987): 1355.

11. Larry Gostin and William Curran, "AIDS Screening Confidentiality and the Duty to Warn," *American Journal of Public Health* 77 (March 1987): 364.

"Here we are at an international AIDS conference. Yesterday a woman came up to me and said, 'May I have two minutes of your time?' She said, 'I'm asking doctors how they feel about treating AIDS patients.' And I said, 'Well, actually I'm not a doctor. I'm an AIDS patient,' and as she was shaking hands, her hand whipped away, she took two steps backward, and the look of horror on her face was absolutely diabolical. Now for that to happen at an international AIDS conference where you're going to meet people with AIDS is, well, I really don't know, but let me say this to all people who are PWAs, Don't be sad, don't go out there and cry all the time and mope around and be sad, be happy, live the rest of your life that you've got left, spend it to the fullest."

U.S. Women and HIV Infection

P. Clay Stephens, P.A.

Women are inadequately provided with HIV services and education and are differentially denied access to these. Divisions of race, ethnicity, economic class, and religion, among others, are compounded by sexual discrimination within each of these categories.

Review of current data on women with AIDS reveals that the reporting methods used convey a false impression that women are not at significant risk. Moreover, the persons indirectly affected by AIDS are predominantly women — mothers, sisters, partners, family members, teachers, and human service workers. Thus, AIDS is more of a women's issue than the statistics imply.

Women, as a gender-defined class, face major cultural obstacles to service, beginning with their characterization as "vessels of infection and vectors of perinatal transmission." Women are considered not as individuals worthy of attention, but merely as sources of the infection of others, that is, men and children.

Examples of barriers to service, of SOP (standard operating procedure), are explored through focusing on specific groups of women and their concerns: the unique peri-treatment issues of women intravenous drug users and their minority status among male users; the inability of mainstream health promotion campaigns to adequately address the gender differences within the minorities; the disregard for the reproductive rights of the mother in the rush to protect the fetus from HIV infection, and the lack of supportive care for the woman who chooses to continue her pregnancy; the blame placed on women prostitutes for "heterosexual spread," hiding the reality of their risk level and obstructing their utilization as models and instructors of risk-reduction activities; and the hostility and twin burden of sexual discrimination and homophobia directed toward lesbians (including those working in AIDS service organizations), which deny these women the ability to access and eliminate their own risk, if any.

The last section of the article explores gender-specific approaches to service delivery and proposes formats for change.

The opinions expressed herein are the personal opinions of the author and do not necessarily reflect the policies of the Massachusetts Department of Public Health.

P. Clay Stephens, P.A., is the coordinator of AIDS Resource Development for the AIDS Program at the Massachusetts Department of Public Health. She was previously involved in clinical HIV research at the Fenway Community Health Center in Boston and is a volunteer with the AIDS Action Committee of Massachusetts. Ms. Stephens has presented both nationally and internationally on women and AIDS.

The bulk of HIV-related services and education in the United States has been aimed at persons whose sex is consensual, whose use of drugs is recreational, and whose language is English; who have the resources to seek and choose their source of health care and counseling; and who have enough control over their own life and their family's lives to make the changes necessary to prevent infection, or to prolong their life and the quality of that life if they do become infected.

The people not yet reached are those whose sex is not or is only marginally consensual; for whom drugs are a lifestyle; who have diminished literacy; who are separated from the dominant culture by racial, ethnic, economic, and religious differences; who do not have access to the health care deemed standard in this society; and who, owing to institutionalized discrimination based on race, sex, and economic class, are not in control of their own and their family's future.[1]

This is not an accident. Most of the AIDS service organizations and the local, state, and federally funded services that followed were initiated by the gay male community or were a result of the lobbying efforts of that constituency. Beset both by a strange disease and by the effects of homophobia, this community began by taking care of its own. Although gay and bisexual men still represent the largest portion of persons with AIDS (PWAs),[2] these agencies have now included services for the full range of those affected by HIV infection. In January 1986, Richard Dunn, executive director of Gay Men's Health Crisis (GMHC) in New York City, described that organization's original client profile as a thirty- to thirty-five-year-old, middle-class, employed, white, gay male earning $35,000 or more per year. By late 1985 the typical GMHC client was a Black or Hispanic, twenty-two- to twenty-nine-year-old, unemployed, possibly Spanish-speaking, IV-drug-using mother of two.[3] In other words, a woman.

Outside the New York/New Jersey area, the change has been less dramatic but is still evident. Realizing that in most instances there would be few others ready and able to care for these nongay and nonmale groups, the AIDS service organizations (ASOs) have created minority and intravenous drug user (IVDU) programs within the scope of services originally designed for gay and bisexual men. Yet the flavor of the early orientation lingers. Programs developed for "single"[4] middle-class white men simply do not fit persons outside these bounds, however well intentioned these programs may be.

Whether speaking of women as a class, as a portion of those persons using IV drugs, or as members of the minority communities or other HIV-affected groups, they do not fit into the services designed for men belonging to these latter communities. The situation is aggravated by the realization that a woman seeking HIV-related services is usually seeking services for her children or other family members as well. (The persons and story described in the following vignette, and in the other vignettes throughout this article, are real; the names and identifiers have been changed to protect confidentiality.)

> Two babies, John and Marcus, tumble over one another, sharing toys, bottles, and occasionally their grandmother's lap. Portia's daughter died six months ago, leaving behind the twins and three older children. Portia feels very lucky that her grandchildren are well and that she has been able to keep them together. The oldest child, Nevita, has been having problems at school. The nurse at her new junior high insisted that she show proof that she is free of HIV infection even though her mother became infected from a transfusion she received after the twins were delivered.

From the perspective of cultural and racial minorities, Mario A. Orlandi discusses the "barriers to intervention experienced by population subgroups when the majority is targeted."[5] Design of prevention strategies must include recognition of the following:

Language — failure to appreciate health promotion messages when language or symbols are used that are not understandable or are misunderstood by the subgroup;

Reading level — using printed materials that are too sophisticated or beyond the reading level of the subgroup members;

Models — using endorsements for the health promotion campaign from prominent individuals or organizations that are not well known to the subgroup members:

Inappropriate messages — using motivational messages that are not salient to subgroup members;

Motivational issues — the fear that the primary motivation for the health promotion campaign is the desire to control the subculture, robbing from it the specific practices that have historically defined it;

Inappropriate target — the belief that the health promotion campaign is worthwhile, but that the designers never really intended the subculture to participate or to benefit;

Welfare stigma — the tendency to view the health promotion campaign as a "handout" and to avoid it as a matter of pride;

Perceived responsibility — the attitude that the campaign deals with subject areas and life choices that concern the family and the individual, not the public health establishment;

Relevance of health promotion — the belief that more pressing concerns such as poverty, crime, unemployment, and hunger should be addressed prior to the health promotion campaign;

Entropy — the tendency for subgroup members to perceive themselves as powerless or helpless when confronted with the enormous economic and sociocultural barriers and to express a lack of motivation to engage in self-improvement activities.[6]

While Orlandi's material was developed to assist in targeting minority health promotion activities, the concepts outlined should be utilized when the target groups differ from the majority by gender or economic class, or both. To fully appreciate the obstacle to service for women affected by HIV infection, it is necessary to understand just who these women are. As of February 1, 1988, the number of women with AIDS, ARC, and demonstrated HIV infection was estimated to be between 189,550 and 379,100. Among the 3,791 women with CDC-defined AIDS,[7] the primary routes of infection are their own needle sharing during intravenous drug use and sexually acquired infection from partners who are themselves intravenous drug users.[8] Other women have become infected through blood transfusions prior to screening of the blood supply in 1985; use of blood products or components, or both, prior to screening and heat treatment begun in 1985; and as partners of infected men. A woman could become infected through sexual contact with another woman if a sufficient amount of blood or body fluids was exchanged. As of February 1988, however, no woman with an AIDS diagnosis had been infected in this manner. (Women-to-woman transmission will be discussed later in this article.)

While the proportion of women among persons with AIDS (PWAs) in the United States has ranged consistently between 6 and 7 percent, it is important to recognize that women constitute a total of 27 percent of the population of PWAs in those groups into which a woman can be placed, that is, all groups except gay and bisexual men and intravenous-drug-using gay and bisexual men. Further, this figure is on the increase, having been 22 percent in the fall of 1987. As only full-blown cases of AIDS are reported in the United States, estimates of the population of women with ARC and HIV seropositivity are derived from seroprevalence studies and are confirmed by demographical information from alternative test sites (ATSs), clinics, AIDS service organizations, hotlines, and so on.

The demographic distribution in children with AIDS parallels that of infected women. Although the number of children with CDC-defined AIDS is relatively small — 789 as of February 1, 1988 — the number of children infected may be as much as ten to fifty times greater.

Women at risk for HIV infection include intravenous drug users and other needle sharers and/or unprotected sexual partners of men using intravenous drugs; and unprotected sexual partners of gay and bisexual men, of men infected through blood or blood products prior to 1985, or of male residents living in areas where HIV infection is considered endemic.

The groups of women just described are often the only ones discussed in AIDS articles and programs. However, the largest group affected by the HIV epidemic are those women responsible for the direct or indirect care of persons with HIV infection. Included are mothers, wives, sisters, and other female family members providing care in home and hospice situations throughout the course of infection up to and including death. Involved in the medical setting, and thus at risk of HIV infection, are physicians, nurses, ancillary

Table 1

Massachusetts Females by Age and Race*

Age	White No.	White %	Minority No.	Minority %	Total No.	Total %
Below 13	4	3%	7	6%	11	9%
13–19	0	0	0	0	0	0
20–29	15	13	15	13	30	26
30–39	17	15	34	30	51	44
40–49	5	4	4	3	9	8
50–59	6	5	2	2	8	7
60 plus	5	4	1	1	6	5
Totals	52	45%	63	55%	115	100%

*In this table, race is not broken down beyond minority status. This is due to the need for confidentiality and is done wherever a specific identifier is under 5 total. Thus, "minority" includes Black, Hispanic, Asian/Pacific Rim, native American/Alaskan native, and other/unknown.

Source: Jeanne M. Day, AIDS epidemiologist, AIDS Program, Massachusetts Department of Public Health.

Table 2

Infection by Risk Behavior or Route, Massachusetts and U.S., as of February 1988

Risk Behavior/Route	Massachusetts				United States			
	Male		Female		Male		Female	
	No.	%	No.	%	No.	%	No.	%
Gay/bisexual male	725	72%			3,369	70%	—	—
Gay/bisexual male using IV drugs	43	4			3,858	8	—	—
Intravenous drug user	131	13	47	45%	6,961	15	1,916	51%
Hemophiliacs	15	1	1	1	499	1	20	1
Heterosexual contact	58	6	38	37	948	2	1,110	29
Transfusion recipients	17	2	13	13	793	2	413	11
Undetermined	24	2	5	5	1,248	3	332	9
Subtotal	1,013	100	104	100	7,676	100	3,791	100
Totals, Male and Female		1,117	100%			51,467	100%	

Source: Jeanne M. Day, AIDS epidemiologist, AIDS Program, Massachusetts Department of Public Health.

Table 3

Massachusetts Cases of Adult and Pediatric AIDS by Race and Sex in Comparison with Total U.S. Cases as of February 1988

		Massachusetts		U.S.		Massachusetts
		No.	% of Sex	No.	%	% of U.S. Cases
White:	Men	738	72.8%			
	Women	48	4.7			
	Pediatrics	8	0.7			
	Subtotal	794	78.3%	31,460	60%	2.52%
Black:	Men	180	17.7			
	Women	45	4.4			
	Pediatrics	9	0.8			
	Subtotal	234	23.0%	13,177	25%	1.77%
Hispanic:	Men	90	8.8			
	Women	10	1.0			
	Pediatrics	>5*	—			
	Subtotal	100*	9.9%	7,135	14%	1.40%
Other/unknown**	Men	5	0.5			
	Women	1	0.1			
	Pediatrics	4*	0.4			
	Subtotal	10	1.0%	484	1%	2.06%
Totals:	Men	1,013	—			
	Women	104	—			
	Pediatrics	21*	—			
	Total cases	1,138	—	52,256	100.0%	2.18%

*This total is, as indicated, less than 5 and therefore not listed. The children in this category, if any, are listed in the undesignated ("other/unknown") group in an effort to protect confidentiality.

**"Other/unknown" includes but is not limited to Asian/Pacific Islanders, native American/Alaskan natives, those cases outside these categories included to protect confidentiality, and those cases where a racial factor was not known.

Source: Jeanne M. Day, AIDS epidemiologist, AIDS Program, Massachusetts Department of Public Health.

Figure 1

Pediatric AIDS Case Distribution, February 1988

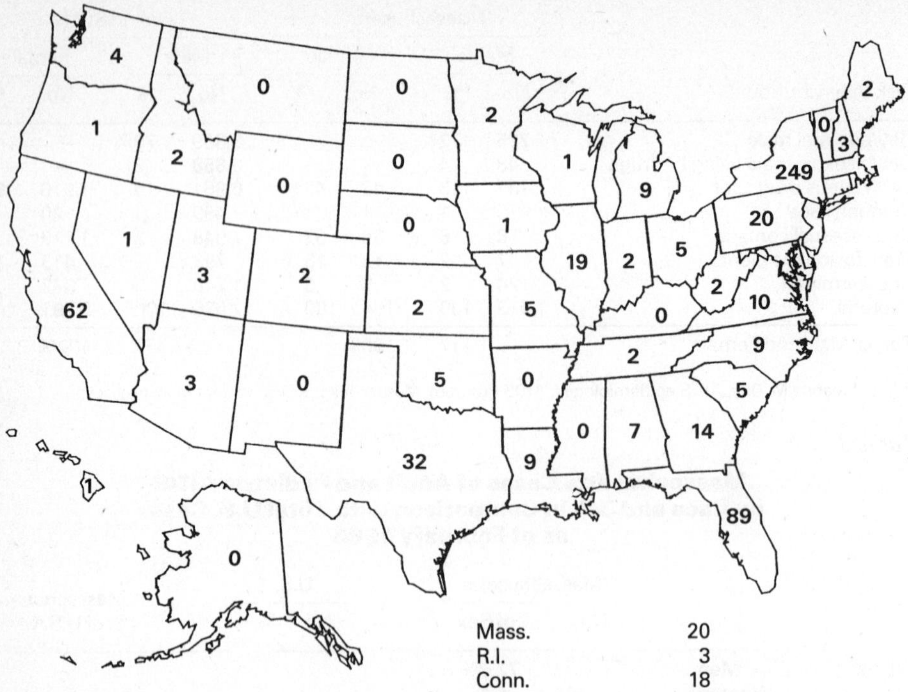

Mass.	20
R.I.	3
Conn.	18
N.J.	103
Del.	2
Md.	20
D.C.	10
Guam	0
Trust Territories	0
Puerto Rico	30

Source: AIDS Weekly Surveillance Report — United States, AIDS Program, Center for Infectious Diseases, Centers for Disease Control, Atlanta, Ga., 1 February 1988.

and accessory personnel, social workers, and custodial and other institutional workers. Persons involved outside hospitals and clinics include hospice workers, home health aides and other home care staff, and visiting nurses. As women predominate in all helping professions, simple mathematics indicate that women provide the bulk of medical, home, and family care for persons with AIDS in the United States.

> Karen is a thirty-eight-year-old ICU nurse at a regional medical center. She works full-time, lives alone, and has just been hired to administrate the AIDS unit when it opens in sixty days. She says she has never been so challenged in her nursing career as she has been working with HIV-infected patients. She is never seen without a journal under her arm. Her smile widens as she tells you that when the epidemic is over, she would like to live in Florida or some other warm place. Karen has had difficulty staying warm since she was diagnosed with her first bout of PCP [*Pneumocystis carinii* pneumonia] just two months after her hemophiliac husband died.

As in other helping professions, educational and outreach workers in both public and private AIDS organizations are predominantly women, as are teachers, media specialists, and cultural, religious, and community service organization members serving the larger community in attempting to reduce the spread of HIV infection.

In a larger sense, it is women who perpetuate and teach cultural norms and who are central to the passage of those norms through child-raising activities, teaching professions, and social service activities. Women must be seen as targets of AIDS education within their instructional roles. They must be trained in the basic information as well as in techniques that will allow them to pass this information on to those around them.

Recognition of the role of women in the struggle to stop the spread of HIV infection should not be read as a belittlement of the efforts of the gay male community. Gay and bisexual men and the organizations they have formed were the first to address the issue of AIDS and as such have led the larger community in its attempts to understand the needs of PWAs and the social and political ramifications of the epidemic. The goal is, rather, to bring to light the contribution of women and to examine the burden placed on them by this disease.

What little attention has been given to women affected by HIV has been inappropriate, offensive, and a perpetuation of negative stereotypes. In Washington, D.C., at the Third International Conference on AIDS (June 1987), women were repeatedly characterized as "vessels of infection and vectors of perinatal transmission,"[9] often by the same researchers who offered in their own work the suggestion that one must be sensitive to the differences of the particular male subculture within which their research was being conducted.

The danger of "vessel and vector" thinking is not only the personal and group insult delivered, but the blindness demonstrated and sanctioned therein. This results in lack of care, inappropriate services or no services at all, and inadequate funding — if any — for research and medical care. What begins as a phrase of epidemiological shorthand becomes a society-wide policy. Most of the problems are not new; they are simply viewed through another set of distorted lenses. AIDS is a paradigm for the condition of women within our society.

> Ellen lives in a small Maine community with her husband and three children, ages six, eight, and twelve. In the spring of 1983, she underwent surgery and received one unit of blood. She is a forty-mile-a-week runner and works full-time as a librarian. In October of 1986 she was notified by phone that the donor of her blood transfusion had developed AIDS and that she should be tested. She is antibody-positive. Her husband is negative and has remained so. She has since developed ITP and has to quit running, no longer works because of her fatigue, and has been on steroids for five months in an attempt to slow the drop in her platelets. She describes her life as working full-time to stay well and complains about the amount of work she must do to keep her various physicians in contact with one another and informed of new advances in HIV-related ITP treatment.

It is difficult to speak of the group of IVDUs as a community, since they are not self- or internally organized. The group has not yet come together to respond to the threat of HIV infection. Most services have been and will continue to be delivered by outsiders, whether social service personnel or recovering or ex-users who are working in their former communities.

As a group, IVDUs have a male:female ratio of 3:1 or 4:1; are undereducated and under- or unemployed; live in urban areas; are frequently members of a minority, possibly non- or minimally English-speaking; have low levels of literacy; are not available to the media; are involved in criminal behaviors aside from their drug use; and are members only of the street corner society and the drug underground.[10]

Women within this group are additionally segregated by their responsibility for family members (male partner(s), children, parents) and by their own pregnancies; are even less likely than their male counterparts to be English-speaking; are less press available; and are more likely to be working in the sex industry for drugs or money. Women are therefore involved in criminal behavior and activities and are at risk of interaction with the criminal system as well as with the welfare/social service systems.[11] The latter connection is often perceived as negative, owing to the power of social workers to remove children from their mother's custody or to interrupt the mother's financial aid as a punishment for various infractions. Even if employed, women often work at minimum wage or in unprotected occupations. Women's salaries continue to represent only 64 percent of men's wages,[12] thus furthering their poverty and alienation.

Very little research has been done on the pre-, intra-, and post-treatment differences between men and women. In preparation for a study of impaired female physicians, Carolyn A. Martin and G. Douglas Talbott conducted a survey of the literature on women and chemical dependence.[13] Although prepared for a particular class of women, their findings apply directly to women intravenous drug users. They noted:

- Women often began drinking later but sought treatment earlier, therefore accumulating fewer years of problems with drugs and alcohol. . . .
- Women's abuse is more likely tied to precipitating adult crisis. . . .
- Women have fewer persons involved in their life-support systems. Women, in fact, are often the support system for their families.
- Women have fewer financial resources.
- Women have fewer employment opportunities.[14]

Women in treatment also differ greatly in that they are in therapy singly or in small groups (unless able to enter a women-only program); are often housed separately from the male participants in inpatient settings and halfway houses; and frequently leave treatment either before completion or otherwise earlier than men, owing to family or financial pressures. Martin and Talbott wisely comment that the underlying realities "may be true for women in general — whether or not chemically dependent."[15] Upon closely observing the Georgia Impaired Physicians Program, the authors made note of intra-treatment problems facing women. Again, the setting is different, but the outcome of their review speaks directly to women intravenous drug users.

Most group treatment concepts utilize peer groups to deal with feelings, to refashion distorted beliefs, to develop nonchemical coping skills, and to establish new peer norms. Over 1,000 males but only 39 females entered the Georgia program between 1975 and 1986. While this may obviously represent problems of identification, intervention, and referral as well as the low proportion of women in the ranks of physicians, it also means that virtually no women entering the program were enrolled with true, that is, female, peers. Further, the confrontational methodology utilized may have been diametrically opposed to the needs of these women, in that women often entered already in touch with their feelings and needing to integrate diverse issues and pressures. The males conversely entered very much out of touch and needed to break down barriers and recognize diversity in themselves through techniques such as confrontation and encounter. Women's goals in treatment were as follows:

1. to trust the treatment concept and staff;

2. to open themselves to others; and

3. to cope with the realities of return to the community:

   a. that — although recovered — women drug users are seen as "worse" than male drug users, and

   b. that no matter how successful treatment was, women would return to a profession in which they encountered hostility and would remain a minority.

Martin and Talbott repeatedly, without naming it as such, point out the sexism and sexual discrimination that women physicians — and all women users — will continue to face before, during, and after treatment. They therefore developed a list of tasks for the treatment and recovery of women users:

1. Provision of women-only groups for the discussion of sexual and spiritual issues.

2. In groups of professional women, dealing openly with the lack of trust in each other engendered by constantly being in the minority.

3. If lesbian women are involved, provision of ground rules enforced for their safety in discussing lifestyle issues. Lesbian groups would be ideal.

4. Recognition that no treatment can change women's experience of their environment as hostile but can offer coping skills and the ability to recognize trustworthiness and support when available from women peers.

To put this in more explicit terms, there is the adage in the alcoholism treatment community that nine out of ten wives stay with their alcoholic husbands but nine out of ten husbands leave their alcoholic wives. This appears to be true in the IVDU treatment community as well. Treatment will not change these circumstances, but it is hoped that each individual woman will leave capable of coping with these stresses without having to resort to substance dependence and with the support of other women living and coping successfully with the same pressures.

Reproductive rights take on new meaning when applied to the issues of HIV infection. Often seen as a shorthand for the availability of abortion, the term *reproductive rights* is actually the umbrella concept of freedom of choice, supported by complete and bias-free information. Applied to HIV infection, it is the right of an infected or at-risk woman to obtain unbiased, factual, and up-to-date information about birth control, safer sex techniques, pregnancy, pregnancy outcome for herself and her child, and full access to supportive perinatal, pediatric, and abortion services. It is further the right of the individual woman to make her own reproductive choices and to have access to support both for her decision and for its outcome.[16]

It is not sufficient to offer the best of information and counseling and then send a woman out alone to seek care in a hostile environment. Unfortunately, early in the epidemic some abortion clinics demonstrated the same reluctance to serve HIV-infected women as did other types of medical facilities. Those clinics which did serve these women often marked charts visibly, insisted on ''spacesuit'' infection control measures, served the HIV-infected woman last during the clinic session, and kept her away from other women having procedures, thus denying her peer support.[17] Other clinics simply refused to serve any women who, by medical and sexual history, might be at risk of HIV infection. This was accomplished by stating that their clinic was not medically equipped or staffed to serve the HIV-infected woman and by providing a ready referral. Happily, instances of this policy are on the decrease, as the concept of universal precautions has become accepted and as the Centers for Disease Control (CDC), medical organizations, and associations have drafted policy and infection-control standards. What has not changed as readily is the attitude of the clinic staff, which often does not recognize that the HIV-infected woman, unlike the bulk of their clients, may be seeking termination not of an unwanted pregnancy but of a wanted pregnancy that was actively sought and that she has chosen to terminate upon learning of her infection and the possible outcomes. This situation, like that of the woman carrying a Down's syndrome child, has forced a review and subsequent change in the counseling and support offered to the HIV-infected woman in the abortion setting.

> Carol is twenty-seven, the mother of two infected children, ages two and one. She used IV drugs for a short time in 1982. She was the first known HIV-positive woman to deliver at a large urban New England hospital. After her Caesarean delivery, she and her baby were left unassisted in her room, and her meals and the baby's bottles were left on the floor outside her door. Social workers, standing gloved and masked in the doorway, berated her for ''giving her baby AIDS.'' Two years later, she and both children are doing very well. She delivered her second child at the same hospital in a warm and caring environment. Between the births she had ''starred'' in a training film for delivery room nurses dealing with HIV infection. She shared her first experience so that other mothers would not have to go through such rejection. The social workers came by during her second hospitalization to apologize and stayed to become friends.

The woman who is both HIV-infected and pregnant and who chooses to continue her pregnancy also finds it difficult to obtain adequate prenatal and delivery services that are supportive of her decision. Even if she is able to locate a clinician who has both an understanding of HIV infection and the personal ability to support her choice, she is still faced with discrimination and hostility from the other staff members. More than once, a receptionist or other ancillary staff person with access to the chart has accused a woman of willfully killing her baby with AIDS. Other women, having made the choice to continue the pregnancy, find themselves questioned repeatedly about their decision right up to the legal limit of availability of abortion. Some have even been offered the chance to abort in the third trimester only because of their HIV seropositivity.

This situation is difficult enough for the woman with the personal and financial skills to control the nature and quality of her health care. For the women most at risk of HIV infection, that is, women of color, women intravenous drug users, and women of lower socioeconomic status who may not share the language and culture of the individuals delivering counseling and care, the results are as reprehensible as those of the early seventies, when women of color and non-English-speaking women were being sterilized without consent.

This only confounds the situation of women who already have little or no access to adequate medical care during their pregnancies and whose attempts to obtain that care are met with hostility, discrimination, and disregard.

This does not occur simply at the health care delivery site but at all levels, including public policy. In early 1985, a Black physician, speaking during the question-and-answer portion of a public health issues conference, stated that "no Black children should be born until there exists a cure for AIDS." Yes, he was responding to the devastating effect of AIDS-related illnesses on the community he represented, but as the Black women in the audience responded, "No Black babies means genocide, whether we do it to ourselves or whether they do it to us."[18]

> Doralina is struggling to tell her eleven-year-old son that she is ill and may not live through the year. He knows she has been tired and regularly sees the family doctor but he thinks she will be well soon. Every time she gets up the courage to tell him that she has AIDS and was infected by her boyfriend, who died last year, she stops. She remembers the AIDS jokes, and the derisive laughter floating up to her bedroom last summer as her son and his friends sat on the stoop.

Add the burden of current intravenous drug use to the situation, and the institutionalized hostility deepens. The typical drug treatment program does not take into account the reality that women care for children and other family members, nor does it consider that in comparison to men, women have less income and less insurance coverage for participation in drug rehabilitation programs, or that they may be pregnant at the time of seeking services. In fact, a great number of women see pregnancy as a time and a motivation either to become drug free or to go on methadone. Long waiting lists characterize drug rehabilitation and detoxification programs. Even entry into such a program does not solve a woman's problems. Once in, she must try to avoid any situation or circumstance that might cause her to leave. But not every woman can. For instance, let's suppose that a woman who has been on a waiting list for many months to enter a methadone maintenance program is notified that she may now begin treatment. Having placed her children in the care of her mother, she enters the program and is doing well as a resident, but then learns that one of her children has become ill. In order to meet the needs of that child, she may have to leave the program, even though doing so could jeopardize her chances of returning. Reentry might involve penalties — such as increased chores and delayed or withheld privileges — or being placed again at the bottom of a lengthy waiting list. This can happen and has happened even to pregnant women, who are thereby forced back onto street drugs.[19] Other women find that in order to have their rehabilitation program paid for by the state or local government, they must give up or sign off custody of their children; if a woman should subsequently leave the program, regardless of the reason, her children may be taken from her.

As the result of these and other instances of standard operating procedure (SOP), the very women who need the services most are prevented from obtaining them. Social commentators have remarked that SOP will kill us all, and the statement may never have been so true as in the fight against AIDS.

> Thea is a family practitioner who has for many years shared a practice with another GP to allow her time to work both medically and politically with women working in

the sex industry. With the AIDS epidemic came an increased involvement in the sharing of safer sex techniques and a concentration on the civil rights of sex workers. Later this year, she will leave her current practice to join that of another friend, which has become exclusively HIV-oriented. She will continue her political work and has begun a support group for family practitioners working with PWAs.

Even the most enlightened and exceptional programs can be handicapped by rules and regulations. In The Hague, the Netherlands, a needle exchange program operates between 1:00 and 5:00 in the afternoon, Monday through Friday. In Great Britain, heroin prescriptions for registered addicts are available Monday through Friday. On Friday, when the addict receives a three-day dose, it is usually taken or sold immediately, thus putting the addict back on street drugs for the weekend.[20, 21] In the United States, safer sex information is printed in slick brochures, clinical language, and, for the most part, only in English. AIDS service providers can be and are prevented by their funding sources from using vernacular; printing explicit materials; providing condoms, dental dams, and needle cleaning supplies;[22] mentioning abortion as a reproductive option; referring to birth control services;[23] speaking about sex or drugs to anyone under age eighteen;[24] discussing same-sex and nonmarital sexual activities; or offering alternative or non-Western medical treatment options.[25] Individuals and agencies can be forced to spend as much time justifying their services as they do delivering them. Creativity is stifled by a funding process that is both lengthy and ornate. Individuals, groups, and associations informally delivering services are often passed over in favor of established agencies even though they have no hands-on AIDS experience.

HIV counselors have related cases in which women clients have listed other infected or at-risk women as their only possible source of infection. Numerous letters in medical journals have postulated this route, but none of the letters, as written, withstand scrutiny.[26]

Prior to 1985, the word "AIDS" or the thought of HIV infection was rarely, if ever, associated with the word *lesbian.* This invisibility stemmed both from the lack of recognition of women's contribution to AIDS service organizations and from the conspicuous absence of lesbians from the Centers for Disease Control Risk Group list. The fall of 1985 was the beginning of a new era of recognition: lesbians were proclaimed to be "God's chosen children"[27] and to be free of any fear of HIV infection. As with most stereotypes, this proclamation was no blessing. Half the lesbian community celebrated their "immunity" by continuation of all sexual and drug-related behaviors without scrutiny, while the other half wondered, "If we are so free, why do we feel so bad?"[28] Thus began a conflict that continues to the present: how to educate the lesbian community about the realities of HIV infection without creating hysteria; how to be recognized by gay men and the heterosexual community without inviting further homophobia and discrimination; and how — within the gay community and the AIDS service organizations — to address the misogyny and oppressive behaviors directed at women. The resolution of this conflict is hampered by the dismal lack of understanding of lesbian sexual practices and the social consequences of living a lesbian lifestyle.

Within the lesbian and gay community, gay males are the prime targets in AIDS public education activities sponsored by AIDS service organizations. Male educators often regard lesbian risk as trivial compared to their own, or, as mentioned above, nonexistent. Lesbian sexuality — and women's sexuality in general — is perceived as boring at best and contemptuous and disgusting at worst.[29]

By 1988, the seventh year since the recognition of the syndrome, only eight women with AIDS have identified themselves as lesbians; two other women identified themselves as engaging exclusively in same-sex activity.[30] All of these women are or were intravenous drug users or transfusion recipients whose sexual identity and practices had nothing to do with their route of infection. As the number of CDC-defined adult AIDS cases in the United States was 51,467 as of February 1, 1988, the total lack of woman-to-woman transmission of infection is profound.

It must be remembered, however, that in the United States only cases of full-blown AIDS are reportable; thus, if there are any cases of ARC or HIV seropositivity in lesbians, there is no documentation of them. Personal communications and letters to medical journals have filled this gap. Lesbian health care workers and AIDS service providers have discussed two sets of lesbian partners in which one woman was infected through IV drug use and her partner became infected through significant contact with the other's menstrual blood.[31] Additionally, a letter to the *Journal of the American Medical Association* in December 1986 attempted to document woman-to-woman transmission via "traumatic sexual activities." This particular case was originally reported by Sabatini and Hirschman in the 1984 *AIDS Research Journal.*

Marea Murray exhaustively dissected the *JAMA* letter and the original report in the July 31, 1986, edition of the Boston newspaper *Bay Windows.* This same analysis appeared in *Gay Community News,* another Boston publication, the following month. Murray concluded that the newly infected woman had a much greater chance of having been infected by her two male sexual partners than by her woman partner, given the dates of appearance of symptoms. The point is not to argue "medical" events, but to note that the researchers' lack of understanding of female/female sexual activity led them to discount behavior that has led to transmission many times over in favor of behaviors that, though exotic to these physicians, have yet to be shown to be more than a theoretical risk. Murray further pointed out the following:

> Lesbians do need to consider our own behaviors and decide for ourselves, between ourselves, with our partners whether to engage in safer sex and which behaviors that might include as well as what changes we wish to make (if any). No one is immune here and as women and lesbians (or bisexuals) we are the least likely groups to be addressed, considered, or informed about how to be safer.[32]

A lesbian is at risk of HIV infection, as is any woman, only to the extent of her risky behavior. Her identity is neither protective nor condemning. Once again it becomes clear that it is particularly important to discuss specific practices rather than personal sexual/political identity and that the discussion must be free of prejudice toward particular sexual activities.

> Claire is bored, lonely, and disgusted. Last night she met a nice woman at the alcohol/chemical free women's dance and invited her home for the night afterward. After a cup of tea, Claire explained to Shirl that she needed to use safer sex. Shirl got upset — practically screaming — calling her "stupid, paranoid, and male-identified" for thinking that two women could transmit HIV to one another. "I thought you were strange when you said you volunteered at the AIDS project," she said when she was asked to leave. A recovering needle user, Claire hopes someday to meet a woman who understands and believes safer sex is the right thing to do. Until then, she'd rather be lonely.

Actual infection, however, is not the only risk this epidemic brings to lesbians. AIDS phobias have contributed to an increase in discrimination, gay-bashing, and an organized assault on the civil rights of the entire homosexual community, lesbians included.

Lesbians are often the recipients of this backlash in that the media has not until recently discussed HIV infection in broader than "gay" terms. Hearing this term repeatedly, the general public does not distinguish between lesbians and gay and bisexual men.

The recently experienced increase in homophobia and violence is dramatic. In a Boston gay-bashing incident in early 1987, the defendants excused their attack on two young lesbians by stating that they thought the "girls" were "faggots."[33] This was offered as a legitimate apology, as if to say that their actions would have been excusable if the "girls" had actually been "faggots."

Situations such as these have led some individuals to discuss the safety of "out" lesbians, especially those living in small communities or in neighborhoods where bashing has occurred. The repeal or failure of passage of civil rights laws, the reinstitution of sodomy laws or defeat of repeals, and the continued struggle over child custody, foster care,[34] and adoption have led women to believe that the heady time of gay and lesbian rights which followed Stonewall[35] is over.

The AIDS epidemic is not occurring in a vacuum, but in the laboratory of society and culture. Thus, this same homophobia has caused some AIDS service organizations that had begun as grassroots responses to the crisis to "become a business"[36] and attempt a single-focus response. While concentrated effort can be laudable, it is ironic that most of the struggles that are dropped in favor of AIDS-only activities are those which affect women's lives: reproductive rights; child-care provisions; birth control and abortion; foster care and adoption; the Equal Rights Amendment; welfare; and health care. While some of the single-issue impetus stems from the misguided concept that if the gay-run agencies "behave" they will continue to be funded, the stance is based partly on a disinterest in and lack of knowledge of women's issues and is held together by internalized and institutionalized homophobia within the service agencies themselves.

> Harriet was infected by her bisexually active husband. She had known about his attraction to men for years. She and Ted had a wonderful relationship, two great teenagers, and a wide spectrum of professional and personal friends. The instant that they heard about the sexual transmission of AIDS, Ted stopped his risky behaviors with men and Harriet and he limited their own sexual activity to safer practices. When the HIV antibody test became available in 1985, they both tested antibody-positive. Ted now has ARC and Harriet is asymptomatic. Both volunteer their professional skills to the local AIDS service organization.

From the beginning of the epidemic, prostitutes have been implicated in the spread of AIDS. Sex workers are often the first ones blamed and the first to be restrained physically or legally during spread of a sexually transmitted disease.[37] Prior to the availability of HIV antibody testing, prostitutes were predicted to be the main source of AIDS spread into the "general population," and as such were listed among the groups at high risk. Forgotten were the thousands of male IVDUs and their sexual partners among the "general population." Also forgotten were the ranks of heterosexually identified men living comfortable lives in the cities, suburbs, and countryside, replete with wives, children, jobs, and churches, who have same-sex encounters on business trips, over weekends, or at sex shops/movie houses. Prostitutes were not listed to notify them of their own risk, but to place the rest of the community on notice that, as always, one must avoid wicked women if one desires to stay clean.[38]

With the advent of the HIV antibody test, evidence has begun to accumulate that, indeed, the exchange of money does not spread AIDS. Diane Richardson states in *Women and AIDS:*

> Studies suggest that "unless a prostitute injects drugs she is unlikely to be infected with HIV. Although only a minority of prostitutes are IV drug users, some women who are "on the game" use prostitution as a way of getting drugs or money to pay for drugs. In New York, for instance, injecting drugs is reported to be most common among the group of prostitutes known as streetwalkers. It is estimated that in the United States about 10–20% of prostitution involves street prostitutes. These are women who pick up their clients on the street rather than through, say, an escort agency. As a high proportion (some estimate as many as half) of the city's injecting drug users are believed to be infected with the virus, this may explain why some street prostitutes in New York, and cities like it, are reported to be at risk.[39]

Richardson goes on to delineate the confounding issues of race and economics:

> A large number of street prostitutes are working class and black women. While this is partly related to poverty, it is also due to the racism which prevents black prostitutes from working indoors in brothels and casinos, or for escort agencies. It is street prostitutes who, because they are more "visible," have particularly suffered from increased harassment . . . one result of blaming prostitutes for spreading AIDS.[40]

Rarely is concern for the prostitute herself mentioned outside the women's and feminist press. Most outreach projects have been designed to keep the sex worker from infecting others rather than from becoming infected herself. Heterosexual transmission studies have attempted to document female-to-male transmission and thus permanently afix blame. Robert R. Redfield, M.D., has repeatedly blamed women for transmission of HIV infection to men, and, thus, for infection among military men. After his article appeared in 1985 in the *Journal of the American Medical Association,* many people began to dispute his premises. Priscilla Alexander writes in *Sex Work:*

> A series of letters have been published in *JAMA* disputing [Redfield's] findings for a variety of reasons, including the consequences of admitting to homosexual activity and/or IV drug use in the military. Interestingly enough, when the United States Army tested fifteen prostitutes near a US Air Force base in Honduras and found that six of the women were seropositive, and then claimed the study as proof that prostitutes were infecting GI's, Redfield disputed their claim. He said that the direction of transmission was more likely to be from the GI's to the prostitutes, because none of the women in the study used IV drugs.[41]

Few have recognized sex workers for what they are: a multifaceted community of women — and men — who, through their provision of sexual services, are experts at sex. By concentrating on the street worker — the woman most likely to use IV drugs, most likely to be a partner of a male IVDU, and most susceptible to economic pressure from her customers to not use a condom — the media and others have ignored the larger population of sex workers. It is this group that can serve as "sex experts" and assist in the design of relevant safer sex materials for the larger community. It is this group of women who can, working together with AIDS service organizations, design projects that will educate and support street workers so that they can institute safer sex guidelines and avoid the risks of needle use and sharing of those needles. Again, Richardson sums this up well:

> In many ways it is ironic that prostitutes have been scapegoated for AIDS. Contrary to popular belief, prostitutes are among the best informed as to how to protect themselves and others from sexually transmitted diseases, including AIDS. After all, it makes good business and health sense for them to know. While it is a common assumption that prostitutes spend most of their time engaging in high-risk sex with their customers, few studies exist of what men specifically pay prostitutes to do for them.[42]

In Africa, prostitutes are being used as sex educators in a condom-use campaign aimed at married heterosexual couples.[43] In the Netherlands, the women of Red Thread and Pink Thread, organizations of sex workers and women working with and in support of sex workers, respectively, organize condom-use campaigns among "window" prostitutes and help women to find work only in those brothels which support condom use.[44] In California, wine, cheese, and safer sex materials are served to working women during educational sessions held in the "trick hotels," and the women leave with condoms and other safer sex equipment.[45]

> Jacqueline does not consider herself a prostitute but occasionally refers to her lunchtime activities as "hooking." She earns $250.00 a day performing oral sex on ten to fifteen "johns" cruising in their cars during the noon hour. She always uses a condom, placing it on their penis with her mouth. The john rarely knows it is in place until after his climax. Still she worries about AIDS, wondering how she would support her kids and her disabled brother without this income. Pretending to her family that she is a secretary, she spends a great deal of time reading in the public library. Lately she has read more about HIV infection and is not amused at the blame placed on sex workers. "So why don't the police arrest johns who try to pay us girls more to skip the rubber?"

Women, as a class defined only by gender, are as varied, as different as can be imagined. What we share is the experience of living in a society that systematically denies our reality, or world view. It is not sufficient simply to provide child care at every AIDS meeting and service if we can't get to the meeting because of economic, class, educational, cultural, and language barriers. The situation requires an overhaul of the very basic concepts of health care and social service. In planning for the future, it is imperative to struggle against these old ways of being and to ensure that changes are made in the manner and style of service delivery. Each program must incorporate the following concepts or activities:

1. Women's caucuses should be established to design, implement, and monitor all women's AIDS/HIV services and projects. Minority women should constitute at least 51 percent of these caucuses.

2. All written and audiovisual material must be culturally sensitive, and should ideally be produced by members of the community at which the material is aimed. The material must be composed in language and vernacular that are understood by the community and must take into account the level of literacy of the target group. Cultural roles must be respected,

and material must be made accessible to those persons, especially women, who occupy specific modeling roles. These materials must be available to an individual without causing him or her to be identified as personally "AIDS-concerned" by other members of the neighborhood or community. Moreover, not all members of a particular group are identical. Materials should reflect, for instance, the differences between Hispanics on the East Coast who have come from Puerto Rico and those on the West Coast who identify as Chicano. Terminology, religious orientation, roles, role models, and many other determinants may vary.

3. Projects for education and risk reduction should follow the same guidelines as those listed in item 1 above. Additionally, funding should be in the hands of the communities affected, enabling persons to work within their own community. Assistance should be available at the governmental funding level to assist new community groups, organizations, agencies, and associations that previously have not received large-scale funding so that they can equip themselves with the knowledge and expertise necessary to administer these projects.

4. Materials and equipment needed for risk reduction should be readily available at no cost and in a manner (place, time, and situation) which is supportive of their use. This includes a broad range of personal sexual risk-reduction materials, such as condoms, dental dams,[46] and spermicide as well as IV-drug-related materials, such as bleach, water, and clean needles and syringes ("works"). Gloves, face masks, plastic barriers, needle disposal containers, and other equipment that contributes to the home and community-level care of infected individuals must similarly be available.

5. Women must have readily accessible entry into drug and substance abuse programs that are designed around the concerns and issues of women and that provide child care or incorporate the family unit into the care facility program. A wide range of programs must be made available so that a woman can choose to protect herself and her family from HIV infection *now* and yet choose to deal with aspects of her drug dependence at a later date. No longer can we require a woman — or a man — to come to grips with addiction as a condition of access to life-saving HIV risk-reduction materials.

6. Custody, adoption, and foster care procedures and regulations must be revised to allow a woman the right to designate who will care for her children, and in what manner, at her death or the point at which she cannot provide care herself, while allowing her to retain custody up to that point.

7. Antidiscrimination laws concerning HIV infection, risk of HIV infection, and testing must be enacted and enforced. Antidiscrimination laws

pertaining to sex, race, ethnicity, and language must be enforced to provide access to vital information and services for disenfranchised groups. Public health regulations and reportable disease regulations must be applied carefully and with the recognition that confidentiality is relative[47] and that anonymity is optimal. Public accommodations and employment nondiscrimination clauses must be enforced.

8. Same-sex sexual practices, sex in exchange for money, and IV drug use must be decriminalized so that individuals engaging in these practices can come forward and seek care without constraint.

9. Shelters, halfway houses, residences, and hospices must be available in every community for women and children. Children in AIDS-affected families who are themselves uninfected must receive appropriate support and hospice services, as do their infected siblings and other family members. The family unit must be protected and supported even during the course of disintegration under the weight of HIV infection. The family members should not be forced to separate from each other in order to receive services.

10. School curricula concerning HIV infection must be developed for all school levels to alert children of the effects of AIDS and its strains on our communities and to provide them with personal risk-reduction information. Moreover, as infected children, born of infected parents — not only children who are hemophiliacs or transfusion recipients — will be attending school in increasing numbers, these curricula can pave the way toward inclusion by their peers in all school activities while also teaching the concepts of infection control in both a home and school setting.

11. Communities must be helped to provide HIV-specific services to the citizenry, but must also integrate HIV-infection awareness into every level of community activity. Each service must be available to each citizen in an appropriate and sensitive manner, whether or not that person is HIV-infected.

12. Participation in medical research and access to experimental treatment and drugs must be increased for women. Research efforts must not continue to focus on women only in their reproductive capacity.

Finally, more individuals and groups must broaden their focus to include the struggle for civil rights, health care, and support for women, people of color, IV drug users, lesbians, children, gay and bisexual men, and all those threatened by HIV infection.

> Sherry is seven years old. Her mother and her little brother died last year. She doesn't know what happened to her father. She goes to the same school she has always attended but lives with her grandparents a few blocks from her old house. Most afternoons she stays inside after school. The kids in the neighborhood think she will make

them die just like her mom and her baby brother. Her only playmate is eight-year-old José. His mother has AIDS, so he isn't afraid to be around her.

While many ills of society must continue to be addressed, there remains but one overriding agenda: the halting of the AIDS epidemic and the end of the discrimination that has furthered its spread and increased the suffering of our entire community.

Notes

1. It is the intention of the author to accord the communities of women — and men — addressed herein the recognition and respect they deserve. Thus, each reference to a specific community, the lesbian, gay, Black, women's, and so on, was capitalized as an indication of that recognition. Most of these capitalizations have been removed in the interest of stylistic consistency with the rest of this journal. Might this, though small, be a part of the SOP (standard operating procedure) that diverts us from validating the lives and world view of others?

2. *AIDS Weekly Surveillance Report — United States,* AIDS Program, Center for Infectious Diseases, Centers for Disease Control, February 1, 1988.
3. AIDS and Public Policy Conference, New York City, January 1986.

4. Gay and lesbian couples have yet to receive the status and recognition accorded heterosexuals. Thus, gay men are listed as single in most discussions of demographics. Pertinent to this article is the fact that, regardless of relationship status, gay men rarely have sole custody and responsibility for children.

5. Mario A. Orlandi, "Community-Based Substance Abuse Prevention: A Multicultural Perspective," *Journal of School Health* 56, no. 9, November 1986, 394.
6. Ibid., 397.
7. *AIDS Weekly Surveillance Report — United States,* February 1, 1988.
8. Ibid.
9. "Open Letter to the Planners of the International Conference on AIDS," International Working Group on Women and AIDS, Washington, D.C., June 1988.
10. Sam Friedman and Don Des Jarlais, "AIDS and the Social Organization of Intravenous Drug Users," presented to the American Anthropological Association, Philadelphia, December 1986.
11. P. Clay Stephens, P.A., "Politics of Women and AIDS," Women and AIDS Conference, Boston, October 1986.

12. United States Department of Labor, 1987. Please note the increase from 59 cents for every male dollar earned.

13. Carolyn A. Martin and G. Douglas Talbott, "Special Issues for Female Impaired Physicians," *Journal of the Medical Association of Georgia* 75, August 1985, 483–488.
14. Ibid., 484–485.
15. Ibid., 485.
16. P. Clay Stephens, P.A., "Reproductive Rights and AIDS," Women and AIDS Conference, Boston, October 1986.
17. David Polando, personal communication, May 1986.
18. AIDS and Public Policy Conference, New York City, January 1986.
19. "Sarah," personal communication, August 1987.
20. Michael Adler, editorial: "AIDS and Intravenous Drug Abusers," *British Journal of Addiction* 81, 1986, 307–310.

21. D. Colin Drummond et al., "Replacement of a Prescribing Service by an Opiate-Free Day Programme in a Glasgow Drug Clinic," *British Journal of Addiction* 81, 1986, 559–565.

22. Judy Spiegel, "Addictaphobia in AIDS Client Advocates," National Lesbian and Gay Health Foundation Conference, Washington, D.C., March 1986.

23. In roundtable discussions with ATS (alternative test site) counselors and HIV educators, these restrictions have been the most troublesome.

24. Hotline counselors are required, in many cases, to inquire about the age of the caller before answering explicit questions or mailing out explicit sexual risk-reduction guidelines.

25. Spiegel, "Addictaphobia in AIDS Client Advocates."

26. Debbie Law, speaking as a member of a panel entitled "Lessons from the Recent Past: What Gay Men and AIDS Service Providers Might Learn from the Women's Health Movement." Moderated by Urvashi Vaid and presented by Debbie Law, Veneita Porter, Suzann Gage, and Suzanne Farr, National Lesbian and Gay Health Foundation Conference, Los Angeles, March 1987.

27. Marshall Forstein, M.D., AIDS and Mental Health Conference, Boston, May 1986.

28. Suzann Gage and Lisa Tackley, "Lesbians: STD's, AIDS, and Safer Sex," National Lesbian and Gay Health Foundation Conference, Los Angeles, March 1987.

29. Veneita Porter, speaking as a panel member, "Lessons from the Recent Past."

30. George Seage, M.P.H., senior AIDS epidemiologist for the Boston Department of Health and Hospitals, personal communication, June 1987.

31. Participants, "Lesbians Working in AIDS Organizations," National Lesbian and Gay Health Foundation Conference, Los Angeles, March 1987.

32. Marea Murray, letter to the editor, *Bay Windows*, 4, no. 31 (July 31, 1986).

33. *Gay Community News*, "News Notes," August 1986.

34. In Massachusetts in 1985, two foster children were removed from the home of a gay male couple. There were no problems with the placement; the removal occurred solely on the basis of the couple's sexuality. Regulations were then passed requiring that placement in traditional families be given priority, thus essentially eliminating the possibility of a placement in the home of any single person or any gay or lesbian couple. A state advisory committee later recommended that this restriction be lifted. The governor has yet to act on the recommendation. The matter is currently in the courts.

35. Stonewall, a drag bar in New York City, has given its name to the riots that marked the beginning of the Gay and Lesbian Rights Movement of the last twenty years.

36. David Polando, HIV counselor, Portsmouth Feminist Health Center, Portsmouth, N.H., personal communication, May 1986.

37. Vern Bullough and Bonnie Bullough, *Women and Prostitution: A Social History,* Prometheus Books, Buffalo, N.Y., 1987.

38. Marjo Meyer, M.D., "Red Thread and Pink Thread," National Lesbian and Gay Health Conference, Los Angeles, March 1987.

39. Diane Richardson, *Women and AIDS,* Methuen Press, New York City, 1988, 43.

40. Ibid., 43–44.

41. Frederique Delacoste and Priscilla Alexander, *Sex Work,* Cleis Press, Pittsburgh, Penn., 1987, 254.

42. Richardson, *Women and AIDS,* 44.

43. "AIDS in Developing Nations," roundtable discussion, Third International Conference on AIDS, Washington, D.C., June 1987.

44. Marjo Meyer, M.D., "Red Thread and Pink Thread."

45. Gloria Lockett, "Women and AIDS," Homosexuality, Which Homosexuality Conference, Free University, Amsterdam, the Netherlands, December 1987.

46. A dental dam is a square of latex approximately six by six inches, typically used during dental procedures as a barrier. As condoms are useful only for sexual activities involving a penis or a penis-shaped sex toy, individuals have used dental dams as a safer sex barrier during oral-genital female-receptive and oral-anal sexual contact.

47. Although medical and professional ethics regulate confidentiality, and although some states, such as Massachusetts, have HIV confidentiality laws or regulations, the protection is only as good as the individuals and agencies participating. There exists, as well, a tension between the duty to warn and the obligation to honor confidences in the medical arena. Anonymity is preferred, in that with no identifying information there can be no breach.

Additional References

Women and AIDS Clinical Resource Guide. San Francisco AIDS Foundation, 1988.

Cindy Patton, *Sex and Germs: The Politics of AIDS.* South End Press, Boston, Mass., 1985.

Barbara Smith, editor, *Home Girls: A Black Feminist Anthology.* Kitchen Table: Women of Color Press, New York, N.Y., 1983.

Accounts of an Illness: Extracts

Ron Schreiber, Ph.D.

The following pieces, with an introduction by the author, are from a work in progress entitled John, *to be published in the fall of 1988 by Hanging Loose Press and Calamus Books, New York City. In this work, Ron Schreiber, John's lover of nine years, writes a chronicle of a terminal illness from diagnosis to death.*

John MacDonald, Jr., was born in Dorchester June 10, 1951; he died in Holbrook, his parents' home, November 5, 1986. John graduated from Holbrook High School, attended Northeastern and graduated from the University of Hawaii with a degree in marine biology. He had done various things in his teens and 20s, since he was kicked out of his parents' home by his father when he was 15 (for being gay). He'd done a nightclub act in New York, cut demo records, modeled, worked as a geisha in Kyoto for three months. He worked for some years for New England Telephone Company and for many years for Winston Flowers on Newbury Street in Boston. He arranged the flowers for the 100th Anniversary of the Boston Pops. But his passions were plants — he planted whole gardens, grew orchids and camelias — and animals — he had three chows and two shih-tzus, five cats, a blue-and-gold macaw and many lesser birds and fish. He'd been cross-pollinating flowers since he was five.

— Ron Schreiber

Dr. Ron Schreiber is chair of the English Department at the University of Massachusetts at Boston.

protocols

so now the test is back:
positive. no surprise.

"maybe that qualifies you
for a protocol," I say.

"I'll get disability,"
John says, either way

he's qualified. he'll be
home in two days — medication

oral. Dr. Tagliaferro
mentioned "control groups,"

an easier term than protocol.
but John doesn't like the

idea of being used as a
guinea pig. or the possible

side effects, which, he says,
could kill him.

but what
if he says yes? is hope
a chimera without even a

gold ring in its nose?
or is it possibility, slowly

creeping through a crack in
the stone door, wriggling

its slimy body into a
kind of tentative life?

4/16/86

your life

right now it's all I care about
& you're going to lose it

(wrong head, I know, but it's
late & I'm scared & tired).

first there's your health: I
want you to have it. you were

exhausted & sun-dazed when I
brought you back from the hospital

— after stopping to get your drugs —
& you were sleeping when I called

downstairs just now. I am tired
beyond anything my body tells me

is fatigue. & when you're sick,

when I look into your tired, lovely
eyes, I want you well. right now

I'm trying to find the railroad cap
I lost on the long flight wait

in Florida last winter (when I was
there & you were home & healthy)

& put it on my head firm & screw it
on. I want you to get back your

health or at least its shimmering
surface. right now.

4/18/86

Sunday morning 4/20/86

John got out of the hospital Thursday morning. We did not know whether he'd be able to leave or not, since his white blood count was low Wednesday night, and they had to get the results of another blood test Thursday morning. They called the lab for results, and got them at 10. OK— so we left.

The sun hurt his eyes coming home. We stopped at the pharmacy to pick up his drugs, and they were expensive: over $100. for four prescriptions. When we got home he was very tired and he was nauseous again, but John noted that his first day out was bad the first time he came back from the hospital, two weeks ago.

When John came upstairs Friday morning, I was momentarily elated: he must be better, I thought. But that was not the case: his fever had returned, the rash had begun again, and he was very weak. While he lay on my bed, I kept trying to reach his doctor, who was not in yet. The intern, Steve Boswell, called about an hour later, and told me to bring John in. Then, as John was walking down the stairs, the phone rang again, and this time it was Nettie Tagliaferro, his doctor, and she said to bring John in.

He was very bad when we reached the emergency room, and I was unwilling to leave until I thought he would be all right. I left about 11, and went into work, as I had done the day before. This time they will keep John two weeks, although apparently the new drug they are using could be administered on an outpatient basis; we would come in for an hour every day. But John does not want that, and I don't think I could stand it.

When I talked to Steve Friday afternoon, he asked me how I was doing. — Not very well, I said, though also, — as well as can be expected, I think. I asked Steve whether it was life-threatening this time, and Steve said no, not this time. We talked a little about protocols. — I want to be with John when he dies, I said. Steve assured me that they would call me right away if anything should happen.

But this time they think it will be all right. We don't know yet what the side effects of this drug will be. Probably we will have to wait ten days and then find out. So far, whenever there are potential side effects, John gets them. They just have to keep trying new drugs. Probably the rash, though, is not a side effect (though it could be), but another opportunistic disease.

Last night I slept nine hours, from 9 to 6; I had also fallen asleep in the afternoon. I am still tired this morning. I hope I can use each weekend to recuperate, for my job is very busy. This is only the second day of a three-day weekend, so I can't tell yet whether the weekend will be long enough. I may have to live with this fatigue. But that is not so difficult as what John has to do, which is to live with his various illnesses and side effects as long as he wants to, as long as he can.

back in

Saturday I waited for the plumber
all morning, & he came at one, but

I'd left the door open & visited
you in the morning. yesterday I

came by twice, & in between got
potting soil so Sue could put up

the plants we'd ordered & dog &
cat food for your larger animals.

today I'm waiting for the extermi
-nator & trying to read the book

I'm teaching tomorrow. when I come
by this afternoon it will be mask

& gloves & paper gown again, not
because you're contagious but for

fear of what I might bring in,
your white count down again.

we'll relate to each other as if
you're living, we said, but this

way it's hard; you in the hospital
& very sick, your whole attention

focused on your body & your illness.
sure, you're living, but I get left

out of the equation, except for job
& chores, the structure of routine,

& thinking of you, thinking of you
all the time.

4/21/86

moving towards memory

what scares me most is that the
virus often goes to the brain.

such a sharp mind, tongue like
a razor, but beard now unshaved

for weeks. then, yesterday (so
soon), John could not remember

the end of a sentence he'd begun.
at noon, when he seemed to be

miserable from the blood samples
of the morning; in the evening

when his left arm was swollen.
it's happening fast, but this

part is — now at least — more
gentle than I'd expected, like

waking from calm sleep, too
early to be able to piece

sentences together, or remember
what it was one wanted to say.

4/22/86

still alive

he slept through the night:
four to eight — no pain

when he sleeps. I slept:
eight to eleven; eleven

to three; three to four;
up at six. worked.

typed two documents,
played solitaire. mailed

letter at the corner
store, where I got cig-

arettes but no paper
(they didn't have one).

came back. played soli-
taire. till John screamed

just now, & I gave him
a morphine capsule.

he's on his stomach.
wet? I don't know; I

didn't turn him over.
I love you, he said.

I'd said that to him
first, and — let it go now;

I'm all right. I *am*
all right, whatever

that means. it means
ready. & I told him so

& he understands me. it's
time for the others to

tell him too.

10/25/86

10/29/86

I tried, last weekend, to convince John's sister Nancy and his parents, John & Lucille, to give John the peace & the encouragement to die. With Nancy it was clear; she could not wish it. His father said, "We don't think that way. It's God's will." "Fine," I said, "but let John know that you accept it either way." No luck. I lost the argument.

I did convince his mother, who is a home health aide, to come both weekend days. I was glad Lisa was not available. When I was out on errands Saturday morning, a decision was made to which I was asked to acquiesce: that John would go home with his mother (to his mother) in Holbrook. "That's what John wants," they said. And "we had been thinking about it, but we didn't want to say anything until Johnny said something." Not to me either, who had no notion what they had been thinking about. (The house queer; the house nigger. He's done his job — back to the family into which he was born.)

How could I tell what John wanted. He has been alert these last three weeks only for visitors. To Lisa he says, "I want to die." Sometimes that's what he says to me. Friday night he slept 16 hours. 20 hours Sunday night, when his family had gone.

Tuesday morning I was able to determine that John does want to go. The result is OK with me. We've done our closure really. We love each other.

It's Wednesday now, 9:30. His parents will be here soon. Lisa is here now. Gail has just arrived. I'm doing a laundry. The ambulance is coming at 11 to take John to his parents' home.

how did it end?

when they carried John out of the
house (on his way to Holbrook) he

looked up at me as they put him in
the ambulance & screamed "Ron! Ron!

Ron!" then they closed the doors,
his mother with him, & drove off.

what happened next?

John went to Holbrook, where they
set him up in a hospital bed. On

Thursday I visited. the nurse
asked me to help her turn John over,

though his mother was there, & trained,
as I was not. by Saturday his mother

was less helpless, more in charge.
his father was pleased to have John

(who was not queer, who had acknowledged
Jesus) home & smiling at him.

what else happened?

Wednesday morning, before his family
arrived to take him "home," John said

to Lisa: "look after Ron because my
family surely won't."

how did it end?

I visited the third time on Tuesday,
& spoke with John. when I left the

room to drive home, Nancy went in,
but John had already fallen asleep.

11/4/86

how did it end (2)?

I wasn't there. twice before
— when John was home with me —

he'd slept a long time: 16
hours, 20 hours. the second time

I'd called Lisa — how do I know
if he's died? I asked. & she told me.

I was at a meeting when the call came.
Mary, my secretary, came in & signaled

to me. I knew what it was.

Gail was there. his mother was there.
John had not awakened but Gail was

talking to him. "I have to go in
ten minutes," Gail said. & then

John's hand went limp as she held it.
John's mother did not realize, though

she held his other hand. "he's gone,"
Gail said. & he is.

11/5/86

Ron Schreiber's poems first appeared in *Radical America*'s "Facing AIDS," a special issue devoted to AIDS. Copies of this issue are available for $3.95 from *Radical America*, 1 Summer St., Somerville, MA 02143. A subscription to *Radical America* is $15 per year.

AIDS Public Policy: Implications for Families

Elaine A. Anderson, Ph.D.

Much has been written about the AIDS crisis in the past few years. However, relatively little of this discussion has focused on AIDS as it may affect families. This report emerged from the 1987 Groves Conference on Marriage and the Family. It is a version of the chapter on public policy in AIDS and Families *(ed. Eleanor Macklin, Hayworth Press, forthcoming, summer 1988), prepared by the conference's Task Force on AIDS and Families. The book details the probable impact of AIDS on individuals, families, and communities and delineates the implications for relevant professionals, organizations, and public policy. Those individuals who participated in writing portions of the chapter on which this article is based are acknowledged at the end of the article.*

AIDS policymakers at all levels should consider the manner in which their efforts may affect the ability of the family to perform successfully its vital roles and functions. Ideally, policy concerning AIDS should be designed to strengthen and protect the family's contribution, not to debilitate or weaken it.

Because of the stigma attached to the disease, as well as its deadly nature and enormous health care costs, policy concerning AIDS treatment and care has an unusual potential to make a negative impact on the family — to encourage families to cast out those members stricken with the disease, and to generate feelings of distance and alienation among family members.

Professionals who are concerned with the impact of AIDS and AIDS policy on family functioning must ask a critical question: How will the proposed policy affect the ability of the family to carry out its important functions in our society?

Guidelines for AIDS Policymakers

The following guidelines and principles should be employed by persons assessing the potential family impact of any proposed legislation related to AIDS, and should be included in any policy considerations.

Dr. Elaine A. Anderson is assistant professor of family and community development at the University of Maryland at College Park. She teaches and writes on social and health policy as they affect families.

1. Families should be broadly defined to include, besides the traditional biological relationships, those committed relationships between individuals which fulfill the function of family.

2. It must be remembered that the effects of policy concerning AIDS prevention, treatment, and care will be experienced by people whose lives usually have implications for a number of other individuals and groups. Family systems theory considers each family member, and the family as a unit, as parts of a larger interactive social system. This interactive systemic view of society suggests that events and feelings in the life of one family member overlap and influence those of the other family members and in turn affect their ability to perform in other life arenas. AIDS, therefore, has an impact not only on the individual and the family system, but also on the broader emotional, sexual, educational, religious, political, legal, health care, work, and economic systems with which the family and its members intersect.

3. The family may take a variety of forms. No single model of family functioning can be used to gauge the effects of AIDS policies, because no standard prototypical American family exists today. Families differ with respect to religion; locus (urban/rural, region of the country); social class; educational level; ethnicity/race; and numbers of parents, children, and grandparents. Responsible strategies for rural families living with three generations under one roof, for example, may produce undesirable outcomes when applied to low-income, inner-city, single-parent families.

4. The influence of a family member with AIDS reaches across generational and geographic boundaries. People with AIDS may also be parents, children, grandparents, siblings, aunts, uncles, lovers, or teachers; eventually, they will be ancestors. Over time, people move from one family form to another. When they move to a new family form, they may pick up new functions. The changing needs over time, of the individual within each family form, must be reflected in policy.

5. AIDS policies should be designed to strengthen families and foster the support that families can provide. Policy development should be conducted with the intention of calling upon the positive, integrative potentials of American families.

6. AIDS policy should take into account the myriad threats that the disease poses to the stability of the family, and should strive to protect and bolster family durability to address those threats.

7. Families have important functions within a broad continuum of health care related to AIDS. Families are important links in the chain of intervention, whether it be at the level of education and prevention or diagnosis, care, and treatment.

8. The family has a particularly important role in AIDS prevention. Families can teach and encourage preventive strategies.

9. The family's traditional role as caretaker and care giver should be fostered by policies that deal with the care and treatment of people with AIDS. Removing the family from this vital caretaking and care-giving role, or making its cost prohibitive — both emotionally and financially — may result in persons with AIDS becoming wards of the state or additions to the indigent homeless population.

10. AIDS policy should strive to support the integrity of the family. In general, whenever a family is available to a person with AIDS, the plan of choice would be to foster that support with psychosocial and financial assistance. Because providing care to a loved one with AIDS can quickly deplete the resources of a family, policies for care and treatment of AIDS, by augmenting the family's financial and emotional resources, should enable a family to continue to be the major source of care.

11. In addition to responsibilities, families have important rights that need to be protected. The family has the right to participate in decision making regarding such issues as testing, residence, and treatment, as well as the right to privacy, confidentiality, and protection from discrimination and disclosure. These rights will be discussed later in this report.

Any policy decision, on any specific issue, can have an effect on the family. Policy decisions may be made at several levels of policymaking, as follows.

Typically, when one thinks of policymaking, *government policymakers* come to mind. Usually these are federal or state officials. However, policy decisions are made at other levels as well. *Communities make policy* decisions. The school board decides whether or not to close a local school; these same policymakers may review and approve the content of the courses our children are taught. *Professionals* within a range of settings *make policy* decisions. These settings may include our place of work, the businesses we use, or the health facilities we need. Within all of these settings, professionals are making policy decisions that affect the lives of individuals and families. Finally, *families* also make *policy decisions* on how they will run their daily lives. These decisions include such things as what children will be taught within the family, who does what, and how money is spent.

Specific Policy Issues

The following discussion addresses some major policy areas related to AIDS and the family. It is organized around the four levels of policy decision making just discussed: government, community, professional, and family. Only those levels of policy decision making which are most relevant are included in the discussion of each policy area.

Social Science Research

In the relatively short time during which we have been aware of HIV and its linkage to the disease syndrome known as AIDS, significant research has been conducted on the biomedical aspects of the disease. Many important areas of research continue to need support.[1]

The social science research needs that fall within the scope of this report are discussed below.

Government policy. Given the potential magnitude of the impact of HIV, epidemiological research at a national level must be expanded. It is especially important that there be support for the epidemiological studies of "lower risk" populations as well as of the "high risk/higher incidence" groups. Such efforts would facilitate the development of a more complete data base, allowing more accurate predictions of spread of the disease and a better understanding of the etiologic factors involved. This could begin with baseline data collected through recommended voluntary, anonymous testing centers and through anonymous randomized samples in other settings.

An ongoing nationwide study of sexual behavior and epidemiology needs to be established. In recent years, less and less financial support has been provided for researchers to study human sexual behavior and patterns. If we are to develop educational programs to change the sexual behaviors that contribute to the spread of HIV, we must know more about the epidemiology of these behaviors.

More knowledge about the dynamics of human interaction will probably be the cornerstone of any concerted effort to change behavior patterns. Little research has been conducted on the relationship between human behavior, HIV infection, and AIDS. The development of healthy human relationships through the progression of temporary sexual relationships, dating and courtship, and partnering, marriage, and parenting needs to be understood further so that the interaction between HIV infection and changes in the development of relationships and the family can be appreciated.

Also needed is longitudinal research with a life-span perspective. In other words, we do not fully know how the presence of this virus will change the ways in which people seek dating partners and potential lifetime companions or marriage partners. We do not know how this virus will change the prevalence of extramarital affairs, nor do we know how the knowledge of such affairs might affect the well-being and future of a particular marital dyad. Finally, we know little about how AIDS will affect a couple's decision whether to have children. All of these issues, which focus on different stages of relationships and family development, present important questions. Following relationships over the course of time is important in our understanding of human behavior. This information likewise is important in the development of the best educational tools for preventive programs.

In addition, social science research efforts must be enhanced to assess (1) the relationship between stress, depression, the knowledge that an individual has tested HIV-antibody-positive, and the open expression of his or her health status; (2) the effect of the virus on the central nervous system; (3) the relationship between fear and the public's ability to appropriately respond to AIDS; and (4) elimination of the discrimination that often arises when changes in behavior become necessary. Research efforts must emphasize the coordination of the psychosocial and medical needs of the population.

Any discussion identifying prevention as the cornerstone of our current response to AIDS assumes that we have developed the educational programs that can encourage change in behavior. Additional research and development funds are necessary to improve the current educational programs and to promote new programs that will reach target groups and provide the necessary information in an appropriately sensitive manner. Evaluation of effectiveness is important for all social science research, but for AIDS educational programs, it is paramount. AIDS educators should receive both training and evaluation.

A coordinated plan to develop research/treatment programs for persons with AIDS needs to be consistent with the continuum of care concept. It is important to recognize that those persons who test positive for HIV antibodies fall within a continuum of care that is widely inclusive. For example, individuals who have been diagnosed as having AIDS have a different set of health care needs than asymptomatic individuals who have just learned that they are seropositive.

Finally, family impact analysis should be incorporated into our research protocols. Families may be affected in two major ways as a result of AIDS. First, their ability to fulfill the typical functions of most family units may be impaired or altered; second, the structure of the family may change as a consequence of the virus, or different structures of the family may respond to the impact of AIDS in different ways. Policy recommendations must take into account both their intended and unintended consequences for families. Once a sound data base has been established, we will have better information to use in prevention strategies and public education.

Education

Education is currently the most powerful weapon in the war against AIDS. Obstacles to the development of effective treatments and vaccines, as well as the possible discovery of additional viruses related to HIV, make it clear that prevention is essential to the public health. Dramatic reductions in unsafe practices among gay men indicate that people can and do alter their behavior when they are convinced that it is important to do so. For these reasons, an increased commitment of resources to the task of public education is strongly recommended.

Government policy. Effective education requires federal support and funding. Only with greater commitment to education at a national level can standards be established and adequate resources be marshaled to ensure preventive education for all citizens.

A federally supported program should collect the most current scientific information. U.S. government plans to establish a clearinghouse to disseminate this scientific information rapidly and directly to all agencies and organizations requesting it should be supported. This clearinghouse should not function as a censor of unpopular scientific ideas; rather, it should encourage the dissemination of all relevant AIDS-related research.

A federally coordinated and funded effort should be mounted to educate health care professionals and providers, as well as lay providers and informal alternative care givers such as family members, on all AIDS-related issues relevant to their own health and that of their patients — including the emotional impact on the family. Primary and secondary school teachers also must be trained to provide sex education and health education. Such a program must support research and development related to effective teaching and must provide for the establishment and evaluation of a wide range of educational programs.

The following principles are essential to the effectiveness of education programs within a community.

Community policy. All children have a right to be informed adequately so that they can protect their own health and safety. AIDS education should be placed in a context of health and sex education, which should be part of every school curriculum at all levels. It is imperative that children learn about problems such as AIDS within the context of a healthy understanding of sexuality, reproduction, and responsible sexual behavior. Problem-oriented approaches to education can generate new problems. Therefore, a good sex education curriculum for all children should precede education regarding AIDS and other sexually transmitted diseases.

It is essential that love, commitment, trust, honesty, caring, and other similar values be taught. It is important, for example, that students be taught that if they become HIV-infected they should not knowingly infect others. But AIDS should not be used as an excuse to erase the progress made by the "sexual revolution" during the past quarter century. Most Americans are not prepared to return to the sexual repression of an earlier era, and it is urgent that we work to safeguard the healthy advances made in our attitudes toward human sexuality.

Education programs should avoid an antisexual bias. Using AIDS education as justification for promoting such biases presents a number of serious dangers. Foremost among these is the possibility that sexual repression promotes the establishment of relationships in which unsafe sex may be more likely to occur. Furthermore, sexual repression inhibits the development of love, respect, and communication with potential sexual partners. And these are the qualities of relationships which facilitate the practice of safer sex.

AIDS education must be grounded in the latest research on relevant topics. This includes social science and epidemiological research as well as biomedical data. Finally, all education programs should support creativity and innovation. Traditional teaching methods may not be the ones best suited to AIDS education, for a variety of reasons; for example, many at risk may be suspicious of authority or may be functionally illiterate. Individuals affected by AIDS and ARC are often willing to share their experiences and newly gained understanding with young people. A personal connection with individuals who have AIDS, as opposed to the use of abstract teaching materials, is especially powerful in helping people to face their own feelings about AIDS. This in turn may lead to positive, dramatic changes in behavior.

Family policy. Parents should be encouraged to participate in the development and implementation of programs directed at children. Special programs that educate parents should be supported at local, state, and federal levels. Such programs can enable parents to be constructive forces in school programs and can help them to supplement school education with home education. Involving all those who may be affected by AIDS, whether they are parents, schools, or members of high-risk groups, is important in any preventive education program in order to dispel myths, quell fears, and forestall discrimination.

Discrimination

The United States today stands at a crossroad. AIDS is only a part of the total epidemic. Fear, lack of understanding, and bigotry have already caused at least as much disruption in the lives of affected persons as has the disease itself. The by-product of this AIDS-related fear, lack of understanding, and bigotry has been discrimination on virtually all levels against persons with (or perceived to have) AIDS, ARC, or HIV infection.

For example, employers have fired employees who have, or who are suspected of having, AIDS, ARC, or asymptomatic HIV infection. Some employers have required employees to take the HIV antibody test. As AZT and other experimental drugs prolong the life span of persons with AIDS, the number of affected individuals in the workplace will climb rapidly. While a few progressive companies have developed explicit policies protecting the rights of their employees with AIDS, most have not. It is likely that the workplace will become the most prevalent arena for AIDS-related discrimination in the near future.

Landlords have evicted, or sought to evict, persons with AIDS from their homes or apartments. In New York City, it is estimated that hundreds of persons with AIDS or severe ARC are homeless, and are forced to live in shelters, on the streets, in the subways, and in the parks. In such environments, they often become victims of violence, theft, lack of privacy, and multiple opportunistic infections. Some landlords have refused to make repairs or provide essential services, such as heat and hot water, for tenants with AIDS. AIDS service and research organizations have themselves been subject to discrimination on the part of unscrupulous landlords who have refused to rent office space or who have charged exorbitant rents.

Insurance companies have required a negative HIV test result for acceptance among many applicants, have refused to cover treatment costs for persons with AIDS or severe ARC, and have terminated coverage even when the patient had no prior knowledge of his or her HIV infection. Many ambulance and ambulette drivers, physicians, psychiatrists and psychotherapists, dentists, hospital cleaning and food preparation staff, laboratory technicians, and physical therapists have refused to help or assist persons with AIDS. Among nearly five hundred funeral homes, a recent study by the Gay Men's Health Crisis in New York City was able to find only seventy-six that were willing to be listed as accepting deceased persons with AIDS without charging excessive rates.[2]

Perhaps most alarming of all has been the dramatic increase in AIDS-related violence directed against gay men and lesbians. The National Gay and Lesbian Task Force has documented a fourfold increase from 1985 to 1986 in the United States in verbal abuse and threats where AIDS is frequently mentioned and in the overall number of homicides. In that one year, physical assaults increased 64 percent while police-related activity increased 72 percent.[3] Even though much of the violence comes from male teenagers, no school district in the country has initiated an educational campaign to curb it. These varied examples point to the importance of addressing AIDS-related discrimination as it affects the family. It is difficult to develop policies for the benefit of the entire family if one member is suffering from such severe stigmatization.

Government policy. There is a need for a policy on AIDS at the national executive level. That policy should include the strongest possible statement against AIDS-related discrimination in every area. The policy should be highly specific in order to avoid ambiguity, and should ban AIDS-related discrimination in employment, housing, prisons, hospitals, schools, nursing homes, insurance coverage, funeral homes, ambulance and ambulette services, health and mental health care services, day care facilities, and any other area where it might occur. However, until a national policy on AIDS is formulated, all state and municipal governments should develop their own legislation to combat AIDS-related discrimination.

State and municipal human rights commissions should develop an AIDS division that would handle only AIDS-related discrimination cases. An ombudsman should actively evaluate patterns of discrimination in various industries and services, such as funeral homes. This cannot be done unless the budgets for human rights commissions are augmented.

Community policy. Fair housing laws should be amended to address AIDS-related discrimination. Persons with AIDS or HIV infection should not be excluded from renting or purchasing an apartment or house, nor should they be evicted from their premises. Many of these individuals are part of a functional family unit. Discriminating against the person with AIDS or HIV infection also prohibits their loved ones from obtaining suitable housing, or may force a family to separate. Family members and lovers of the deceased should not be evicted from the house or apartment following the death of a person with AIDS. Construction of new housing for homeless persons with AIDS or HIV infection is urgently needed.

Professional policy. Employers should be prohibited from firing, not hiring, or limiting the work of persons with AIDS or HIV infection, provided that such persons can reasonably perform their job. No one should be required to take the HIV antibody test as a condition of ordinary employment, nor should an employer be allowed access to any record indicating that an employee has taken an HIV antibody test — or to the results of such a test. AIDS education workshops should be conducted in the workplace for both management and employees. Sexual orientation or race should not be a presumption of HIV seropositivity, and employment decisions should not be based upon such considerations. The ability of persons with AIDS or HIV infection to provide for themselves economically is important for several reasons. First, being active and busy can positively affect one's mental health. Second, many insurance policies won't cover AIDS-related illness; thus, money is needed to pay the health care bills. Third, many persons with AIDS or HIV infection also have family members who are economically dependent upon them.

The federal government will inevitably have to provide economic assistance through catastrophic health insurance coverage or some co-insurance plan, at least for persons with AIDS or severe ARC. In the meantime, health insurance companies must be prohibited from discriminating on the basis of HIV infection or risk-group membership. They must not be allowed access on any level — governmental or through health care professionals — to HIV antibody test results, and they must not be allowed to require HIV testing for enrollment purposes.

Hospitals and nursing homes should provide compassionate, nondiscriminatory care for persons with AIDS. An ombudsman at each hospital should be appointed to monitor the care of AIDS and severe ARC patients. Hospitals and alternative test sites should create strong links with existing community-based AIDS social service organizations. As with all institutional settings, hospitals and nursing homes should encourage involvement by family members, lovers, and friends of the patient.

Family policy. AIDS-related discrimination has occurred in schools, in prisons, in other institutional settings, and — most poignantly — in the home. For example, the New York City Commission on Human Rights reported that a grandmother called, wanting to know where she could take the HIV antibody test. She had two children: a son who was gay and whose lover had recently died of AIDS, and a married daughter with two children. After the death of her son's lover, the woman had visited her son, and her daughter subsequently refused to allow her to visit her grandchildren, because she feared they would become infected. The woman was heartbroken and wanted to take the HIV antibody test to prove to her daughter that it was safe for her to visit her grandchildren.[4] Fear, lack of understanding, and bigotry often take their greatest toll in the home. The American family, in all its diverse forms, must be supported and strengthened under such adverse conditions.

Treatment

The need for effective delivery of health services to persons with AIDS presents health care policymakers in both the public and private sectors with compelling and difficult challenges. Providing health care to an increasingly debilitated chronic population with a limited life expectancy is an enormously complex task, unprecedented in its capacity to tax our existing system. The issues involved include access to and the appropriate delivery of care and treatment; the recruitment of sufficient and well-trained health care personnel; the provision of adequate numbers of beds in hospitals, long-term care facilities, and other settings; and the underlying, difficult matter of financing this care.

Community policy. It is evident to the health care provider community, including thousands of family professionals in the United States, that the rights, the privacy, and, ultimately, the dignity of persons with AIDS and their families must be respected and manifested. This overarching principle must always be preserved.

Two other important assumptions are made at the outset. First, care and treatment must be provided from a multidisciplinary perspective, using appropriate treatment regimens, biomedical or physiological and psychosocial. Second, an effective and efficient system of care for persons with AIDS must be a coordinated system. For example, care must be integrated between health care programs funded and administered at the local, state, federal, and private-sector levels. Also, care must integrate comprehensive treatment at several levels of service delivery, such as the family unit, the outpatient clinic, the acute care hospital, the extended care facility, and the hospice.

Moreover, medical treatment should be accompanied by care that meets the emotional and psychosocial needs of the person with AIDS and his or her immediate and extended family. For example, housing requirements, employment, and virtually every other system with which the person with AIDS engages must be coordinated at every stage of the illness, with his or her medical needs. These systems change as the illness progresses. Nevertheless, at every stage of the illness, a "systemic" focus must be preserved.

There is an inherent interrelationship between the care and treatment necessary for persons with AIDS and the necessity of providing adequate funds to support this care. The care and treatment that actually are available (and provided) will be determined by available funds. It also is true that the funds that eventually become available will be determined, at least in part, by the need for care and treatment. These issues seem to be circular, and they are. Nonetheless, it is vital for policymakers to tackle this web in a deliberative fashion. The service requirements must dictate the funding that becomes available, rather than the opposite. It would be catastrophic if, in the final analysis, services were determined exclusively by the funds that were available. Thus, a discussion of health care financing for care and treatment of persons with AIDS should be approached from the perspective of the social and medical services that are needed. This inductive approach to policy formation is sensible and serves the public interest.

Professional policy. A network of services for persons with AIDS must be developed and must be integrated to the fullest extent possible within the established health care delivery system. The evolving integrated service delivery must combine the latest biomedical information with an understanding of and sensitivity toward the psychological sequelae of AIDS and ARC. An integrated care system should be staffed by trained health care personnel at every level of the delivery structure, from clerical and support staff to medical staff. They should not only understand the complexities of the AIDS illness pattern, but also be committed to integrate biomedical treatment with psychosocial concerns. One example of a viable conceptual model comes from the burgeoning field of family system medicine. This field integrates both the biomedical and psychosocial with an appreciation of the needs of the family within the context of systems theory. That is, the person with AIDS or ARC is viewed not in isolation from his or her environment, but rather as an active participant influenced by and contributing to the many "subsystems" with which he or she interacts. Another appropriate example is the hospice. Hospice care integrates necessary treatment directed at comforting chronically ill individuals, respects an individual by affirming his or her dignity, and includes an individual's family within the treatment program.

Care and treatment of the person with AIDS or ARC, from this perspective, should take place in the least restrictive and most appropriate setting. A continuum of care setting must also be included in a service delivery plan. The continuum should include, for example, outpatient treatment; partial hospitalization; acute care inpatient settings; after-care facilities; home health care; chronic and long-term care; and hospice care that integrates and coordinates the necessary treatment. AIDS-related care must be provided in a variety of locations.

Many services for persons with AIDS can reasonably be included in outpatient settings. However, as the illness progresses, the continuum of care also must advance to an increasingly acute and then chronic level. It is inevitable that this will be the case for many thousands of persons with AIDS in the years ahead. A service delivery structure must be planned now that will be in place so that the estimated 1.5 million to 2 million Americans who are HIV-positive, a large percentage of whom eventually will manifest some measure of AIDS-related symptoms, will have available to them and to their families the appropriate and necessary care. It is very likely that families will be the site of care for many AIDS patients. We must work now to enable families to provide care in most instances. This challenge is a major imperative to which the health policy community must respond.

Government policy. Governments — local, state, federal, and international — must develop a significantly expanded and targeted health care delivery system for the care and treatment of persons with AIDS. This system must be coordinated with existing health resources in communities. It must be attentive to biomedical developments and sensitive to the psychosocial needs of persons with AIDS and their families, including the right of privacy and confidentiality. The thrust of government-derived health and social policy should be to provide universal access to necessary health services, with regard for the appropriate level of care within a continuum of care. This help should be provided in a nondiscriminatory manner, without consideration of race, sexual orientation, or other criteria affecting civil and human rights and one's ability to pay. Thus, a partnership among business, labor, and government — the private and public sectors — must be formed to ensure that care and treatment are provided.

Considerable discussion and creativity will be entailed in designing an equitable system with sufficient funds to allow for the development and implementation of programs. Certainly, as the prevalence of HIV infection, AIDS, and ARC increases, an evaluation component must also be included within any program. Whichever treatment strategies are selected, they must reflect the varied population at risk, including children, gay men and lesbians, intravenous drug users, and straight women and men.

Children

Policies concerning children with AIDS are particularly complex. All children, by virtue of their age, are dependent and vulnerable. Their parents are presumed to be the natural protectors of their interests. When parents are unable or unwilling to assume this role, others — relatives, court-appointed guardians, social service agencies — must step in. Children at risk of contracting AIDS are in jeopardy in several ways. In the case of perinatal transmission, the mother is by definition infected. If she is not already ill, she is at risk of developing symptoms and eventually dying.

Currently, most cases of perinatal transmission occur in black and Hispanic/Latino mothers.[5] HIV-infected women from these groups are most often either intravenous drug users or the sexual partners of intravenous drug users. They are already bearing the burdens of discrimination and poverty — even without the added weight of HIV infection. Furthermore, in many cases the birth of an infected baby is often the first sign that the mother is infected and that AIDS may already be a threat to family stability. A baby born under these circumstances — infected, perhaps ill, the unwelcome herald of illness in the family, and a member of a group already suffering severe social discrimination — has a poor chance in life.

Articulation of many of the policy issues surrounding children is still on the horizon. Increasing numbers of these children and their families will be affected by policy decisions not yet made. All such decisions must take into account the material and emotional needs of children, the importance of maintaining (wherever possible) a family structure that can support these needs, and adequate social and community services to support the families.

Government policy. At the federal level, sufficient levels of funding should be channeled through state and local agencies to provide needed services. Federal officials can also play a part in reducing fear and stigma by educating the general public about the lack of evidence for casual transmission and the importance of accepting children with AIDS, ARC, or HIV infection in schools and other community settings.

State agencies and city and local governments can play a similar role. They are directly responsible for education, foster care, day care, and health care policies that will affect children and their families. These policies will have to take into account the needs of children and their families, the interests of workers who provide services, and the other funding needs in the community. Local circumstances will dictate specific policies. However, all policies should be designed to fulfill society's obligations to children.

Community policy. Many of the most important policy decisions will occur at the local level. In terms of school attendance, the American Academy of Pediatrics, the U.S. Public Health Service, and the *Surgeon General's Report on Acquired Immune Deficiency Syndrome* stress that casual contact between infected children and their schoolmates is not a risk for AIDS. The surgeon general's report states, "None of the identified cases of AIDS in the United States are known or are suspected to have been transmitted from one child to another in school, day care, or foster care settings."[6] No blanket rules can be made for all school boards to cover all possible cases of children with AIDS, and each case should be considered separately, as would be done with any child with a special problem, such as cerebral palsy or asthma. A good team to make such decisions jointly with the school board would consist of the child's parents and physician and a public health official.[7]

Attendance at day care and placement in foster care present more problems, since infants and preschool-age children do not have the same ability to control behavior and bodily excretions that older children do. However, with adequate staff education and precautions, these children can ordinarily be placed in such settings, as the American Academy of Pediatrics and the Centers for Disease Control suggest.[8] Here too, individualized decision making is central.

Since day care is not a legal right, and since most day care is offered through private institutions and individuals, it is particularly important that governmental agencies monitor the policies of these agencies to make sure that children with AIDS, ARC, or HIV infection are not systematically excluded.

Two problems require particular attention: confidentiality, and consent for testing. Because information about a child's serostatus can have devastating consequences if it becomes known to people other than those who have direct responsibility for the child, special care must be taken to protect confidentiality. The question of who has a legitimate need to know this information must be discussed thoroughly and carefully, with special consideration given to the circumstances that prevail. All those who are deemed to have a need to know must be made aware of their responsibility to keep this information confidential.

Testing for entry to day care raises other issues. Adults are ordinarily given the opportunity to give a voluntary, informed consent to HIV antibody testing. This process includes information about the test and the interpretation of the results, whether they are negative or positive. Parents and guardians should have the same opportunity to give consent for a child, or to decline testing, if they fully understand the reasons that the test may be considered appropriate. Counseling is essential not only for adults who are being tested, but also for those who bear the responsibility for a child's welfare.

Another aspect of consent is the question of whether foster parents should have information about a child's serostatus before they agree to take the child. Practice in this area is divided; some agencies refuse to screen children or to divulge this information to prospective foster parents; others will do so on request. Some foster parents understandably wish to have this information, both in deciding whether to commit their emotional and other resources to a particular child and in planning their own child-care procedures. However, policies should be constructed in ways that will give potential foster parents complete information about risks and outcomes while not unduly discouraging them from taking on this responsibility. At the same time, the issue of liability for a foster care agency must also be considered. Children with AIDS, ARC, or HIV infection are particularly dependent on foster care. This avenue of family support should not be closed to them by virtue of their infection.

If it is impossible to place some children with AIDS, ARC, or HIV infection in foster care, day care, or schools, appropriate alternative facilities must be devised to give such children as normal an existence as possible. However, these alternative facilities should not be considered the first choice for placement.

Professional policy. Professional education and training must include information about pediatric AIDS, ARC, and HIV infection and the most up-to-date treatment and research protocols. Education is particularly important for health care, day care, and other workers who will have direct contact with infected children. The risk of their becoming infected through working with these children is small, but it does exist. Workers must be trained in appropriate infection control measures. In addition, the extraordinary stress of dealing with infected and dying children must be recognized in professional training. Persons who have had experience in pediatric oncology may be able to provide advice to those who are involved in developing appropriate stress reduction and anti-burnout programs.

Family policy. All members of a family are affected when a child has AIDS, ARC, or HIV infection. The birth of such a baby may place a severe strain on a marriage or other relationship. Uninfected siblings may also suffer deprivation and stigmatization, and may worry about their own health or that of their mother or father. The family focus on the infected child may alter family dynamics and functioning. Family members who may be brought into the situation should be aware of these far-reaching effects. Professional family therapy should be available to assist families in adjusting to the situation and in providing the best care for all members of the family.

Risk Reduction

Membership in a risk group does not cause AIDS; risk behaviors do. An HIV-negative male couple who have been together in a monogamous relationship for the past ten years and who do not inject drugs are not at risk for AIDS. Not who you are, but rather what you do and with whom creates the problem.

Government policy. The U.S. Department of Education should take the lead in providing and funding a massive AIDS risk-reduction program directed specifically at the various sociocultural subpopulations throughout the United States. Condoms, spermicides, and literature on AIDS should be made available at no cost or on a sliding-fee scale upon request. Television, radio, newspapers, magazines, and other media should be utilized. The messages should be easily understandable, explicit, and not moralistic. It is the responsibility of the federal government, in concert with state and local officials, to educate the American public about AIDS. Punitive measures, such as quarantine, mandatory HIV antibody testing, and travel restrictions, may only drive persons most at risk for HIV infection underground. Efforts must be made to reduce the stigma of AIDS, not to enhance it.

Community policy. Specifically, the needs of some of those groups who have been most affected must be addressed. The dignity of millions of gay men around the world should be maintained. The families of gay men should be encouraged to become supportive in these most difficult times. State and municipal governments should be encouraged to put an end to AIDS-related discrimination. From the perspective of risk reduction, society should be especially supportive of two gay men living together in a monogamous relationship. It should, however, be kept in mind that monogamy (or abstinence) is not for everyone, and that safer sex practiced with extreme caution with more than one partner is a more responsible alternative than not practicing safe sex with one infected partner.

Prostitution will not be stopped by AIDS, but its risks can be minimized. Prostitutes should be educated about the use of condoms and spermicides during vaginal intercourse, and about refraining from anal sex. Legalization of prostitution, by permitting greater regulation of the practice, would lead to increased safety both for prostitutes and their clients.

Intravenous drug users should be encouraged to stop using drugs. Many more drug rehabilitation centers and methadone programs must be established to meet the demand for treatment. For those who cannot stop shooting drugs or who lack the desire to stop, needles and syringes should be distributed to terminate the practice of sharing "works." "Shooting galleries" — gathering places where drug users congregate to share drugs — should be closed throughout the United States. Intravenous drug users must become better informed about disinfectant practices. More important, the social conditions that lead to intravenous drug use should be improved. Unemployment, illiteracy, poverty, racial discrimination, inadequate housing, and troubled families are underlying causes of widespread intravenous drug use. These social problems must be addressed and corrected.

Persons who are in jails and prisons also are at higher risk for HIV infection. More extensive health and psychosocial therapy must be made available in these institutions. Many of these individuals are part of families to whom they will return. Enhancing health and safety opportunities, as well as the availability of counseling for incarcerated individuals, will also enhance and protect the future care of their family members. Condom distribution in jails and prisons, along with safer sex information, may protect the health of many individuals, as well as their families and society. Increased opportunities for conjugal visits might also decrease the frequency of high-risk sexual behaviors.

Professional policy. Voluntary HIV testing should be encouraged, particularly for (1) individuals who are not practicing strictly safer sex at all times, unless they have been in an exclusively monogamous relationship for at least a decade; (2) women who wish to have a child; and (3) persons for whom not knowing their status has become more anxiety-provoking than knowing for certain would be. It is absolutely essential that HIV testing be anonymous or confidential. A "confidential" HIV test result that is entered onto the named individual's computerized medical file at a hospital, clinic, physician's office, or laboratory is not confidential at all.

It is important that blood and blood products continue to be carefully screened for HIV. Blood should also be screened for HIV-2 and possibly other newly discovered retroviruses. Support services for hemophiliacs and their families are also necessary, since a large percentage of hemophiliacs became infected before blood screening and heat treatment of Factor VIII were introduced. Within this population, adolescent hemophiliacs need special attention. Not only do these adolescents have to be able to cope with their potentially life-threatening health condition, but they also are attempting to handle the normal sexuality concerns of adolescence. Adolescent hemophiliacs and their families need help to address the sex questions of an adolescent in the special context of AIDS for hemophiliacs.

All risk-reduction efforts should be supportive. Family members, lovers, and friends should be encouraged to be involved in all activities affecting the HIV-infected person. All of the aforementioned recommendations should have funds made available for the social services, education, and research essential for their implementation. A well-planned and well-developed financing mechanism must begin to be implemented immediately if we hope to responsibly meet this public health care crisis.

Financing

The impetus for a health care delivery system to assist persons with AIDS and their families must be service delivery needs, not available funds. This principle is particularly important in the design of a health care delivery system for persons with AIDS, where the needs will quickly exceed the available resources. Extending national health benefits for catastrophic coverage regardless of age should be considered. Such an extension would eliminate the necessity for many persons with AIDS or severe ARC to face destitution if inadequately insured. AIDS must be viewed in the context of other diseases and social problems; thus, the broadest solution to the financing question lies in some form of national health insurance. The model for financing discussed in this article is but one among many alternatives.

Government policy. Envisioned as a system for financing the care and treatment of persons with AIDS and their families is a partnership between the private sector, principally through employer-based health benefit programs, and government funding. Evidence increasingly shows that the cost of providing necessary treatment for persons with AIDS is extraordinarily high. AIDS, a long-term illness, becomes chronic and requires substantial, labor-intensive, long-term care. In combination, these factors are very costly. It is likely that the expense of care and treatment for persons with AIDS will become a significant drain on our private-sector health benefit plans, on the government, and even on our entire economy. For example, Scitovsky and Rice estimated that the direct costs of providing health care to persons with AIDS rose from $630 million in 1985 to over $1.1 billion in 1986.[9] The direct costs will continue to rise, so that by 1991 they will exceed $8.5 billion. Economists have estimated that by 1991, *aside from* the staggering medical costs of the illness, the AIDS epidemic will have cost our nation over $55 billion in lost personal income and other such factors.[10] Now is the time for both private industry and our government to design financing projects that will provide necessary funds at the required fiscal levels.

Private-sector health benefit plans, whenever available, should provide coverage for persons with AIDS, but this cannot be the exclusive coverage. Ten to 15 percent of the U.S. population — 37 million Americans — are covered by individual and small group insurance plans; another 37 million have no health insurance at all.[11] These two groups represent a disproportionate number of persons at high risk for AIDS. Intravenous drug users often are uninsured, and many members of the gay male community appear to be self-employed, therefore more likely to be enrolled in individual or small group plans and subject to stricter underwriting criteria. Health benefit plans should not discriminate against persons with AIDS or HIV infection by denying or limiting coverage. Rather, private-sector plans must continue to provide coverage to the limits of their allowed benefit structures, with the federal government providing a re-insurance or "stop-loss" form of backup protection. In the partnership that is envisioned here, the government would invest in the care and treatment of persons with AIDS or HIV infection, yet not assume the entire financial burden for these services. Some policymakers are suggesting that there be a federally mandated "tax" on health benefit premiums to provide funds to assist with the financing of needed services for persons with AIDS or ARC. Consideration should be given this idea, with appropriate regard for the rights, privacy, and dignity of persons with AIDS or ARC. It may be a viable approach to the issue of financing.

The political context within the Congress, with which the current discussion rests, must be the now popular notion of catastrophic health insurance. During the 100th Congress, proposals have been debated to create a catastrophic program for the nation's largest health benefits program, Medicare. It is entirely appropriate for the question of care and treatment of persons with AIDS or ARC to be linked to this concept, if not to the specific proposals that are being considered.

Catastrophic health coverage is designed to insure an individual and his or her family for serious and costly events beyond their control — events that they could not predict, such as a serious illness requiring lengthy hospitalization and long-term care. This is the situation with AIDS. Advocates support the development of a system of catastrophic care coverage which includes persons with AIDS or ARC. The system envisioned would be parallel to the hospice program, a system of care for terminally ill patients which was affirmed by Congress in recent years and which is now included within the benefit structure of Medicare. However, a health care financing program for persons with AIDS need not be included within Medicare. This is a possible structure, yet other structures should be considered by the Congress, the federal Health Care Financing Administration, and other institutions.

Recognizing that many persons with AIDS do not have insurance, the federal government, in partnership with private industry and local and state governments, should initiate and fund a program that would reflect level of need yet permit autonomy in the selection of health care services. Assuming that treatment protocols will increasingly become standardized, and that the number of experimental procedures will increase, persons with AIDS or HIV infection must remain free to choose from whom and where they wish to receive health care services. With a voucher system, a person with AIDS or ARC could take his or her benefit to any government-sanctioned treatment setting.

In this model, a person with AIDS or ARC who had insurance would first need to use and exhaust all benefits provided through his or her own private health benefits program. It is possible that the government would, in a yet undetermined manner, assist by subsidizing such care. This would be the "means test" component of the program: the use of available benefits. In addition, there should be some mechanism for co-payment by an individual who has sufficient resources to afford a reasonable co-payment. However, it is not recommended that a co-payment provision become a part of any means test if such a provision is to become a deterrent or barrier to care and treatment.

Therefore, the central part of a program to finance and provide care and treatment for persons with AIDS or ARC would be coordinated and heavily funded by the federal government, with some assistance from both state and local governments. The most effective system might be one in which the federal government would develop and then apply a series of criteria for different levels within appropriate continuum of care settings providing care and treatment for persons with AIDS or HIV infection. At each level of a continuum of care, appropriate criteria would be developed. This process must involve input from all of the relevant constituencies, including both consumers (persons with AIDS or HIV infection and their families) and health care providers. Care for persons with AIDS or ARC must be systemically integrated within the established health care delivery system. Standards must be developed to guarantee that those settings providing care to persons with AIDS or HIV infection have the facilities and staff available to provide necessary services of the very highest quality. A network of service delivery settings throughout the nation may evolve which has met federally sanctioned criteria for providing care and treatment to persons with AIDS or ARC. It is probable that most of the needed facilities already exist. These extant facilities can be combined with newly developed facilities to form the federally sanctioned, but not federally administered or directly controlled, settings. This plan is parallel to the federal approval program qualifying hospitals to receive reimbursement from the Medicare program.

Such a system would be expensive to develop and administer. It would, however, provide a framework for a collaborative system of care that could be positioned over the next few years to meet the needs of persons with AIDS or ARC. It would allow for universal access to care. However, there are problems with the design. First, a bureaucratic superstructure would be created. Also, this type of reimbursement structure would be complex, with funding based on chronicity and factors relevant to actual costs of care at different developmental stages of the virus. Moreover, given the size and complexity of such a structure, confidentiality would be difficult, but not impossible, to maintain. Further, this model could unintentionally create a network of AIDS and HIV infection treatment centers that would suffer from discrimination of many types.

Despite these possible criticisms, it is a fundamental responsibility of government to assure the availability of and access to necessary and appropriate health care services. The model described provides a vehicle for the federal government to fulfill its responsibility of providing needed health care services for persons with AIDS or ARC. Neither private industry nor government alone can carry the burden.

Summary

Sufficient fiscal resources must be made available by federal and state government, together with private-sector services, to fund necessary research, education, and training. Therefore, funds must be made available to continue basic and applied research, including both biomedical and psychosocial research, with appropriate attention to social and behavioral science. It would be a tragic error for social and behavioral science research to be sacrificed in favor of biomedical research. Both perspectives of inquiry are necessary.

Funding for education and training must include targeted efforts directed at three groups: individuals at high risk; professionals who may become involved with the care and treatment of persons with AIDS; and the general public. Educational and training efforts must be systematically developed and well funded. Prevention, through careful practices or elimination of high-risk behaviors, could slow the spread of the epidemic. Proper education and training offer our best chance at prevention. These tasks collectively — research, education, and training — must be funded through both existing programs of support and newly developed programs. Funds should be made available from both the public and private sectors.

The authors who contributed to this article are Elaine A. Anderson, Ph.D., assistant professor, Department of Family and Community Development, University of Maryland; Diane Beeson, Ph.D., associate professor, Department of Sociology and Social Services, California State University; Douglas A. Feldman, Ph.D., executive director, AIDS Center of Queens County, Inc.; Mark R. Ginsberg, Ph.D., executive director, American Association for Marriage and Family Therapy; Carol Levine, executive director, Citizens Commission on AIDS, New York City; Robert M. Rice, Jr., Ph.D., executive vice-president, Family Service America; Steven M. Vincent, Ph.D., Psychology and Outpatient Counseling, St. Cloud Hospital, St. Cloud, Minnesota; and Deborah Weinstein, M.S.W., executive director, Foundation for the Scientific Study of Sexuality.

Notes

1. See Institute of Medicine/National Academy of Sciences, *Confronting AIDS: Directions for Public Health, Health Care, and Research* (Washington, D.C.: National Academy Press, 1986).
2. Kay Glidden, "Funeral Home Resource List Survey," by Gay Men's Health Crisis in New York City, Office of Ombudsman, Robert Cecchi, Fall 1986.
3. *National Gay and Lesbian Task Force Newsletter* (Washington, D.C.: National Gay and Lesbian Task Force, March 1987).
4. *New York City Commission on Human Rights: Report on Discrimination Against People with AIDS* (November 1983–April 1986): 1–47.
5. Martha T. Rogers, M.D., et al., "AIDS in Children: Report of the Centers for Disease Control National Surveillance, 1982–1985," in *Pediatrics* 79, no. 6 (June 1987): 1008–1014.
6. U.S. Department of Health and Human Services, *Surgeon General's Report on Acquired Immune Deficiency Syndrome* (1986): 23–24.
7. Committee on Infectious Diseases, American Academy of Pediatrics, "School Attendance of Children and Adolescents Infected with Human T-Lymphotropic Virus Type III/Lymphadenopathy-Associated Virus," in *Pediatrics* 72, no. 3 (1983): 430–432.
8. Committee on Infectious Diseases, American Academy of Pediatrics, "Health Guidelines for the Attendance in Day-Care and Foster-Care Settings of Children Infected with Human Immune Deficiency Virus," in *Pediatrics* 79, no. 3 (March 1987): 466–469.
9. See Anne A. Scitovsky and Dorothy P. Rice, "Estimates of the Direct and Indirect Costs of Acquired Immunodeficiency Syndrome in the United States, 1985, 1986, and 1991," in *Public Health Reports* 102, no. 1 (January–February 1987): 5.
10. Ibid.
11. See Peter S. Arno, Ph.D., "Private Health Insurance and the AIDS Epidemic: Distributing the Economic Burden," paper presented at the Annual Meeting of the Association for Health Services Research, Chicago, Illinois (June 15, 1987).

When I was first diagnosed, I was very worried about what my family was going to think, my friends, just people in general, and I was real sad and guilty and then I thought, you know, who is the most important person, you know, is it the president, is it Mother Teresa, is it the pope? It's not. It's yourself. Each individual person. There's no reason why you should be alive unless you're the most important person in the world to yourself. And you've got to live your life accordingly and enjoy it to the fullest or it's not worth living."

AIDS Initiatives in Massachusetts: Building a Continuum of Care

Nancy Weiland Carpenter

The Health Resource Office was officially established within the Massachusetts Department of Public Health in August 1985 to coordinate policy, education, research, and service response to the AIDS epidemic, and to focus attention on the social and economic impact of the disease. The actual work of the office was begun earlier, in October 1983. This article reviews the activities of the Health Resource Office from October 1983 through June 1987 in allocating resources for AIDS and ARC programs and services. It then describes the conceptual model that evolved during this period for the continuum of services needed to reduce HIV transmission and to provide services to those who are infected and ill.

In October 1983, the Massachusetts Governor's Task Force on AIDS, appointed by Governor Dukakis, held its first meeting. At that time, there were 33 known cases of AIDS in the state. By December 1987, 1,174 cases had been reported in Massachusetts. The Task Force was comprised of individuals from the sectors of medicine, clinical research, epidemiology, public health, state and local government, and the legislature. Meeting on a monthly basis, it worked under the governor's mandate to guide the state's education, policy, and service response to the AIDS epidemic.

The Health Resource Office was formally established in the Massachusetts Department of Public Health (DPH) in the summer of 1985 to define public policy regarding the AIDS epidemic and to guide response to the myriad of health, social, and economic concerns it had raised. The Health Resource Office worked with the AIDS task force to ensure that policies developed to guide social interaction with those infected with human immunodeficiency virus (HIV) were based on medical and scientific evidence, not on fear and ignorance.[1] The office has also been responsible for administering a program of research support; conducting extensive education and in-service training programs through its staff of health educators and through funding support provided to the AIDS Action Com-

Nancy Weiland Carpenter is director of patient policy at the Massachusetts Hospital Association. She was director of the Health Resource Office within the Massachusetts Department of Public Health from the fall of 1983 to the summer of 1987.

mittee of Massachusetts; and allocating resources for needed health and social services. Case surveillance and the state-sponsored anonymous HIV testing and counseling programs have been administered separately, through the Department of Public Health's State Laboratory Institute. As well, a ten-bed inpatient AIDS unit has been established at the DPH's Lemuel Shattuck Hospital by DPH staff at that facility.

Four goals were endorsed by the AIDS task force in June 1986 and were used by the Health Resource Office to guide resource allocation activities. These goals were as follows:

- to continue to support research in an effort to find a cure and an effective treatment
- to increase the availability of direct services to people with AIDS
- to further pursue reduction of the spread of HIV through education and outreach
- to maintain the state's commitment to providing the leadership and guidance necessary to ensure care and compassion for those who are stricken with this illness

Massachusetts AIDS Research Program

In Massachusetts, state funds for efforts to deal with AIDS first became available in the beginning of the 1985 fiscal year, which ran from July 1, 1984, through June 30, 1985. Concern about the safety of the blood supply resulted in a $1.5 million appropriation by the Massachusetts legislature to support research into the cause, prevention, surveillance, methods of treatment, and cure of AIDS in order to protect the public health. (The antibody test to screen the blood supply for exposure to HIV was not available until the middle of that fiscal year, and was not approved for actual use by the Federal Drug Administration until April 1985.) Lacking an administrative precedent within the state purchase-of-service contracting rules for supporting research, the Health Resource Office devised a mechanism to award research funds via a Request for Proposal (RFP) process. The Massachusetts AIDS Research Council was convened by Bailus Walker, Jr., then commissioner of the Massachusetts Department of Public Health and chairman of the AIDS task force, to make recommendations for funding on the basis of a peer review of submitted applications. Although the Massachusetts Governor's Task Force on AIDS included some of the nation's leading experts on AIDS research, it was deemed necessary to convene a distinct body to allocate research funds in order to avoid conflicts of interest if task force members applied for support.

The Request for Proposal identified two categories of funding support: (1) pathogenesis and treatment of AIDS, and (2) epidemiological, social, and behavioral factors associated with AIDS.

The first category was intended to provide support for laboratory or clinical investigations, or both, into the basic science of the disease, including its cause; mechanism of infectivity and relationship to other illnesses; mode of transmission in the blood supply and methods to assure its protection; and other avenues of investigation with potential for increasing knowledge of the disease, preventing its further spread, and treating or curing those already infected.

The second funding support category was intended to identify (1) social and behavioral precursors to the disease and methods of intervention to prevent its continued spread, and (2) new approaches to the management of patients with AIDS and those infected with the virus.

Twenty proposals were funded in FY'85. Prior to the start of FY'86 and FY'87, the progress of funded projects was reviewed by the Massachusetts AIDS Research Council and recommendations were made for continued support on the basis of (1) an assessment of the progress that had been made during the previous contract period, and (2) the proposed activities to be pursued during the next funding cycle. By FY'87, eleven of the original projects were still being supported. Contracts to continue the eleven projects were renewed for the first six months of FY'88 (through December 1987) without review by the research council.

Ongoing administrative concern with justifying state support of AIDS research has centered on the need to find the appropriate focus for state funds in this ever changing arena. In order to ensure that state AIDS research priorities are appropriate and are not duplicative of national or other state efforts, an inventory of new funding sources (primarily federal funds) acquired by state-funded AIDS researchers since the award in FY'85 of the initial Massachusetts research support was identified as a priority in FY'87 for the following fiscal year. As well, identifying new areas for research was considered an appropriate focus for state efforts. These concerns were scheduled for consideration during the latter part of FY'88. Also, it was anticipated at that time that a new Request for Proposal would affect FY'89 AIDS research allocations.

Community Resources and Services

In June 1986, the Massachusetts Governor's Task Force on AIDS endorsed the "Massachusetts Department of Public Health FY'87 AIDS Resource Allocation Plan."[2] Its purpose was to establish priorities for directing resource allocation efforts. Development of the plan was the result of information about community service needs which had been obtained by the Health Resource Office from a variety of sources.

In response to complaints and anecdotal information from providers, patients, and advocates about barriers to home care services experienced by people with AIDS, the Health Resource Office, during the fall of 1985, had conducted an informal assessment of physicians, hospital discharge planners, visiting nurses, and home health providers in an attempt to pinpoint the underlying reason(s) impeding access to service for this group. The information that was sought ranged from estimates of the number of people with AIDS who had been referred for service and of the actual number served to an assessment of how the home care needs of patients with AIDS differ from those of patients with other infectious or chronic diseases. Information was also sought regarding increased need for staff training and supervision, as well as reimbursement barriers to patient service.

In an effort to obtain more specific information on the service needs of individuals ill with AIDS or showing signs and symptoms of HIV infection, the position of community resource specialist was established in the Health Resource Office to document gaps in service for individual clients as a basis for targeting resources.

The first community resource specialist was hired in the winter of 1986 to work in the Boston area, where most of the state's patients with AIDS live. Though an employee of the Department of Public Health, the community resource specialist was placed half-time at the AIDS Action Committee's office in order to ensure her familiarity with client concerns and her availability for assisting AIDS Action Committee client service workers in their efforts to manage the most difficult-to-serve clients and obtain services for them. It was felt that because the community resource specialist was an employee of the Department of Public Health, some of the complexities of working through the bureaucracy might be reduced by capitalizing on personal relationships already established between staff in public agencies and by exerting an influence on administrative rules and procedures that might be found to hamper access to services. Three additional community resource specialists were hired by the end of FY'87 and were placed in targeted areas around the state, including Springfield, Worcester, and Barnstable County.

In addition to providing valuable information about the impediments experienced by patients with AIDS in their efforts to obtain access to entitlements and services, the community resource specialist is also in a position to document gaps in the availability of services as well as the need for new service entities within the spectrum of a comprehensive continuum of care. Information and inferences provided by the community resource specialist, in conjunction with those provided directly by the AIDS Action Committee and other sources, have been used as the basis for establishing priorities for resource allocation.

Expanding Home Care Services for AIDS Patients

With the need for expansion of home care services identified as a priority, a strategy for allocating resources to increase services and access to them was developed. An important principle guiding this program-development activity was that expanding the existing array of services that comprise the health care system (with modifications where necessary) to include services to AIDS patients was preferable to the creation of new service entities specifically for AIDS care. Under this principle, new services and program models would be developed when no other appropriate service existed. Following this principle would ensure that to the greatest extent possible, AIDS care would be financed through the current third-party reimbursement structure, leaving new resources available to fill gaps in the service spectrum. Clearly, the problems of access, that is, efforts to obtain services without insurance or with inadequate insurance coverage, would not be resolved by this approach; however, it was felt that the AIDS appropriation was not intended to address the universal concerns of the uninsured or underinsured.

Accordingly, the first step in devising a strategy to affect home care support involved (1) determining what impediments to the delivery of AIDS care were being experienced by existing service providers; (2) gathering recommendations on how best to target resources to alleviate access barriers and increase services; and (3) developing a programmatic and fiscal focus as a target for new funding initiatives. Over a period of several weeks during July and August 1986, meetings were held with representatives from Massachusetts visiting nurse agencies, hospice programs, home care agencies, trade association representatives, and others knowledgeable in the areas of community services and the needs of AIDS patients. More than fifteen meetings were held.

As a result of information gathered from these meetings, from talks with client services staff and with the supervisor of the volunteer "buddy" program at the AIDS Action Committee, and from a review of recent articles on AIDS home care, a model program was described for delivering home care services to patients with AIDS.[3] This program description was then incorporated into the Request for Proposal issued to community agencies that were providing home support services. A maximum obligation of up to $50,000 a year was noted as available to selected agencies for use in expanding their operational capacity to deliver AIDS care. These funds were not intended for use as entitlement funding for individual patients.

The RFP stated the intent to select agencies for funding which clearly indicated their commitment on behalf of using additional operational support to expand their capacity to deliver services. Funds were to be used to support direct care staff, supervisory or support staff, or staff whose services were not covered through third-party reimbursement. While other expenses might also be appropriate for state support under this program, priority was to be given to agencies that evidenced a strong commitment to use additional state resources to enhance or expand care for AIDS patients, in conjunction with maximizing third-party reimbursement for those patients with coverage.

In addition, the RFP noted that criteria for funding included the need for statewide allocation of resources; delineation of the geographic distribution and clustering of diagnosed cases of AIDS throughout the state; and an estimation of the expected demand for client services in the proposed program's service area.

Home Health Initiative Program Components

The definition of a comprehensive home care program outlined in the RFP reflected two concurrent perspectives: that of the patient and that of the agency.

Patient needs. When a diagnosis of AIDS is made, hospitalization is usually required for testing and treatment. At the termination of the hospital stay, the patient is faced with decisions about further treatment and care. By its nature, AIDS is a disease that may incorporate a wide range of treatment and various modes of care. Much of this care and treatment can take place in an outpatient setting or in the home, provided that the appropriate services are in place. The care may range in type from the aggressive and curative to the palliative and respitive. To provide this range of care, the RFP noted that the following should be available:

- A primary care giver (a family member, a significant other, or a mutually agreed upon person)
- A home health aide
- A medical consultant
- A skilled nurse (up to twenty-four hours per day)
- Physical, occupational, and speech therapists
- A volunteer or "buddy" (to prepare meals, run errands, and provide psychological support)
- A social worker/case coordinator
- A counselor/chaplain (to provide bereavement and spiritual counseling)
- A psychiatric consultant (to provide neurological evaluations/staff training on central nervous system [CNS] involvement)

The RFP stressed that to benefit the AIDS patient, a consistent and cohesive provision of care throughout the illness is imperative. This can most successfully be accomplished through a team approach, engaging the services of the persons in the preceding list, or through provision of a consistent person to act as an advocate during the course of the illness, such as a social worker, nurse, or volunteer.

Agency needs. When a home care program is viewed from the agency perspective, a different set of issues is identified. AIDS patients have demanding physical ailments and a host of psychosocial problems. The infections associated with AIDS are usually multiple. There may be central nervous system involvement, with or without other diagnosed infections, which further complicates care.

Enabling a patient with AIDS to remain at home in the community requires the commitment and creative use of staff and resources by care givers and providers. Assurance of a comprehensive and consistent type of care for AIDS patients requires a multidisciplinary team approach. An essential component of any program is a detailed plan for the provision of emergency care and after-hours consultation, based on a prescribed protocol. The RFP recognized that in some agencies each of the identified components of the team might already exist; for other agencies, it might be necessary to identify other resources in the community in order to create the team. The team consists of the following providers:

- Homemaker/home health aide
- Nurses
- Social workers
- Therapists
- Medical consultant
- Psychiatric consultant
- Bereavement counselor
- Volunteers
- In-service training and support professionals

With a conceptual model devised and described in the RFP, copies were issued to all visiting nurse, hospice, and home health agencies in the state. In all, forty-three RFPs were distributed. Thirteen agencies responded, and eight were selected for funding to begin in January 1987. The contracts for these eight programs were renewed in FY'88 for $50,000 plus an increase for cost of living according to state purchase-of-service guidelines.

Residential Facilities

From documentation gathered by the community resource specialists as well as from ongoing discussions with providers, the AIDS Action Committee, and other patient advocates, it is clear that the need for housing resources for patients with AIDS is an overwhelming problem. During the course of the disease, the individual who is ill may have one or several acute episodes of illness requiring inpatient hospitalization in an acute care facility. Upon release from the hospital, the individual may return home and live in the community, though often in an increasingly debilitated state. Patients who are single, living alone, and unable to maintain an income may find it necessary to leave their apartment or house and live with relatives or friends. If this is not an option, then these patients may become dependent on advocacy resources.

In Massachusetts, the AIDS Action Committee maintains several houses that persons with AIDS or AIDS-related complex (ARC) may use in accordance with the policies and stipulations of the committee. Some of the individuals seeking housing are unable to comply with the house rules. These houses are not staffed; they are managed by the persons residing in them, with support from the AIDS Action Committee's housing supervisor. Therefore, individuals with active substance problems, central nervous system involvement (AIDS dementia), or other difficulties that may be disruptive to residents in the house are impossible to place in these facilities.

Recognizing that alternatives were needed for these individuals and that the state must assume more responsibility in meeting these needs, the Health Resource Office sought to develop a prototype staffed residential facility for use by individuals with AIDS or ARC. During FY'87, a facility was actually opened under contract to the Commonwealth of Massachusetts.

After obtaining permission to use a house on the property of the Western Massachusetts Hospital in Westfield, one of the Department of Public Health hospitals that had recently become vacant in accordance with new state rules regarding the use of such property, the Health Resource Office identified a local human service agency and requested its involvement in developing the facility and managing it as a residence for individuals with AIDS. Under a contract negotiated with the Jewish Family Services of Greater Springfield, a program for housing up to five persons in a facility staffed twenty-four hours per day was implemented. Individuals housed in the facility may be in a transitional phase and can live in the house until stabilized, or they may be unable to leave, in which case they will live in the house until the terminal phase of their illness.

A unique feature of the program at Western Massachusetts Hospital is its eighteen-bed palliative care unit, in which AIDS patients residing in the house may elect to be placed during the final stage of illness. Duplicating this model, particularly in the Boston area, will be difficult, owing to the lack of available property and the high cost of an appropriate site.

The need to find an appropriate residential setting for children who are ill with AIDS or ARC and whose parents are unable or unwilling to care for them was addressed during FY'87 through a joint venture between the Massachusetts Department of Public Health and the Boston Department of Health and Hospitals. By December 1987, twenty-four cases of pediatric AIDS had been reported in Massachusetts.

Using space owned and operated by the City of Boston, a contract was negotiated between the Boston Department of Health and Hospitals and the Massachusetts Department of Public Health to house four children in a twenty-four-hour staffed facility, with social worker and nurse practitioner time included to ensure continuity of care for the patients. While preference is given to placing these children with family members or in foster care, the pediatric residence assures that children will not be forced to remain inappropriately in an acute hospital bed until more suitable arrangements can be made.

During FY'87, while plans for the Western Massachusetts Hospital facility and the pediatric residence were under way, attention was directed to the plight of individuals with previous mental health histories who were homeless and had become infected with HIV. It was recognized that these persons posed special problems and that placements for them were at times impossible to secure. The staff of the Health Resource Office convened representatives from the City of Boston, the Robert Wood Johnson Health Care for the Homeless Project, the Pine Street Inn, the Lemuel Shattuck Hospital homeless shelter, and the AIDS Action Committee to address the growing concern about these individuals. Using documentation of several cases that fell into this category, the community resource specialist outlined the contacts that had been made and the steps taken to try to find an appropriate service for these persons. The role of the Department of Mental Health in caring for them was considered as an additional concern. Several issues were raised in this context by the Department of Mental Health, including (1) whether it was able to ensure appropriate infection control precautions; (2) whether the patients would be more appropriately assisted by a medical service than in a Department of Mental Health facility, since their dementia was the result of organic disease and could not be expected to be responsive to traditional psychiatric interventions; and (3) whether the mental conditions experienced by AIDS patients were irreversible and therefore not the proper focus for the Department of Mental Health.

In addition to concerns about these patients, issues were raised about finding an appropriate placement for individuals with HIV infection who were homeless or actively using drugs or engaging in prostitution, or a combination of these. After consideration of the legal, social, economic, and ethical implications of these complex situations, it was felt that two objectives required an immediate response. Individuals with these complex social and medical problems needed to be placed in an environment that met their basic needs and that was conducive to helping them understand their infection and the need to observe infection control precautions at all times in order not to infect someone else; and a public response was needed to provide resources and an appropriate service for this difficult-to-serve population.

Building the Continuum of Care

In allocating resources in the midst of a crisis as large and overwhelming as the AIDS epidemic, a major tension arises, stemming from the need to have in place a plan of action based on future projections of need while at the same time responding to the call for immediate action. State funds are allocated for a one-year period. Funds not spent during that time are usually reverted. Not only does this raise concerns for the next year's allocation, but in addition, advocates are likely to attack politically sensitive administrators for their lack of action during a crisis.

In recognition of these factors, the Health Resource Office pursued a dual course of action. While working to assess unmet need and develop a process and structure for establishing priorities for funding, the office undertook simultaneous efforts to allocate existing resources to those areas where there was a consensus of need. These latter efforts have been described above. What follows is a description of the conceptual model for a continuum of care which was developed by the Health Resource Office and which was presented to the Massachusetts Governor's Task Force on AIDS, to be used in developing a five-year plan.[4]

Many of the health, social, and emotional support services needed to respond to the growing number of AIDS patients in the Commonwealth are already in place. However, their distribution throughout the Commonwealth may be uneven. The model is most useful as a basis for discussion among community leaders as they assess their own preparedness for addressing AIDS prevention and care.

Prevention

Preventing the transmission of HIV is the only currently available method of curtailing the epidemic. Therefore, the first component on the continuum of AIDS care consists of education and outreach services so that those who are at risk of exposure can be alerted to their risk status, assisted in obtaining additional information, and supported in changing risky behaviors.

Providing simple factual information is an important part of prevention efforts. This includes directions to services; notification of educational programs, including television and print media efforts, public programs, and special advocacy events; and resources for further information or assistance.

Awareness education is also an element of AIDS prevention activities and is intended to provide substantial information about the virus; its effect on the body's immune system; the meaning of antibody status and blood tests; current medical interventions; transmission of the virus; and methods to prevent exposure.

The third focus of AIDS prevention activities is risk-awareness education. This is intended to reach those individuals whose behaviors place them at high risk for exposure to the virus, and it includes specific knowledge of how to prevent initial infection and transmission of HIV.

The fourth category of the prevention component is training and in-service education. Through the efforts of the Health Resource Office staff, a trainer-of-trainer model has been pursued to ensure that health and social service professionals throughout the state are well versed about AIDS and that they incorporate AIDS awareness and education into their programs and client meetings.

Clinical Transition

The second component on the continuum of AIDS services is referred to as clinical transition. This is intended to help those individuals who may have been exposed to the virus and who require access to medical, social, and support services for detection and treatment and for the provision of care. Counseling and testing are critical pieces of this component.

Patient Care Services

An individual who is in fact infected with HIV will require patient care services, the third component on the continuum, during the course of his or her battle with the disease. In order to provide the full spectrum of services, both hospital- and community-based services will be needed.

Medical evaluation for seropositive adults and children, and diagnosis for those who are symptomatic, should be available in a variety of settings, including community-based medical practices and hospital outpatient and inpatient services.

Physicians from a range of specialities and in a range of settings should be well versed in HIV infection, as should other health providers.

Hospital services need to be appropriately distributed throughout the state, with the capability to treat the array of medical, neurological, and emotional problems experienced by those with HIV infection. As well, inpatient units capable of treating both the medical and psychiatric manifestations of the illness are a critical part of patient care services.

Community-Based System of Care

The fourth component on the continuum is a strong community-based system of care. This will enable those who are ill to remain at home as long as possible when not in an acute phase of the illness. A strong home health care service, able to provide nursing care and homemaker services as well as help with activities of daily living, is essential. Specialized care that includes IV therapy and other medical services will enable patients to stay out of the hospital for longer periods of time.

A full range of housing resources is going to be needed to support the individual's capacity to maintain maximum self-sufficiency during the course of illness. As well, specialized housing needs exist for particularly vulnerable persons, such as those with children or persons with central nervous system infections. Housing needs include emergency shelter; independent living in shared, group, or single-family housing; and supervised housing.

Other specialized services may need to be adapted or developed for treatment of those at high risk of exposure to HIV. Of particular concern is the need to develop services for intravenous drug users who seek to eliminate needle use, but these services must also address immediate methods for reducing the drug user's potential exposure to the virus. The existing system of drug treatment programs represents a critical element of the community-based system of care. These programs need to be expanded and supported in order to intensify AIDS prevention efforts.

Public Health Policy and Planning

The fifth and final component of the continuum consists of the public health and research efforts needed to continue to address surveillance and monitoring, treatment, and policy development and implementation. Consensus of thought may not always be achievable among persons whose professional or advocacy experience has dealt with the complex issues of providing care and service to those who are ill with AIDS or ARC. The role of government, therefore, is important in forging strong partnerships wherever possible on the federal, state, and local levels among government, physicians, health and social service providers, and concerned and compassionate volunteer organizations such as the AIDS Action Committee to ensure that debate and discussion on the issues are focused and directed toward specific goals. The preceding outline of a continuum of care, it is hoped, will provide a focus for that effort.

Community-Based Development of a Continuum of AIDS Services

With a conceptual model in place which defines the services needed to prevent transmission of HIV and to provide care for those who are infected and ill, it is essential to form community networks of public health officials, health and social service providers, medical personnel, and community leaders, with particular emphasis on those community leaders who represent high-risk groups, educators, the media, and elected officials.

Initially, an assessment of the impact of the epidemic in the community will need to be made. Using epidemiological information from the state, including a breakdown of cases by risk factor, an understanding of the community risk potential can begin to be made. Through conversations with community leaders and service providers, an estimate of the number of individuals at high risk for exposure can be developed. Working with epidemiologists, a projection of case load can be developed as a benchmark for future planning efforts.

Using the conceptual model as a basis for discussion among the community leadership, an assessment of the applicability of the model to the individual community can serve as the beginning of a dialogue on a range of AIDS-related issues. As a focus for discussion, the conceptual model allows the provider community to be fully involved from the beginning and underscores the crucial concept that to be effective, AIDS planning and program development must be based on scientific and medical evidence, not on the community's fear and lack of knowledge.

Once the community's leadership shares the concept of the components needed to provide a continuum of care, an assessment of the services currently available in the community can be conducted. Information obtained as part of this effort will include the location of services; the capacity for care; barriers to care, such as a waiting list, residency requirements, language barriers, cost, and other factors; planned changes, such as expansion or relocation; sources of support; community sensitivities, and so on.

Conducting a comparison of existing services with the conceptual model will indicate to a community where gaps in service exist. Factoring in epidemiological projections for expected case load by risk group will help in determining priorities for resource allocation, which in turn will lead to decisions on whether to develop a new service or expand an existing one. In some instances, though a gap in service may be evident, a community may determine that since there is little need for that particular service, no resources or planning effort will be directed toward filling the gap.

Once priorities have been established, new resources can be sought through a range of means, including the efforts of individual providers to seek new funds; local initiative to attract state or federal resources; and advocacy to expand third-party coverage for specific services.

Community-based planning must work in tandem with state policy and with resource-allocation initiatives. Through increased information on community needs and priorities, state initiatives can better serve local communities in their efforts to prevent transmission of HIV and to provide care for those who are ill.

Notes

1. Massachusetts Governor's Task Force on AIDS, *Massachusetts Governor's Task Force on AIDS Policies and Recommendations,* Massachusetts Department of Public Health, January 1987.
2. The FY'87 resource allocation plan was the subject of a June 1986 memorandum from Bailus Walker, Jr., then commissioner of the Massachusetts Department of Public Health and chairman of the Massachusetts Governor's Task Force on AIDS, to the members of the task force.
3. The articles on AIDS home care referred to here were published in *Caring, AIDS and Home Care* 5, no. 6 (National Association for Home Care, Washington, D.C., June 1986).
4. The Health Resource Office document describing the conceptual model for a continuum of care was entitled *AIDS Policy Initiatives: Planning for Future Research, Education and Service Needs,* Massachusetts Department of Public Health, April 23, 1987.

Call to Action: A Community Responds

Larry Kessler
Ann M. Silvia
David Aronstein
Cynthia Patton

This article will examine the early formation of the AIDS Action Committee of Massachusetts, and what it has become. It will examine particular philosophical and organizational conflicts, some unique to AIDS organizing, that have influenced the direction the group has taken. It will try to tease out some of the factors that have made the organization successful in delivering services, providing education, and affecting city and state policy. It will also examine some of the unresolved conflicts that threaten the organization.

The AIDS Action Committee of Massachusetts (AAC) began as a "rap group" in November 1982. By 1987, it had grown into an advocacy and service organization with a $3 million budget; thirty-three staff, with funding for fifteen more pending; seven hundred active volunteers; and a national reputation. Welding strategies from social justice movements to concepts from social service management, the organization created a vision and structure to guide decision making through a complicated medical and political crisis that continues to unfold at lightning pace. The AAC has become a credible resource and an essential participant in community, city, and state AIDS policy development.

There were no chapters in textbooks which told us how to build an organization that could respond to a contemporary epidemic. Especially challenging were these two requirements:

1. balancing the needs of those diagnosed with AIDS or ARC with broader community issues related to the AIDS crisis, and

2. maintaining professional services and a grassroots volunteer base.

The authors are affiliated with the AIDS Action Committee of Massachusetts, where Larry Kessler is executive director; Ann M. Silvia is director of the Education Department; David Aronstein is director of Client Services; and Cynthia Patton is consultant for Special Projects.

While the conflicts inherent in these aims are faced by many volunteer-based organizations, several factors gave them unprecedented significance. AIDS is a new, incurable, infectious disease linked in the public's mind with controversial social practices. Preexisting racism, sexism, homophobia, and fear of addicts hindered the vision and actions of the agencies most needed to mount a rapid response to AIDS and the accompanying epidemic of fear. Those who first volunteered their time and talents risked accusation that they were members of the hidden minorities first affected by AIDS, and thus faced possible discrimination by offering of themselves. Patterns of prejudice obscured the line between realistic public health concerns and political opportunism that allowed repressive social agendas against the minorities first affected to cloud issues of testing and quarantine and of funding and allocation of medical and social resources.

Preconditions of AIDS Organizing in Boston

AIDS organizing in larger cities began within the existing predominantly gay male communities. Boston's gay and lesbian community was well organized and was perceived as a viable political constituency with recognizable issues, institutions, and leaders. There were important institutions with nearly a decade of service to the community: Fenway Community Health Center (FCHC), a gay-oriented health center; Gay and Lesbian Counseling Services (GLCS), a mental health center; *Gay Community News (GCN)*, a nationally distributed newspaper; and Gay and Lesbian Advocates and Defenders (GLAD), a gay legal organization with strong ties to mainstream civil liberties groups. There were several more locally oriented newspapers, and dozens of groups, from athletics clubs and professional and business fraternities to religious groups and political caucuses, many linked to state or national organizations.

In 1982, Boston had a mayoral liaison to the gay and lesbian community and would soon have an openly gay male city councillor and other openly gay and lesbian appointees to city human rights commissions and social service departments. The community infrastructure and the links with the liberal city government provided channels for communication within and outside the gay and lesbian community. There was a wide base of professional politicians and grassroots organizers expert in working within the gay and lesbian community and interfacing with government agencies. And yet, despite the large number of city agencies and community groups that could have taken on AIDS as a primary issue, most were reluctant: Fenway Community Health Center came closest, perhaps because AIDS was initially most obviously a medical problem.

Recognizing a Need

The AAC formed out of disparate organizational and individual foci of concern. Concern in Boston, a secondary epicenter, grew from observing what was happening in New York City (the nearest primary epicenter), which was overwhelmed with hundreds of cases in 1982, when Boston had fewer than a dozen.

The rap group that was the beginnings of the AAC was offered by two mental health providers at the Fenway Community Health Center. The AAC's current executive director, Larry Kessler, who early emerged as a leader and in August 1983 became the first staff person, joined the group in January 1983. Key people from other parts of the gay and lesbian community joined over the next year and formed the first steering committee, operating as a subcommittee of the FCHC board of directors. The AAC functioned as a special project of the FCHC board until 1986, long after it had equaled and surpassed FCHC in size and budget.

Early organizers saw the AIDS crisis as similar to other social issues — there was an identifiable group with a need, who would be overlooked by mainstream society and systems and who faced isolation, stigma, and discrimination. Many of the problems that became crystallized with AIDS — poor organization of health care, fear of minorities, too few funds for human needs — are deeply entrenched aspects of American society. It became clear that personal contact and grassroots organizing could improve the position of those most affected by AIDS and could provide a basis for political education that could encourage some to tackle the broader issues shaping the AIDS crisis.

Founding members also believed that a volunteer response would meet both the needs of the diagnosed and the needs of volunteers who came with an urgent desire to quell their fears by gaining information and expressing their concern through action. Becoming a volunteer was also an opportunity to provide an experience of community, perhaps for the first time, for these members of the stigmatized subcultures.

The AAC mission statement grew out of simple statements by members about their concerns and experience. In 1982–83, most media reports expressed the isolation and discrimination faced by people with AIDS (PWAs). Simple and evocative observations such as "it seems most important to support the people with the diagnosis because the whole world is against them" were translated into the first mission of support. There was a tremendous fear of men with AIDS within the gay male community, so the emerging AAC assumed the role of befriending and supporting those diagnosed both in that community and in medical/social service institutions.

Second, AAC members observed that their fears had lessened once they learned facts about AIDS and discussed their worries with people who took them seriously. The mission of education was to duplicate that experience for others.

Third came advocacy, which concerned wresting a response from agencies that should have been concerned with AIDS but that were doing nothing. Advocacy initially focused on procuring federal and state money for research. In the early years of organizing, no cause had been identified (human T-cell lymphotropic virus type III [HTLV-III], now called human immunodeficiency virus [HIV], was identified in 1984), and it was hoped that AIDS would be quickly and easily cured.

Finally, outreach was defined as getting out the word that the AAC had answers and resources. The first major outreach project was the hotline, which today is part of the Education Department. Outreach was initially defined simply as making it possible for people to find the AAC.

In choosing projects, the AAC chipped away at an iceberg of ignorance, apathy, and denial. The added responsibility of coping with the anxiety of those at risk would come later, when people were better educated and realized that they, too, might be at risk for AIDS. Anxiety moved from group to group as different sectors of society came to understand their relationship to AIDS. Anxiety in Boston's gay male community began in about 1984 and peaked in mid-1986, with continuing effects through other groups and agencies.

Needs Defined for Education and Services

The potential agenda of the AAC was immense. The emerging leadership pushed for projects that had a high probability of success in order to give the group an opportunity to see how members worked together, build a sense of confidence and cohesiveness, and establish credibility outside the group. The philosophy that emerged was volunteer involvement in practical projects of doing for others — either through direct service to PWAs or through defined projects like letter-writing campaigns and media watchdogging, producing educational materials and events, fund-raising, and organizational development (personnel and documentation).

The AAC formed subcommittees to accomplish each of these activities, with chairs serving as the steering committee. Serving on the steering committee were also FCHC board members and other "at large" members, invited because of their particular expertise or their tenure with the group. Policies developed in 1985 recognized subcommittee chairpersons through an election process by members of the subcommittee. Subcommittees that provided direct service functioned best and maintained a shared sense of purpose. Committees like education and media had a series of internal conflicts over strategy as well as conflicts with the steering committee over policy.

The early steering committee members were mainly liberals — with a few radicals and conservatives — who came from social service or community organizing backgrounds, with experience in democratic and collective group structures. The AAC sought a decision-making process that maximized participation and allowed time both for business and emotional support.

The line between business and support was not always easily drawn. Early members provided direct service and also performed other, less tangible functions. People brought strong emotions — grief, a sense of injustice, anger, fear, discouragement, incredulity — to the business of the organization. The wide range of emotional needs and the importance of attending to the social and political realities underlying the emotions are problems unique to building a volunteer organization to address AIDS.

The fact that many people doing AIDS organizing — gay men — were apparently "at risk" made it difficult to prioritize conflicting needs as strategies and programs were created. Of the two different approaches that emerged for understanding AIDS work, one now predominates in AAC organizational philosophy. The dominant view holds that in order to maintain the perspective necessary to set priorities, volunteers and staff should view their work as doing for others, a form of altruism well articulated in Catholic service movements, which strongly influence the executive director.

The second philosophy, drawn from liberation movements — including gay and black liberation — tried to engender a self-interest by encouraging people to perceive that their communities and friends were under attack, even if they personally were not involved with or did not know someone with AIDS. This view saw AIDS work as community building, linking these efforts with past and future projects in the respective communities.

Both ideas continue to inform decisions within the organization. Volunteer subcommittees represent both views as well as combinations of the two. Client Services tends to articulate the dominant idea, while the Education Department strongly reflects the second philosophy. The differing strategies used in each department permit a stable compromise between the two ideas: while they generate conflict over organizational strategies, they often lead simultaneously to novel solutions. On balance, the organization prioritizes immediate aid to those who are directly affected by a diagnosis or fear of a diagnosis, while setting less clear-cut funding and staffing policies for projects aimed at decreasing the number of future cases or future impediments to services.

Client Services: Professionalism in a Community of Difference

By 1985, the AAC was offering a mix of direct services, provided through volunteer subcommittees and some staff members. A staff mental health coordinator was hired to organize the services offered by these subcommittees. The coordinator soon saw the need to make a distinction between which services the AAC would provide directly and which it would advocate the provision of by existing agencies in the affected communities and in the health care system at large. The AAC wanted services provided in a manner consistent with its philosophy but knew that financial limitations would not permit it to become a full-service medical and social service agency. Mental health was subsumed under Client Services, which gave overall direction to the conglomerate of direct services, eliminated duplication, and provided professional accountability.

The current staff of Client Services consists of a coordinator of advocacy; six staff advocates; a coordinator of mental health and support groups; a holistic health coordinator; a buddies coordinator; and a housing coordinator. Newly funded positions include staff to develop additional public- and private-sector housing, mental health services, and home care services.

The department employs a case management model, drawn from mental health/social work agencies. Social workers serve as advocates who coordinate the care and support network for person(s) with AIDS/person(s) with AIDS-related complex (PWAs/PWARCs). They combine professional social worker skills with a mandate to ensure that services be provided with sensitivity to the prejudices faced by the affected minorities and with sensitivity to the particular stigma of an AIDS/ARC diagnosis.

Until this consolidation, the AAC had developed organically, trying to match the volunteer's need to provide help with the needs of those diagnosed with AIDS or ARC. Much more so than in other kinds of volunteer agencies, individuals volunteered out of a need for ongoing support, information, and at potential cost of being perceived as "gay." Although a study conducted at Gay Men's Health Crisis in New York shows that volunteers perceive their motives as altruistic, volunteers in fact describe concerns for their community and a sense of empowerment through action that are more characteristic of social justice motivations.

The AAC was faced with structuring direct and concretely defined services to PWAs/PWARCs and creating a place for volunteers with a range of needs and motivations. Creating an accessible structure for volunteerism was seen as providing a form of support — a service — to the worried well. The professional and lay services offered generally matched the services needed by those diagnosed and their families, friends, and lovers.

The buddy program retained its structure of peer supervision by tenured buddies who continued to provide companionship and practical help services to PWAs/PWARCs. The buddy program is modeled on a hospice concept, modified to meet the needs of people who, because of social stigma, may have diminished family and community ties.

The evolving volunteer hierarchy and the new professional hierarchy were retained and function in parallel. The interlocking structure of the two hierarchies permits professional accountability where needed as well as a grassroots-style support network that empowers the volunteer within the decision-making process. This solution provides the visible, professional accountability required by professional associations and funding sources while retaining a strong base of community involvement with real input into the AAC.

Simultaneously with the reorganization of Client Services, the AAC was separately incorporated as a 501-c(3) nonprofit, and a board of directors was formed. The first board was created in January 1987. The steering committee became a coordinating committee to supervise the volunteer function of the organization. The board is intended to take legal responsibility for the organization and set policy. The coordinating committee helps maintain volunteer input by creating a volunteer hierarchy that trains volunteers and promotes leadership. Recently, the key decision makers expressed the view that volunteers should work adjunctly to staff, rather than as staff enacting the will of a membership, as they do in some organizations. Though some have seen this as a move to decrease volunteer decision making, others believe it still allows volunteer input through the volunteer hierarchy, while recognizing that full-time staff are best situated to make day-to-day decisions. The extent to which the coordinating committee and board will project policy that the staff must follow is still at issue, and will be worked out only as the board finds its place and gains operational credibility with both staff and active volunteers.

While Client Services streamlined through developing a case management model, care has been taken to ensure that different styles of providing direct service are maintained. The mental health coordinator oversees a variety of groups whose services range from support to therapy and makes sure that clients have access to individual therapy or to goal-based groups such as stress management. In addition, the holistic health coordinator can refer clients to nontraditional therapies such as acupuncture, special diets, or movement classes which are adjunctive to their other medical care.

The AAC has also maintained strong ties with the National Association of People with AIDS (NAPWA) and works with Boston People with AIDS (BPWA) to foster a sense of empowerment for PWAs. The AAC has provided both financial and technical assistance to both groups and strives to allow the groups to determine their own priorities without imposing the agenda of people involved in providing services.

Refining Professional Services

In consolidating professional services and providing a clearer arena for community involvement, the AAC had to reach certain policy decisions by 1986. Among the most important were the following:

- The AAC does not provide professional treatment services — including medical, mental health, holistic health, legal, or other such services. Instead, advocates create and supervise the PWA/PWARC's network of services by referral. Advocates make certain that inpatient and outpatient services are coordinated, that home care planning meets the special needs of those with this unprecedented illness, and that clients understand and avail themselves of other AAC groups or activities as they wish.

- Institutionalization of the department director and advocates is an acknowledgment that group decisions are not possible in direct service administration.

The narrowing definition of what would be provided by the AAC allowed for a more coherent approach to services, but also generated resentment among some volunteers whose input into the organization was diminished. Although the intent of the parallel volunteer and staff structure is to maintain volunteer input throughout the organization, this has not been fully worked out in practice. The novel structure is still supported by members of the organization; they hope to better delineate communication and policy definition within the interlocking structures. The interaction between volunteer subcommittees and paid staff works better in some instances than in others.

The AAC became a new kind of organization: there were mainstream groups willing to work with gay and lesbian clients and groups formed with a primarily gay and lesbian client base. The AAC was also the first major group in Boston to come out of the gay and lesbian community with a commitment to serve nongays. Thus, from its inception the AAC was committed to providing services to all PWAs/PWARCs and their family or friendship system. It was difficult to be sensitive to the varying needs of people from different communities and backgrounds in designing programs and literature. In addition, intravenous drug users, women, and minorities were more likely to question the authority of professionals than were white, middle-class gay men, who dominated early AIDS organizations and who believed that the government and the medical establishment could be quickly reformed to meet the needs of the AIDS crisis. The AAC retains the open style and values of the gay and lesbian community, although the internal culture of the organization has evolved to incorporate many kinds of differences.

When impediments to service arise, it is often difficult to know whether they stem from fear of AIDS or from the older stigmas faced by most PWAs — homophobia, racism, sexism, disdain of drug use. Some believe that working through AIDS will help eliminate these prejudices, while others believe that good AIDS strategies require directly confronting the preexisting problems. The AAC seeks to keep the need of the PWA/PWARC and the aim of social justice separate within the organization: when clients are prevented from getting services because of homophobia, sexism, racism, or other biases, then that battle is fought in that case. The AAC does not want clients to become causes célèbres, although some PWAs have chosen to pursue legal battles or to publicize their difficulties. No general effort is made within Client Services to attack social problems that impinge on PWAs/PWARCs. The leadership believes that political and legal advocacy are best handled by other groups that advocate for the rights of gays and lesbians, IV drug users, or women or minorities.

The AAC believes that the best way to ensure quality services to all PWAs/PWARCs is to work with medical and social service delivery systems to make changes that meet the varied social, legal, medical, and psychological problems faced by PWAs/PWARCs, who necessarily come from different backgrounds and bring different needs. Staff are being hired to develop new programs within the public and private sectors to address the specific and emerging needs of all PWAs/PWARCs.

Education Department: Speaking the Right Language

The first two paid education staff members were a health educator, hired in late 1984, and a hotline coordinator, hired soon afterward. These two positions were subsumed under the Education Department in the fall of 1985, when an education director was hired. Today, the department has four health educators working with target populations, with funding available for four more. There is an administrative staff person, with funding for a second. A communications expert who will organize print media will soon be hired. Three volunteer subcommittees — Education, Hotline, and Minority Concerns, each comprised of a dozen task forces — work with health educators to staff the hotline, which operates twelve hours per day during the week, six hours on Saturday, and four hours on Sunday.

Since the inception of the AAC, groups have requested speakers and AAC health educators (volunteers from a wide range of backgrounds), often accompanied by a PWA, to give talks. As the level of awareness about AIDS has risen among citizens and health organizations, and as AAC programs have proven effective, the Education Department has become increasingly involved in the development of programs within certain settings or aimed at specific target audiences — for example, helping the Visiting Nurse Association organize a conference.

Limitations in funding and staff affect every program at the AAC, but especially the Education Department, because it is difficult to neatly define projects. Client Services can use the projected number of cases and statistical breakdowns of people served to define and evaluate specific projects. The Education Department must use more difficult tests of efficacy to define less tangible targets. What constitutes education, and who must be educated? How can projects address nuances of culture and prejudice? How many people can be grouped in a target audience without homogenizing an AIDS message to the point of meaninglessness? How specific can a pamphlet be without alienating subgroups within a target audience?

The consultative approach, in line with the organizational philosophy of promoting thoughtful response from existing agencies, has permitted other groups to educate some audiences while reserving for AAC educators hard-to-reach or newly discovered target groups. This has generally widened the range of effectiveness for the AAC. It has also enhanced the credibility of AAC staff and has permitted them to become involved in the early stages of policy and curriculum development, decreasing the need for "re-education" of well-meaning but ill-informed groups. AAC input is seen as vital to any programming about AIDS: media and organizations seek AAC approval and participation because the AAC educational programs are viewed as innovative and successful.

Targeted Education and Outreach Emerge

Disseminating the knowledge and techniques hammered out over the past few years, the Education Department continues to expand and experiment with new programs. These include a street corner outreach program aimed at IV drug users and prostitutes; "safety net" home education parties for gay men, soon to be made available to women considered to be at high risk; "hot, horny, and healthy" safer sex workshops; a program to distribute compact bleach bottles and information on cleaning drug works; efforts to install condom vending machines in gay bars; and a recent ad campaign called "The Road to Summer Fun," which utilizes road signs and attractive men in hard hats to convey safer sex concepts. Although not everyone is comfortable with every program, educators are perceived as experts in designing effective targeted messages.

As time passed, the AAC recognized a need for broader impact through exposure of the AAC philosophy in media reports. The "general public" is more likely to get AIDS information from television or radio than to attend a seminar on AIDS. Consultation by the Education Department with the media, including three major local television and some local radio stations, provides media messages with AAC input and gives this information a legitimacy that an AAC program alone might not have. If radio and television personalities talk freely about AIDS, then citizens will view discussion of the topic as permissible.

The Education Department maintains a mix of educators who are responsive and committed to particular communities. This diversity helps ensure that AIDS messages are sensitive to the underlying social issues that increase the difficulties of PWAs/PWARCs from different cultures. The department recognizes that many agencies offer factually correct AIDS information, but that some agencies include messages that differ from the AAC's attempt to be nonjudgmental and sensitive to cultural meanings. The AAC has defined a set of concepts which it believes must be adhered to if AIDS educational material is to be effective. AAC printed materials and talks rarely address underlying social issues didactically, except in challenging stereotypes. However, great attention is paid to the language used to talk about risk behaviors and about people whose communities may have a high incidence of them. Risk behaviors — drug practices and certain sexual practices — are understood by the AAC as acts promoting social cohesion in subcultures. As such, risk behaviors have specific meaning and importance in the lives of individuals who engage in them. AAC messages are designed to inform about the dangers of some practices and suggest changes that reduce risk while promoting positive self-image.

AAC educational messages focus on risk behavior rather than on risk groups: overemphasis on groups can inflame prejudice and may prevent accurate risk assessment on the part of those who engage in risk behavior but who do not identify with the "risk group" as defined by the Centers for Disease Control or as self-defined by some communities.

This creates a paradox that requires sophisticated targeting: gay men or IV drug users, for example, who self-identify as part of the gay male or drug subculture may be best educated by material that makes reference to the details of subculture life. However, homosexually active men or IV drug users who do not perceive themselves as part of a subculture may well become hostile to a message that equates their behavior with a stigmatized group. They may reject the idea that they are "gay" or an "IV drug user" and may not make an accurate risk assessment. These people need a message that encourages risk reduction while remaining neutral on what engaging in those behaviors may mean to others in society.

The AAC's success in formulating these sensitive messages is due to involvement of staff and volunteers who understand the workings and language of various subcultures. These culturally sensitive educators — who may or may not have traditional health education training — are expert at identifying the subtle language choices that make the difference between a credible AIDS message and one that is ignorant or insulting.

Acknowledging Cultural Diversity

The AAC believes that attitudes about AIDS and attitudes toward minorities work hand in hand: undoing misconceptions in one diminishes prejudices in the other. For example, overcoming fear about AIDS makes it easier to care for or befriend a PWA and thus to acknowledge different cultures. The opportunity to work with groups of people who may have been feared as a result of social prejudice allows a health care worker or friend to separate AIDS fears from social prejudices. This kind of education has been extremely liberating for friends, families, and coworkers who may previously have been uncomfortable with a gay man or an IV drug user. Effective education about the disease and subtle, positive messages that combat prejudice allow people to move past stereotypes and fears that may have been immobilizing or that may have prevented them from being compassionate toward those directly affected by AIDS.

The AAC educational philosophy is designed to articulate a range of messages under the umbrella of AIDS information. The Education Department believes that ultimately people will not understand the complex issues surrounding AIDS unless they are informed about the preexisting social problems.

The Education Department further recognizes that AIDS work done within and by the communities first affected — IV drug users and gay men — provides a model for other communities and for society at large. Gay men have made important subcultural and personal changes that have decreased the rate of HIV transmission. The anxiety, embarrassment, and fear caused by efforts to negotiate safer sex are similar regardless of gender or sexual preference. Educators incorporate the experience of gay men and their sexual community in sex education for heterosexuals. Educators also use the gay community's experience of death and grieving as a model for others and as a challenge to the general denial of mortality issues in American society.

The AAC also teaches people to be knowledgeable health care consumers. Drawing on the self-help movement, a long-standing countertrend to U.S. big medicine, the AAC has developed patient guidelines for asking good questions of medical providers. The involvement of lay educators from communities at risk challenges the notion that only doctors can provide good information and reinforces the belief that patients have a right to comprehensible answers. An important message in AAC literature is that individuals can and must take responsibility for their health and for AIDS prevention, and that AIDS awareness is a positive act of self-determination.

Whenever possible, the Education Department engages PWAs/PWARCs as speakers to give accounts of their experiences. The importance of meeting and shaking hands with a PWA who has a feared disease and who also may be a member of a stigmatized social group cannot be overestimated. This personal contact provides another layer of education — it makes those in an audience responsible for their attitudes toward a real individual. The message that people who have met a PWA take back to their friends and families may be one of the most powerful factors in changing attitudes about the disease, especially for people who have not had the experience of personally knowing someone with AIDS.

Fund-raising: Building a Sound Financial Base

Because the AAC grew out of grassroots organizations, its first fund-raising efforts consisted of small-scale events and direct mailings within the Boston community. It was sometimes difficult to involve bars and social clubs in fund-raising activities, given the denial of the seriousness of AIDS and the belief that the mention of AIDS would turn customers away. Resistance also occasionally came from other community organizations, which were afraid that AIDS fund-raisers would deplete their funding base. In 1983, asking the society at large to help fund this nascent organization working primarily with homosexuals and drug users needed to be done diplomatically and cautiously.

From the beginning, the AAC saw fund-raising as a three-part project: raise needed funds, provide educational opportunity, and afford a sense of participation in the effort to fight AIDS. The first major fund-raising event had an additional purpose: to consolidate morale and give organizers a concrete project that could realistically be accomplished.

That event was a major fund-raising and public relations success. It brought in $25,000 — an unheard-of sum in the history of Boston gay and lesbian fund-raising in 1983 — and provided for those attending both a good time and a "good feeling" of being part of a community trying to help itself. The value of the good feeling was immediately obvious: new volunteers made contact with the committee during fund-raising events, and media coverage put a compassionate face on a disease mostly reported in abstract scientific accounts or sensational stories.

As the AAC undertook educational projects and as PWAs met with apathy and discrimination, the need for money became urgent. There were pamphlets to be printed and phones to be installed. There were emergency loans to be made to people thrown out of their homes and food to be bought for those having difficulty working their way through the welfare system. There were wheelchairs to rent and funerals to pay for. The requests for money were difficult to prioritize, and as paid staff were hired, it was hard to decide which positions were immediately necessary and which committees could make do without paid staff backup.

The AAC attracted experienced fund-raisers early on, in part because of personal connections between committee members and people in the business community, and partly because some excellent fund-raisers had loved ones who had died of AIDS early in the epidemic. The need to raise money, combined with the accessibility of compassionate, experienced fund-raisers, allowed the AAC to aim for larger events and campaigns that would attract both gay and straight donors. The first large-scale event outside the gay male community was the ArtCetera Auction, first held in 1985. This was soon followed by several benefit concerts sponsored by the Boston branch of Saks Fifth Avenue and by local radio and television personalities.

At the same time that major fund-raising became possible outside the gay and lesbian community, more state and federal monies became available. The City of Boston had early given small grants to the AAC, and altogether, governmental monies made up about 40 percent of the AAC budget.

The organization's financial experts were aware of the need to keep a diversified funding base, and pursued private foundation money and in-kind donations, as well as continuing annual versions of several highly successful events, such as the art auction, the pledge event called "Walk for Life," and a fall gala.

In many organizations, the function of fund-raising seems remote, even opposite in values, from the other educational or services tasks. However, fund-raising at the AAC continues not only to raise money, but to integrate the missions of the AAC with financial realities. More so than some other major AIDS organizations, the AAC has combined the quest for a broad range of funding sources with high-profile education, group morale building, and a sense of participation on the part of those who attend or work on events. The fact that money is being raised for AIDS is not obscured, and the opportunity to educate is not deferred to another occasion. Fund-raising as a department provides an excellent model for integrating volunteers and paid staff. Those who have decided to devote their time to AIDS fund-raising are committed to the goals of the organization, using their personal skills to create successful events. Although many people perceive those doing fund-raising as personally remote from the daily realities of AIDS work, in fact, they share the passion for AIDS work with other kinds of staff and volunteer buddies.

The AAC of Tomorrow

The AAC is an exciting and frustrating organization for those inside and out. The current board is acutely aware of its mission to project a vision that guides the organization through the difficult years ahead, when the pressures to serve, advocate, and set policy — for the AAC and for society — will only increase.

The board has set two priorities: define better how the components of the organization work together, and determine how the AAC can best relate to communities of color, who are now becoming the emergency arena in the AIDS crisis. The board plans to accomplish these goals through meetings outside the regular twice-monthly business format, which allows members to take a hard look at the organization and at themselves. The board will try to look at the issues and policies of the current AAC and determine whether these offer the best way to accomplish the mission.

Defining a relationship with communities of color for the predominantly gay and white AAC will be an organizational challenge and an opportunity to break down social barriers. The AAC could become a microcosm for a more compassionate, pluralistic society, in which each person's unique background enriches the organization and is not lost to mainstreaming. The AAC has experience with respecting and incorporating cultural differences, but a visionary cooperation between racial and sexual minorities will demand yet more. The delicate balance between "doing for others" and promoting community self-interest will loom large as the AAC works in communities of color that have their own political ideology and power infrastructure.

The AAC must balance cultural sensitivity with the urgency within communities of color, who currently have the highest percentage increases in spread of HIV and AIDS/ARC diagnosis. The AAC must come to grips with what the experience of the gay and lesbian community has been so it can share that experience with minorities who face other forms of oppression. It must define what it is capable of and experienced in providing, and it must be prepared to learn from the communities with whom it forms a partnership to combat AIDS.

Conclusion

The special historical conditions that determined the exact inception of the AAC include a liberal city government; significant existing ties between the gay and lesbian community and city social service agencies; a commitment on the part of government officials to deal with the AIDS crisis in a nondiscriminative way and to listen to the experts within the affected communities; the presence of long-standing medical, social, and psychological organizations within the gay and lesbian community; active gay and lesbian community news media and known locations for community contact; proximity, but not centrality, to the epidemiological center of the epidemic; and large numbers of teaching and research medical facilities in the area. But these conditions do not fully explain why the AAC has continued to evolve to meet the needs of the many communities and individuals that need support and education.

The AAC has a unique ability to adapt to new circumstances and confront internal conflict compassionately. Its quiet commitment to grassroots-organizing techniques and to understanding the special needs of different kinds of people affected by AIDS has enabled it to keep sight of its mission — to support, educate, advocate, and reach out. The success of the AAC derives from the commitment of the leadership and volunteers to listen to the many voices in need, and to keep focused on AIDS as the central concern. Where other groups have become enmeshed in either playing or avoiding politics, the AAC has achieved a balance between doing its work and making the necessary demands of a system fundamentally perplexed by AIDS and its social ramifications. The AAC has also achieved a level of fund-raising success unmatched in any similarly sized city — in part because of committed and experienced fund-raisers, and in part because the organization established credibility and a compassionate face early in its existence.

The history of the AAC provides a model of community resistance and compassion: it is the story of a group coming to understand the disaster that has befallen it, and to project its unique subcultural values to create a selfless yet self-defined movement to help itself and others. The members of the AAC who reflect on this experience are well prepared to learn about and overcome their own prejudices toward other affected groups and to continue to inform others about the prejudices they face.

The AAC will face more challenges in the years ahead, as AIDS continues to be a medical and social problem of unpredictable dimensions. Once a small, collectively oriented group of volunteers, and now a large, nonprofit corporation with dozens of staff and hundreds of volunteers, the AAC is adaptable because everyone involved is committed to making a difference in the lives of all people in any way affected by AIDS. It will continue to be an innovative organization carefully treading the line between bureaucracy and grassroots movement. The openness and willingness of individual staff and volunteers to look inside themselves and share their emotional and practical experience should militate against organizational stagnation. Whatever strategic errors are marked against the AAC, the sheer vision and willingness to struggle through a difficult crisis will write as heroes the many men and women who have been its members and staff.

"I'm a New Yorker, I'm a city boy. But like most city boys in New York, in the summertime, I went down south—to my grandmother's farm, and every so often, my Aunt Sweet, who lived to be one hundred and sixteen, Aunt Sweet would say, 'You children, you all stop playing and come in here.' And we would go in and she would be humming and singing a song, and every once in a while she would pull up her dress and she would show the scars from plantation life. And I realize I am one who came from that. AIDS can't do a* damn *thing to me."*

Politics and AIDS: Conversations and Comments

Interviews Conducted by
Steven Stark

As AIDS has emerged as a medical and social concern, it has become a political issue as well. In a series of interviews, we asked some leading authorities for their opinions on how AIDS is emerging as a political issue, particularly during the campaign of 1988. In all cases, the comments that follow represent an edited version of their remarks. Those participating were Ronald Bayer, director of the Project on AIDS and the Ethics of Public Health at the Hastings Center; William Schneider, resident fellow at the American Enterprise Institute; Jonathan Handel, a gay activist and a member of the Cambridge, Massachusetts, Human Rights Commission and the AIDS Task Force for the City of Cambridge; Stanley Greenberg, president of the Analysis Group, a national Democratic polling firm with offices in Washington, D.C., and New Haven, Connecticut; Denise McWilliams, director of the AIDS Law Project for the Gay and Lesbian Advocates and Defenders in Boston; William Shannon, professor of journalism and history at Boston University and a columnist for the Boston Globe; *and Barbara Whitehead, a social historian and a consultant with Public Policy Associates in Chicago. Steven Stark, a Boston writer, conducted the interviews for this piece.*

Stark: In terms of the 1988 election, do you see AIDS emerging as an issue in this campaign?

Whitehead: Well, it's going to be harder and harder to ignore AIDS, because it carries a head count. The death toll does keep rising. And along with that are the costs associated with AIDS, so that eventually its place on the public agenda is going to expand as the costs grow. I saw an article that said in Massachusetts the cost of AIDS will equal the entire Massachusetts Medicaid budget this year. That means it's going to be harder and harder simply to ignore.

But it goes beyond that. AIDS is the ultimate social issue; if you wanted to go to the drawing board and invent some kind of social problem that triggered a host of other disturbing or important social issues, you couldn't do

Steven Stark is a free-lance writer.

AIDS is to talk about an underclass, to talk about drug abuse, to talk about sex education.

Shannon: AIDS will not emerge as an issue during the primary stage, but I think it will next autumn. I think a Democrat, particularly when campaigning in areas like New York City and San Francisco, which have a large gay population, will make the point that the Reagan administration was very tardy and delinquent in coping with the crisis.

But is it a cutting issue? Not at the moment. On the scale of one to ten, with ten being the most important, I think that except in certain communities like San Francisco I would put it down at two or one.

It hasn't made an impact yet. I think it will. But not by 1988. I think most heterosexual people have — after the initial panic — screened it out of their mind, deny it as a real threat to themselves. So the heterosexual cases would have to increase dramatically in number before the broad voting public would decide an election on that basis.

Bayer: I don't think that the issue will emerge as a challenge to what the government has done so far in terms of funding, and the clear evidence is that the response has been woefully inadequate. But the issue will emerge from the right flank, from people suggesting that we haven't done enough in terms of repressive measures — why aren't we screening more people mandatorily, why have we allowed civil libertarians and the gay lobby to set the political agenda on this issue. That's my concern. I think it's substantiated by the kinds of things we hear even from the center of the Republican Party in terms of "much wider" mandatory screening.

The issue is one that could be easily politicized. There is an enormous amount of anxiety that is generally kept under wraps. But when the appropriate moment arises, that anxiety will express itself. Last year, for instance, it took a huge effort on the part of a broad coalition in California to defeat the LaRouche amendment, though they defeated it very handily. About 70 percent voted against the amendment. However, it took enormous exertion, and the entire establishment of California was opposed to it — the health establishment, the media, the TV networks, and political figures.

Despite the fact that this was an amendment backed by someone who is widely thought to be politically paranoid, it was able to get 30 percent of the vote. I take that as a sign that there are many people out there whose anxieties could be mobilized in a way that would be socially disastrous.

Greenberg: AIDS is a big public health issue. It is not yet a political issue, and I think it will become one only if parties or presidential candidates choose to try to shape it as such. At the moment I'm not sure that is happening.

Handel: It's an issue but only barely. If you watch the debates you will see one question on AIDS and I think that there is both a positive and a negative to that. I think that on the one hand the candidates are really afraid of the issue and they are afraid of how it is going to play. On the other hand, given who a lot of these candidates are, it's a positive that we are not getting even more negative.

Moreover, the health community has been so united in its approach to AIDS and its insistence that discrimination is not appropriate that it would be hard for right-wing candidates to stand up there and say some of the things they might be inclined to say.

McWilliams: AIDS doesn't seem to be taking on anywhere near the significance that I think it should. Candidates are coming out with fairly vague, broad statements when they bother to mention it at all. I think there has been very little thoughtful analysis or debate.

There are a variety of reasons for this. Part of the problem is that to date there is still the perception that it is a disease of marginal types of people. People see it as a disease of homosexuals, IV drug users, poor people — constituencies that traditionally politicians felt no compelling need to address. I think it also raises the sorts of issues that this society has never dealt with well. We have never dealt well with the issue of sex. We've dealt even less well with the issues of homophobia and racism. And we are doing an abysmal job of addressing addiction in this country. AIDS doesn't come by itself, it comes with all these other issues. So in a sense it is almost all of our failures packaged into one word.

Stark: Do you see AIDS breaking down as a partisan political issue?

Whitehead: It hasn't yet. But if Bob Dole says that he wants the Republican Party to be a party that embraces an ethic of caring, is he going to include AIDS? Does he mean to talk about people with AIDS and their families? Or when Mike Dukakis says we need to have opportunities for all people, does he mean to include AIDS patients and their families, that they should stay in the work force as long as possible? This is something that all candidates will have to address.

Schneider: There are several different issues. There's testing, which I think will become an issue principally for people on the right fringes of the Republican Party, who are demanding more rigorous screening and testing. There's funding, which is an issue on the left, where there are many groups demanding more research and educational funding. But I think that basically, for most of the broad middle of the electorate, the issue isn't all that important. Of course, it's a serious issue; they want more funding; they want more testing; they want the government to do something more about it. But it's not that divisive an issue. I don't think you're going to see leading Democratic or Republican candidates divided on it.

It's an issue that everyone is concerned about, but there's a kind of broad consensus. The broad consensus is, Do whatever is necessary to rid society of this plague. People take it very seriously. But it isn't an ideological issue. The issue really has a kind of ideological meaning only to the groups on the left and the right, who insist on interpreting it in moralistic terms.

Greenberg: People don't view it as a narrow interest-group-based issue. I believe there would be very strong public resistance to politicizing the issue. There's been very strong positive response to congressmen who have mailed out educational information, but I believe that candidates who sought to use this issue as a way of trying to link Democrats to homosexuals would find a public that was unreceptive to that position. I also believe that the president did try with the AIDS testing issue to see whether they could turn this into something that paralleled the drug testing issue.

What we have found in our polling is that drug testing has not caught on as some kind of test of people's commitment to a conventional family life or sexual preferences. The public supports AIDS testing, but mainly as a public health matter that would benefit society and benefit individuals who are afflicted. But there is no evidence that they use it as some kind of litmus test on social issues or family issues. In addition, the health professionals have become so deeply involved in this question that I think it's become very difficult to turn it into a partisan issue. Health professionals have been very cautious about universal AIDS testing, and that's made it difficult for elected officials to try to shape the issue in a way that would offer political advantage.

Stark: If a presidential candidate asked you for advice and in boldly political terms said, "I want to say the right thing but I also want to say the politically beneficial thing," what would you tell him?

Whitehead: I think AIDS offers a real opportunity for politicians if only they would see it as such. If people are looking at political candidates for signs of character, and if character is defined as telling the truth and facing facts and showing courage and gutsiness in the face of long odds, then what better issue is there than AIDS? I think a model here is C. Everett Koop, the surgeon general. He has stood out as probably the only public figure who's willing to talk directly and clearly and in a factual way about what AIDS is and what it is not. If we're talking about moral leadership, then that's my definition of true moral leadership.

I think that's the challenge for the candidates. I would tell someone that it's a good opportunity for leadership. They should use it.

Shannon: I would tell them that it's a very serious public health problem. I should preface it by saying that this question is so complicated and potentially so serious that a candidate would do best to handle it in as truthful, direct, and responsible a manner as possible. This is a case where being too clever would probably not serve any purpose. I think the only voters who are going to be deeply agitated are two sets of voters. One is homosexuals, who are not going to vote for a conservative Republican candidate in any case, because of the Reagan administration's record on gay rights. At the other extreme are fundamentalist Christians, who are unlikely to vote for a liberal Democrat on any issue. So I think the votes to be won or lost are few. I then would simply have him say that it's a very serious public health issue, that we have to have extensive testing for public health reasons so that we can track the progress of this disease and know the shape of the enemy we're fighting. But if we are to do that, we also have to have stringent protections like the Kennedy bill now pending in Congress to protect the rights of all persons who are tested.

Then, second, in addition to all the other fiscal problems we have, we have to start planning for how our medical health insurance programs are going to cope with what is a totally new and staggeringly expensive burden, one that strikes people who are normally not health risks at all. I've seen estimates that by the early 1990s the cost of caring for AIDS patients will be anywhere from eight billion to thirty-eight billion.

I would also add a third group that the issue might influence, aside from gay men and fundamentalists, and that is blacks and Hispanics, because this disease seems to hit with higher incidence among them than the general population. Now, coming from a strictly political point of view, those groups have a poor voter registration and voter turnout record, but nevertheless insofar as you are appealing to blacks and Hispanics and want to have an issue beyond the standard ones to appeal to them, you could stress the importance of health care for them, because many of them have no health insurance.

Schneider: I would advise the candidate to say, when asked about the issue — or to announce on his own initiative — that the United States government will do whatever is necessary and reasonable to rid society of this plague — that we have to increase education, quite clearly, that we have to be realistic about the risks involved, that we have to support funding where there is any indication that it will be productive. I think a candidate has to indicate that he takes the issue very seriously.

In fact, they have handled it very reasonably. As I say, it's principally those on the left and right of American politics who insist on a confrontational position. I think once the crisis became evident the government has been very seriously concerned and attentive. It took a while for people to understand the dimensions of the crisis. A great deal of headway has been made. Obviously, there's always more that can be done. But considering that the disease has not yet spread widely outside the male homosexual and intravenous drug user communities — and it simply has not spread widely in these communities — I think the government has been quite responsible in its approach to the problem.

Stark: Let me ask a broader question. To take it out of the domain of just electoral politics, in defining politics broadly, how do you see AIDS changing the American body politic?

Whitehead: One of the distinguishing characteristics of polity, almost since the beginning, and one of the reasons that Americans believe they're exceptional, is that we have been an extraordinarily optimistic and self-confident people. This is a young country, and our social confidence is a resource. AIDS is a great threat to social confidence in this country for a couple of reasons. Postwar American medicine, with its successes in conquering disease, had a lot to do with bolstering a sense of social confidence. It's been a realm where Americans could demonstrate their individuality, their innovative methods. Much like the space program, it's been a carrier of a sense of progress. When we think about AIDS, not only is it a disease that metaphorically fragments the society, but also you have to think about what's happening to the medical establishment itself.

There used to be a broad consensus in the postwar period about what doctors were and what they should do, who patients were and what they should be, and what hospitals were and what they should do in the community. All of that is being called into question. In a sense, we could become very European, and the optimistic American outlook could become tragic very quickly. Broadly speaking, I think AIDS has that effect.

AIDS also creates a kind of wall of suspicion. You have to know someone's history and we know so little of each other's history. Everyone who enters a hospital or a dentist's office is now treated as if they are potentially infected.

It's a little bit bleak. And then there are movies like *Fatal Attraction.* One of the reasons that it has become such a box office success is that it is not only about old-fashioned morality or about a backlash against career women, it's about the penalties of intimacy with a stranger. And that's the message of AIDS as well. I think we just can't trust each other. We make fewer assumptions about people whom we don't know well, and in contemporary society, none of us know each other very well.

I would like to be optimistic. I would like to tell you that I feel optimistic. But I don't think that there's anything, at least in the history of the way that we have dealt with AIDS to this point, that would encourage optimism. However, I don't think it's too late.

I don't think it's too late to have people begin acting collectively to deal with this.

And I think it's a tremendous opportunity for the candidates, for one or more, to show real courage and leadership. People seem to focus on the economy and whether candidates have the courage to step foward and talk about tax cuts, but an equally good test of their capacity for leadership is the AIDS issue. We need more Koops out there right now. It's remarkable to me that he has been the only public figure who has been talking the way people should talk about this issue.

Schneider: I have been struck, having read the polls on this for a number of years, about the rationality of people's responses. While of course one will always find evidence of irrationality and hysteria in the public, the fact is, people have behaved very reasonably. There is no real evidence of any antihomosexual hysteria emerging out of it. If I had to describe the public's view of gay men in a single word as a result of this crisis, I think it would be sympathetic. They are concerned, they are a little confused about the messages they are getting. If you watch the news or read the newspapers, you get two very different and conflicting messages. One of them is, Panic, ten million Americans are going to die, and the other is, Don't panic, because the disease is very hard to catch and you shouldn't be alarmed about casual contacts or allowing people carrying the AIDS virus in the workplace or in the schools. It's a very conflicting message. It's a very difficult message to sort out and I think the public has been quite responsible about it, and that's one of the reasons that most politicians don't want to inflame the issue.

Bayer: I don't have a good answer. As the numbers mount even further, as they most certainly will in the next three to four years, especially in places like New York, San Francisco, LA, and Miami, I think that the impact is going to be quite profound. I think the sheer magnitude of living in communities where large numbers of relatively young people are dying will have a profound effect. The other thing that's going to happen is, as the color of people with AIDS gets darker, within relatively cosmopolitan communities, it will have an interesting impact. Up until now, rather than provoking an hysterical homophobic response, I think what in fact has happened in places like New York and San Francisco is that there has been an integration, or at least a consultative relationship established, between gay male leaders and the political establishment that ten or fifteen years ago would have been unthinkable.

But the attitude will be very different with addicts. Whatever efforts have been made to expand the notion of how a humane and decent social system responds to a disease like this will take on a very different quality when it's black and Hispanic addicts that are being dealt with. I think, for instance, the issues of physicians' refusals to treat patients with the infection will grow, and a tendency to think about creating special hospitals will intensify, not so much to meet the needs of AIDS patients as to create separate places where these people — or "those people" — are taken care of. I cannot help but feel that a hospital made up primarily of black and Hispanic addicts with AIDS would be a very grim place. It would not be the designated ward in San Francisco General Hospital.

It depends, of course, very much on the pace of scientific progress. We are used to being able to deal with acute situations rapidly, with some degree of dispatch in our culture, and unless there are quite dramatic developments in medicine in the next few years, one of the things that American culture is going to have to come to grips with is a sense of its own limits or powerlessness in the face of things like this epidemic. I think that will have a profound cultural impact. Teaching people a sense of restraint and also a sense of their own limits will not be easy. I think you can get people to appreciate the fact that we can do a great deal to limit the spread of this epidemic but that we can't stop it and that we should think in terms of the long haul. I think those are going to be very critical challenges.

Greenberg: AIDS has been incorporated into the list of indicators that there are big problems on the horizon, that there is some kind of social decay, that the country's off on the wrong track. AIDS has become part of a bundle of things that give you a reason to fear the future. Drugs fall into that category, trade deficits fall into that category, divorce rates fall into that category, and AIDS is part of that list. It suggests that one needs to be anxious about the future. So I think it does reinforce a mood in the country that is fairly pessimistic.

Overall, there is an electoral environment in 1988 which would favor a change in leadership away from the incumbent leadership to new leadership. Under normal circumstances, that would favor the Democrats. Wherever you go in the country, there is a pretty strong majority that say the country's off on the wrong track, and AIDS is part of that mood. That is conventionally the response — let's throw out those in office and let's bring in a new crowd to try to get the country off in a good direction. Those are the kinds of numbers that were evident when Jimmy Carter was thrown out in 1980.

AIDS is one of those reinforcing elements that say we're just not dealing with the kinds of things that are going to create enormous problems for our kids and enormous problems for us in the years ahead.

Handel: I think the gay male community conceives the world differently now. The effect of AIDS in the gay and lesbian communities has been striking. I think that the story of AIDS that is by and large untold and underreported is the incredible work that the gay male community has done in forming organizations, in helping its own and crying out in the wilderness for many years when there wasn't any real attention to this disease. The effect has been that a lot of people who were not political, or people whose economic interest ran counter to their interest as gay people, speaking particularly of white gay men, affluent white gay men, have become a lot more politicized. I keep hearing from people who are saying, I am angry, what I am seeing about AIDS makes me angry, the death of my friend makes me angry, the march on Washington uplifted me, you know, I am getting involved.

Outside the gay male community, it's a different story. The nongay communities have not been affected by AIDS in nearly the same compelling way that the gay male community has. I don't think there has been much of a sort of drawing together in these communities as a result of AIDS.

McWilliams: Well, I think AIDS has several potential implications. I think the issue is going to create enormous pressure on people, if not for quarantine then at least to ghettoize the problem. I think it has the real potential to develop a scapegoating mentality — you know, your taxes wouldn't be so high if it weren't for this, for example, or, our medical system wouldn't be quite so strained but for these immoral sorts of people. I think it has enormous implications for how people deal with employment situations. For instance, even though in this state the use of the HIV antibody test for employment purposes is prohibited, there are attorneys in businesses across the country who make the argument that they should be allowed to use the test because that is going to have a direct impact on the employee benefit package they can offer their employees.

I think it also has real serious implications for people in unions, because obviously again you are going to get into the ghettoizing mentality, that they-are-dragging-all-of-us-down type of thing. And to put it mildly, unfortunately that is the tack that we seem to be following. You know, a situation like this calls for all the wisdom and compassion we can muster, and we're getting very much mired in this traditional us-them mentality.

Stark: Well, related to that, let me ask you another question. About a year ago if you looked at the media, and I guess using that as a measure of what is on people's minds, AIDS seemed to have been a much bigger issue. Correct me if you think I am wrong, but if that is true, why has it seemed to recede somewhat, do you think, in the past nine months to a year?

McWilliams: In this country, we have a notoriously short attention span and, particularly, where there have not been that many new, dramatic developments on AIDS. I think our reporting is not the type that is geared to taking a long hard look at an issue. It's much more the glitzy sort of headline approach. We just haven't had that many glitzy headlines coming out lately. Second, I think people are getting tired of it. It is interesting that if you look at the history of how the media has covered this issue, how much it has been the search to find and portray the innocent victim of AIDS. Right now I think we are down to children. It is interesting to note that the news coverage that has been out there has been around the children of IV-drug-using parents.

Handel: Prior to Rock Hudson, the disease got very little attention, and the quality of attention that it did get was pretty marginal. It was a gay disease and it was a scare story every now and then. We've really got a system that encourages very episodic attention to issues, and that applies to Iran, the Contras, AIDS. With AIDS a lot of the hot news pegs sort of disappeared.

Stark: Anything else you want to add?

Greenberg: The only other thing I would add is that wherever we've done this research — and this includes work in the South — people want government to take charge on this problem, they want control of AIDS, they believe the government has to play a very affirmative role and they believe the Reagan administration has been pretty indifferent. They don't believe they politicized it but they think they've not used the government to take charge. They believe there was no leadership to deal with this issue. And it reinforces the feeling that nobody's in charge.

Handel: I thought one of the striking stories about AIDS about a year ago was what I thought of as the tale of two Arcadias, I guess because there is Arcadia, Florida, where a kid with AIDS was ostracized or some of the kids were ostracized, not allowed to go to school, and the mayor was one of the first people to pull his son or daughter out of school and help start or encourage the fear. And at exactly the same time, apparently, there was a kid, a school-age kid with AIDS in Arcadia, Illinois, who had no problem going to school, he had incredible community support, which I guess is a counter-example to what I've said before about communities pulling together. And the question to me is why in Arcadia, Florida, did the darkest side of American politics rule and the darkest side of the American character, the fear and ignorance, and in Arcadia, Illinois, it was sort of the most exalted and the best that you hope for in this country. I don't think there are quick answers to that. I think that honest answers to a question like that go to the socioeconomic levels of the community and education and courage on the part of particular politicians and educational and religious leaders in the community; they really go in some sense to the quality of life in the community. But it was a striking sort of study in contradiction.

Covering the Plague Years: Four Approaches to the AIDS Beat

James Kinsella

AIDS reporting has changed dramatically since 1981. But it was not until mid-1985, when Rock Hudson was diagnosed with the disease, that media outlets began playing the epidemic as a story of major proportions.

Because almost no major media institution embraced the AIDS story as an important issue, coverage of the epidemic was often the result of a reporter's initiative. Consequently, the connection the individual journalist had with the epidemic became a much stronger influence on what appeared in the news and on what Americans knew about the crisis than in any other recent major health story. This article examines how four prominent journalists covered the disease.

The reporting by the San Francisco Chronicle's *Randy Shilts, a gay man seemingly aligned with a political faction in the city's homosexual community, reflected that affiliation. Jim Bunn, a heterosexual reporter for KPIX-TV in San Francisco, worked hard to get the word out about the possibility of an epidemic sweeping the entire population. The* New York Times's *Dr. Lawrence Altman viewed the epidemic from his perspective as a traditional medical doctor — maintaining a professional distance from the tragedy. And National Public Radio's Laurie Garrett, a scientist as well as a heterosexual woman politically in touch with the gay community, took a compassionate, informed stance.*

Almost all the coverage of these journalists had discernible policy impacts.

More than any other major modern story, AIDS has challenged basic journalistic methods and ethics. None of the mainstream media covered the disease as thoroughly as they had covered similar health crises, such as the swine flu scare and Legionnaires' disease in the mid-seventies. When AIDS first appeared — identified as a disease affecting homosexual men exclusively — almost no newsroom editor considered the story worth covering. After all, it did not seem to be affecting the larger population, as swine flu threatened to, or a socially acceptable group like middle-aged war veterans, as Legionnaires' disease did. Those editors who gave reasons for not covering the AIDS story most

James Kinsella, editor of the editorial pages at the Los Angeles Herald Examiner, *is the author of* Covering the Plague, *a critique of American media's reporting of the AIDS epidemic. It will be published by Rutgers University Press in the fall of 1989.*

often reasoned that news about homosexuals would not interest the great majority of "family newspaper" readers. Media interest did not increase when discovery was made of the next AIDS-affected group — users of nonprescription intravenous drugs.

There were, of course, other obstacles to covering the story appropriately. For instance, it is often not in the best interest of scientists to talk to journalists about their ground-breaking work, since researchers want their papers to be published first in scientific journals that can place a professional imprimatur on their findings. And, for the most part, AIDS is not a television story. Many patients do not want to be photographed, as the effects of the disease are so debilitating. Furthermore, few media outlets have journalists on staff who are specifically trained to cover the complex beats of science and medicine. But even the political stories of the epidemic got short shrift. Again, most editors — and reporters — were not interested in covering a disease affecting social outcasts. As a consequence, AIDS coverage in the early years was almost always a result of a reporter's individual initiative.

Because the AIDS beat was considered unimportant in the journalistic institution, few of the recognized processes that were used for traditional political stories or even medical stories affecting traditional groups were available to cover the plague. And in the beginning, there was a dearth of reliable information on the disease, on how it was spreading and whether it could be stopped. So when AIDS was allowed to be covered, the individual reporter who took an interest and worked to develop an understanding of it had great influence over what was published or broadcast. The story behind the story of the AIDS epidemic, therefore, is a highly personal one.

This is made clear by analyzing the work of most of the major figures who covered the crisis from mid-1981 to mid-1985, before the story became mainstream with the AIDS diagnosis of actor Rock Hudson. Four of the best examples are the *San Francisco Chronicle*'s Randy Shilts; Jim Bunn, now working with the World Health Organization while on leave from KPIX-TV in San Francisco; the *New York Times*'s Lawrence Altman; and National Public Radio's Laurie Garrett.[1]

These journalists did more than tell the story. Their biases and backgrounds helped shape it. Their very different approaches describe the spectrum of journalistic response to the crisis: from Shilts's politicized reporting to Bunn's health education approach, from Garrett's compassion for the victim to Altman's concern for the scientist. With at least three of these four reporters, the tack they took in describing the epidemic had measurable public policy implications.

Randy Shilts: The Politicized Reporter

To walk the streets of San Francisco's Castro district is to feel the cozy compactness of a Thornton Wilder village gone gay. The streets are peopled largely by homosexual men and lesbians, the bustling businesses are bars and trendy clothing stores, and the flags flying high from the carefully renovated Victorian buildings are the rainbow pennants of the gay liberation movement. It is to this hometown that Randy Shilts has returned a hero.

The author of *And the Band Played On,* the best-selling book about the first six years of the AIDS epidemic, has been ridiculed, reviled, even ostracized by some of his fellow homosexuals for his reporting on this community for the *San Francisco Chronicle* and other publications. Now, as he strolls these streets, he is stopped by strangers who want to let him know what a great job he has done.

Shilts, thirty-six, does deserve praise for his dogged work in uncovering the improprieties of federal policy regarding the epidemic. He gained access to the federal government's files by using the Freedom of Information Act, and he managed to discover the truth about huge funding needs and inadequate requests within the federal agencies responsible for AIDS programs.

But Shilts did most of his influential reportage on the local level, telling the tale of how gay politics and City Hall pressure molded San Francisco's public policy on AIDS. It was a story he knew intimately. Shilts had come to San Francisco in the mid-seventies, at the height of the sexual liberation movement that was attracting tens of thousands from across the country — and the world — to the sexually tolerant city. As a young, openly homosexual journalist interested in covering the issues in this community, he could not have picked a better news town. He covered the campaign and election of the nation's first openly homosexual city official, Harvey Milk; he reported on the battle over the state's Briggs Initiative, which would have reinstated part of California's abolished sodomy law; and he was on the front line when Milk and San Francisco's mayor George Moscone were gunned down by Dan White. When Shilts was hired by the *Chronicle* in 1981 to cover the city's gay community, the reporter brought his contacts and his alliances. At the top of both those lists were members of the Harvey Milk Gay Democratic Club, the organization devoted to promoting the martyred politician's vision of pragmatic politics.

In the spring of 1983, with 1,279 cases of AIDS reported in San Francisco, most of them homosexual men, the Milk Club decided the pragmatic thing to do was to convince homosexuals to stop having unsafe sex. A first step in that effort was to target meeting places where casual sex flourished, specifically, San Francisco's gay bathhouses.

Shilts's ties to San Francisco's homosexuals and the *Chronicle*'s commitment to covering that financially and politically powerful community are the two reasons the newspaper has almost always been on the cutting edge of AIDS news. And the *Chronicle*'s coverage served as an impetus for the other local daily, the *San Francisco Examiner,* to follow the story closely. The importance both newspapers placed on the epidemic had a clear impact on City Hall and on private citizens: San Francisco led the nation in developing and funding care facilities and educational efforts.

But because of his personal power, Shilts also influenced the policies more than a reporter should. Shilts covered the Milk Club's attempt to get safe-sex warning signs posted in the bathhouses and detailed the subsequent waffling on the issue by the city's public health director. But then he became part of the story. In a June 1983 cover story in *California* magazine, two free-lance journalists quoted Shilts as lashing out at those gay politicos — including Milk Club opponents — who, he believed, were denying the seriousness of the AIDS problem and trying to keep it under wraps. The piece drew howls of protest from many San Francisco homosexuals, who claimed Shilts's criticisms were an attempt to undermine the campaign of a candidate for supervisor whom the Milk Club was not supporting. The reporter already had been tainted by his ties to the Milk organization — a relationship solidified by writing a book on its founder and by forming friendships with the club's leadership. To defend himself against these outcries of bias, Shilts agreed to take part in a documentary on the issue, to be produced by a local television station.

By this point Shilts had personalized the story. He admitted there were certain results he wanted. Frightening his fellow homosexuals into safe sexual behavior was one of his goals. He tried throughout 1983 and 1984 to get his editors to run his stories on the dire consequences of promiscuous sex on Friday — before gay men hit the bars or baths on the weekend. He understood the risks involved for homosexuals participating in unsafe sex.

He was now witnessing some of his acquaintances facing the death sentence of an AIDS diagnosis. And he was aware that he, too, could be at risk. After all, he had been sexually promiscuous himself; indeed, he had even worked in a bathhouse during college.

His personal history was the most important factor propelling him to embrace the battle against the bathhouses, and his side eventually won. After a divisive municipal battle, with Public Health Director Dr. Mervyn Silverman vacillating on the issue, the bathhouses were closed in the fall of 1984.

In light of other pressing AIDS issues, such as providing adequate education and handling the increasing case loads of patients, the media concentration on the baths is a troubling example of overexposure. The issue could not, and should not, have been consciously avoided by Shilts or any other journalist, but the battle over the bathhouses drowned out any reasonable debate over the public health issue. Indeed, Dr. Silverman, a career public health official, eventually resigned under fire, partly because of a heated situation created by Shilts's coverage. The way in which Shilts personally embraced the story helped not only to define what was important but also to dictate the news.

Furthermore, focusing on the bathhouses as though *they* were the primary sources of infection tended to discount the more basic problem — changing individuals' sexual behavior. Although anonymous sex at the baths undoubtedly contributed to the epidemic, the most important factor was the mores of the gay culture, resulting from centuries of sexual oppression and denial which encouraged promiscuity and unsafe sex. Shilts and the *Chronicle* helped breed a false sense of security for those gay men who had never visited the baths and who would not. For a city that defined the appropriate response to AIDS, the bathhouse controversy was nothing but an embarrassment. And Shilts's role in that public policy debacle should give journalists pause.

Jim Bunn: Journalist as Health Educator

Since his college days at Oklahoma City University, Bunn had known he had a desire to save the world. It started when he organized a candlelight vigil following the Kent State shootings in 1970 in order to defuse the student anger and avoid violence on campus. And thirteen years later it would manifest itself in his AIDS reporting.

TV station KPIX–San Francisco had an interest in covering the epidemic years before most broadcast outlets took AIDS seriously. That was in part because the station was based in San Francisco and in part because Art Kern, KPIX's general manager, was convinced AIDS would be the story of the decade.

When Bunn came to the station in 1983, he "discovered" the epidemic for himself. He went to a press conference held by the local blood bank, which left many questions unanswered: Without a test for the disease, how could anyone be sure transfusions weren't spreading AIDS? Were San Franciscans in danger from the blood supply?

He had been able to overlook the epidemic in his previous job as assistant news manager at a Connecticut station, but as a reporter in San Francisco he could not disregard the fact that large numbers of people were dying from AIDS. Hundreds of locals already had been diagnosed, and doctors said thousands were probably harboring the disease without any signs of illness yet. Bunn had been at KPIX only a month before he was asked to do a San Francisco–based series on the disease to run in the fall "sweeps," one of the regular periods during which the audiences of local TV news stations are measured. He scrambled to fill the huge holes in his understanding of AIDS and coaxed the budget-minded management into sending him on the road. "You can show the audience you're making a commitment to the coverage," he argued. He traveled to the Centers for Disease Control in Atlanta, Georgia, to research facilities in Washington, D.C., and to hospitals in New York.

But for an audience of 5.2 million viewers, the reach of KPIX in the Bay Area, AIDS was little more than San Francisco's problem. The general suburban viewer did not care much about news that affected the city's urban homosexual men and was not likely to be impressed with a TV station's commitment to covering such stories.

Making the average viewer in the hugely diverse television audience care about AIDS became Bunn's biggest challenge. First, he had to overcome his own inhibitions about tackling a disease that was at the time affecting mostly homosexual men. Bunn is a heterosexual, married family man; he fits the bill of a Midwestern TV personality, pleasant to look at, reassuring, sincere. Yet he has an edge to him, and the threat of AIDS making its way into the heterosexual population was his current obsession.

In one of his first jobs in journalism, working for a radio station in Oklahoma, he had learned that the most gripping stories were about individuals. So he began telling the stories of individuals with AIDS: those who had lost their jobs, had lost their insurance, and were unable to get disability from the federal government. Not surprisingly, Bunn focused on gay men in the beginning. But to increase the impact of his reporting — that is, to draw the attention of a broader audience to information about the disease — he also put women and children with AIDS on the screen.

Employing such dramatic methods is an understandable urge for broadcasters, who are probably more concerned about demographics than their newspaper reporter counterparts. But in this case, the ploy led to a distorted perception of AIDS sufferers. According to the Center for Media and Public Affairs, in recent depictions across the country of those with the disease, heterosexuals were eight times more likely to be shown than homosexuals, although there are about eight times more homosexual AIDS sufferers than heterosexual. Similarly, females make up about 14 percent of the recent televised depictions of AIDS patients but represent only 7 percent of the national total AIDS cases.[2] But Bunn was driven to warn his viewers about what he believed was the coming onslaught. He put his attention to institutionalizing KPIX's AIDS coverage.

The idea was hatched over lunch between a KPIX producer and a volunteer at the San Francisco AIDS Foundation. It grew into "AIDS Lifeline," the most impressive public education campaign produced by any single news outlet — and perhaps the most successful. Bunn argued to the station's management that such an investment would pay off in larger audiences, since Bay Area viewers would know they could turn to KPIX for information on the epidemic as it grew. The station's current general manager, Caroline Wean, claims that this was not the impetus for agreeing to push ahead with the project. And in the beginning, extra resources were not devoted to "AIDS Lifeline"; money was simply rerouted from other areas of the station. Looking back, it is clear to Wean and others on the money side of the station that the effort made sense, if just in terms of prestige for KPIX.

"AIDS Lifeline" incorporated Bunn's daily reporting and the station's special series on the disease. It also included educational pamphlets, produced in conjunction with the AIDS Foundation and sent across the country. "AIDS Lifeline" broadcasts have appeared on stations throughout the United States and have been picked up by universities as well.

In 1986, Bunn and his colleagues at KPIX won the prestigious Peabody Award for their public service effort in creating "AIDS Lifeline." So strong is Bunn's commitment to educating the masses about the threat of the disease that he has since moved to Geneva, to work with the World Health Organization's AIDS information campaign. The reporter intends to return to KPIX. Indeed, the station is paying his salary at WHO, as its contribution to the international effort to stop the epidemic.

The impact of the work done by Bunn and KPIX is not entirely clear. The station undoubtedly influenced City Hall, as did the *Examiner* and the *Chronicle,* and it can take some of the credit for the politicians' quick and compassionate response. KPIX's educational campaign, in coordination with the San Francisco AIDS Foundation, also helped change unsafe sexual behavior among the city's gay male community. Surveys from mid-1983 to 1987 show significant shifts in the sexual habits of San Francisco's homosexual men, the population that some researchers believe has made the most dramatic change in lifestyle since the onset of AIDS.[3]

The effect "AIDS Lifeline" has had on the heterosexual population is much less apparent. As in most other parts of the country, sexually transmitted disease among heterosexuals is on the rise in the Bay Area. But only in San Francisco does AIDS remain almost exclusively a gay male problem. Some 97 percent of those with AIDS in the city are homosexual men; in most parts of the country, they make up only 60 to 70 percent of those with the disease.[4]

From a public health educator's perspective, those data pose some tricky questions. Should education efforts be aimed at the general heterosexual population? Or should the target be the heterosexual minority population, the next group expected to be affected? And shouldn't the majority of local resources continue to go toward influencing homosexual behavior, since homosexual men are still the largest risk group in San Francisco? These are questions KPIX has to consider, now that it is in the business of health education. Such issues put constraints on journalists, whose primary responsibility is to report what is new rather than to target their reporting toward specific ends.

Just as Shilts played a political role in AIDS coverage, Bunn assumed a public health authority's role. In so doing, he had the opportunity to mold the news to fit a policy goal: making every viewer aware of the threat the epidemic posed. In itself, that role has positive effects. San Franciscans are better informed because of Bunn's efforts. But his emphasis on getting the information out to all people by showing a disproportionately large number of women and children could very well have a negative backlash. It is now known that AIDS is far less of a threat to the non-drug-using heterosexual population than first believed. Some listeners might feel that KPIX has misled them and that any AIDS prevention is unnecessary or that KPIX information cannot be trusted.

In trying to push a media message, the journalist runs the risk of distorting the news. Bunn's aim was certainly not mischievous — indeed, his work is highly laudable. But the approach raises questions about the role of the journalist in a crisis.

Lawrence Altman: The Detached M.D.

He is one of the most educated science reporters in the nation: Harvard undergraduate, Tufts Medical School, a fellowship in epidemiology at the Centers for Disease Control in Atlanta, residency at the University of Washington. His comprehensive reporting of the Legionnaires' disease outbreak in Philadelphia a decade ago has been cited as one of the reasons the cause was found so quickly. The scientists working on the case knew they were under severe scrutiny by the *New York Times,* which meant the rest of the press was soon to follow. Altman, fifty, did write one of the first articles on AIDS that appeared in the major media, following the *San Francisco Chronicle* and the *Los Angeles Times*. But he was extremely slow to follow up on the news. More than most journalists, Altman reflects the institution for which he works. An eighteen-year *Times* veteran, his paper has inculcated most of its traditional journalistic standards in him. For the most part, the news that's fit to print happens in centralized places, such as state capitals and government institutions; and it happens to white, middle-aged males. The pressure against covering minority groups in a sophisticated and comprehensive way is best exemplified by the *Times*'s style book. Only in the summer of 1987 did the paper's editors finally drop the prohibition against the word *gay* to describe homosexuals, years after the *Los Angeles Times* and the *Washington Post*, the *Times*'s chief news rivals, had accepted the term.

But Altman's reporting is not only influenced by the *Times*'s institutional norms; his perspective is also a product of his medical training. Thus it is not surprising that when in late June 1981 scores of doctors in New York City were concerned about the rapidly spreading Kaposi's sarcoma and *Pneumocystis carinii* pneumonia, Altman did not come to the story until the CDC put out its *Morbidity and Mortality Weekly Report* on the subject in the first week of July.[5] "Rare Cancer Seen in 41 Homosexuals" was placed on page A20 in the July 3, 1981, edition. Altman described the new infections as far from a frightening phenomenon: it was an outbreak, he wrote, with "as much scientific as public health importance because of what it may teach about determining the causes of more common types of cancer."[6]

As the epidemic rampaged through Manhattan's gay male communities, Altman continued to look to the CDC for his leads: the first 41 cases reported, next the first 107 cases, and then 335 cases. In all, the *Times* ran seven stories in the first nineteen months of the epidemic, none of them on the front page. While reporters covering AIDS for the *San Francisco Chronicle*, the *Boston Globe*, and on National Public Radio were describing the impact AIDS was having on the lives of individual sufferers, most of them homosexual men, Altman took a different tack in his column, "The Doctor's World." The January 3, 1984, article largely by-passed the patients at the hospital Altman visited and focused on the issues physicians were struggling with:

> If, despite the odds, one of the physicians or others on the staff did come down with AIDS, he or she could inadvertently become a martyr to medicine, possibly offering the vehicle by which the cause of AIDS would be determined.[7]

What he omitted — any mention that the hundreds of patients who already had passed away might have contributed to medical knowledge — says more about his bias than what he included. Altman's connection to the CDC also seems to have had an effect on his reportage. The best example is his coverage of the international scramble to gain credit for discovery of the AIDS virus. The Pasteur Institute in Paris had come up with a possibility named lymphadenopathy-associated virus months before Dr. Robert Gallo at the U.S. National Institutes of Health began preparing his findings on human T-cell lymphotropic virus type III. But the French had gotten almost no U.S. press. At home Gallo had been battling with the CDC over issues of research control — and the CDC itself had been working with the Pasteur Institute on discovering the cause of AIDS.

Altman's coverage is professional overall and indicative of the high-quality newspaper for which he works. Yet his own background — a *Times* man, a doctor — defines his connection to the AIDS story. Specifically, he chose largely to ignore the crisis in the gay male community for the first critical months.

The public policy consequences of Altman's news choices cannot be minimized. The *New York Times,* arguably the United States' paper of record as well as a news leader for media outlets across the country, can move bureaucratic mountains in both Washington, D.C., and New York. Conversely, it can chill almost any issue simply by ignoring it. The feeble response of New York and Washington in the early years of the epidemic gives witness to that power.

But the *New York Times*'s poor early coverage since has been replaced with particularly strong reporting. From the social to the political, the medical, and the scientific, the newspaper has perhaps the single best coverage of any print medium in the United States. The *Times* cannot take all the credit for the new concern shown by the federal government, but the paper's intense recent reporting on the issue has focused national debate more than the coverage of any other media institution.

Laurie Garrett: Compassion and Science

Garrett, thirty-seven, is no political ingénue. She got her first experience when she dropped out of the University of California, Santa Cruz, to work full-time for the antiwar movement in the spring of 1970. The United States had invaded Cambodia, escalating the conflict in Southeast Asia. Shortly after came the Kent State shootings. If the Johnson administration's deceit about Vietnam made cynics of even the most traditional reporters, the nation's young became downright hostile. The youth of that period who went on to become journalists themselves, like Laurie Garrett, often have been those most suspicious of government policy. But suspicion was not the only thing Garrett garnered from her activism. In the 1970s, to be a political organizer, and to be successful at it, meant understanding coalition building. In northern California, that meant being plugged in to the gay community, a burgeoning power in San Francisco politics. Garrett came to rely on those connections a decade later in her post as West Coast correspondent for National Public Radio. Her impressive science credentials — she was pursuing a Ph.D. in immunology at the University of California, Berkeley, before devoting herself to journalism — and her political background made her the best-informed journalist covering AIDS in the early years.

NPR was one of only a few media outlets that broke the story on Kaposi's sarcoma among gay men, on July 3, 1981.[8] It was the best medium for separating reality from the fiction of overblown optimism in the first drug trials for treating AIDS. And Garrett was one of the few journalists who knew enough about politics and science to question the official government line in 1983 that adequate funding was being provided for the fight against the epidemic. But no amount of sophistication or experience could prepare Garret for every aspect of AIDS reporting.

She had confronted death before — first her mother's lingering struggle with cancer and then her brother's losing battle with diabetes. Now the list of deaths she had to deal with — of both friends and acquaintances — was expanding as the epidemic rolled through San Francisco. By 1987, when she covered the epidemic in Newark, New Jersey, and met Sylvia in a local hospital, Garrett felt death-weary. A petite Puerto Rican woman in her early thirties, Sylvia was facing not only her own impending death from AIDS, but that of her daughters, aged five and seven, both of whom had contracted the disease. Garrett's coverage of the crisis in Newark, including segments on Sylvia's family, is powerful and effective. Garrett's sensitive questioning and her emotion-filled pauses speak volumes about this reporter, who has become extraordinarily affected by the human aspect of the epidemic.[10]

The impact of her first-rate coverage is difficult to discern. NPR's audience is very diffuse, though the network does count among its listeners a large number of powerful political leaders. Perhaps more important is the model of journalist that Garrett offers to her colleagues and to younger professionals. She is, like Shilts, a reporter who has a connection to the community in which AIDS news first broke; who has the strong technical underpinnings to understand the science involved, as Altman does; and who, like Bunn, has a very strong commitment to educating the public.

Although she clearly has compassion for those she is covering, she maintains a distance from the politics involved. That separation suggests something more than the vaunted objectivity that U.S. journalists claim to prize so much; it indicates instead a certain independent perspective on the issue. This is not to say that Garrett is completely unbiased — she is too politically aware for that. But she does not actively play a role in the news, which is one reason her reporting on the epidemic has been so effective.

What We've Learned

Looking back over the last seven years, it is obvious that the media in the United States came too late and gave too little to covering the AIDS crisis. As a result of the media's failure to warn the public and government about the epidemic, thousands who might otherwise have avoided infection have died or are suffering from the disease.

It is not the job of journalists to act as public policy manipulators, but it is their responsibility to cover the news in a sophisticated and modern manner. To do so requires understanding that the news — the events that affect our lives — happens not just in the mainstream communities or those pockets of cities on which newspapers and broadcast outlets focus their coverage. News happens in gay ghettos, black communities, Hispanic barrios.

AIDS is increasingly becoming not a disease of white, middle-class homosexual men. It is now making its way into Third World America. Major metropolitan dailies throughout the nation have reached out to cover their outlying communities in a more sophisticated manner, but they also need to cover other communities within their cities. This coverage is not approached with traditional journalistic techniques: attending the Tuesday board meeting, quoting the titular leader. Instead, it requires a much more astute sense of trends as well as a feel for community.

The four models of coverage discussed here suggest the kind of reporter who will successfully cover the AIDS crisis. Such reporters will not only be in tune with the diverse communities that the disease affects, but also will be equipped with a basic knowledge of science to understand the nature of the viral beast, a sense of duty to those people they report on, *and* compassion.

The media institution itself will have to change to accommodate a broader range of techniques in disseminating information. The reporter is only one conduit. Members of the editorial page should recognize their responsibility to educate readers not only on the political and moral issues of the day, but also on the health realities that increasingly face communities. Family papers and broadcast outlets will have to avoid the squeamishness that has resulted in their creating phrases such as "exchange of bodily fluids" to mask perfectly appropriate words such as *semen, ejaculation, penis, vagina,* and *intercourse.* Some progress has been made in this area, especially at major media institutions, but U.S. editors have a long way to go. None of these suggestions require a radical departure from the current mission of many broadcast and print outlets: serving as a community record and providing news in the public interest. The recommendations, however, do necessitate that publishers, owners, editors, and reporters take another look at just how they are fulfilling that mandate.

As the world's geopolitical dimensions shrink, those groups which used to be considered "fringe" will play increasingly larger roles. AIDS has made Americans aware that there is more to the world than they had imagined. From Africa's jungles to Europe's cities, from prostitutes to the wives of middle-class businessmen, from the veins of junkies to the bodies of our children, we are all more intimately connected than we may care to admit.

Robin Nagle, a graduate student at Columbia University, provided research for this article.

Notes

1. The profiles of Shilts, Bunn, Altman, and Garrett are a result of intensive analysis of their work as well as extensive interviews with reporters, editors, and producers familiar with their coverage. I have also interviewed Shilts, Bunn, and Garrett, at length, by phone and in person.
2. Center for Media and Public Affairs, "The AIDS Story: Science, Politics, Sex and Death," *Media Monitor* (December 1987), Washington, D.C.
3. Several published and unpublished studies indicate this change: "Designing an Effective AIDS Prevention Campaign Strategy: Results from the First and Second Probability Sample of an Urban Gay Male Community," published by the San Francisco AIDS Foundation, 3 December 1984 and 28 June 1985; and Leon McKusick et al., "Reported Changes in Sexual Behavior of Men at Risk for AIDS," *Public Health Reports* 100, no. 6: 622, 628.
4. Interview with Centers for Disease Control, Atlanta, Georgia.
5. "Kaposi's Sarcoma and Pneumocystis Pneumonia Among Homosexual Men — New York City and California," *Morbidity and Mortality Weekly Report,* July 4, 1981.
6. Dr. Lawrence Altman, "Rare Cancer Seen in 41 Homosexuals," *New York Times,* 3 July 1981.
7. Dr. Lawrence Altman, "Making Rounds: AIDS Rooms," *New York Times,* 3 January 1984.
8. Laurie Garrett for National Public Radio, "High Incidence of Cancer in Homosexuals," San Francisco, 3 July 1981.
9. Laurie Garrett for National Public Radio, "Newark AIDS Cases Getting Out of Control," Newark, New Jersey, 7 May 1987.

New Hampshire: The Premarital Testing Debacle

Susan D. Epstein

In 1987, the New Hampshire Division of Public Health Services had a bill introduced in the legislature to improve contact tracing and establish statewide public education on HIV infection, transmission, and disease control. This article traces the bill, and issues surrounding the bill, through the legislative process and focuses on an unexpected intervention by the governor through a proposed amendment to add mandatory premarital testing. Its conclusions offer advice to other states on how best to avoid political exploitation of AIDS/HIV issues.

By the summer of 1987, the AIDS issue in New Hampshire had become devoted to everything but AIDS. It revolved around presidential preferences, a governor's show of strength, and legislative grandstanding. Substantive progress in curbing the further transmission of the virus through education, testing, and behavioral changes had been stymied. How did this issue become so hotly politicized in New Hampshire? Can our sister New England states learn from our experience? Can the issue be better handled?

This article will trace a benign bill from its inception through its demise in the legislature. It will illustrate how the absence of a plan and of consensus can leave this sensitive issue open to political exploitation.

Late in the summer of 1986, top staff in the Division of Public Health's Disease Control Bureau met with the agency's deputy director to ask for any available money to deal with AIDS. The Division's AIDS program was, and still is, financed entirely through federal funds granted for services to the high-risk population: male homosexuals, hemophiliacs, intravenous drug users, and their partners. The number of seropositive AIDS tests was beginning to climb steeply, and transmission had begun to move into the general population. Like many other rural states, New Hampshire had had a slow start-up on AIDS, but recent test results had indicated that the rate was escalating rapidly. The Division was without resources — staff, supplies, equipment, expense money — to deal with this rise.[1]

Susan D. Epstein, who holds a master of public administration from the University of New Hampshire, served as deputy director of the New Hampshire Division of Public Health Services from 1982 to 1987.

To carry out its work with the high-risk population, the Division had hired one health educator, one nurse, a part-time laboratory person, and a part-time secretary. Other Disease Control staff had been diverted to deal with the ever expanding cries for help with the disease, and staff energies were stretched dangerously thin. The number of positive tests in 1986 was projected to quadruple from 1985.[2] No other resources could be redeployed.

The Disease Control staff had other concerns besides money. Through a network of volunteers at five clinic sites and physicians around the state, word had already come back: instances of confidentiality breached, patients attempting suicide after receiving a positive initial test result over the phone, hasty and illogical local policies implemented to deal with fear of AIDS. The Division had received entreaties from local and state prisons, the state's reform school, its mental hospital, drug abuse units, private and public hospitals and specialty hospitals, police units, schools, insurance companies, and others for help in developing policies and guidelines for staff, patients, customers, travelers, and inmates. Nowhere in state law was the Division authorized to take these initiatives, and nowhere had the legislature or the governor made clear whose job it was to handle all the issues around AIDS.

The Bill

Following consultation with the director and the commissioner of the Department of Health and Human Services, a bill was drafted to outline the duties of the Division in dealing with the disease. The governor's staff was notified that an AIDS bill would be added to those bills coming from Public Health. A small AIDS task force, chaired by the commissioner, received the preliminary draft. The chairpersons of both House and Senate Health Committees were notified, as was the state's health/medical community.

Public Health had only three weeks to prepare the bill for submission for a September deadline. The Division felt that the bill should address the duties assigned to Public Health as well as issues relating to those duties, but not tackle those other areas which have been affected by AIDS, such as housing, labor, employment, and civil rights. The Division also determined that the bill would address disease prevention and disease control issues for AIDS but would not discuss those at high risk and the specifics of transmission. In other words, sex, homosexuality, and drug use were not mentioned.

The bill filed in the fall had six major components:

1. The Division of Public Health Services was authorized to develop AIDS-education materials for schools, colleges, health care providers and institutions, state agencies, business and industry, the media, and the public.

2. The Division was to assist all these groups in developing policies and programs to deal with AIDS.

3. The Division was to conduct laboratory testing for HIV infection already in place, but was authorized to certify outside laboratories to conduct further testing and reporting.

4. A highly specific informed-consent provision was included to combat the increasingly prevalent practice of testing someone's blood for HIV without the person's knowledge, a practice leading to some tragic responses.

5. A tight confidentiality plan was included to safeguard test results. Confidentiality provisions were backed up with penalties and liability provisions.

6. A total of $339,000 was requested for FY'88 and $325,000 for FY'89, virtually doubling the size of the existing program.

Strategy

The strategy for the bill was based on the assumption that it would take its hardest hits in the financial area, given the New Hampshire State Legislature's traditional reluctance to fund new programs. Further, the Division assumed that the purpose of the bill was so inoffensive that little if any restructuring would be done with its substance.

With this logic, the Division requested sponsors from four key sources: several House sponsors from the House Health and Human Services Committee; one member from House Appropriations; and on the Senate side, Elaine Krasker, the new chairperson of the Senate's Health and Welfare Committee, who was to play a pivotal role, and two members of the Senate's powerful Finance Committee; Sen. Frank Torr and Sen. Ed Dupont, the new majority leader. With support in Appropriations, and with the assurance of key conservative votes to add to more liberal votes in Senate Finance, the Division hoped to pave a smooth passage. The legislative plan had been fashioned by Sen. Elaine Krasker, a seasoned representative and a former Democratic whip in the House, newly elected to the Senate. Through her efforts, Representative Ramsay and Senators Torr and Dupont joined the team.

Legislative Process

The bill was well received at a large hearing before the House Health and Human Services Committee. Chairman Matthew Sochalski had placed some key committee members as sponsors on the bill, in addition to the committee's six-term ranking Democrat, Rep. Marion Copenhaver. A subcommittee headed by a retired pediatrician, Rep. Robert Wilson, met to iron out some of the major issues raised in the committee hearing.

A major point of contention was the penalty provision, aimed at anyone who breached confidentiality concerning a patient tested for HIV infection. For obvious reasons, representatives of the New Hampshire Medical Society and the New Hampshire Hospital Association wanted the provision deleted. The subcommittee needed to weigh their plea against that of the Coalition of Gay and Lesbian Rights (CAGLR), which argued that without this legal protection, they would refuse to be tested. The recommended version was a compromise, maintaining the penalties but stipulating that a person must "purposely" violate confidentiality in order to have them apply. A section was added, requested by the corrections commissioner, to permit testing without informed consent in prisons and mental institutions when the testing would be necessary to place and manage the individual within the facility. A troublesome section specifying at what age a minor's parents must be told of test results was deleted, permitting other statutes already on the books to apply. Having been amended but still intact, the bill sailed through the House Health and Human Services Committee and, some weeks later, through House Appropriations. The issue of mandatory testing was not raised.

By the time of the appropriations hearing, concerns that the bill's budget would be diced up had vanished. Those who had raised concerns about substantive issues in the bill had their concerns dealt with by the compromises in committee. Appropriations was supportive and sent the bill back to the full House, where it passed on a voice vote.

Then the bomb dropped. The director of Public Health Services received a call on Monday, April 6, from the governor's legal counsel, indicating that the governor was going to hold a press conference on the AIDS bill on the following day and warning the director not to "shoot [them] in the foot." There had been no prior discussion with the director of Public Health Services or with his boss, the commissioner of Health and Human Services. There was no indication as to what the governor was planning to say, and no request for opinion from Public Health — not even an invitation to attend the press conference. Several phone calls ascertained that neither the bill's sponsors nor the medical community had been consulted.

On Tuesday, April 7, a staffer from the Division, armed with a tape recorder, went to the governor's press conference to find out more. At the conference, the governor, flanked by the Speaker of the House and the president of the Senate, Republicans all, said he planned to introduce an amendment to the AIDS bill which would require AIDS testing before couples would be permitted to marry. He indicated that the amendment would reinstate the old syphilis premarital testing requirement, since it could serve as a legal precedent for requiring HIV testing. He repeated several times that AIDS was a legal issue, a political issue, a civil rights issue, but not a medical issue. Finally, to the distress of Public Health staff who had been struggling for three and a half years to quell the spread of the disease, he noted that his measure was a start and a small beginning.[3]

Of the many questions from the press that followed, only one raised the prescient issue. Veteran State House reporter Donn Tibbetts, of the *Manchester Union Leader*, asked, with due respect to the state's three foremost political leaders, where were the medical people who supported or requested this measure. Governor Sununu simply repeated his claim that AIDS was not a medical issue.[4]

If AIDS had not been a political issue before the governor's press conference, it became one immediately afterward. Legislative sponsors, including Reps. Marion Copenhaver, Trudy Butler, Larry Chase, and Robert Wilson, as well as Senator Krasker, were incensed. The state medical society hastily called together the infectious disease physicians, who prevailed upon the society's Executive Committee to oppose the measure. At Public Health, which had been muzzled by orders not to shoot [the governor's office] in the foot, press calls were passed to the governor's office, and the Division's role in working on its highest priority bill ended.

Press reaction to the proposed premarital testing plan included criticism from medical specialists and no comment from Public Health.[5] The governor then announced that he would veto the bill unless it came to his desk with his premarital amendment included.[6] Some local reporters picked up on Vice President George Bush's statement, made a day after Sununu's to *USA Today*, supporting premarital testing and remarked on the coincidence, as Sununu serves as Bush's campaign chairman in New Hampshire.[7]

Criticism of the proposed amendment by the medical community was swift and damning. Using data from Public Health's current testing, the critics pointed out that of 22,000 people who would be required to be tested, only 2 would turn out to be truly positive. All the other people who tested positive — 218 — and their families and friends, would go through hell in that interval between the first positive test and the ultimately negative result. Critics questioned why a low-risk group, monogamous couples already committed to a long-term sexual relationship, should be compelled to be tested. The medical community voiced concerns about the premise that premarital testing for syphilis would be reinstated. The law mandating premarital syphilis testing by the state had been repealed in 1981; there had not been a positive test for over five years.[8]

The governor's threat to veto the AIDS bill if it arrived without his amendment drew indictment from newspapers around the state. The *Concord Monitor* headlined its editorial "Cross Power Play" and chastised the governor for "playing a deadly game of chicken with the Legislature."[9] Dr. Miles McCue, a member of Governor Sununu's handpicked Task Force on AIDS, editorialized in the *Boston Globe* that the mandatory testing proposal was "reckless with regard to its ignorance."[10] Even the *Manchester Union Leader*, the only statewide daily newspaper, generally supportive of Sununu, criticized the governor's "browbeating politics."[11] The press also reported, in a limited way, a "man on the street" sense from the public which indicated a measure of public support for mandatory premarital testing. There seemed to be low recognition of the distinction between consequences of confidentiality leaks for syphilis and AIDS. A breach of confidentiality concerning AIDS causes more than embarrassment. At the present time, it can threaten the loss of one's housing, one's employment, life insurance, health insurance, and potentially one's medical and dental providers. The absence of a public education program — as the bill would have provided — left the public unable to debate the merits of the very issue that had been placed between the bill and its passage.

The New Hampshire Medical Society's Infectious Disease section moved to convince its Executive Committee to take action with the governor. The society directed its action to two fronts: first, to try to deal directly with Governor Sununu, and, second, to try to kill the amendment when it was introduced in the Senate. A meeting between the governor and a group representing the medical society proved inconclusive, and the society's efforts were then directed toward the upcoming hearing in the Senate where the premarital amendment was to be introduced.

In both the House and the Senate some of the debate over the premarital testing plan began to center around which presidential aspirants supported it. Bush supporters, Kemp and Dole supporters, lined up on the side of their candidate to show their relative strength. Having dared the legislature to defy him, the governor's supporters and opponents, Republican and Democrat, fell in line. Having neglected to take any strong positions or to initiate any action in the first four months of the six-month legislative session, and having placed himself firmly in a box on this issue, Governor Sununu had to rally the House and Senate leadership to hew to his position.

The first draft of the amendment was issued from the governor's legal counsel only hours before the Senate hearing was to be held. A copy had to be leaked to Public Health. The draft amendment by the governor's office would have gutted the money needed for education and contact tracing by using most of it for premarital testing. It breached confidentiality and eliminated pre- and post-test counseling. The process for testing and test-results reporting was replete with dead ends. As the result of conversations between the attorney general's office and the Speaker's office, the amendment had been completely rewritten by April 28, the day of the Senate hearing. Provisions were added to allow the testing to be self-supporting, the syphilis provision was quietly deleted, and some of the procedural issues were clarified.

The Senate hearing on April 28 was chaired by Sen. Elaine Krasker, the leading Senate sponsor of the bill. Of the many speakers that morning who addressed the committee, only one urged the adoption of the governor's/Speaker's/Senate president's amendment: an Ernest Schapiro, representing Lyndon LaRouche.

One speaker after the next urged the committee to pass the bill as it arrived from the House and not to include the governor's amendment. The director of the New Hampshire Civil Liberties Union argued that the state would be unable to prove it had a compelling reason to require the invasive procedure of drawing blood, because the state could do nothing with the results of that test; it couldn't offer a cure, stop the marriage, or prevent conception. Dr. James Kahn of Deerfield warned the committee that "many of the people we need to reach are socially ostracized, medically indigent, and otherwise disconnected." He pointed out that these are not the people who are already accepting enough of society's norms to be getting married.

At the close of the hearing, the committee unanimously passed the bill without the premarital amendment. The bill came to the full Senate for a vote on May 5, having been through the Senate Finance Committee without a hearing, and it was there that the governor's staff went to work. They leaned on senators for hours, making promises and threats, "bullying and bartering some members into changing their positions," according to the *Concord Monitor*.[12] On a roll call vote, the bill passed 13 to 11 with the premarital provision attached.

Headed for Conference Committee to resolve the dispute (or kill the bill, as Conference Committee must have unanimous votes and acceptance by both chambers), the pressure increased with the approaching deadline in the Senate. The deadline for bills and committees of conference reports to be heard on the floor of the Senate was May 15. In order to hear a bill or report after that date and vote on it, the House and Senate required a two-thirds vote to suspend the rules.

The Senate vote on May 5 left ten calendar days to have conference committees appointed by both chambers, have the committees meet, deliberate, and concur, and have both houses accept their version of the bill. By this time, national newspapers were reporting on the issue, including the *New York Times* and the *Wall Street Journal*.[13] The debate was being heard as well from the Cabinet in the White House, where Surgeon General Koop and Education Secretary Bennett were evidently arguing over AIDS testing and AIDS education.[14]

At Public Health, an eerie kind of calm had settled in. The state budget bill was headed into Conference Committee; other Division bills were in their final stages of negotiation; press teams roamed the halls; but Division staff had no comment and made only the most necessary, and briefest, forays out.

Since the House had passed the bill without the premarital amendment and the Senate had passed the bill with the amendment, the House Speaker and Senate president appointed a Conference Committee. Despite their position in support of premarital testing, both leaders appointed members on both sides of the issue.

The group met in the basement of the State House, in the cramped offices of Senator Krasker. A fire in the Legislative Office Building days earlier had left many legislators "homeless" and had destroyed a great many files. The Conference Committee, after some rousting about, voted to include a sanitized version of the premarital testing plan. They added funds to conduct the testing so as not to have the costs of the testing be taken from the main AIDS bill. They also worked out a timing mechanism for reporting to town clerks that a couple had taken the test such that the town clerk would not be able to deduce who had had a positive test. Both Senator Krasker and Representative Copenhaver made it clear they didn't much like having to include even a sanitized premarital provision, but they were concerned that the bill would not prevail without it.

On May 13, just two days before the Senate deadline, the Senate approved the Conference Committee's report on a voice vote. The Conference Committee report then had to be adopted by the House.

That day, Representative Copenhaver called the other sponsors, and Public Health, to say she just could not sign the report. She indicated that she would fight against the Conference Committee report on the floor.[15]

She then went to the members of the House one by one and explained why it would be wrong to include the premarital provision. She argued the impropriety of the governor's having introduced an amendment after the bill had already been passed by the House; she talked about the anguish of those testing positive who eventually are found to be negative, and graphically depicted the plight of couples and families with their weddings on hold and their reputations ruined. She dared the House members to stand up for what she knew to be right, in spite of possible retribution from the governor and the wishes of their own Speaker. Other House sponsors worked the floor with her, letting members know that they had not been consulted, that the testing was expensive and would yield few positives, that even the U.S. Surgeon General had written to say that mandatory premarital testing was a poor solution.

The House, in an emotional session, rallied to Representative Copenhaver's call and rejected the Senate's version, with a roll call vote of 136 yeas to 165 nays. Then, in a show of strength, the House voted 157 to 138 to convene a new Conference Committee, with instructions that they consider the bill only on the basis of the House-passed version, that is, *without* the premarital provision. The Speaker replaced Marion Copenhaver on the new Conference Committee, but included members who had strongly and eloquently supported the House position. This gesture of support for the House's position, although it was antithetical to his own stance, earned him respect from his colleagues, as he had promised to listen to the House's voice when elected Speaker.

A first moral crusade had been fought and won. A second Committee of Conference on the AIDS bill was to then convene in some haste. The May 15 deadline for bills and reports on the Senate floor had passed; therefore, a two-thirds majority vote would be required to suspend the rules and allow a bill to be voted on. The House had locked itself into a tight position, making negotiation difficult. Sen. Edward Dupont, the new Senate majority leader, was a conferee, and he represented the Senate president. A small room had been located on the first floor of the State House. It was packed and hot, and press were in attendance. A unanimous vote was needed or the bill would die.

Senator Dupont opened by roundly criticizing the House for sending in conferees whose hands were tied. He talked about how committed he was to the premarital testing, indicating that, as an original sponsor of the bill, had he known then what he knew now, the bill would have been introduced with the provision included. He voiced the plea that had been used over and over by the Speaker and Senate president, that "if only one baby is saved by this," then the amendment is worth it. He said he would compromise by allowing anyone who was phobic about needles to be excused from the test by an order of the court. The House members indicated that this really did not represent much of a compromise.

Representative Kerk, a new conferee and House member, proposed an alternative that had been discussed earlier with some of the medical society physicians. Why not, he suggested, have a mandatory premarital questionnaire, and allow people to elect to take the test if they answered yes to some of the questions. Senator Dupont went off to seek guidance on this idea, and returned later to say that it was unacceptable.

An emotional burst from Rep. Ednapearl Parr brought the issue to a head. Why, she shouted, did they demand to test "innocent people" when they should be testing drug addicts and homosexuals and — In a level voice, Senator Krasker silenced her by saying, "Ednapearl, they are *all* innocent. There are no guilty people in this."

In the quiet that followed, Senator Dupont explained that this was exactly why the premarital group would be so useful. It was precisely their "innocence" that meant their subjection to mandatory testing would open the way for mandatory testing of "other groups." He did not elaborate. After another break to receive instructions, he returned and announced that he would sign the Conference Committee report without the premarital provision included. But, he added, he would fight its entry onto the floor, and block the necessary two-thirds vote. He concluded, "I have the votes."

This, then, was the plan. If Dupont could indeed block the bill's entry onto the floor, the bill would technically die in Conference Committee. No senator would actually have to vote against the AIDS bill, and the governor would not have to fulfill his threat of a veto.

However, in his last plea, Dupont had revealed the purpose of the governor's amendment. It was clear now why the amendment had been proposed, why the governor had called it "a start, a small beginning," and why he had repeated that this was a legal issue, a civil rights issue, a political issue, but not a medical issue. For indeed, if you can mandate testing of a low-risk group, even when the results of that test cannot be used by the state for any purpose, then it is a first step to begin testing of *any* group, especially any group that those in power find unacceptable. Using AIDS as a mechanism to curtail a group's civil rights is certainly a legal issue and a political issue, not a medical issue. But it is exactly this use of medicine to achieve results that have nothing to do with health that is most distressing.

On May 19, Senator Krasker's motion to suspend the rules and allow the AIDS bill to be heard on the floor failed in a 12–12 Senate vote, and the bill died.

Conclusion

HIV testing is an issue ripe for distortion and political manipulation. Because so much is not known, and since much that is known has not been clearly enunciated, there is widespread public fear. To this is added a growing distrust of the health care community's truthfulness in assessing the real risks of AIDS. Suspicion that medicine is deliberately understating the risks of transmission and is wrong in its assessment that HIV infection cannot be transmitted through casual contact makes public education a particularly difficult endeavor.

In New Hampshire's experience last year, the problem stemmed from too little education of the public and elected officials to permit genuine debate and unbiased consideration of the AIDS issue. For our sister New England states, the issue by now may be not too little information, but too much. There are many voices talking, authoritatively, about AIDS testing, and the public and media have little to help them sift through the morass of speculation, hyperbole, and fact. The New Hampshire experience had three bad long-term consequences: (1) it left scarred relationships between decision makers, making future planning difficult; (2) it further confused, and therefore frightened, an already wary public; and (3) by killing the bill, it delayed care, counseling, and public education for at least one year — one year longer for the disease to spread among a poorly informed public.

To avoid New Hampshire's debacle, our sister states need to build a central coalition whose "voice" is reasoned and whose membership represents a broad spectrum of respected medical and community organizations. Without such a coalition, politicians and some media will exploit conflicting opinions and further erode the public's confidence that it is receiving honest information. In concert with governors, a central coalition should establish a plan that considers all the many ramifications of AIDS and HIV infection with respect to states and lays out concrete actions. Then, and only then, should the doors be opened to introduce legislation. A well-informed coalition and a well-informed governor can prevail upon legislators to withhold bills until they have been educated and brought into the fold. With legislative, gubernatorial, and coalition support, bills have not only a better chance of passage, but also a better chance of producing useful information for press and public to consider. Harassment and discrimination have no place in the consideration of disease-control measures. We can and must do better.

Notes

1. "AIDS in New Hampshire," pamphlet, New Hampshire Division of Public Health Services, May 25, 1987.
2. Ibid.
3. Press Conference, Governor John H. Sununu, April 7, 1987.
4. Ibid.
5. Miles John McCue, M.D., "Premarital AIDS Testing Misdirected," *Boston Globe*, April 19, 1987; James B. Kahn, M.D., "The State Would Be Ill-Served by Premarital AIDS Testing," *Concord Monitor*, May 12, 1987.
6. "Governor Won't Sign Bill Unless Mandatory Amendment Stays: Sununu Lobbies for AIDS Tests," *Manchester Union Leader*, May 7, 1987.
7. "Bush Backs Mandatory Marriage AIDS Test," *Manchester Union Leader*, April 9, 1987; "Politics of AIDS," editorial, *Concord Monitor*, April 10, 1987.
8. Aaron Zitner, "AIDS Test: Doctors Doubt Value of Sununu's Plan," *Concord Monitor*, April 9, 1987.
9. "Cross Power Play," editorial, *Concord Monitor*, May 12, 1987.
10. Miles John McCue, M.D., "Premarital AIDS Testing Misdirected."
11. "AIDS Squabble: Bickering Over Testing Goes On," *Manchester Union Leader*, April 30, 1987.
12. Aaron Zitner, "AIDS Testing: Governor Accused of Forcing Issue," *Concord Monitor*, May 6, 1987.
13. "Forced AIDS Tests; Then What?" editorial, *New York Times*, June 7, 1987.
14. "Evans and Novak," syndicated column, *Manchester Union Leader*, April 30, 1987.
15. Ben Stocking, "Foes of AIDS Tests Plan Fight in the House," *Concord Monitor*, May 14, 1987.

[illegible] We can ask [illegible] to [illegible].

Notes

1. "AIDS in New Hampshire," New Hampshire [illegible]

[illegible]

3. [illegible] conference, [illegible], April [illegible]

4. Ibid.

[illegible]

[illegible]

7. [illegible] AIDS [illegible]

8. [illegible]

9. [illegible] May [illegible]

10. [illegible] March [illegible]

11. "AIDS [illegible] Testing [illegible]"

12. [illegible]

[illegible]

10. [illegible]

[illegible]

The Big One: Literature Discovers AIDS

Shaun O'Connell

Among the works discussed in this essay:
An Intimate Desire to Survive, by Bill Becker. 31 pages. Dorrance & Company, 1985. $5.95.
Epitaphs for the Plague Dead, by Robert Boucheron. 47 pages. Ursus Press, 1985. $5.95.
A Cry in the Desert, by Jed A. Bryan. 235 pages. Banned Books, 1987. $9.95.
The World Can Break Your Heart, by Daniel Curzon. 241 pages. Knights Press, 1984. $6.95.
Safe Sex, by Harvey Fierstein. 112 pages. Atheneum, 1987. $15.95.
"The Castro," in *Cities on a Hill: A Journey Through Contemporary American Culture,* by Frances FitzGerald. Simon and Schuster, 1986. $19.95.
As Is, by William M. Hoffman. 97 pages. Vintage Books, Random House, 1985. $3.95.
Plague: A Novel About Healing, by Toby Johnson. 250 pages. Alyson Publications, 1987. $7.95.
The Normal Heart, by Larry Kramer. 123 pages. A Plume Book, New American Library, 1985. $6.95.
To All the Girls I've Loved Before: An AIDS Diary, by J. W. Money. 188 pages. Alyson Publications, 1987. $6.95.
Facing It: A Novel of AIDS, by Paul Reed. 217 pages. Gay Sunshine Press, 1984. $7.95.
And the Band Played On: Politics, People, and the AIDS Epidemic, by Randy Shilts. 630 pages. St. Martin's Press, 1987. $24.95.
Men on Men: Best New Gay Fiction, edited by George Stambolian. A Plume Book, New American Library, 1986. $9.95.

> Not stability but a sequence of sharp alterations and abrupt oscillations in existing balances between microparasitism and macroparasitism can therefore be expected in the near future as in the recent past.
>
> —William H. McNeill
> *Plagues and People*

In *Illness as Metaphor,* Susan Sontag insists that illness is *not* a metaphor. "The most truthful way of regarding illness — and the healthiest way of being ill — is one most purified of, most resistant to, metaphoric thinking."[1] By such logic, illness exists in its own autonomous realm; illness insists upon an original response. When Henry James suffered a stroke in 1915, he heard a voice exclaiming, "So here at last is the distinguished

Shaun O'Connell is professor of English at the University of Massachusetts at Boston; he teaches and writes on Irish and American literature.

thing!"[2] So, too, should we understand illness — particularly the collective illness that is called plague — as a distinguished, incomparable thing.

However, Sontag grants, "it is hardly possible to take up one's residence in the kingdom of the ill unprejudiced by the lurid metaphors with which it has been landscaped."[3] Suffering from cancer, in the 1970s, Sontag attempted to clarify, if not control, her condition through an analysis of the disease and its implication, just as many writers would, in the next decade, turn their attention to AIDS and its ominously intensifying reverberations. In times of crisis, the attraction of metaphor, the root of all artistic expression, is too powerful to resist, though the dangers associated with the imposition of ready-made verbal constructs upon new crises are well expressed by Sontag. Her book, principally on the literature of cancer and tuberculosis, is, then, a proper first, oblique step in confronting the unimaginable threat posed by AIDS. *Illness as Metaphor* serves both as a warning against the reckless use of metaphor and, paradoxically, as a tribute to the powers of many writers' imaginations, including her own, to name and contain, at least in words, the disease that ravishes them and their loved ones and that threatens everyone. There is a natural inclination to confront mystery with metaphor, as though words could tame. Even when words fail, metaphor can articulate the imagination of disaster, as does Lear, near the end, his mind and his language reeling:

> There is the sulphurous pit, burning, scalding,
> Stench, consumption. Fie, fie, fie! pah, pah!
> Give me an ounce of civet; good apothecary,
> Sweeten my imagination. There's money for thee.[4]

The myths of TB and cancer have served many purposes, Sontag discovered. Both have been seen as diseases of passion, though lately cancer has also been understood as a result of repression.[5] The diseased have been separated for special metaphoric attention; they have been invested with sinfulness, their disease interpreted as punishment, or they have been granted special poetic powers, their disease seen as evidence of the medieval humor, melancholy, or the "romantic agony" of the nineteenth century.[6] Alternatively, the diseased have been seen as innocent victims of foreign invasion by the Other: alien occupiers from outer space are blamed or alien members of the society are imagined. "Massacre of Jews in unprecedented numbers took place everywhere in plague-stricken Europe of 1347–48, then stopped as soon as the plague receded," writes Sontag.[7] Finally, illness has long been used as a measure of the health (spiritual, moral, political) of the society in which disease occurs, the infected "body politic."[8] All of these tropes, long established in the literature of TB and cancer, have been appropriate and have been applied to the AIDS crisis. The sudden impact of AIDS has sent writers reeling, grasping for long-standing verbal formulations, groping for original rhetorical powers to meet the challenge. It is no surprise, then, that many literary responses have been inadequate: formally repetitive or rhetorically hyperbolic. Still, some writers have succeeded in finding new structures of understanding and apt verbal equivalents to describe the crisis.

In 1969, after long-repressed tensions broke to the surface in Belfast, Seamus Heaney realized that "the problems of poetry moved from being simply a matter of achieving the satisfactory verbal icon to being a search for images and symbols adequate to our predicament."[9] So, too, have writers begun to search for images and symbols, metaphors of understanding, to do justice to AIDS, the "distinguished thing" that has become a plague of our time.

In the age of AIDS, a sense of *before* pervades the collective consciousness. In *Safe Sex,* a play by Harvey Fierstein, a character says, "'Now' will always define us. Different times. Too late. At last we have Safe Sex."[10] For those who came of age before the 1960s, the period of sexual liberation had been a long time coming. As Philip Larkin wittily put it in "Annus Mirabilis,"

> Sexual intercourse began
> In nineteen sixty-three
> (Which was rather late for me) —
> Between the end of the *Chatterly* ban
> And the Beatles' first LP.[11]

By the 1980s, that go-with-the-feeling period seemed distant, even innocent, like fading pictures of those confident, stoned young men and women making love in the mud of Woodstock or those other eager young men, out of the closet, fresh from provinces of the republic and finding sex in the bathhouses of San Francisco or Manhattan. A *triste* of nostalgia for lost splendor in the grass characterizes much of the literature of love and sex in our day. This tone of poignant recollection is similar to Larkin's regretful look back at the young men who marched off to certain death in 1914: "Never such innocence again."[12] Remembrance sweetens the imagination. Randy Shilts, writing on the AIDS crisis in *And the Band Played On,* puts it this way:

> Before. It was the word that would define the permanent demarcation in the lives of millions of Americans, particularly those citizens of the United States who were gay. There was life after the epidemic. And there were fond recollections of the times before. Before and after. The epidemic would cleave lives in two, the way a great war or depression presents a commonly understood point of reference around which an entire society defines itself. Before would encompass thousands of memories laden with nuance and nostalgia. Before meant innocence and excess, idealism and hubris. More than anything, this was the time before death. . . . Nothing would ever be the same again.[13]

Good-bye to All That, the title of Robert Graves's at once nostalgic and ironic memoir of World War I, might well serve as a description of much of the literature of the 1980s, particularly that literature which responds to AIDS, most of which emerges from or describes the male homosexual community.

However, some fiction about male homosexuality avoided the AIDS issue by focusing upon matters of recognition and roles, particularly within the American family. David Leavitt's novel, *The Lost Language of Cranes,* for example, represents a movement into mainstream publication and acceptance of literature about male homosexuals: father and son confront their gay identities within a traditional family structure in a pre-AIDS era. [14]Leavitt places homosexuality at the heart of the American family, but he does not deal with the divisive effects of AIDS. Paradoxically, AIDS would, for some, enlarge the concept of family.

Though plays and novels that are directly about AIDS lend themselves less easily to such happy endings — for the AIDS victim always dies — even in this genre heterosexual harmony is sometimes reaffirmed. In *Intimate Contact,* an English drama presented on cable television in the United States, a husband contracts AIDS — "the big one, the really big one," as his friend calls it — from a prostitute. However, the wife figure, Ruth, who represents the response of uninfected citizens, is the center of the drama, which traces her evolution from outrage to involvement in AIDS education; eventually, she enlists in the struggle against the disease that has infected her wayward husband.[15] In the popular literature of the AIDS era, terror of transmission of the disease through sexual contact sometimes teaches heterosexual couples that there is good in the old, monogamous ways. More subtle works convey more complex messages.

At the same time, the mass media was trying to have it both ways. Men and women, seized by sudden lust, still strip-searched each other with reckless abandon on movie and television screens. Quick, down-and-dirty sex still had its appeal, for, as A. M. Rosenthal put it, "AIDS is a lousy love story." Hollywood and television were reluctant to surrender their hot-to-trot stereotypes.[16]

For all that, in 1987 other popular and serious dramas and fictions reflected a gradual realization that AIDS had changed the artistic landscape of imagination: significantly, if not utterly. Even formerly randy James Bond is now monogamous in the latest film about this fantasy figure, *The Living Daylights.* Sgt. Christine Cagney, who frequently slept around in the television series *Cagney and Lacey,* was off sex in the new season until the program's creators could figure out what to do with her. "For the first time in the history of the show, I am stymied," said its executive producer, Barney Rosenzweig.[17]

Others were undaunted by the challenge. CBS presented a docudrama, *An Enemy Among Us,* and ABC has an After School Special planned. Soap-opera creator Agnes Nixon promised cautionary story lines on AIDS in her serial *All My Children.*[18] In prime time, condoms, which until recently were a taboo item on television, were freely and righteously passed around, to prevent disease. In the late 1970s, Dan Wakefield, creator and story consultant for the television series *James at 15,* quit the show when network censors cut out his euphemism for the word "condom." Wakefield had wanted James to say he should be "responsible," but NBC wanted no reference to birth control devices. AIDS has changed all that. "It took AIDS to free up information on birth control," said Peggy Charren, president of Action for Children's Television.[19] "These are the concerns real people are having," said Terry Louise Fischer, co-creator of the NBC *L.A. Law* series, "and to ignore that on a socially conscientious show just wouldn't wash."[20]

The deaths in 1987 of director and choreographer Michael Bennett, who created *A Chorus Line,* and off-Broadway innovator Charles Ludlam, who founded the Ridiculous Theatrical Company — both men died at age forty-four — symbolized the devastation of AIDS-related deaths in the theatrical world. In a column in the *New York Times,* Fran Lebowitz offered a dozen illustrations under the general heading "The Impact of AIDS on the Artistic Community." In one epiphany of mortality, she recalls a telling moment when she was on the phone with a friend, trying to make plans to leave town; flipping through her appointment book, she heard herself saying, "Well, I have a funeral on Tuesday, lunch with my editor on Wednesday, a memorial service on Thursday, so I guess I could come on Friday, unless, of course, Robert dies."[21]

If he had AIDS, Robert, sooner or later, would surely die. AIDS, a fatal disease with no cure, an expanding epidemic, strained the imagination. In late 1987 it was estimated that there were nearly fifty thousand AIDS cases in the United States, with almost half of the victims already dead.[22] However, as staggering as those figures were, the uncertainty of the extent or prospects of AIDS infection was even more frightening. Surgeon General C. Everett Koop said he did not know how many were infected: it could be anywhere between 1 and 4 million! "Those estimates are based on very shaky evidence," Koop said. "We just don't know." Nor could the extent of AIDS be forecast with any accuracy. Health

Commissioner Stephen C. Joseph of New York City said, "The hardest thing for the public, for all of us, is that we desperately want certainty. But there just is no certainty on most of these issues, except that we face an enormous toll of illness and death."[23] Mystery intensified anxiety.

Faced with the unknowable, responsible commentators reached for analogies to awe. In a guest column written for newspapers that served his constituents, Rep. Chet Atkins (D–Mass.) took his text from Albert Camus's novel *The Plague.* "There have been as many plagues as wars in history," wrote Camus, "yet always plagues and wars take people equally by surprise." Then Atkins, as have many other writers on AIDS, invoked the Black Death of the fourteenth century, which killed a quarter of Europe's people; the smallpox outbreak in the eighteenth century, which killed some 400,000 Europeans; the influenza epidemic of 1917–18, which killed 20 million; and other modern scourges caused by typhus and polio.[24] Stephen Jay Gould, in an essay on the "ordinary natural phenomenon" of epidemics, went for The Big One in shaping an analogy adequate to the occasion of AIDS: "The AIDS pandemic, an issue that may rank with nuclear weaponry as the greatest danger of our era, provides a more striking proof that mind and technology are not omnipotent and that we have not canceled our bond to nature."[25]

Like the Great Depression in 1930 or the Vietnam War in 1968, AIDS was moving to the center of the national consciousness in 1987. In such a context, passages from William H. McNeill's *Plagues and Peoples* are instructive, in that they remind us of the pattern of plagues which has shaped human history, particularly "when an unfamiliar infection attacks a population for the first time. . . . The Black Death of the fourteenth century was the chief example of this phenomenon, and the cholera epidemics of the nineteenth century constitute a second, far less destructive, but more recent and better-documented instance."[26] So, too, would AIDS stir debate over proper artistic response.

During the economic depression of the 1930s, literary figures debated art and politics with vigor. Commenting on one of these spats, between novelist Thornton Wilder and Mike Gold, editor of the *Daily Worker,* Edmund Wilson wrote, "It has now become clear that the economic crisis is to be accompanied by a literary one."[27] That is, Wilson implied, literary values are shaped by cultural crisis.

During the early days of World War I, Henry James struggled to come to terms with the horror of European warfare. Though he had long had what he described as an "imagination of disaster," nevertheless he was astounded by the surprise of warfare on such a vast scale. Looking across the Channel from Rye toward France, James wrote to an old friend in August of 1914,

> Black and hideous to me is the tragedy that gathers, and I'm sick beyond cure to have lived to see it. You and I, the ornament of our generation, should have been spared this wreck of our belief that through the long years we had seen civilization grow and the worst become impossible. The tide that bore us along was then all the while moving to *this* as its grand Niagara — yet what a blessing we didn't know it. It seems to me to *undo* everything, everything that was ours, in the most horrible retroactive way — but I avert my face from the monstrous scene. . . . The country and the season here are of a beauty of peace, and liveliness of light, and summer grace, that make it inconceivable that just across the Channel, blue as *paint* today, the fields of France and Belgium are being, or about to be, given up to unthinkable massacre and misery.[28]

This luminous passage shows James simultaneously realizing and articulating the shock of the new.

In *The Great War and Modern Memory,* his study of the writers of World War I, Paul Fussell suggests that the realization of disaster had the effect of substituting irony for grand rhetoric. That is, the war crisis was accompanied by shifts of concern and emphasis for writers. Writers of that era tried, like James, to avert their gaze from the monstrous scene, to retreat into conventional literary formulation. Fussell: "The point is this: finding the war 'indescribable' in any but the available language of traditional literature, those who recalled it had to do so in known literary terms."[29] Writers saw what they were coded to see and described what they saw and thought they understood in conventional language and familiar forms. However, as time passed and realization deepened, other writers came to terms with the conceptual and aesthetic implications of the Great War. "Thus the drift of modern history domesticates the fantastic and normalizes the unspeakable. And the catastrophe that begins it is the Great War."[30] Eventually the dominant mode of understanding becomes *irony.*[31] The literature of AIDS has ranged from irony to sentimentality, from realism to fabulation, from redundancy to originality.

Gradually, the belletristic writing on AIDS has come to terms with the cultural and literary implications of the disease. The sudden appearance of AIDS challenges the abilities of our imaginations to *know.* Writers in various fields and forms have registered their surprise in many ways. The literature of the AIDS era is high-minded, didactic, and direct, though also often comic. This literature documents and articulates a major shift of consciousness which accompanies the disease. Much of the writing that responds to AIDS, literature that describes its effects upon the male homosexual community, is raw, unpolished, angry, contentious, as though shouting might break through the walls of ignorance and indifference surrounding the affected. As we might expect from writings on such a horrific topic, much of the fiction on AIDS presents simple characterizations, types who embody positions in didactic designs, and predictable themes: insistence that attention must be paid to AIDS victims, for we are all, directly or indirectly, AIDS victims. (Many writers urge the use of the more oblique description "person with AIDS," but there is no way to deflect the power of AIDS to create victims.) Many works of fiction on AIDS have the feel of thinly disguised autobiographical testimonies: cries in the gathering darkness. No doubt, in time, given the projected progress of the disease and the growing sophistication of those who seek to translate its implications into art, we will have a distinguished literature on the topic, as we have, say, on the Holocaust. There is yet, however, no work of fiction on AIDS to match Leslie Epstein's novel on the Holocaust, *King of the Jews* (1979), a work that mixes modes, comic and tragic, that deals with personal and ethnic identity — what is a Jew? — in complex and subtle ways, a novel that is sustained by a fully articulated sense of irony.

The best literature on AIDS is found in the theater, for several reasons. Not only has the world of the theater been shaken by the disease, but the theater has long been the proper medium to bear bad tidings in artful designs to affected communities in times of crisis. As the early Abbey Theatre sought to raise Irish consciousness and mobilize its energies; as the Group Theater sought to articulate Depression grievances before audiences of the grieved; so too does AIDS theater seek, sometimes in wonderfully inventive fashions, to shock its audiences with the recognition of its human bond with those stage characters who suffer and find symbolic triumphs over AIDS. However, worthy works on AIDS appear, with increasing frequency, in a variety of other forms: journalism, poetry, and fiction.

In the midst of crises — wars and other disasters, natural and man-made — the documentary impulse is strong. One of the most insightful records of the effects of AIDS upon the male homosexual community can be found in Frances FitzGerald's *Cities on a Hill.* Her book examines several utopian or visionary subcultures in America, ranging from Florida's Sun City to Jerry Falwell's Liberty Baptist Church in Lynchburg, Virginia. Her study of the gay male community focuses on the Castro, an area of San Francisco where, in the mid-1970s, homosexual men established their own cultural identity, and where they eventually, in the 1980s, saw their lives and community divide under the threat of plague. FitzGerald approaches her subject with the eye of a cultural anthropologist, aware of the shifts in values and alterations of sensibilities which accompany this decade of change. Men had traveled far, geographically and personally, to come into their own sexual identities — which often meant sexual promiscuity in the Castro's gay bars and bathhouses — only to discover that they had to adapt to a scourge that challenged their personal and community existences. Suddenly, "the Castro became a city of moral dramas — dramas that involved not only the victims but their lovers, their parents, and their friends." The Castro, then, became an allegorical landscape; its citizens were passionate pilgrims who had to confront the new implications of their actions.

> In the Castro those who had spent a good part of their lives in the struggle against the sexual taboo now had to acknowledge that the sexual liberation they had fought for so strenuously — and on which they had laid their claims of being the avant-garde of a national revolution — had deadly consequences. What was more, they had to face the fact that they were giving the disease to one another.[32]

Life in the Castro changed when its residents acknowledged this *memento mori* in their midst. It is estimated that between 1981 and 1987, 2,030 people, almost all of them gay men, died in San Francisco, nearly 10 percent of the nation's AIDS fatalities.[33] After much intense debate, the baths, and many other establishments that catered to homosexual men, closed; their former patrons were dead, had fled, or were chastened. A report in the *New York Times* cites a young man, on Castro Street, holding a gay newspaper: "It's full of obituaries for people you know and ads for mortuaries, crematoriums and lawyers who warn you to write a will. I'm weary of grieving."[34] At the same time, others in the Castro community were made tougher, more resilient, and more humane by the presence of death in their midst.

By far the most comprehensive and moving work of journalism on the AIDS crisis, Randy Shilts's *And the Band Played On* is driven by similar impulses of grief, protest, and the celebration of courage and heroism among those who fought the good "fight for acceptance and equality, against ignorance and fear," first in establishing a gay male community and later in protesting that the Reagan administration and state and local agencies were criminally negligent in dealing with the killing disease.[35] Where FitzGerald had placed the life and death cycle in the Castro in the context of other fringe communities in American culture, Shilts's massive and impassioned book, which catalogues nearly a decade of the growth of the disease and the recognition of its threat, establishes AIDS and its implications at the heart and soul of American life.

Shilts structures *And the Band Played On* on a time line of ever increasing dramatic occasions; ironic juxtaposition sets the AIDS crisis in relation to major public events in American life. For example, at the bicentennial celebration in New York City, in 1976, tall ships from fifty-five nations brought sailors, some of whom may have been carrying the AIDS virus, to America. In November 1984, Ronald Reagan, who had never spoken out on AIDS, was reelected president, an occasion upon which Shilts casts a cold eye. "When claiming victory on election night, President Reagan told a cheering crowd, 'America's best days lie ahead.' It was during the month of Reagan's reelection that the nation's AIDS caseload surpassed 7,000."[36] Shilts notes that by the time Reagan tentatively spoke out on AIDS, in mid-1987, 36,058 Americans had been diagnosed with the disease and 20,849 had died.[37] The two Americas portrayed in *Band* — Reagan's myth of morning in America and the dark night of the soul created by AIDS — are traced in lines that, eventually, converge.

And the Band Played On is at once a chronicle — jump-cuts intersect moments of medical research, political in-fighting, and case histories of those affected — and a polemic, a work of vivid advocacy journalism, an indictment of national bigotry. Shilts details the various ways in which Americans respond to what some of them ironically call "gay cancer."[38] Some showed a stunning insensitivity. For example, columnist and former Nixon adviser Patrick Buchanan, in 1983, thought the diseased got what they deserve. "The sexual revolution has begun to devour its children," wrote Buchanan. "And among the revolutionary vanguard, the Gay Rights activists, the mortality rate is highest and climbing. . . . The poor homosexuals — they have declared war upon nature, and now nature is exacting an awful retribution."[39] Most politicians, particularly in New York and Washington, tried to ignore the problem, until the news of Rock Hudson's illness, in 1985, drew public attention and shifted sympathies sufficiently to make AIDS a safe topic for political discourse. Throughout the crisis, medical institutions reacted with confusion, denial, territorial bickering, and occasional courage. People continued to die, mystified, terrified, often bravely, sometimes ignobly. Particularly fascinating is Shilts's tracing of the florid sexual career and finally horrid death of Gaetan Dugas, an airline steward from Canada, who was one of the first North Americans diagnosed with AIDS. Knowing he was infected, Dugas continued coupling in bathhouses; after sex he would taunt his partners, telling them they too would surely die. After sexual encounters, Dugas would turn on the lights, point to the purple lesions on his chest, then say to his shocked lover, "Gay cancer. Maybe you'll get it too."[40] Poe's gothic story "The Masque of the Red Death" had turned real.

> There's no doubt that Gaetan played a key role in spreading the new virus from one end of the United States to the other. The bathhouse controversy, peaking so dramatically in San Francisco on the morning of his death [March 30, 1984], was also linked directly to Gaetan's own exploits in those sex palaces and his recalcitrance in changing his ways. At one time, Gaetan had been what every man wanted from gay life; by the time he died, he had become what every man feared.[41]

Yet Shilts celebrates more than he denigrates. Particular praise is reserved for social activists. Shilts praises Cleve Jones, famous for his memorial marches in San Francisco in memory of Harvey Milk, member of the city's Board of Supervisors and gay rights activist, and George Moscone, the city's mayor — both of whom had been killed by a deranged politician; later, Jones founded the Kaposi's Sarcoma Research and Education Foundation. Shilts also praises Larry Kramer, writer and organizer of Gay Men's Health Crisis in New York City. It was Kramer's article in March 1983, "1,112 and Counting," argues Shilts, which "irrevocably altered the context in which AIDS was discussed in the gay community and, hence, in the nation."[42] Kramer attacked the medical community, especially the Centers for Disease Control, for its hesitancy; the political community, particularly Mayor Ed Koch of New York, for its callous disregard; and the gay male community, for its refusal to change its ways: "Unless we fight for our lives we shall die. In all the history of homosexuality we have never been so close to death and extinction before. Many of us are dying or dead already."[43]

When the novelists and playwrights examined those who suffer, directly or obliquely, from AIDS, they too found enormous strengths. Occasionally these writers match and surpass, in fiction, poetry, or drama, the level of conviction and sense of crisis achieved in documentaries. Whatever the form, some writers who emerge from the gay male community to tell the story of AIDS have the authenticity and the passion of some Holocaust testimony, from Anne Frank to Elie Wiesel. "I had the energy to do my book because I'm gay," Randy Shilts told *Newsweek.* "AIDS wasn't somebody else's problem. I live every day with the knowledge that friends will be dead in five years. I had to write the book, or go crazy."[44]

Larry Kramer was goaded by the epidemic to move from form to form until he discovered the best way to portray and convey its pain and importance. His novel of male homosexual life in New York City and Fire Island in the 1970s, *Faggots,* had stirred attention for its graphic description and its theme: that the lives of these men centered too much on sex and too little on love. As we have seen, Kramer turned to polemical journalism and political organization in response to the AIDS crisis in the early 1980s. Having exhausted himself and his effectiveness in those forms, he had an epiphany of renewed mission in a visit to Dachau, in 1983. There, he was impressed that the camp had been opened as early as 1933. "They were killing Jews, Catholics, and gays for eight years and nobody did a thing."[45] Suddenly, Kramer knew what he had to do, so he returned to the United States and wrote a play, *City of Death,* about the AIDS epidemic in New York City in the early 1980s, a play that he eventually titled *The Normal Heart.*[46]

This play, which had its premier in New York City at the Public Theater in April 1985, brought the AIDS crisis to community attention and translated its tensions into dramatic terms with clarifying insistence. The elaborate, alarmist set for *The Normal Heart* made Kramer's point as effectively as its language. A wall count of AIDS cases was displayed, the number of the dead updated during performances. Another wall graphic cited options American Jews had during World War II: to fight government indifference to the Nazi camps openly or to work secretly from within. The play insists that it is futile to try to work from within a system that tolerates genocide. Another wall graphic showed a list of names in the manner of the Vietnam Memorial in Washington. Stage setting, then, places the AIDS crisis within the larger context of our era's many victims.

People were affected by Kramer's play, as perhaps only a theater audience can be, for drama, at its best, involves audiences in an ancient ritual of recognition and purgation. In the theater, if not in life, we occasionally transcend differences, feel joined as a group. The play was widely praised: one critic said it did for the AIDS epidemic what Arthur Miller's *The Crucible* did for the McCarthy scare of the early 1950s.[47] The comparison is apt, for Kramer, like Miller, dramatizes an era of social crisis in documentary fashion, with arias of prose-poetry inserted for moments and messages of heightened effects. Miller's brotherhood theme in *All My Sons* is repeated in an exchange between Ned, the play's gay protagonist who resembles Kramer, and Ned's brother, Ben, who has never been able to accept Ned's homosexuality.

Ben.	My agreeing you were born just like I was born is not going to help save your dying friends.
Ned.	Funny — that's exactly what I think will help save my dying friends.[48]

Finally, Ben does accept Ned as he is; Ben even attends a pseudo-wedding, performed by Dr. Emma Brookner, an AIDS researcher, between Ned and his lover, Felix, who is dying of AIDS. In the play, Ned separates from Mickey, who represents erotic celebration, to care for Felix, who represents one effect of that style of open sexuality. Kramer's point: that gay men should leave bathhouse encounters, where they use each other's bodies, and learn to care for each other.

Mickey.	What are you, a closet straight?
Ned.	Mickey, more sex isn't more liberating. And having so much sex makes finding love impossible.[49]

The Normal Heart seeks to shock its audience into an understanding of AIDS: politicians (particularly Mayor Koch) are excoriated for inaction; gay male leaders are criticized for pushing liberation instead of politicking for the right to marry; and the straight audience is shamed for its detachment from those who are affected. Kramer, like the Clifford Odets of *Waiting for Lefty,* breaks through the barrier between drama and audience when he has Dr. Brookner deliver an impassioned monologue to an invisible doctor, in the audience. She, like Kramer, is addressing us. "We are enduring an epidemic of death," she says.[50] "Attention must be paid," she might insist, as did Linda Loman in Miller's *Death of a Salesman.* Linda was speaking of Willy Loman, but her words effectively address the cautionary themes of the literature surrounding AIDS. "He's not to be allowed to fall into his grave like an old dog. Attention, attention must be finally paid to such a person."[51] Larry Kramer conveys a similar message, though he has not yet achieved the authority of Miller's language and the imaginative power of Miller's dramatic structure.

The AIDS epidemic increasingly is a challenge to the imagination's capacity to make credible its threats. Reporters found it hard to conceive; in a series on AIDS in the *Boston Globe,* for example, Judy Foreman said this:

> If an enemy of humankind had set out to design the most terrifying, insidious biological agent imaginable, he could hardly have done better — or worse — than the AIDS virus.[52]

Some creative writers were driven to construct horrific visions of a plague-ridden, fascist future; others, as we see, were driven to drama by the memories of historical horrors.

William M. Hoffman's play, *As Is,* opened at the Lyceum Theater in May 1985. Hoffman, like Kramer and so many others who seek to understand and articulate into art the AIDS crisis, used the Holocaust as an apt analogy.

> I knew intellectually that the epidemic was *not* the Holocaust, but I had no other experience of mass death and public indifference and brutality to compare it with.[53]

Dramatically far more adventurous than Kramer's *Heart,* Hoffman's *As Is* sets out to break the psychic barrier of the proscenium arch, which safely separates audience from the onstage drama. As Marshall W. Mason explains in the Production Note to *As Is,* actors remain onstage throughout the performance in choral testimony, to witness as a community the events of the play in which they do not participate as characters. The audience must not be kept from feeling "safe" from this subject, so the actors of the "chorus" must act as a bridge between the fictional characters and the real theater events, and also as an unconventional kind of "threat" — keeping the audience aware that entertaining as the play may be, the subject is deadly. The desired effect is to assist the audience in a catharsis, as they are required to contemplate our common mortality.[54]

As Is, then, is an exemplum: it illustrates a moral point. The audience here too bears witness so that we may acknowledge our common humanity with the suffering stage characters. As in *The Normal Heart, As Is* presents a straight man who overcomes his repugnance and hugs his gay brother. As in *The Normal Heart, As Is* presents an extended monologue, by a hospice worker, who stresses the courage and style of a dying AIDS victim who affirms his diminishing life by having his nails painted.

As that anecdote illustrates, Hoffman is sly in conveying his message, while Kramer is blunt. *As Is* uses all the resources of the modern theater — quick shifts of scene, tone and time shifts, lighting, character ambiguity — to make its point: artfulness is affirmation of the spirit in a time of crisis.

Above all, Hoffman draws us into his play and elicits our sympathy through humor. A TV announcer gives exposition on the disease, then Clone 1 and Clone 2 enact gay male dating bar rites that ignore AIDS:

Clone 2. Thought you were this guy Chip I met here on Jockstrap Night.
Clone 1. Haven't been here since the Slave Auction.[55]

A black humor sustains the courage of his characters, who reveal a jaunty elan in the face of death. Saul, who is standing by his afflicted lover, Rich, finds another common analogy for AIDS, but gives it his own wry twist:

I feel the disease closing in on me. All my activities are life and death. . . . [Bars and clubs] remind me of accounts of Europe during the Black Plague: coupling in the dark, dancing till you drop. The New Wave is the corpse look.[56]

Unlike Kramer, Hoffman includes a strain of nostalgia for the days of open sexual expression. Perhaps the diaries of British playwright Joe Orton, which revel in sleaze, inspired this ironic reflection by Rich: "God how I love sleaze: the whining self-pity of a rainy Monday night in a leather bar in early spring. . . . God, how I miss it."[57]

Such passages qualify the sentimentality that is always built into the situation of early death. Rather than put off the general audience, such recollections of lost days of lust authenticate and humanize characters who are caught in a lethal fate that tests their capacities to love before it kills them. Hoffman validates his audience's need to express grief and gives voice to their desire to deflect that grief through laughter.

Harvey Fierstein's play *Safe Sex* dramatizes the AIDS crisis with rare wit and imagination. Two young men, Ghee and Mead, teeter on opposite ends of a giant seesaw, discussing their relationship. Mead accuses Ghee of using AIDS to withdraw from commitment: "You're not scared of AIDS, you're scared of sex."[58] Ghee takes a larger view, noting the shift in consciousness that has taken place in the public attitude toward homosexuals ("We were Gay. Now we're human."), yet mourning the old days of reckless passion: "We can never touch as before. We can never be as before."[59] In *Safe Sex,* which premiered in January 1987 at the La Mama ETC, in the East Village, Fierstein caught a moment with the quick clarity of a Walker Evans photograph. As he said in his preface to three one-act plays, "So new is the world from which I address you that nothing in these plays can be assumed common knowledge. So new is the concept of safe or unsafe sex that I still can't accept its reality. I believe these plays have a great deal to say about who and what we are."[60] After the premier of *Safe Sex, New York Times* theater critic Frank Rich agreed: "At La Mama, the theater had become a temple again, offering the temporary illusion — and, with AIDS, it is most definitely an illusion — that there's at least some safety in numbers."[61]

Kramer's *Heart,* Hoffman's *As Is,* and Fierstein's *Safe Sex* (all published plays) present different strategies for responding, humanly and theatrically, to the AIDS crisis. Many more AIDS plays have been produced, particularly in New York. On Broadway, Stuart Spencer's *Last Outpost at the End of the World* portrays AIDS and its multiple effects. Off Broadway, Robert Chesley's *Jerker, or the Helping Hand* dramatized the safest sex, while Alan Browne's *Beiruit* portrayed the effect of AIDS on heterosexuals. In a *New York Times* article on these plays, Don Shewey concludes,

> These plays are significant in that they assert the theater's ancient function as a public forum in which a community gathers to talk about itself. What's happening onstage and what's happening in the audience is sometimes so similar that the script seems to disappear.[62]

Poetry on AIDS tends to be traditional in form and moral in intent: direct and didactic. Robert Boucheron, in *Epitaphs for the Plague Dead,* invokes Tennyson's *In Memoriam* as his model. Boucheron draws his technique — testimonies from those killed by AIDS — from Edgar Lee Master's *Spoon River Anthology,* Thornton Wilder's *Our Town,* and A. E. Housman's *A Shropshire Lad,* works by writers who also composed epitaphs as dramatic monologues. Boucheron's volume, however, owes more in form than in achievement to those predecessors. Rather than devise a new form to fit this new threat to our health and consciousness, Boucheron has forced a contemporary horror into the rigidities of Victorian verse, all the better to instruct. Still, some of his poems convey the shock of sudden awareness of the threatening ways of this plague, as in "Epitaph for an Innocent":

> I got it from my mother's breasts,
> unknowing, as an infant sips.
> She got it from my father's lips,
> conceiving in my interest.
>
> He got it lying still in bed,
> his arm connected to a sack
> that, as a hemophiliac,
> he needed any time he bled.
>
> A small, unhappy family,
> we shared more than a common cold.
> For my part, the sum is soon told:
> nine months I lived, dying in three.[63]

In another collection of AIDS poetry, *An Intimate Desire to Survive,* Bill Becker keeps a diary in poetic form during the eighteen months in which he suspected he had contracted AIDS. Both poets obey a documentary impulse: Boucheron moves through a range of characters for his AIDS chronicle, while Becker moves through time. Becker, too, dramatizes the plight of the victim who cannot imagine what has happened to him. Like Job,

Becker asks, "Why me?"[64] However, Becker poses his questions and finds his working metaphors in more original poetic forms, which, in turn, convey more complex impressions, as does this entry of choppy lines and patterned associations which records the disease cycle, "5 Feb 85":

The body collapses
into itself
Structured demolition
surface unseen
Candid eruption
doing havoc on nerve
Nuclear fission
on a human scale —

Cellular chain reaction
An immunity implosion
Self interest
Self pity
Schizophrenic optimism
Relapse — [65]

Poetry in the AIDS crisis is commemorative and dedicatory, written in memoriam. It is the verbal equivalent of the "performance art" emblem displayed at the October 1987 gay rights march on Washington: a giant quilt, composed of three-by-six-foot, hand-made panels, each containing the name of a person who had died of AIDS. More than two thousand names were recorded, from forty-eight states and five nations, on the Names Project, which covered an area equal to two football fields.[66] Like the Vietnam Memorial wall nearby, this quilt recorded and preserved in artful arrangement the names of victims of a war few wanted to fight. The Vietnam War, however, is over, its body count complete, while the number of AIDS crisis victims is still climbing. Some poets have enlisted in the war against AIDS.

Fiction on AIDS can be loosely grouped in two categories: first, horrific cautionary tales of fascist responses to the AIDS crisis: dystopias, in the manner of *1984,* in which writers posit scenarios of massive retaliation against homosexuals by a society — set some time in the near future, or in the reconfigured immediate past — which seeks a Final Solution to the plague; second, documentary, largely autobiographical records of case histories of persons with AIDS, along with the ramifications of the disease for the victim's immediate family and loved ones. In *Plagues and People,* William H. McNeill makes the distinction between external and internal threats to man's survival: "One can properly think of most human lives as caught in a precarious equilibrium between the microparasitism of disease organisms and the macroparasitism of large-bodied predators, chief among which have been other human beings."[67] The social and science fiction fantasies on AIDS move from lethal microparasites, fostered by the AIDS virus, to speculations upon the form of lethal macroparasites: those who seek the Final Solution against AIDS through elimination of its carriers.

The AIDS crisis has stirred fears — paranoia, unfounded hysteria, justly founded anxieties — in the male homosexual community over social isolation and retaliation. Testing for AIDS was advocated by the Reagan administration; some police wore masks in the presence of male homosexuals; and a Florida boy with AIDS was assaulted, his family's house burned. Where will all this lead? Two novelists, Jed A. Bryan and Toby Johnson, fear they know.

Bryan's *A Cry in the Desert* imagines a "pogrom" against male homosexuals in Nevada, in the early 1980s, a genocide that began with AIDS testing.[68] It is an insistent example of message literature. As Bryan notes, in a brief preface, "the message is clear. AIDS is not a *gay plague.* It is a very real danger to us all."[69] The novel is driven and sustained by a sense of threat and betrayal. Its epigraph is from Luke (21:16), a passage that could serve as the epigraph for many illustrative works on the AIDS crisis.

> And ye shall be betrayed both by parents and brethren and kinfolk and friends; and some of you shall they cause to be put to death.[70]

Bryan construes Luke's text into a wild parable. Alfred Botts, himself a repressed homosexual, heads up Project ERAD (Emergency Research and Development), on two thousand acres of Nevada desert, near a nuclear plant, and works for a new Emergency Quarantine Act, under which he seizes homosexuals, then brings them to ERAD, where they undergo experiments, then are eliminated. Botts is aided by the Reverend Theophilis Stokeswood, a radio minister, who preaches on the scourge of God: AIDS as God's punishment against male homosexuals. Industrialist Kurt Stakl bankrolls Botts's research project, hoping to patent an AIDS cure through which he seeks world control! Arrayed against this powerful triumvirate are a few journalists, doctors, and others who are fighting for the rights of homosexual men. Incredibly, despite many lurid assaults — one homosexual man is nailed to a cross, another is dehydrated to death! — this group of citizens, working together, brings down Botts and his nefarious associates. *A Cry in the Desert* is a model of improbable fiction.

So too is Toby Johnson's *Plague: A Novel About Healing.*[71] Johnson, a psychotherapist who has worked with AIDS victims and has sought to educate the public about preventive measures, contrives an equally unlikely, melodramatic parable of warning. Like Bryan, Johnson sees his fantastic story — the planned use of nuclear weapons against AIDS carriers — as reasonable. "The projections for the resolution of the plague that haunts us in 1987 are reasonable extrapolations of current medical fact."[72] Set in "Early Autumn, in the Possible Near Future," *Plague* imagines evil men, Dr. Strangeloves and Dr. Frankensteins, who are repressed homosexuals; they manipulate the crisis, developing and withholding an AIDS antidote so that they can seize money and power. Arrayed, once again, against them are various high-minded gay males who struggle within encompassing plots. The AIDS crisis, in this dystopia, reveals the homophobic depths of American culture: "Curiously, at the very heart of this discussion was the notion that pinko-leaning homosexuals were undermining American morality."[73] AIDS, we are told, allows fag-bashing fascists to come out of the closet and do their damndest, though they, in turn, are done in by noble gay males and their fellow travelers. While all literature tends toward mythic reductions, these fictions tend toward the simplifications of comic strips.

Though one can easily understand the sense of psychic dread that motivates the writing of *A Cry in the Desert* and *Plague,* it is difficult to take them seriously as analyses or as predictive models. In both works, AIDS is seized upon to settle old scores — hostility to homosexual men comes from those who repress their own homosexual inclinations — and imagine fantastic political scenarios, in the manner of the suspense fiction of Robert Ludlum, Ken Follett, or Tom Clancy. But then, it might be argued, until recently AIDS itself would have seemed to most people an imaginative extravagance, a science fiction.

Jed A. Bryan and Toby Johnson have tried to think about the unthinkable in implausible but haunting fictions. Voices crying in the wilderness don't have perfect pitch!

It is as difficult to plot a plausible mystery on the AIDS topic as it is to contrive happy endings for an AIDS story, for the same reason: because persons with AIDS die. As soon as a lesion appears, sadly, we know the rest of the story. Some writers, as we have seen, shift readers' attentions to plots against homosexual men either by the disease itself or by those who want to gain wealth or power through their extinction. Other writers take the AIDS story head-on, without embellishment or imaginative contrivance. They resort to plain-style prose and accessible plots to bear witness to the devastation of AIDS. Either these writers are dying or their loved ones have died. Their books are records that implicate the reader in the victim's suffering and in the impact of the victim's suffering upon his lovers, his friends, and his family. Most of these autobiographical works avoid artful indirection: they make their claim for the victim's humanity with the blunt insistence of a heart's cry.

J. W. Money's *To All the Girls I've Loved Before* has the artless authenticity of dying words, for that is just what they are: brief, self-reflective essays written, during March 1986, while the author suffered high fevers that kept him up at night.[74] He wrote his entries on the bathroom floor to keep from disturbing his companion. This, then, is a version of prison literature, though the author was to be released from his sentence only by death. Many of Money's reflections — notes, memories, whimsies, farewell missives, and thank-you notes — are not on AIDS, but on music, fashion, people, and places he has loved. He thanks his mother for introducing him to opera; she died of cancer at age forty-three, the same age he would contract AIDS. He recalls his crushes on media stars: Bette Davis, Natalie Wood, and Joan Baez. He tries to construe his life as an allegory in a stiff, jingly poem about Prudence and Folly. He, of course, assumed the role of Folly, who "was last seen somewhere near the docks" with a sailor.[75] That is, he blames himself for AIDS, but defends his choices. "I have AIDS in part, because I was promiscuous. I'm not complaining: If God's punishing me, He's certainly allowed me to have a lot of pleasure." At that point, words fail Money and he invokes a sentimental song to speak for him: "Kiss the day goodbye, and I won't regret what I did for love."[76]

J. W. Money died in October 1986. His lover, who had stood vigil over him during his illness, died a few months later. All that remains is this fragmentary, flawed, but moving work, written in feverish conviction, when he knew that time was running out.

In *The World Can Break Your Heart,* Daniel Curzon tells the familiar story of a sensitive young man (Benjamin Vance) who grew up in a tough environment (Detroit), with a sense of his difference and a need to discover his own place in the wider world: "I'm gonna be a movie star like Sonja Henie!" declares the boy.[77] Though he is shamed by adults and Catholic clergy, Benjamin accepts his identity as a homosexual, then goes to Hollywood in search of fame. There he meets gay men who celebrate their sexuality: "Leave Detroit behind, sweetie," says one.[78] Benjamin learns to turn tricks, but, when one of his partners contracts AIDS, Benjamin quickly grows up; he learns love and compassion. Here, as in other AIDS-related literature, the disease concentrates the mind upon Final Things and intensifies the humanity of those affected. As in Money's commitment to writing during his last days, Curzon's Benjamin affirms art over deteriorating life: "Life may be a 'long disease', as Hamlet said. But a work of art, I see now, is the cure!"[79]

Of course, this asks too much of art. In *The Renewal of Literature,* Richard Poirier questions the powers and responsibilities of literature to address the problem of culture. "Literature is a very restricted passage into life, if it is one at all."[80] At its best, said limited powers, *The World Can Break Your Heart* is not the best art: the novel seems hasty, episodic, undeveloped, with no detailed sense of its Detroit and Hollywood settings. In form, it is a conventional novel of coming out with the consciousness of AIDS tacked on, as Curzon's own words imply: he dedicates his novel "to all straight readers so that they will know what it felt like to grow up gay and for all gay people so they won't forget."[81] Still, this novel follows the pattern of direct appeal for the sad plight of those who struggle to accept and have accepted their sexual identities only to discover that their lives are threatened by AIDS. These writers are correct in insisting that this story must be told and told again, whatever the effects or achievements of their art. Fiction, too, as Auden said of poetry, "survives in the valley of its saying."[82]

Paul Reed's *Facing It: A Novel of AIDS* is a romance of sorts, with a love story in the foreground and AIDS looming in the background. In the summer of 1981, Andy Stone, a handsome young worker for gay rights in Manhattan, grows ill. His macho father rejects his dying, homosexual son. Andy finds support from his elected, gay male "family." His lover, David, is ennobled through suffering. A writer for various gay presses, David had been "waiting for something to write about, something worth the effort; he knew inspiration would hit him in time."[83] Andy's illness and the wider threat of AIDS give David a worthy personal mission and a significant public topic for his writing. He investigates the AIDS disease, in search of explanations. David finds some dedication in the medical profession but also uncovers much callousness — "Fags are big news nowadays, and dead ones are even better news," says one calculating researcher — and evil.[84] As in *A Cry in the Desert* and *Plague,* the villain in *Facing It* is a closet homosexual man. Dr. Arthur Maguire won't release funds for the dedicated Dr. Branch's research: "What with the homosexual element and all — well, it's all delicate and avoidable," says Maguire.[85] It turns out that obese Maguire had been Kinder-Mann's lover in medical school, that he had used a woman, Carolyn, who later became Branch's rich wife, as his cover. However, now Carolyn threatens Maguire with exposure if he does not release funds. That is, the novel descends to soap opera villainy and intrigue to make its point. In *Facing It,* the AIDS crisis renews the bonding not only of gay male lovers but of this married couple. Like every other work in the genre, this novel sets out to raise the consciousness of its readers and to renew the covenant between gay men, even in the face of AIDS. The disease is, it seems, a great teacher as well as a great killer.

The most subtle and moving fiction on AIDS that I have read appears in George Stambolian's anthology *Men on Men: Best New Gay Fiction.*[86] Despite its flaunting title, many stories in this anthology do more than celebrate coming-out parties for young men, though that pattern appears. As Stambolian notes, AIDS-era fiction is likely to be even more controversial, particularly descriptions of sexual practices. "This situation partly explains why many stories involving erotically unrestrained behavior are now habitually set in the years preceding the advent of AIDS."[87] It is the turn away from scenes of explicit sexuality and the turn toward mature and eloquent confrontation with disease, death, and the effects of death upon the living which distinguish these stories. Paradoxically, but justly, as the gay male community suffers its Holocaust, its fiction has increasingly been accepted by mainstream publishers and readers. Gay male literature has gone past the stage of either justifying itself to American straight culture or shocking the bourgeoisie; rather, at its best, it portrays characters who are confronting the meaning of their lives and the mystery of death.

John Fox's "Choice" is a poignant tale of a gay antihero, Jimmy Abooz, who suppresses his lusts out of the fear of AIDS, though his caution has so far protected him and given him a wry humor. "He doesn't know a single person with AIDS and hopes he never does. . . . The previous summer he wore shorts almost every day to show off his lesion-free legs."[88] Still, he does not know which way to turn. He still does not get along with his family, though they drink chi-chis (piña coladas with vodka) together during a dreary Christmas day. Jimmy, weary of his family, afraid of sexual encounters, stays in his room, alone. "He decided to start saving for a video-cassette player so he could watch porn videos in the privacy of his own home."[89] Fox catches the AIDS-era state of personal paralysis: isolation and masturbation.

The central character in Edmund White's "An Oracle" resists changing his life. Though he has buried his lover, Ray feels "dying would be easier than figuring out a new way of living."[90] In Greece, Ray reads Homer, weeps over Achilles' death, and confronts his own fragile mortality. "He thought it very likely that he was carrying death inside him, that it was ticking inside him like a time bomb but one he couldn't find because it had been secreted by an unknown terrorist."[91] Still, he cannot keep his hands off a local boy. However, no longer able to see other men as sex objects, Ray falls in love with the Greek boy, who, wary of involvement, rejects him. The old wanton ways of Ray's gay days are long gone.

In Andrew Holleran's fine story "Friends at Evening," mourners gather for the funeral of Louis, an AIDS victim. Louis is a symbolic figure who stands for all the friends and lovers they have lost. Unlike Clifford Odets's Lefty or Samuel Beckett's Godot, chimeras of hope and rescue, Holleran's Louis presents only an occasion for mourning. The narrator gathers Louis's friends for the occasion. One cites Walt Whitman: "It is enough to be with friends at evening."[92]

The gathering turns into an extended elegy. "We're all going, in sequence, at different times. And will the last person please turn out the lights?" says one mourner.[93] Another, who refuses to detach his identity as a homosexual man from sexual practices, complains, "*The wrong people are dying.*"[94] The city has become a cemetery through which this group of sad men passes, like a funeral procession. "More Than You Know" serves as their plaintive theme song: "Oh how I'd die. Oh, how I'd cry, if you got tired and said good-bye."[95] Romance is gone. Yet their friendships are intensified and narrowed, their lives reaffirmed in their ceremonial mourning.

In Sam D'Allesandro's "Nothing Ever Just Disappears," a survivor grieves for his lost lover in similarly plaintive yet oddly affirming terms. "Someone said the pain would go away, but I'm not sure that's where I want it to go. It's how I feel him most sharply."[96] In Robert Ferro's "Second Son," a tough antiromantic note is struck when a son dying of AIDS wards off his father's bluff reassurances. "The bottom line is that there's no cure," the wise child tells his stunned father.[97] The wise children of AIDS have much to tell us all.

The literature of AIDS, then, is

- divided between conflicting impulses: realistic and antiromantic or satiric and fantastic;
- more concerned with death than sex, though nostalgic for the lost old days of wine and roses;

- family-centered, whether that means a reconciliation with the victim's biological family, the affirmation of one's elected family, or both: fellowship and family renewal in the face of death are the constant themes of these works;
- antibourgeois; evil and indifferent men from the social establishment exploit the crisis;
- self-reflective: these works raise questions about the nature, form, and substance of gay male literature and ask members of the male homosexual community to question what it means to be gay;
- committed to the proposition that most victims and their loved ones are ennobled through suffering;
- intensely, bleakly humorous; thoughtful, inward, plaintive, eloquent; often artless or excessive;
- cautionary: AIDS affects us all; no man is an island.

The AIDS crisis has already produced a considerable body of literature, though not yet a great work of art. In a provocative survey, Daniel Harris dismisses most recent gay male fiction. "It's a literature caught in limbo between the hell of outlandish grotesques and the heaven of recipes and salads, one twisted and misshapen by its own extreme ideological tensions."[98] Certainly it is true that AIDS has shaken the identity of the gay male community, but Harris's objections to new gay male literature are excessive.[99] Though much of the literature that responds to AIDS — most of which emerges from or studies the male homosexual community — is pedestrian, repetitious, or special-pleading, all of it resonates with the shock of recognition of the power of AIDS to alter our collective consciousness, to change *all* our lives. Some writings on this topic are achieved works of literature: the journalism of FitzGerald and Shilts; the plays of Kramer, Hoffman, and Fierstein; the fiction of Holleran and a few others who have raised gay male literature from the celebration of uncloseted sexuality to the level of a requiem. AIDS literature will expand and, in time, will find its genius, as AIDS increasingly finds its place at the center of the American mind.

On Tidy Endings, Harvey Fierstein's brief play, is the most successful treatment of the AIDS crisis in literature which I have read. It meets the challenge of incorporating the horrific fact of AIDS — *memento mori,* masque of death, plague — in a drama that, without resort to theatrical tricks, teaches us how to see, prods us to feel our way to new levels of understanding. In the play, a recent widow, Marion, confronts Arthur, her deceased husband's lover, in the cooperative apartment in which Arthur had cared for Collin, the man they both loved, who has died of AIDS-related disease. Marion had sent her son, Jim, away before her meeting with Arthur, who is hurt that the boy blames him for Collin's death. Marion and Arthur are each wary and jealous. "He died in my arms, not yours," cries Arthur.[100] They bicker over mementos of Collin: a teapot that had been given to Collin and Marion as a wedding gift, though Arthur tells her it is a replacement for the burnt-out original, bought by Collin and Arthur in the Village. Marion and Arthur cannot acknowledge each other. They savage each other so thoroughly that, at last, nothing is left but compassion. Arthur tells Marion of Collin's final moments.

Arthur. Marion, you've got your life and his son. All I have is an intangible place in a man's history. Leave me that. Respect that.
Marion. I understand.[101]

Here Marion comes a long way, from the role of the conventional, aggrieved wife, to stand before and understand her dead husband's lover. Moved by his pain, she asks Arthur how he is. Arthur is not infected, he says, but when he asks how *she* is, Marion admits that she has AIDS antibodies in her blood. No one, then, is free from the threat of infection, so no one can remove himself/herself from the human family, which has no choice but to stand together in the face of this awesome threat.

Marion calls her son, Jim, back into the room and insists that the boy tell Arthur what his father had told him. Reluctantly, Jim speaks:

Jim. He said that after me and Mommy he loved you the most. . . . And that I should love you too. And make sure that you're not lonely or very sad.
Arthur. Thank you.[102]

At the end of *On Tidy Endings,* Marion and her son are on one side of a door; Arthur is on the other side. That separation symbolically acknowledges the social division between those who choose either heterosexual or homosexual relationships in America. However, the real story of Fierstein's fine play is that doors have been opened and thresholds of understanding have been crossed between different kinds of people who have been affected and infected by a family death caused by AIDS. Indeed, AIDS, in this play, knows no barriers; it has forced characters to acknowledge each other's humanity and to accept each other's love. The common threat posed by AIDS may redefine and restore our idea of the American family.

Larry Kramer drew the title of *The Normal Heart* from W. H. Auden's poem "September 1, 1939," a poem that also embodies Kramer's theme, the theme of most AIDS literature, in one memorable injunction: "We must love one another or die."[103]

Notes

1. Susan Sontag, *Illness as Metaphor* (New York: Vintage Books, 1979), 3.
2. Henry James, cited in F. W. Dupee, *Henry James* (New York: William Morrow & Co., 1974), 250.
3. Sontag, *Illness as Metaphor,* 3.
4. William Shakespeare, *King Lear,* ed. G. Blakemore Evans, in *The Riverside Shakespeare* (Boston: Houghton Mifflin Co., 1974), 1286–87.
5. Sontag, *Illness as Metaphor,* 20–21.
6. Ibid., 25.
7. Ibid., 69.
8. Ibid., 71.
9. Seamus Heaney, "Feeling into Words," in *Preoccupations: Selected Prose 1968–1978* (New York: Farrar, Straus, Giroux, 1980), 56.
10. Harvey Fierstein, "Safe Sex," in *Safe Sex* (New York: Atheneum, 1987), 58.
11. Philip Larkin, "Annus Mirabilis," in *High Windows* (New York: Farrar, Straus and Giroux, 1974), 34.
12. Philip Larkin, "MCMXIV," in *The Whitsun Weddings* (Great Britain: Faber and Faber, 1964), 28.

13. Randy Shilts, *And the Band Played On: Politics, People, and the AIDS Epidemic* (New York: St. Martin's Press, 1987), 12.

14. David Leavitt, *The Lost Language of Cranes* (New York: Alfred A. Knopf, 1986).

15. John J. O'Connor, "'Intimate Contact,' Devastation of AIDS," *New York Times,* 6 Oct. 1987, C18.

16. A. M. Rosenthal, "No Way Out," *New York Times,* 10 Oct. 1987, A35.

17. Barney Rosenzweig, cited in John M. Wilson, "How AIDS is Affecting Films, TV," *Boston Globe,* 2 Aug. 1987, A1.

18. Ibid., A10.

19. Dan Wakefield, "Teen Sex and TV: How the Medium Has Grown Up," *TV Guide,* 7 Nov. 1987, 5.

20. Terry Louise Fisher, cited in Daniel B. Wood, "AIDS Now Affecting Lives of Fictional Characters," *Boston Globe,* 23 June 1987, 67.

21. Fran Lebowitz, "The Impact of AIDS on the Artistic Community," *New York Times,* 13 Sept. 1987, 22.

22. Loretta McLaughlin, "The Spread of A Modern Plague," a review of Randy Shilts, *And the Band Played On, Boston Sunday Globe,* 25 Oct. 1987, B13.

23. Bruce Lambert, "Numbers Don't 'Add Up': AIDS Forecasts Are Grim — And Disparate," Week in Review, *New York Times,* 25 Oct. 1987, 27.

24. Rep. Chet Atkins, "AIDS — The Modern Plague," (Mass.) *Sudbury Town Crier,* 10 Sept. 1987, 8.

25. Stephen Jay Gould, "The Exponential Spread of AIDS Underscores the Tragedy of Our Delay in Fighting One of Nature's Plagues," *New York Times Magazine,* 19 April 1987, 33.

26. William H. McNeill, *Plagues and Peoples* (Garden City, N.Y.: Anchor Books, 1976), 3.

27. Edmund Wilson, "The Literary Class War," in *The Shores of Light: A Literary Chronicle of the Twenties and Thirties* (New York: Farrar, Straus and Young, 1952), 539.

28. Henry James to Rhoda Broughton, 10 August 1914, in *The Selected Letters of Henry James,* ed. Leon Edel (Garden City, N.Y.: Anchor Books, 1955), 214–15.

29. Paul Fussell, *The Great War and Modern Memory* (New York: Oxford University Press, 1975), 174.

30. Ibid., 74.

31. Ibid., 35.

32. Frances FitzGerald, "The Castro," in *Cities on a Hill: A Journey Through Contemporary American Culture* (New York: Simon and Schuster, 1986), 88–89.

33. Robert Lindsey, "Where Homosexuals Found Haven There Is None Now with AIDS," *New York Times,* 15 July 1987.

34. Ibid., Bart Levin cited.

35. Shilts, *And the Band Played On,* 601.

36. Ibid., 495.

37. Ibid., 596.

38. Ibid., 165.

39. Ibid., Patrick Buchanan cited, 311.

40. Shilts, *And the Band Played On,* 198.

41. Ibid., 439.

42. Ibid., 245.

43. Ibid., Larry Kramer cited, 244.

44. Randy Shilts, cited in Jim Miller with Pamela Abramson, "The Making of an Epidemic," *Newsweek,* 19 Oct. 1987, 93.

45. Larry Kramer, cited in Shilts, *And the Band Played On,* 358.

46. Shilts, 381.

47. Ibid., 556.

48. Larry Kramer, *The Normal Heart.* With an introduction by Andrew Holleran and a foreword by Joseph Papp (New York: New American Library, 1985), 70.

49. Ibid., 60–61.

50. Ibid., 109.

51. Arthur Miller, *Death of a Salesman,* in *Arthur Miller's Collected Plays* (New York: Viking Press, 1963), 162.

52. Judy Foreman, "The Revolution in Immunology: How AIDS Virus Wreaks Its Havoc," second of three articles, *Boston Globe,* 19 Oct. 1987, 1.

53. William Hoffman, *As Is* (New York: Vintage Books, 1985), xiii.

54. Ibid., xx.

55. Ibid., 25.

56. Ibid., 11–12.

57. Ibid., 32–33.

58. Fierstein, *Safe Sex,* 42.

59. Ibid., 57.

60. Ibid., preface, xi.

61. Ibid., Frank Rich, cited on dustjacket.

62. Don Shewey, "AIDS on Stage: Comfort, Sorrow, Anger," *New York Times,* 21 June 1987, H5.

63. Robert Boucheron, "Epitaph for an Innocent," in *Epitaphs for the Plague Dead* (New York: Ursus Press, 1985), 32.

64. Bill Becker, "1 Feb 85," in *An Intimate Desire to Survive* (Bryn Mawr, Penn.: Dorrance & Co., 1985), 27.

65. Ibid., 30.

66. Susan Wilson, "Giant 'Quilt' Commemorates AIDS Victims," *Boston Globe,* 16 Oct. 1987, 102.

67. McNeill, *Plagues and Peoples,* 5.

68. Jed A. Bryan, *A Cry in the Desert* (Austin, Tex.: Banned Books, 1987), 121.

69. Ibid., preface.

70. Ibid., epigraph.

71. Toby Johnson, *Plague: A Novel About Healing* (Boston: Alyson Publications, 1987).

72. Ibid., preface.

73. Ibid., 184.

74. J. W. Money, *To All the Girls I've Loved Before: An AIDS Diary* (Boston: Alyson Publications, 1987).

75. Ibid., 7.

76. Ibid., 18.

77. Daniel Curzon, *The World Can Break Your Heart* (Stamford, Conn.: Knights Press, 1984), 44.

78. Ibid., 189.

79. Ibid., 241.

80. Richard Poirier, *The Renewal of Literature: Emersonian Reflections* (New York: Random House, 1987), 5.

81. Ibid., dedication.

82. W. H. Auden, "In Memory of W. B. Yeats," in *The Collected Poetry of W. H. Auden* (New York: Random House, 1945), 50.

83. Paul Reed, *Facing It: A Novel of AIDS* (San Francisco: Gay Sunshine Press, 1984), 30.

84. Ibid., 105.

85. Ibid., 76.

86. George Stambolian, ed., *Men on Men: Best New Gay Fiction* (New York: New American Library, 1986).

87. Ibid., introduction, 8.

88. Ibid., 25.

89. Ibid., 36.

90. Ibid., 342.

91. Ibid., 347.

92. Ibid., 92.

93. Ibid., 95.

94. Ibid., 105.

95. Ibid., 112.

96. Ibid., 131.

97. Ibid., 298.

98. Daniel Harris, "La Cage au Dull," *Boston Review* (December 1987): 14.

99. See Richard Blow's article, "Those Were the Gays," *New Republic* (2 Nov. 1987): 16.

100. Harvey Fierstein, "On Tidy Endings," in *Safe Sex,* 92.

101. Ibid., 104.

102. Ibid., 111–12.

103. W. H. Auden, "September 1, 1939," in *The Collected Poetry of W. H. Auden* (New York: Random House, 1945), 57–59.

Resources and Services:

For People with AIDS, ARC, or HIV Infection, Their Families, and Friends

This section lists state-sponsored and other testing sites and indicates those that allege to provide anonymous testing. Readers should be aware that there are differing definitions of "confidential"—in one case we were told that the testing was confidential but that state regulations required the reporting of test results by name.

A sample of programs for each state has also been provided, but this list is by no means complete. Please call the hotline, state or local health department, local gay and lesbian organization, Metropolitan Community Church in your area, or one of the national listings if you wish to

- get information on whether testing in your area is anonymous or confidential, free or provided for a sliding-scale fee
- find out whether there is a local group more suited to your needs than those listed here

Other useful directories are issued by some of the national organizations listed here. Those published by the National AIDS Network, the National AIDS Information Clearinghouse, and the U.S. Mayors' Conference may be particularly helpful.

Alabama

State Services:

AIDS Program **(205) 261-5016**
Division of Disease Control
Alabama Department of Public Health
State Office Building, Room 662
434 Monroe Street
Montgomery, Alabama 35130

Testing and counseling; risk-reduction education and outreach; speakers' bureau; printed materials.

AIDS Prevention Program **(205) 471-7322**
Alabama Department of Public Health
University of Southern Alabama Medical Center
2451 Fillingim
Mobile, Alabama 36617

Coordinates statewide education programs. Publishes directory.

Local Services:

Birmingham AIDS Outreach, Inc. **(205) 322-4197**
P.O. Box 550070
Birmingham, Alabama 35255

Helpline **(205) 322-0757**

Information and referrals; education, counseling and support groups; speakers' bureau.

The AIDS Task Force of Alabama **(205) 933-9110**
P.O. Box 55703
Birmingham, Alabama 35255

In-state AIDS helpline **1-800-228-6069**

Community education; risk-reduction workshops; network of direct services and advocates.

Mobile AIDS Buddy Program **(205) 476-9142**
P.O. Box 6968
Mobile, Alabama 36660

Counseling; support groups; other services.

Mobile AIDS Support Group **(205) 690-8167**
Mobile County Health Department AIDS Control
251 N. Bayou Street
Mobile, Alabama 36602

Testing and counseling; social service; financial assistance.

Mobile AIDS Support Service **(205) 342-5092**
Unitarian Universalist Fellowship
P.O. Box 16341
Mobile, Alabama 36616

Information and crisis hotline; counseling; support groups.

Montgomery AIDS Outreach **(205) 284-2273**
P.O. Box 5213
Montgomery, Alabama 36103

AIDS Helpline
Monday through Friday 6:00–9:00 P.M.

Hospice of West Alabama **(205) 345-0067**
2123 9th Street
Tuscaloosa, Alabama 35401

Social and medical support services.

West Alabama AIDS Committee **(205) 345-4131**
West Alabama Health Department
1101 Jackson Avenue
Tuscaloosa, Alabama 35401

Information and referrals; education; counseling and support groups.

Alaska

State Services:

Alaska AIDS Program **(907) 561-4406**
Department of Epidemiology
Division of Public Health
Department of Health and Social Services
P.O. Box 240249
Anchorage, Alaska

Testing and counseling; health and risk-reduction education; technical assistance; in-service training.

Local Services:

Anchorage STD Clinic **(907) 343-4605**
P.O. Box 19-6650
Anchorage, Alaska

Testing and counseling; information; education.

Alaskan AIDS Assistance Association | **(907) 276-4880**
417 West 8th Avenue
Anchorage, Alaska 99501

In-state hotline **1-800-478-AIDS**

Information and referrals; speakers' bureau; printed materials; buddy program; volunteer network and training.

Anchorage Neighborhood Health Center **(907) 258-7888**
1217 East 10th Street
Anchorage, Alaska 99502

Testing and counseling.

Interior Alaska ASAP (AIDS Service and Prevention) **(907) 452-5005**
c/o SADATP
P.O. Box 405
Fairbanks, Alaska 99707
Ask for Bonnie McCorquodale

Anonymous testing and counseling; direct services; buddy program; support groups; education; outreach.

Arizona

State Services:

Arizona Department of Health Services **(602) 230-5819**
Division of Disease Prevention
AIDS Program
3008 North 3rd Street
Phoenix, Arizona 85012

Anonymous testing and counseling; information and referrals; education; counseling; support groups.

Local Services:

A.R.C.E. Program **(602) 461-2205**
508 West 10th Street
Mesa, Arizona 85201

Hotline **(602) 461-2437**

Information and referral; counseling; support groups; education; speakers' bureau; bilingual services.

Arizona Stop AIDS Project **(602) 277-1929**
736 East Flynn Lane
Phoenix, Arizona 85014

Counseling and support groups; education and risk-reduction programs; information and referrals; bilingual services.

Little Innocent Victims of America Foundation **(602) 843-8654**
4345 W. Shangri-la Road
Glendale, Arizona 85304

Network to locate foster and adoptive homes for babies with AIDS.

Planned Parenthood **(602) 277-PLAN**
5651 North 7th Street
Phoenix, Arizona 85014

Anonymous testing and counseling at various sites.

Phoenix Shanti Group **(602) 265-3884**
P.O. Box 17618
Phoenix, Arizona 85011

Information, education, and referrals; counseling and support groups; buddy program; residency program.

National Women and AIDS Network (WARN) **(602) 256-9276**
402 W. Roosevelt, Suite G
Phoenix, Arizona 85002

Information and referrals; risk-reduction and other education programs; counseling and support groups; speakers' bureau.

Tucson AIDS Project **(602) 322-6226**
151 S. Tucson Boulevard, Suite 252
Tucson, Arizona 85716

Hotline **(602) 326-2437**
Monday through Friday 10:00 A.M.–12:00 noon;
Sunday 7:00–9:00 P.M.

Information; education; referrals; speakers' bureau; counseling and support groups.

Arkansas

State Services:

Arkansas Department of Health **(501) 661-2111**
STD/AIDS Program
AIDS Prevention and Surveillance
4815 W. Markham Street
Little Rock, Arkansas 72205

In-state AIDS hotline **1-800-445-7720**

Testing and counseling; information; referrals; education; speakers' bureau.

Local Services:

Washington County AIDS Task Force **(501) 443-AIDS**
P.O. Box 4224
Fayetteville, Arkansas 72702

Information and referrals; education; counseling and support groups.

Arkansas AIDS Foundation **(501) 663-7833**
P.O. Box 5007
Little Rock, Arkansas 72225

Hotline **(501) 666-3340**
6:30–10:30 P.M.

Information and referrals; education; buddy program; speakers' bureau; housing referrals; civil rights advocacy.

California

State Services:

Department of Health Services **(916) 445-0553**
Office on AIDS
714-744 P Street
P.O. Box 942732
Sacramento, California 94234

Free, anonymous testing at 80 sites. Information; referrals; education.

Local Services:

Bakersfield Gay and Lesbian Information Line **(805) 328-0729**

Los Angeles Hotline **(213) 976-4700**

Kern County AIDS Team **(805) 327-3724**
P.O. Box 30357
Bakersfield, California 93389

Information and referrals.

Aris Project **(408) 370-3272**
595 Millich Drive, Suite 104
Campbell, California 95008

Information and referrals; counseling; support groups.

The AIDS Services Foundation for Orange County **(714) 646-0411**
1685-A Babcock
Costa Mesa, California 92667

Information and referrals; buddy program; counseling and support groups; case management, home health and residence programs.

Central Valley AIDS Team **(209) 264-2437**
P.O. Box 4640
Fresno, California 93744

Information and referrals; buddy program; counseling and support groups.

AIDS Response Program of the Gay and Lesbian Community Center **(714) 534-0961**
12832 Garden Grove Boulevard
Garden Grove, California 92643

Information and referrals.

Families Who Care **(213) 498-6366**
3900 E. Pacific Coast Highway
Long Beach, California 90804

Counseling and support groups.

Project Ahead (213) 439-3948
2017 East 4th Street
Long Beach, California 90814

Information and referral; direct services; buddy program; counseling and support groups.

AIDS Project Los Angeles **(213) 380-2000**
3670 Wilshire Boulevard, Suite 300
Los Angeles, California 90010

Information and referrals; speakers' bureau; counseling and support groups; food, housing, and insurance assistance programs; bilingual services.

Milagros AIDS Project **(213) 725-1337**
El Centro Human Service Corp.
972 South Goodrich Boulevard
Los Angeles, California 90022

Information and referrals; counseling and support groups; case management; bilingual services.

Los Angeles Gay and Lesbian Community Services **(213) 464-7400**
1213 North Highland Avenue
Los Angeles, California 90038

Computerized info service **(213) 854-3006**

Information and referrals; counseling and support groups; testing on site by appointment.

AIDS Project of the East Bay **(415) 420-8181**
400 40th Street, Suite 205
Oakland, California 94609

Information and referrals; speakers' bureau; buddy program; counseling and support programs.

Desert AIDS Project **(619) 323-2118**
Community Counsel and Consultation Center
750 S. Vella Road
Palm Springs, California 92264

Information and referrals; counseling and support groups; assistance in obtaining AZT; testing on site.

Island AIDS Project (IAP) **(714) 784-2437**
3638 University Avenue, Suite 223
Riverside, California 92501

In-state information line **1-800-451-4133**

Information and referrals; speakers' bureau; buddy program; counseling and support groups.

Sacramento AIDS Foundation **(916) 448-2437**
1900 K Street, #201
Sacramento, California 95814

Information and referrals; speakers' bureau; buddy program; counseling and support groups.

San Diego AIDS Project **(619) 543-0300**
P.O. Box 89049
3777 4th Avenue
San Diego, California 92138

Information and referrals; counseling and support groups.

Lesbian and Gay Center of San Diego **(619) 692-2077**
P.O. Box 3357
San Diego, California 92103

Psychotherapy and holistic alternative counseling and support groups.

Mid-City Consortium to Combat AIDS **(415) 751-4221**
1779 Haight Street
San Francisco, California 94117

Outreach and education with IVDU and their partners.

AIDS Health Project **(415) 476-6430**
Box 0884
San Francisco, California 94143

Training to health professionals; counseling and support groups.

AIDS Interfaith Network of North America **(415) 928-HOPE**
2261 Market Street, #502
San Francisco, California 94114

Information and referrals; spiritual and psychological counseling; support groups.

Asian AIDS Project/Asian-American Recovery Project (415) 386-4815
2024 Hayes Street
San Francisco, California 94117

Information; referrals; education; risk-reduction; community outreach. Only group with extensive Asian community focus and program.

Shanti Project **(415) 777-2273**
525 Howard Street
San Francisco, California 94105

Direct services; counseling and support groups.

Stop AIDS Resource Center **(415) 621-7177**
584 Castro Street, Suite 318
San Francisco, California 94119

Information and referrals; risk-reduction programs; community outreach; speakers' bureau.

Women's AIDS Network/AIDS Activity Office **(415) 864-5855**
333 Valencia Street, 4th floor
San Francisco, California 94103

Information and referrals; education programs; speakers' bureau.

National Lawyers Guild AIDS Network **(415) 861-8884**
211 Gough Street, Suite 311
San Francisco, California 94102

Legal information and referrals.

AIDS Services **(805) 681-5120**
Santa Barbara County Health Services
300 San Antonio Road
Santa Barbara, California 93110

Information and referrals; risk-reduction programs; anonymous testing at 5 alternative sites.

Santa Cruz AIDS Project **(408) 427-3900**
1606 Soquel Avenue
Santa Cruz, California 95062

Information and referrals; direct services; speakers' bureau.

Sonoma County AIDS Project — **(707) 527-2247**
3313 Chauate Road
Santa Rosa, California 95404

Hotline — **(707) 579-AIDS**

Information and referrals; anonymous testing by appointment.

San Joaquin AIDS Foundation — **(209) 476-8533**
4410 N. Pershing Avenue, Suite C5
Stockton, California 95207

Information and referrals; case management; buddy program; counseling and support groups.

AID for AIDS, Inc. — **(213) 656-1107**
P.O. Box 69523
6235 Santa Monica Boulevard
West Hollywood, California 90046

Financial assistance.

Colorado

State Services:

Colorado Department of Health — **(303) 331-8320**
STD/AIDS Office
AIDS Education Program
4210 East 11th Avenue
Denver, Colorado 80220

Statewide hotline — **(303) 333-4336**

Testing and counseling; information and referrals; education and risk-reduction programs.

Local Services:

Boulder County AIDS Project — **(303) 444-6121**
P.O. Box 4375
Boulder, Colorado 80306

Information, education, and referrals; counseling and support groups.

Colorado AIDS Project **(303) 837-0166**
P.O. Box 18529
Denver, Colorado 80218

Hotline **(303) 830-2437**

Information, education, and referrals; buddy program; speakers' bureau; food bank; counseling and support groups.

People With AIDS Coalition of Colorado **(303) 837-8214**
P.O. Box 300339
Denver, Colorado 80203

Counseling and support groups.

Connecticut

State Services:

AIDS Program **(203) 566-1157**
Department of Health Services
150 Washington Street
Hartford, Connecticut 06106

Information; speakers' bureau.

Local Services:

AIDS Project Hartford **(203) 247-AIDS**
P.O. Box 6723
Hartford, Connecticut 06106

Counseling and support groups. Volunteers on phone Monday–Friday 6:30 P.M.–9:30 P.M.

Gay and Lesbian Health Clinic **(203) 236-4431**
P.O. Box 2094
Hartford, Connecticut 06145-2094

Multiservice clinic; health education and advocacy; AIDS support networking.

Hartford AIDS Prevention Program — **(203) 722-6742**
Hartford Health Department
Hartford, Connecticut

Bilingual (English and Spanish); HIV and STD counseling and testing; education; individual and community presentations; outreach to high-risk populations. Wednesday and Thursday 9:00 A.M.–1:00 P.M.; Friday 1:00 P.M.–4:00 P.M.

AIDS Project New Haven — **(203) 624-0947**
P.O. Box 636
New Haven, Connecticut 06503

Anonymous hotline — **(203) 624-AIDS**
Monday through Friday 6:30 P.M.–9:00 P.M.

Volunteer, nonprofit organization; all services free of charge; buddy system; counseling and support groups; crisis intervention and risk reduction; education and outreach; speakers' bureau.

AIDS Project — **(203) 426-5626**
P.O. Box 347
Newtown, Connecticut 06470

Support group; counseling; home assistance (professional and volunteer); practical services; speakers.

Norwalk Health Department — **(203) 854-7979**
Mid-Fairfield AIDS Project, Inc.
137 East Avenue
Norwalk, Connecticut 06851

Support groups; speakers; educational materials; referrals; HIV counseling and testing. By appointment: call 8:30 A.M.–4:30 P.M., Monday through Friday.

Stamford Health Department — **(203) 967-2437**
Stamford AIDS Project
888 Washington Boulevard
Stamford, Connecticut 06904

HIV counseling and testing by appointment; hotline; information; referrals.

Delaware

State Services:

Delaware Department of Public Health **(302) 995-8422**
AIDS Program Office
3000 Newport Gap Pike
Building G
Wilmington, Delaware 19808

Anonymous testing and counseling; education; client advocacy; case management and resource coordination.

Local Services:

Delaware Lesbian and Gay Advocates **(302) 652-6776**
214 N. Market Street
Wilmington, Delaware 19801

Anonymous testing and counseling; buddy program; counseling and support groups; housing referrals; bilingual.

Gay and Lesbian Alliance of Delaware **(302) 655-5280**
214 N. Market Street
Wilmington, Delaware 19801

Education and information.

In-state hotline **1-800-422-0429**
Monday through Saturday 11:00 A.M.–11:00 P.M.

District of Columbia

Commission of Public Health **(202) 673-6888**
Office of AIDS Activities
1875 Connecticut Avenue, N.W.
Washington, D.C. 20009

Hotline **(202) 332-AIDS**

Free anonymous testing; two alternative test sites. Education; information; counseling.

Alianza Project—Koba Associates **(202) 328-5700**
1156 15th Street, N.W., #200
Washington, D.C. 20005

Information and referrals; speakers' bureau; printed materials; bilingual; Latin community outreach.

Whitman-Walker Clinic/AIDS Program **(202) 332-5295**
1407 S Street, N.W.
Washington, D.C. 20009

Testing by appointment (call 202-332-EXAM); residential, legal, and social services assistance.

Florida

State Services:

State Health Program Office **(904) 487-2478**
Florida Health and Rehabilitative Services
AIDS Program Office
1317 Winewood Boulevard
Tallahassee, Florida 32301

In-state information hotline **1-800-352-2437**

Anonymous testing and counseling; education; information and referrals; counseling and support groups.

Local Services:

Center One AID **(305) 561-0316**
370 East Prospect Road
Fort Lauderdale, Florida 33334

In-state hotline **1-800-325-5371**

Information and education; speakers' bureau; buddy program; counseling and support groups.

North Central Florida AIDS Network — **(904) 372-4370**
1005-I S.E. 4th Avenue
Gainesville, Florida 32601

Information line — **(904) 37A-IDSO**
2:00–10:00 P.M.

Information and education; speakers' bureau; buddy program; case management; counseling and support groups.

AIDS Project — **(904) 630-3237**
515 West 6th
Jacksonville, Florida 32206

Anonymous testing and counseling; information and education; speakers' bureau; HIV positive medical clinic.

AIDS Help, Inc. — **(305) 296-6196**
P.O. Box 4374
Key West, Florida 33041

Information and referrals; financial assistance.

AIDS Education Project — **(305) 292-6701**
515 Whitehead Street
Key West, Florida 33040

Anonymous testing and counseling; information; education; risk-reduction programs.

Comprehensive AIDS Program (CAP) — **(407) 582-4357**
P.O. Box 3084
Lantana, Florida 33465
and
P.O. Box 1056 — **(407) 996-7059**
Belle Glade, Florida 33430

Anonymous testing and counseling; in-home services; information and education.

Health Crisis Network | **(305) 326-8833**
P.O. Box 42-1280
Miami, Florida 33242

Hotlines
In-state | **1-800-443-5046**
9:00 A.M.–12:00 noon | **(305) 634-4436**
Spanish-speaking | **(305) 324-5148**

Counseling and support groups; information and referrals.

South Florida AIDS Network | **(305) 549-7744**
1611 N.W. 12th Avenue
Miami, Florida 33136

Case management; education; speakers' bureau; bilingual services.

Sarasota AIDS Support | **(813) 951-1551**
1441 State Street
Sarasota, Florida 34236

Hotline | **(813) 951-AIDS**

Information, education, counseling and support groups; buddy program; drop-in center.

Tampa AIDS Network | **(813) 221-6420**
P.O. Box 1062
Tampa, Florida 33601

Information and referrals; education; speakers' bureau; buddy program; counseling and support groups.

Hospice of West Palm Beach | **(407) 582-2205**
444 Bunker Road
West Palm Beach, Florida 33405

Hospice care.

Georgia

State Services:

Office of Infectious Disease **(404) 894-5304**
AIDS Projects
Public Health Division
Department of Human Resources
878 Peachtree Street, N.E.
Atlanta, Georgia 30309

Anonymous testing, free or sliding-scale fee. Information; education.

Local Services:

AID Atlanta **(404) 872-0600**
1132 West Peachtree, N.W.
Atlanta, Georgia 30308

Infoline **(404) 876-9944**

Information and referrals; education programs; counseling and support groups.

Athens AIDS Support Group **(404) 546-0737**
11 Cloverhearst Court 4
Athens, Georgia 30605

Information; counseling; support groups.

First City Networks, Inc. **(912) 236-2489**
P.O. Box 2442
Savannah, Georgia 31401

Information and referrals; newsletter.

Hawaii

State Services:

Hawaii Department of Health **(808) 735-5303**
STD/AIDS Project
3627 Kilauea Avenue
Honolulu, Hawaii 96816

Hotlines:
Oahu **(808) 922-1313**
All other islands **1-800-321-1555**

Anonymous testing and counseling; outreach and education; counseling and support group referrals.

Local Services:

Life Foundation **(808) 924-AIDS**
P.O. Box 88980
Honolulu, Hawaii 96830

Information and referrals; education; speakers' bureau; buddy program; counseling and support groups.

Hawaii Council of Churches **(808) 263-9788**
1300 Kailua
Room B-1
Kailua, Hawaii

Education and information; counseling and support group; healing services held monthly.

Idaho

State Services:

Department of Health and Welfare **(208) 334-5937**
Bureau of Preventive Medicine
AIDS Program
450 West State Street
Boise, Idaho 83720

Testing, free or sliding-scale fee. Information; referrals; education; speakers' bureau; counseling and support groups.

Local Services:

Central District Health Department **(208) 375-5211**
1445 N. Orchard
Boise, Idaho 83704

Information and referrals; education programs; counseling and support groups.

Illinois

State Services:

Department of Public Health **(217) 524-5983**
AIDS Activities Section
525 West Jefferson Street
Springfield, Illinois 62761
Chicago office **(312) 917-4846**

Free or sliding-scale, anonymous testing at 41 test sites. Information, education, and referrals; speakers' bureau.

Local Services:

Gay Community AIDS Project (GCAP) **(217) 351-2437**
P.O. Box 713
Champaign, Illinois 61820

Information and referrals; community education programs; buddy program.

AIDS Foundation of Chicago **(312) 525-9466**
2035 N. Lincoln Avenue, Suite 619
Chicago, Illinois 60614

Information and referral; association of service providers in Chicago area.

AIDS Mental Health Education Project **(312) 908-9191**
303 E. Superior, Passavant 5 West
Chicago, Illinois 60611

Information and referrals; education programs; counseling and support groups.

Chicago House and Social Service Agency, Inc. **(312) 248-5200**
P.O. Box 14728
Chicago, Illinois 60614

Residential referral services.

Howard Brown Memorial Clinic **(312) 871-5777**
AIDS Action Project
945 W. George Street
Chicago, Illinois 60657

Information and referrals; education programs; speakers' bureau; direct services.

Gateway Foundation **(312) 663-1130**
624 S. Michigan Avenue, Suite 1400
Chicago, Illinois 60605

Information and referrals; risk-reduction and other educational programs; treatment center for IVDU and alcohol.

Illinois Alcoholism and Drug Dependence Association **(312) 477-0731**
AIDS Project Office
859 West Wellington Avenue
Lower level
Chicago, Illinois 60657

Information; referrals; education programs and community outreach; training for agency staff; counseling and support groups for drug and alcohol users.

Indiana

State Services:

Indiana State Board of Health **(317) 633-0841**
AIDS Activity Office
1330 W. Michigan Street
Indianapolis, Indiana 46206

In-state hotline **1-800-848-AIDS**

Free testing at 13 sites. Information; education; referral.

Local Services:

AIDS Resource Group (812) 473-2851
111 N. Spring Street
Evansville, Indiana 47711

Information; referrals; education programs; speakers' bureau; counseling and support groups.

AIDS Task Force, Inc. (219) 484-2711
P.O. Box 13527
Fort Wayne, Indiana 46869

Educational and direct services.

Damien Center (317) 632-0123
1350 N. Pennsylvania Street
Indianapolis, Indiana 46202

Support groups; buddy program; emergency temporary housing program.

Iowa

State Services:

Department of Public Health (515) 281-4938
Division of Disease Prevent
AIDS Program
Lucas State Office Building
Des Moines, Iowa 50319

Free anonymous testing at 11 alternative test sites.

Local Services:

Quad City AIDS Coalition (319) 326-8618
605 Main Street
Davenport, Iowa 52803

Hotline (319) 324-8638

Information and referrals; counseling and support groups; speakers' bureau.

Central Iowa AIDS Project — **(515) 244-6700**
American Red Cross
2116 Grand Avenue
Des Moines, Iowa 50312

In-state hotline — **1-800-445-AIDS**

Information and referrals; speakers and printed materials; buddy program; counseling and support groups; information on hospice care.

ICARE — **(319) 351-0140 or**
P.O. Box 2989 — **(319) 338-2135**
Iowa City, Iowa 52204

Information and referrals; training; buddy program; direct services; counseling and support groups.

Johnson County AIDS Coalition — **(319) 351-2726**
c/o Iowa City Crisis Center
321 E. First Street
Iowa City, Iowa 52204

Hotline; 24-hour crisis center — **(319) 351-0140**

Information and referrals; education programs; advocacy; counseling and support groups.

AIDS Coalition of Northeast Iowa — **(319) 234-6831**
2530 University Avenue
Waterloo, Iowa 50701

Information and referrals in conjunction with Red Cross of Waterloo.

Kansas

State Services:

AIDS Program
Bureau of Epidemiology
Department of Health and Environment
Mills Building, Suite 605
109 S.W. 9th
Topeka, Kansas 66612

(913) 296-1500

In-state hotline
Monday through Friday 8:00 A.M.–5:00 P.M.

1-800-247-4101 ext. 333

Testing by appointment at 44 sites. Information; referrals; education; state-supported AZT services.

Local Services:

Kansas AIDS Network
P.O. Box 2728
Topeka, Kansas 66601

(913) 357-7499 or 1-800-365-0219

Information and referrals; speakers' bureau.

First Metropolitan Community Church
1704 S. Santa Fe
Wichita, Kansas 67211

(316) 267-1852

Information and referrals; counseling and support groups; education programs.

Kentucky

State Services:

Department for Health Services
STD Program
275 E. Main Street
Frankfort, Kentucky 40601

(502) 564-4804

Hotline

(502) 546-AIDS

Information and referrals.

Department for Health Services **(502) 564-7112**
Health Promotion Branch
275 E. Main Street
Frankfort, Kentucky 40601

Information and education; training programs for health professionals; printed materials.

Local Services:

AIDS Crisis Task Force of Lexington **(606) 281-5151**
1450 Newtown Pike
Lexington, Kentucky 40511

Information and referrals; education programs; speakers' bureau; counseling; printed materials.

Community Health Trust of Kentucky **(502) 634-1789**
P.O. Box 363
Louisville, Kentucky 40201

Information and referrals; housing services; advocacy; counseling and support groups.

Louisiana

State Services:

Department of Health and Human Resources **(504) 568-5005**
Department of Epidemiology
AIDS Prevention and Surveillance
Room 618
325 Loyola Avenue
New Orleans, Louisiana 70112

In-state hotline **1-800-99A-IDS9**

Testing at 32 sites. Information; education; referrals; speakers' bureau; counseling and support groups.

Lafayette CARES **(318) 265-3066**
P.O. Box 91446
Lafayette, Louisiana 70509

Information and referrals; buddy program; counseling and support groups.

NO/AIDS Task Force **(504) 891-3732**
P.O. Box 2616
New Orleans, Louisiana 70176

Infoline **(504) 522-2437**
Monday through Friday 2:00–10:00 P.M.

Information and referrals; education programs; speakers' bureau; buddy program; counseling and support groups.

Maine

State Services:

Maine Department of Human Services **(207) 289-3747**
Office on AIDS
State House Station 11
Augusta, Maine 04333

Printed and audiovisual material; education for health and risk-reduction; professional conferences; public information events.

In-state AIDS hotline **1-800-851-2437**
(207) 775-1267

Educational referrals and technical assistance.

Maine Department of Education and Cultural Services **(207) 289-5926**

AIDS curriculum development.

Local Services:

AIDS Support Group **(207) 469-7343**
Eastern Maine AIDS Network
P.O. Box 2038
Bangor, Maine 04401

AIDS case management services; public education; support groups; 24-hour phone coverage.

Merrymeeting AIDS Support Services **(207) 729-8727**

Buddy training sessions; Bellevue Counseling Services
Call Wednesday to Sunday.

The AIDS Project (TAP) **(207) 774-6877**
P.O. Box 4096
Portland, Maine 04101

Provides assistance, information, direction, and support.

In-state AIDS information line **1-800-851-AIDS**
(207) 775-1267

Speakers; educational materials; counseling; testing; risk-reduction; support groups; practical assistance; financial assistance; volunteer services/care; AZT Support Fund: direct aid to people using AZT.

Kennebec Valley Regional Health Agency **(207) 873-1127**
8 Highwood Street
Waterville, Maine 04901

AIDS case management services; 24-hour phone coverage.

Maryland

State Services:

In-state hotline **1-800-638-6252**

Department of Health and Mental Hygiene **(301) 225-1255**
Maryland CARES
201 W. Preston Street, 5th floor
Baltimore, Maryland 21201

Testing; information; education and speakers' bureau; counseling and support groups.

Local Services:

AIDS Action Baltimore **(301) 837-9870**
1315 N. Charles Street
Baltimore, Maryland 21201

Direct patient services; financial assistance available; housing and legal advocacy.

Health Education Resource Organization (HERO) **(301) 685-1180**
101 West Read Street, Suite 812
Medical Arts Building
Baltimore, Maryland 21201

Information and referrals; education, outreach and risk-reduction programs; speakers' bureau; printed materials; buddy program; counseling and support groups.

Montgomery County HERO **(301) 762-3385**
100 Maryland Avenue, Suite 240
Rockville, Maryland 20850

Information and referrals; education and risk-reduction programs; speakers' bureau; printed materials; buddy program; counseling and support groups.

Massachusetts

State Services:

Massachusetts Department of Public Health **(617) 727-0368**
Office of Health Resources
150 Tremont Street, 9th Floor
Boston, Massachusetts 02111

Educational programs on AIDS; develops policies; research activities; expansion of services for people with AIDS.

Massachusetts Department of Public Health
AIDS Program/Alternative Test Site Program
State Laboratory Institute
305 South Street
Jamaica Plain, Massachusetts 02130

Coordination of Alternative Test Site Program; statewide AIDS surveillance and analysis of disease trends; technical advice regarding HIV testing.

Information on HIV testing: **(617) 727-9080**

Community Health Resource Specialists

Advocacy; education; resource identification for people with AIDS.

Massachusetts Department of Public Health Office of Health Resources 150 Tremont Street Boston, Massachusetts 02111	**(617) 727-0368**
Massachusetts Department of Public Health HIV Clinical Center, Room H7-393 University of Massachusetts Medical Center Worcester, Massachusetts 01655	**(617) 799-9219**
Barnstable County Health and Environmental Department Superior Court House Barnstable, Massachusetts 02630	**(617) 362-2511, ext. 333**
Massachusetts Department of Public Health Office of Health Resources 91 East Mountain Road Westfield, Massachusetts 01085	**(413) 781-5070**

Hotlines

In-state AIDS Action Line Monday through Saturday 9:00 A.M.–9:00 P.M. Sunday 12:00 noon–4:00 P.M.	**(617) 536-7733** **1-800-235-2331**
AIDS hotline, City of Boston Monday through Friday 8:00 A.M.–4:30 P.M.	**(617) 424-5916**
Gay and lesbian hotline Monday through Friday 6:00 P.M.–11:00 P.M.	**(617) 426-9371**
Hispanic AIDS information hotline Monday through Friday 9:00 A.M.–5:00 P.M.	**(413) 737-2632**
Massachusetts Alternate Test Site Program 24-hour taped information about HIV testing	**(617) 727-9080**
Operation Venus Information about sexually transmitted diseases (STDs) In-state information line Monday through Friday 8:00 A.M.–10:00 P.M.	**(617) 774-7492** **1-800-272-2577**

Local Services

AIDS Action Committee of Massachusetts **(617) 437-6200**
661 Boylston Street
Boston, Massachusetts 02116

Support services for people with AIDS, their families, friends, and health providers; education, printed material, videos; AIDS hotline; speakers.

AIDS Coordinator, City of Boston **(617) 424-4744**
Department of Health and Hospitals
818 Harrison Avenue
Boston, Massachusetts 02118

Cambridge Haitian American Association **(617) 492-6622**
105 Windsor Street
Cambridge, Massachusetts 02139

Fenway Community Health Center **(617) 267-7573**
16 Haviland Street
Boston, Massachusetts 02112

Facility geared toward gay men; medical workups; counseling; HIV testing; education.

Gay and Lesbian Advocates and Defenders **(617) 426-1350**
AIDS Law Project
P.O. Box 218
Boston, Massachusetts 02112

Gay and Lesbian Counseling Services **(617) 542-5188**
6 Hamilton Place
Boston, Massachusetts 02108

Massachusetts Department of Mental Health **(617) 727-8600**
AIDS Task Force
160 North Washington Street
Boston, Massachusetts 02114

Task Forces:

AIDS Project Worcester **(617) 755-3773**
69 Hammond Street
Worcester, Massachusetts 01610
Tuesday through Sunday 12:00 noon–5:00 P.M.

Greater Lawrence, Merrimac Valley: **(617) 475-7610**
Committee for AIDS-Related Concerns
Visiting Nurse Association Home Care Hospice
1 Union Street
Andover, Massachusetts 01810

Provincetown AIDS Support Group **(617) 487-9445**
P.O. Box 1522
Provincetown, Massachusetts 02657

Michigan

State Services:

Detroit Health Department AIDS Project **(313) 876-0980**
1151 Taylor
Detroit, Michigan 48202
Monday through Friday 9:00 A.M.–5:00 P.M.

Free and anonymous counseling and testing by appointment (IVDU walk-ins accepted), 9:00 A.M.–3:00 P.M., Monday through Thursday. Risk-reduction and risk-awareness training for health practitioners; bilingual community outreach program.

Department of Public Health **(517) 335-8371**
AIDS Prevention
P.O. Box 30195
3423 N. Logan
Lansing, Michigan 48909

Testing at 24 sites through county health departments. Information and education; speakers' bureau; training for health professionals and other state employees.

Local Services:

Michigan Organization for Human Rights **(313) 537-6647**
19641 West Seven Mile
Detroit, Michigan 48219
Monday through Friday 9:00 A.M.–5:00 P.M.

Support groups; education and prevention programs; bilingual services.

Southeastern Michigan Gay and Lesbian Information Center — **(313) 345-2722**
940 West McNichols
Detroit, Michigan 48203
and
120 West 4th
Royal Oak, Michigan 48067

Information and referral services, sponsored by Chosen Books.

Wellness House of Michigan — **(313) 342-1230**
P.O. Box 03827
Detroit, Michigan 48203

Residential, housing, and support services.

Wellness Networks — **(313) 547-3783**
P.O. Box 1046 — **1-800-872-AIDS**
Royal Oak, Michigan 48068

Free information and referral, psychological support services.

Minnesota

State Services:

Department of Health — **(612) 623-5698**
AIDS Prevention Services Section
717 Delaware Street, S.E.
Minneapolis, Minnesota 55440

In-state hotline — **1-800-248-AIDS**

Some anonymous test sites; testing at 11 sites. Information; referrals; education programs; training for city and county employees.

Local Services:

Minnesota AIDS Project — **(612) 870-7773**
2025 Nicollett Avenue S. #200
Minneapolis, Minnesota 55404
Monday through Friday 8:00 A.M.–5:00 P.M.

AIDS line **(612) 870-0700**
9:00 A.M.–11:00 A.M. Monday through Thursday;
9:00 A.M.–5:00 P.M. Friday.

Information and referral; education; support groups; residential services; workplace consulting program.

Mississippi

State Services:

Department of Health **(601) 960-7725**
AIDS Office
2423 N. State Street
Jackson, Mississippi 39216

In-state Hotline **1-800-826-2961**

Information and referral; education and workshops; speakers' bureau; printed materials; training for AIDS health educators.

Local Services:

Mississippi Gay Alliance **(601) 353-7611**
P.O. Box 8342 city health line
Jackson, Mississippi 39204 24-hour on-call coverage

In-state 24-hour hotline **1-800-537-0851**

Information and referrals for counseling and testing; education.

Missouri

State Services:

Department of Social Services **(314) 751-6438**
Division of Health
Bureau of AIDS Prevention
1730 E. Elm
P.O. Box 570
Jefferson City, Missouri 65102

Testing at 15 sites. Risk-reduction programs; information and referrals; speakers' bureau; printed materials.

Good Samaritan Project **(816) 561-8784**
3940 Walnut
Kansas City, Missouri 64111
Monday through Friday 8:30 A.M.–5:00 P.M.

Information and referral; volunteer legal advocates; support groups; residential hospice; home health referral; speakers' bureau.

Information hot line **(816) 561-8780**
Monday through Friday 8:00 –10:00 P.M.

National AIDS Teens TAP hotline (Teaching AIDS Prevention) **1-800-234-TEEN**
Monday through Saturday 4:00–8:00 P.M.

Kansas City Free Clinic **(816) 231-8896**
5119 E. 24th Street
Kansas City, Missouri 64127
9:00 A.M.–10:00 P.M. Monday through Thursday;
9:00 A.M.-12:00 noon Friday

Medical outpatient clinic; free testing and counseling by appointment; support groups; information and referral; alternative therapies; education and community outreach; in-home visiting nurses for, e.g., IV therapies.

St. Louis Effort for AIDS **(314) 531-2847**
4050 Lindell Boulevard
St. Louis, Missouri 63018

Information and referrals; speakers' bureau; buddy program; counseling and support groups; education programs.

Montana

State Services:

Health and Environmental Sciences Department **(406) 444-4740**
Health Services Division
AIDS Program
Cogswell Building
Helena, Montana 59620

In-state hotline	**1-800-537-6187**

Free anonymous testing at 9 sites. Information and referral; risk-reduction programs; printed materials; counseling training.

Local Services:

Call city/county health departments for counseling and testing as listed

Billings	**(406) 256-6821**
Bozeman	**(406) 587-0681**
Butte	**(406) 723-3271**
Glendive	**(406) 365-5213**
Great Falls	**(406) 761-1190**
Havre	**(406) 265-5481 ext. 66**
Helena	**(406) 442-3830**
Kalispell	**(406) 752-5300 ext. 343**
Missoula	**(406) 721-5700 ext. 398**

Billings AIDS Support Network **(406) 252-1212**
P.O. Box 1748
Billings, Montana 59103

Information and referral; education for high risk; support groups.

Nebraska

State Services:

Department of Health **(402) 471-2937**
AIDS Program
301 Centennial Malls
P.O. Box 95007
Lincoln, Nebraska 68509

Anonymous testing at 5 sites; information; referrals; education; speakers' bureau; printed materials.

Local Services:

Nebraska AIDS Project — **(402) 342-4233**
3624 Leavenworth
Omaha, Nebraska 68105

In-state hotline — **1-800-782-AIDS**
In Omaha — **(402) 334-4233**

Free, anonymous testing, 7:00–10:00 P.M. Thursday; information and referrals; speakers' bureau; buddy program.

Nevada

State Services:

Department of Human Resources — **(702) 885-4800**
Health Division
AIDS Program of the Communicable Disease Division
505 E. King Street
Carson City, Nevada 89710

Sliding-scale fee for anonymous testing at 16 sites; information and referrals; education programs.

Local Services:

AID for AIDS of Nevada — **(702) 369-6162**
2116 Paradise Road, Suites C&D
Las Vegas, Nevada 89104

Hotline — **(704) 369-5637**

Information and referral; support groups; education; speakers' bureau; community and minority outreach program; residential and financial emergency assistance; buddy program; newsletter.

Nevada AIDS Foundation — **(702) 329-2437**
P.O. Box 478
Reno, Nevada 89504
Information line 6:00–10:00 P.M.

New Hampshire

State Services:

N.H. Department of Health and Human Services — **(603) 271-4477**
Division of Public Health Services
AIDS Program
Bureau of Disease Control
6 Hazen Drive
Concord, New Hampshire 03301-6527

In-state hotline — **1-800-852-3345**

Counseling and testing sites; referrals to physicians and education.

Catastrophic Illness Program (CIP) — **(603) 271-4529**, **1-800-852-3345, ext. 4529**
N.H. Division of Public Health Services
Bureau of Medical Services
6 Hazen Drive
Concord, New Hampshire 03301

Financial assistance available for individuals with AIDS who have Kaposi's sarcoma or other cancers.

Hotlines and Information

State of New Hampshire in-state AIDS Hotline — **1-800-872-8909**
Monday through Friday 8:30 A.M.–4:30 P.M.

New Hampshire AIDS information line — **(603) 224-3341**
Monday, Tuesday, Wednesday 7:00 P.M.–10:00 P.M.

Gay Infoline — **(603) 753-9533**
Referrals, information
Help line — **(603) 225-9000**

Local Services:

New Hampshire Citizens' Alliance for Gay and Lesbian Rights (CAGLR) — **(603) 224-3341**
P.O. Box 756
Contoocook, New Hampshire 03229

Education; conferences and workshops; newsletter.

The Clinic **(603) 749-2346**
Strafford County Prenatal and Family Planning Program
50 Chestnut Street
Dover, New Hampshire 03820

Referrals; education. Anonymous HIV counseling and testing, $15.
Walk-in: Tuesday 5:00 P.M.–6:00 P.M.
By appointment: Monday through Friday 8:30 A.M.–4:30 P.M.

Feminist Health Center of Portsmouth **(603) 436-7588**
559 Portsmouth Avenue
Greenland, New Hampshire 03840

Support groups; education; referral network. Anonymous HIV counseling and testing, $15.
Walk-in: Monday 5:00 P.M.–6:00 P.M.
By appointment: Tuesday.

Dartmouth-Hitchcock Hemophilia Program **(603) 646-5486**
Hitchcock Clinic
Hanover, New Hampshire 03756

Anonymous HIV testing; counseling; risk and family stress reduction; immunologic workups; research studies.
Monday through Friday 8:00 A.M.–4:30 P.M.

Latin American Center **(603) 669-5661**
521 Maple Street
Manchester, New Hampshire 03101

Bilingual community education; translators at HIV testing sites for pre- and post-test and counseling.

Other Services in New Hampshire:

American Civil Liberties Union **(603) 225-3080**
11 South Main Street
Concord, New Hampshire 03301

Referrals of free legal advice to low-income people.

New Hampshire AIDS Foundation (NHAF) **(603) 880-6560**
P.O. Box 59
Manchester, New Hampshire 03105

Financial assistance and counseling; buddy system; support groups; legal referrals and education; newsletter. All services confidential and nondiscriminatory.

New Hampshire Human Rights Commission **(603) 271-2767**
61 South Spring Street
Concord, New Hampshire 03301

Accepts complaints from individuals discriminated against in employment, housing, and public accommodations.

New Jersey

State Services:

Department of Health **(609) 984-6000**
John Fitch Plaza
363 West State Street
Trenton, New Jersey 08625

Local Services:

New Jersey Buddies **(201) 837-8125**
P.O. Box 222
Mahwah, New Jersey 07430
10:00 A.M. –10:00 P.M.

Information and referrals; speakers' bureau; buddy program; support groups and some direct services.

New Mexico

State Services:

New Mexico Health and Environment Department **(505) 827-0090**
Public Health Division
AIDS Prevention Program
P.O. Box 968
Santa Fe, New Mexico 87504

Free, anonymous testing at 20 sites. Information and referral; speakers' bureau; risk-reduction workshops; community outreach programs; bilingual services.

New Mexico AIDS Services | **(505) 266-0911**
124 Quincy NE
Albuquerque, New Mexico 87108
and
129 H West San Francisco Street | **(505) 984-0911**
Santa Fe, New Mexico 87501

Free, anonymous testing and counseling; information and referral; support groups; risk-reduction education; case management; volunteer buddy program; speakers' bureau; cash grant assistance for food and housing.

New York

State Services:

Department of Health **(518) 473-7542**
AIDS Institute
Empire State Plaza
Corning Tower Building
Room 359
Albany, New York 12237

In-state hotline **1-800-541-AIDS**

Testing through community service programs by appointment **1-800-872-2777**
AIDS Drug Assistance Program (ADAP) for, e.g., AZT **1-800-542-2437**

Information; referrals; education; printed materials; training for community service providers.

Local Services:

AIDS Council of Northeastern New York **(518) 434-4686**
307 Hamilton Street
Albany, New York 12210

Local hotline, 7:00–9:00 P.M. **(518) 445-AIDS**

Information and referrals; counseling and support groups; buddy program; educational programs.

Haitian Coalition on AIDS **(718) 855-7275**
50 Court Street, Room 605
Brooklyn, New York 11201

Information and referrals; counseling; home visits; financial assistance.

Western N.Y. AIDS Program **(716) 847-2441**
Buffalo AIDS Task Force
220 Delaware Avenue, Suite 512
Buffalo, New York 14202

Local hotline, 9:00 A.M.–9:00 P.M. **(716) 847-AIDS**

Information and referrals; community outreach and education; speakers' bureau; direct services; counseling and support groups; case advocates program; bilingual: Spanish and signing.

AIDS Resource Center (ARC) **(212) 481-1270**
24 W. 30th Street
New York, New York 10001

Information and referrals; Bailey House residence and scattered-site supportive housing; pastoral care and spiritual support.

Gay Men's Health Crisis, Inc. **(212) 807-6664**
132 West 24th Street, Box 274
New York, New York 10011

Local hotline, 10:00 A.M.–9:00 P.M. **(212) 807-6655**

Information and referrals; direct services.

AIDS Rochester, Inc. **(716) 232-3580**
20 University Avenue
Rochester, New York 14605

Information and referrals; community education and outreach.

AIDS Task Force of Central New York **(315) 475-2430**
P.O. Box 1911
Syracuse, New York 13201

Hotline, 9:00 A.M.–9:00 P.M. **(315) 475-2437**

Information and referrals; counseling and support groups; speakers' bureau.

AIDS Related Community Services (ARC) **(914) 993-0606**
214 Central Park Avenue
White Plains, New York 10606

Info line, Monday through Friday, 9:00 A.M.–9:00 P.M. **(914) 993-0607**

Information and referrals; community outreach and education programs; inservice training for health-care workers; speakers' bureau; risk-reduction programs; counseling and support groups; buddy and case management programs.

North Carolina

State Services:

Division of Health Services **(919) 733-7301**
AIDS Control Program
225 N. McDowell Street
Raleigh, North Carolina 27602

In-state hotline, Monday through Friday, 9:00 A.M.–5:00 P.M. **1-800-535-2437**

Free, anonymous testing through 100 local county health departments. Information and referrals; educational programs for health educators; printed materials.

Local Services:

Western North Carolina AIDS Project **(704) 252-7489**
P.O. Box 2411
Asheville, North Carolina

Tuesday, Wednesday, Friday 1:00–5:00 P.M.; same number is hotline Monday, Wednesday, Thursday 7:00–10:00 P.M. Counseling and referral; speakers' bureau; risk-reduction program; buddy support program; support groups.

Metrolina AIDS Project **(704) 333-2437**
P.O. Box 32662
Charlotte, North Carolina 28232

Monday through Friday 9:00 A.M.–5:00 P.M.; same number is hotline Monday through Friday 7:00 P.M.–12:00 midnight Information and referral; counseling; safer sex workshops; group support and counseling.

TRIAD Health Project — **(919) 275-1654**
P.O. Box 5716
Greensboro, North Carolina 27435

Monday through Thursday 2:00–6:00 P.M. Information and referral; support groups; training and education.

AIDS Control Project — **(919) 733-7301**
P.O. Box 2091
Raleigh, North Carolina 27602

Educational Programs:

Grow AIDS Resource Project — **(919) 675-9222**
P.O. Box 4535
Wilmington, North Carolina 28406

Information and referrals; education and prevention workshops; buddy program; support groups.

Other Services:

Greensboro area hotline, after 6:30 P.M. — **(919) 274-2100**

North Dakota

State Services:

Department of Health — **(701) 224-2378**
Division of Disease Control
AIDS Project
State Capitol
Bismarck, North Dakota 58505

In-state hotline — **1-800-472-2180**

Testing at 10 sites. Information and referrals; education programs; speakers' bureau; printed materials; curriculum development for K–12.

Local Services:

Fargo Community Health — **(701) 241-1360**
401 3rd Avenue, North
Fargo, North Dakota

Information and referrals; counseling; alternate test site.

Ohio

State Services:

Department of Health — **(614) 466-5480**
Bureau of Preventative Medicine
AIDS Activities Unit
246 N. High Street
Columbus, Ohio 43215

In-state hotline — **1-800-332-AIDS**

Contact city health departments for free, confidential testing and counseling, information and referrals, Monday through Friday 8:00 A.M.–5:00 P.M.

Akron City AIDS Task Force — **(216) 375-2960**
City Health Department
177 South Broadway
Akron, Ohio 44308

Cincinnati AIDS Task Force — **(513) 352-3143**
City Health Department
3101 Burnet Avenue
Cincinnati, Ohio 45229

Local Services:

AIDS Holistic Services Program — **(216) 762-7481**
c/o Catholic Service League of Summit
640 North Main Street
Akron, Ohio 44310

Information and referrals; speakers' bureau; in-service training; buddy program; counseling and support groups.

Blacks Educating Blacks About Sexual Health (BEBASHI) **(215) 546-4140**
1319 Locust Street
Philadelphia, Pennsylvania 19107

Monday through Friday 9:00 A.M.–5:00 P.M. Information and referral; counseling, education, and training; projects for IVDU, children and youth, women and AIDS; sliding-scale fees for some services.

Philadelphia Community Health Alternatives (PCHA) **(215) 545-8686**
Philadelphia AIDS Task Force
P.O. Box 53429
Philadelphia, Pennsylvania 19105
Monday through Friday 9:00 A.M.–5:00 P.M.

Hotline **(215) 732-AIDS**

Free anonymous testing; information and referral; education; support groups; buddy system; speakers' bureau; counseling; AIDS library; case management; community and minority outreach.

Puerto Rico

Department of Health **(809) 767-6060**
P.O. Box 9342
Santurce, Puerto Rico 00908

Fundacion SIDA **(809) 728-6169**
Call Box 8347
San Juan, Puerto Rico 09910

Information, education, counseling, buddy program.

Rhode Island

Local Services:

AIDS Clinic **(401) 277-4741**
Rhode Island Hospital
593 Eddy Street
Providence, Rhode Island 02902

Support groups; consultations. Monday through Friday 8:00 A.M.–4:30 P.M.

Amara Resources | **(401) 272-5960**

Amara Resources P.O. Box 3477 Providence, Rhode Island 02909	**(401) 272-5960**

Shelter needs, hospice.

Gay/Lesbian help line	**(401) 751-3322**

Information; referrals 7:00 P.M.–11:00 P.M.

Marathon House, Inc. 131 Wayland Avenue Providence, Rhode Island 02906	**(401) 331-4250**

Focus on IVDUs.

Rhode Island Alliance for Lesbian and Gay Civil Rights	**(401) 861-1269**

Rhode Island CARES P.O. Box 3477 Providence, Rhode Island 02909	**(401) 272-5960**
In-state hotline	**1-800-32CARES**

Counseling; information; referrals.

Rhode Island Division of Substance Abuse Contact: Steve Morris, Director Treatment Alternatives to Street Crime (TASC)	**(401) 464-2091**

Information; counseling; referrals.

Rhode Island Peace Work Project 78 Airport Road Warwick, Rhode Island 02889	**(401) 732-4144** **(401) 464-2091**

Fund-raising for direct care of people with AIDS.

Rhode Island Project/AIDS, Inc. Roger Williams Building 22 Hayes Street, Room 124 Providence, Rhode Island 02908	**(401) 277-6545**

Hotline **(401) 277-6502**

Support group of volunteers for people with AIDS or ARC, their families, and friends; public and professional education.

Tel-Med (taped message), tape #571/AIDS **(401) 521-7120**

Traveling Road Show **(401) 273-7059**
AIDS Information Series

Weekly lecturers at various sites.

South Carolina

State Services:

Department of Health and Environmental Control **(803) 734-5482**
STD Division
AIDS Prevention Project
2600 Bull Street
Columbia, South Carolina 29201

In-state hotline **1-800-322-2437**

Testing at 46 sites. Information and referrals; risk-reduction and education programs.

Local Services:

Palmetto AIDS Life Support Services (four offices)

P.O. Box 12124 **(803) 779-7257**
Columbia, South Carolina 29211

P.O. Box 207 **(803) 577-2437**
Charleston, South Carolina 29402

P.O. Box 1215 **(803) 271-9308**
Greenville, South Carolina 29602

P.O. Box 13542 (803) 665-3435
Florence, South Carolina 29504

Information and referrals; education programs; training to health-care professionals; speakers' bureau; buddy program; counseling and support programs.

In-state info line **1-800-868-7257**

South Carolina AIDS Education Network, Inc. **(803) 736-1171**
2768 Decker Boulevard, Suite 98
Columbia, South Carolina 29206

Information and referrals; education programs; speakers' bureau.

South Dakota

State Services:

Department of Health **(605) 773-3364**
Communicable Disease Program
AIDS program
523 E. capitol
Pierre, South Dakota 57501

In-state hotline **1-800-592-1861**

Testing at 4 sites. Information and referrals; education programs; printed materials.

Local Services:

Sioux Empire Gay and Lesbian Coalition **(605) 332-4599**
Box 220
Sioux Falls, South Dakota 57101

Crisis line **(605) 339-HELP**

Information and referrals; speakers' bureau; printed materials.

Tennessee

State Services:

Department of Health and Environment **(615) 741-7247**
AIDS Program
100 9th Avenue North
Nashville, Tennessee 37219

In-state hotline **1-800-525-AIDS**

Testing at 22 regional sites. Information; referrals; education programs; speakers' bureau; printed materials.

Local Services:

Chattanooga Cares **(615) 265-2273**
P.O. Box 8402
Chattanooga, Tennessee 37411
7:00–11:00 P.M.

Information and referrals.

AIDS Response Knoxville **(615) 523-2437**
P.O. Box 3932
Knoxville, Tennessee 37927

Information and referrals; speakers' bureau; buddy program; counseling and support groups.

Nashville Cares **(615) 385-1510**
P.O. Box 25107
Nashville, Tennessee 37202

Info line **(615) 385-AIDS**

Information and referral; community education programs; speakers' bureau; counseling and support groups; printed materials and video lending library; buddy program; social services.

State Services:

Department of health **(512) 458-7207**
AIDS Division
1100 W. 49th Street
Austin, Texas 78756

Testing and counseling; information and educational programs.

Local Services:

AIDS Services of Austin **(512) 472-2273**
P.O. Box 4874
Austin, Texas 78765

Info line **(512) 472-2437**

Information and referrals; speakers' bureau; counseling and support groups; buddy program.

AIDS Arms Network **(214) 521-5191**
P.O. Box 190945
Dallas, Texas 75219

Case management.

Southwest AIDS Committee **(915) 533-5003**
916 East Yandell Street
El Paso, Texas 79902

Education and direct services; information and referrals; speakers' bureau; counseling and support groups; buddy program; bilingual.

AIDS Foundation Houston, Inc. **(713) 623-6796**
3927 Essex Lane
Houston, Texas 77027

Local hotline **(713) 524-2437**

Information and referrals; education; prevention and other support services; counseling and support groups; buddy program.

Utah

State Services:

Department of Health | **(801) 538-6101**
Bureau of Epidemiology
AIDS Control Program
P.O. Box 1660
Salt Lake City, Utah 84110

In-state hotline **1-800-537-1046**

Testing at 6 sites. Information and education programs; printed materials.

Local Services:

AIDS Project Utah **(801) 359-2438**
P.O. Box 8485
Salt Lake City, Utah 84108

Local hotline **(801) 359-2437**
Monday through Friday 6:00–9:00 P.M.

Information and referrals; community education; counseling and support groups.

Vermont

State Services:

State Department of Public Health **(802) 863-7243**
Division of Epidemiology
60 Main Street, P.O. Box 70
Burlington, Vermont 05402

In-state hotline **1-800-882-2437**
Monday through Friday 7:45 A.M.–4:30 P.M. **(802) 863-7245**

Anonymous HIV and STD counseling and testing, by referral; education and speakers.

Vermont Committee on AIDS Resources **(802) 863-2437**
Education and Services (CARES)
30 Elmwood Avenue
P.O. Box 5248
Burlington, Vermont 05402

Counseling; education.

Vermont Regional Hemophilia Center **(802) 658-4310**
96 Colchester Avenue
Burlington, Vermont 05401

Focus on hemophiliacs and their families; information and education on risk and stress reduction.

Local Services:

Office of Alcohol and Drug Abuse Program **(802) 241-2263**
Department of Corrections
103 South Main Street
Waterbury, Vermont 05676

Information and education.

Virginia

State Services:

Department of Health **(804) 225-4844**
AIDS Program
109 Governor Street
Madison Building
Richmond, Virginia 23219

In-state hotline **1-800-533-4148**

Anonymous alternate test sites. Call hotline for site location. information, referrals, and education programs; speakers' bureau; printed materials.

Local Services:

AIDS Support Group | **(804) 979-7714**
P.O. Box 2322
Charlottesville, Virginia 22902
Monday through Thursday 4:00–7:00 P.M.

Tidewater AIDS Crisis Task Force | **(804) 423-5859**
814 W. 41st Street
Norfolk, Virginia 23508

Info line | **(804) 877-1300** or **440-5400**
9:00 A.M.–9:00 P.M.

Richmond AIDS Information Network | **(804) 355-4428**
1721 Hanover Avenue
Richmond, Virginia 23219

Local hotline | **(804) 358-6343** or **358-2437**
Monday through Friday 10:00 A.M.–10:00 P.M.

Information and referrals; counseling and support groups; community outreach; speakers' bureau; buddy program.

Washington

State Services:

Department of Social and Health Services | **(206) 586-0426**
Office on AIDS
Mail Stop LP-20
Building 14
Olympia, Washington 98504

In-state hotline | **1-800-272-AIDS**

Call hotline or local health department for information on testing. Information, referrals and education.

Northwest AIDS Foundation **(206) 329-6923**
1818 E. Madison
Seattle, Washington 98122

Infoline **(206) 329-6963**

Case management; emergency housing assistance; hospice; education programs.

West Virginia

State Services:

Department of Health **(304) 348-2950**
Office of Epidemiology
Division of Surveillance of Disease Control
AIDS Program
1800 Washington Street, E.
Charleston, West Virginia 25305

In-state hotline **1-800-642-8244**

Testing at 14 sites. Information and referrals; STD education program; speakers and printed materials.

Wisconsin

State Services:

Division of health **(608) 267-5287**
AIDS/HIV Program
One W. Wilson
Box 309
Madison, Wisconsin 53701

In-state hotline **1-800-334-AIDS**

Free anonymous testing at 46 sites. Information and referrals; risk-reduction and education programs; community and minority outreach; curriculum development from 6th grade up.

Wyoming

State Services:

Division of Health and Medical Sciences **(307) 777-5800**
Wyoming AIDS Prevention and Education Program
Hathaway Building; 4th floor
Cheyenne, Wyoming 82002

In-state hotline **1-800-327-3577**

Testing at 7 sites. Information; referrals; education programs; printed materials.

Additional National Listings

AIDS Action Council **(202) 547-3101**
729 8th Street, S.E., #200
Washington, D.C. 20003

National lobbying organization.

American Foundation for AIDS Research **(212) 333-3118**
40 West 57th Street, Suite 406
New York, New York 10019

Centers for Disease Control (CDC) **(404) 639-3311**
P.O. Box 5528
Atlanta, Georgia 30307-0528

COSSMHO **(202) 371-2100**
National Coalition of Hispanic Health and Human Service Organizations
1030 15th Street, N.W., Suite 1053
Washington, D.C. 20005

Policy consultants.

Lambda Legal Defense and Education Fund, Inc. **(212) 995-8585**
666 Broadway, 12th floor
New York, New York 10012

Legal assistance and referrals.

National Association of PWAs | (202) 429-2856
2025 Eye Street, N.W., Suite 415
Washington, D.C. 20006

National Coalition of Black Lesbians and Gays | (202) 737-5276
930 F Street, N.W.
Washington, D.C. 20002

National Gay and Lesbian Task Force | (202) 332-3097
1517 U Street, N.W.
Washington, D.C. 20009

National Leadership Coalition on AIDS | (202) 429-0930
1150 17th Street, N.W., Suite 202
Washington, D.C. 20036

National Lesbian and Gay Health Foundation | (202) 797-3708
P.O. Box 65472
Washington, D.C. 20035

National Minority AIDS Council | (202) 544-1076
714 G Street, S.E.
Washington, D.C. 20003

National Women's Health Network | (202) 347-1140
1325 G Street, N.W.
Washington, D.C. 20005

Public Health Service National Hotline | 1-800-342-AIDS

English and Spanish message.

U.S. Conference of Mayors | (202) 293-7330
1620 Eye Street, N.W.
Washington, D.C. 20001

Women's AIDS Network | (415) 864-4736
c/o San Francisco AIDS Foundation
333 Valencia Street
San Francisco, California 94103

The Women's AIDS Project | (213) 650-1508
8235 Santa Monica Boulevard, Suite 201
West Hollywood, California 90046

Multicounty AIDS Network **(216) 762-8144**
P.O. Box 1523
Akron, Ohio 44309

Information and referrals; speakers' bureau; buddy program; advocacy, civil rights, and medical support programs.

Northeast Ohio Task Force on AIDS **(216) 375-2960**
177 South Broadway
Akron, Ohio 44308
9:00 A.M.–5:00 P.M.

24-hour hotline **(216) 375-AIDS**

Information and referral; support groups; buddy program; education program.

Canton City AIDS Task Force **(216) 489-3322**
City Hall
Canton, Ohio 44702

Information and referral; support groups; buddy program; speakers' bureau; emergency financial assistance.

AIDS Volunteers of Cincinnati **(513) 421-2437**
P.O. Box 19009
Cincinnati, Ohio 45219

Monday through Friday 9:00 A.M.–5:00 P.M.; same number serves as hotline 7:00–10:00 P.M. Monday through Friday and 10:00 A.M. to 3:00 P.M. Information and referrals for greater Cincinnati, northern Kentucky, and southeastern Indiana; STOP AIDS safer sex project; legal and religious referrals; food assistance program.

AIDS Program **(216) 664-2324**
City Health Department
1925 Saint Clair Avenue
Cleveland, Ohio 44114

Information and referrals; education programs; counseling and support groups.

Health Issues Taskforce **(216) 621-0766**
2250 Euclid Avenue
Cleveland, Ohio 44115

Information and referrals; direct client services; education and prevention programs; buddy program.

Columbus AIDS Task Force **(614) 488-2437**
1500 W. 3rd Avenue, Suite 329
Columbus, Ohio 43212

Information and referrals; education programs; buddy program; speakers' bureau; counseling and support groups.

Toledo Area Aids Task Force **(419) 242-4777**
151 N. Michigan, Suite 322
Toledo, Ohio 43613

Information and referrals; education; outreach programs for IVDU; speakers' bureau; HIV screening; family support groups.

Other Services:

Gay hotline, Toledo **(419) 245-9351**

Nova Project (buddy program), Toledo **(419) 244-6682**
3:00–7:00 P.M.

Oklahoma

State Services:

Department of Health **(405) 271-4636**
AIDS Division
1000 N.E. 10th
P.O. Box 53551
Oklahoma City, Oklahoma 73152

In-state hotline **1-800-522-9054**

Free anonymous testing at 6 sites. Information, referrals, education programs; speakers' bureau; printed materials.

Local Services:

Oasis Community Center/AIDS Support Program **(405) 232-5453**
2135 N.W. 39th Street
Oklahoma City, Oklahoma 73112

Info line **(405) 525-AIDS**

Oregon

State Services:

Department of Epidemiology | **(503) 229-5792**
Health Division
AIDS Program
1400 S.W. Fifth Avenue
Portland, Oregon 97201

Free anonymous testing at 27 sites. Information and referrals; education and preventive programs.

Local Services:

Willamette AIDS Council | **(503) 345-8271**
329 W. 13th Avenue, Suite D
Eugene, Oregon 97401

Helpline | **(503) 345-7089**

Information and referrals; education programs; speakers' bureau; counseling and support programs.

Pennsylvania

State Services:

State hotline | **1-800-342-AIDS**

Department of Health | **(717) 787-6436**
AIDS Activities
801 Health and Welfare Building
Harrisburg, Pennsylvania 17120

In-state hotline | **1-800-692-7254**

Testing at 76 sites. Information and referrals; education programs.

Local Services:

Lehigh Valley AIDS Services Center — **(215) 435-6708**
P.O. Box 1656
Allentown, Pennsylvania 18105
Monday through Friday 9:00 A.M.–5:00 P.M.

Hotline — **(215) 433-6708**

Information and referral; support services and groups; buddy program; networking for medical, psychological, religious counseling; in-home nonmedical care services; housing referrals.

AIDS Intervention Project — **(814) 946-5411** — **1-800-445-6262**
P.O. Box 352
Altoona, Pennsylvania 16603

South Central AIDS Assistance Network — **(717) 238-AIDS**
P.O. Box 11573
Harrisburg, Pennsylvania 17108
Monday through Friday 9:00 A.M.–5:00 P.M.

Information and referrals; education; support groups; buddy program.

Lancaster AIDS Project — **(717) 394-3380**
P.O. Box 1543
Lancaster, Pennsylvania 17603

Hotline — **(717) 394-9900**

Monday and Wednesday 12:00 noon–3:00 P.M.; Monday through Saturday 6:00–9:00 P.M. Information and referrals; buddy program; support groups; speakers' bureau; educational programs.

Action AIDS — **(215) 732-2155**
P.O. Box 1625
Philadelphia, Pennsylvania

Monday through Friday 9:00 A.M.–5:00 P.M. Information and referral; case management; support groups; buddy program; education programs; speakers' bureau.